Pearson New International Edition

Orthopedic Physical Examination Tests:
An Evidence-Based Approach
Chad Cook Eric Hegedus
Second Edition

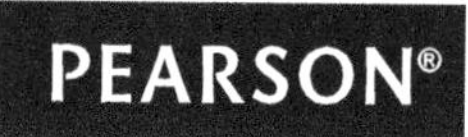

Pearson Education Limited
Edinburgh Gate
Harlow
Essex CM20 2JE
England and Associated Companies throughout the world

Visit us on the World Wide Web at: www.pearsoned.co.uk

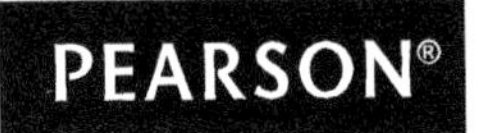

ISBN 10: 1-292-02796-7
ISBN 13: 978-1-292-02796-8

British Library Cataloguing-in-Publication Data
A catalogue record for this book is available from the British Library

Printed in the United States of America

Table of Contents

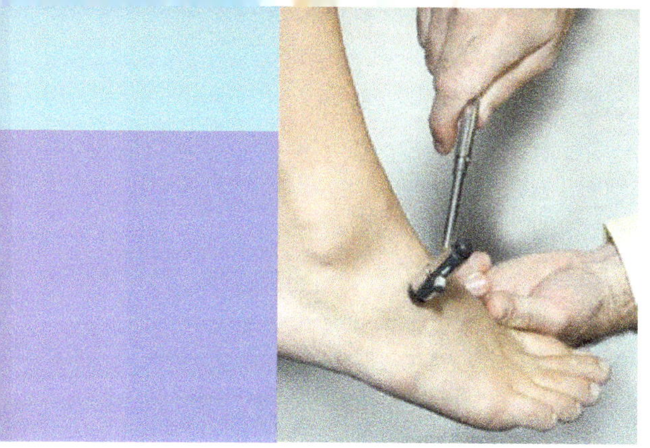

Introduction to Diagnostic Accuracy

Eric J. Hegedus

Introduction

Diagnosis of patients with orthopedic problems is a complex cognitive and psychomotor task that primarily consists of patient interview and physical examination. The patient interview produces the patient history and the range of possible diagnoses. A well-performed history also begins to narrow the range of possible diagnoses.[3,22,35] The physical examination is the next step in the patient encounter and a cornerstone of the diagnostic process. During the physical examination, the clinician uses findings to further modify the probability of the range of diagnoses,[3,30] retaining some, ruling out others, creating a list of impairments, and ultimately arriving at a hypothesis as to the pathology that produced functional limitation and disability.[1,42] We use the term "Physical Examination Tests" to capture diagnostic elements of observation, motion testing, strength testing, accessory motions, palpation, and special tests.

Physical Examination Tests have historically been an integral part of the clinical examination and have great allure for the clinician who may want to simplify the complex diagnostic process or save the patient from expensive, and often painful, imaging and lab tests. Evidence of the magnetism of Physical Examination Tests is obvious in that the rate of publication of these tests continues to accelerate[25] and musculoskeletal textbooks are rife with descriptions of tests.[9,26,33] Unfortunately, many published articles lack sound methodology.[12,23,32] Further, many of the current textbooks[26,33] offer no guidance as to the clinical utility of the test, the reliability with which the test is performed, or the quality of the research evaluating the test, leading the reader to the conclusion that "all Physical Examination Tests are created equal." Clearly, all Physical Examination Tests are not created equal.[31]

Purpose of Physical Examination Tests

Physical Examination Tests exist as part of the overall scheme for the physical examination of the patient. These tests are typically performed at two different time periods: (1) at the beginning of the physical examination as a screening test and (2) toward the end of an orderly examination as a diagnostic test.[42] The purpose of the Physical Examination Test as a screen is to help the clinician rule out some of the many possible diagnoses.[34] As a diagnostic test, the purpose of the Physical Examination Test is to validly differentiate among the few remaining competing diagnoses. These diagnoses are close to each other with regard to nature and severity so the clinician uses the Physical Examination Test to ease any remaining confusion with regard to the condition or disorder.[19]

Regardless of whether the Physical Examination Test is used for screening or diagnostic purposes, the test must be performed reliably by the practitioner or practitioners in order for that test to be a valuable guide during the clinical diagnostic process.[9,40,41] Reliability captures the extent to which a test or measurement is free from error. In reference to Physical Examination Tests, reliability is often used to capture agreement and is subdivided into intra-rater reliability and inter-rater reliability.[38] Intra-rater reliability examines whether the same single examiner can repeat the test consistently while inter-rater reliability captures whether two or more examiners can repeat the test. Both intra- and inter-rater reliability can be represented by a statistic called the intra-class correlation coefficient (ICC). Many Physical Examination Tests have dichotomous outcomes, meaning that the result of the test is either positive (the patient has the pathology) or negative (the patient does not have the pathology). When the Physical Examination Test has a dichotomous outcome, there is a high possibility that two or more examiners will agree by chance alone. The statistic frequently used to adjust for this chance agreement in dichotomous outcome tests is called kappa (κ). Kappa measures the amount of agreement beyond what would be expected by chance alone. Values for κ were categorized and value-labeled in 1976 by Landis and Koch[24] and this categorization remains prevalent today despite its arbitrary nature (Table 1). In order to determine if the Physical Examination Test serves the purpose of being both a reliable and valid screen or diagnostic tool, the test must be examined in a research study and preferably, multiple studies.

TABLE 1 The Value of Kappa (κ) (Adapted from Landis and Koch[24])

Kappa (κ) Value	Explanation
< 0	Poor/less than chance agreement
.01 to .20	Slight agreement
.21 to .40	Fair agreement
.41 to .60	Moderate agreement
.61 to .80	Substantial agreement
.81 to .99	Almost perfect agreement

Research Studies Assessing Physical Examination Tests

Research examining the reliability and diagnostic accuracy of a Physical Examination Test should be of high quality. Unfortunately, the quality of research is an issue that has plagued studies on Physical Examination Tests.[12,23,25,32,40] In an effort to improve the quality of research design in the area of Physical Examination Tests, the quality of publication of Physical Examination Test research, and the critique of that research, the scientific community has produced tools to aide the clinician on all counts.[5,6,27,40] Figure 1 shows a tool developed by Whiting et al.[40] called the Quality Assessment of Diagnostic Accuracy Studies (QUADAS). The QUADAS tool helps the evidence-based researcher detect error and bias in diagnostic accuracy studies, factors which negatively impact study quality.[40] In research terms, the QUADAS tool provides an organized format in which a reader can examine the internal validity and external validity of a study. Internal validity is improved when the research design minimizes bias. External validity is judged by whether the estimates of diagnostic accuracy can be applied to the clinical practice setting. QUADAS involves individualized scoring of 14 components. Each of the 14 questions is scored as "yes," "no," or "unclear." Individual procedures for scoring each of the 14 items, including operational standards

FIGURE 1 QUADAS Quality Assessment Tool. Used with permission from Whiting et al.[39]

Item #		Yes	No	Unclear
1	Was the spectrum of patients representative of the patients who will receive the test in practice?			
2	Were selection criteria clearly described?			
3	Is the reference standard likely to classify the target condition correctly?			
4	Is the period between reference standard and index test short enough to be reasonably sure that the target condition did not change between the two tests?			
5	Did the whole sample or a random selection of the sample receive verification using a reference standard of diagnosis?			
6	Did patients receive the same reference standard regardless of the index test result?			
7	Was the reference standard independent of the index test (i.e., the index test did not form part of the reference standard)?			
8	Was the execution of the index test described in sufficient detail to permit replication of the test?			
9	Was the execution of the reference standard described in sufficient detail to permit replication of the test?			
10	Were the index test results interpreted without knowledge of the results of the reference standard?			
11	Were the reference standard results interpreted without knowledge of the results of the index test?			
12	Were the same clinical data available when test results were interpreted as would be available when the test is used in practice?			
13	Were uninterpretable/intermediate test results reported?			
14	Were withdrawals from the study explained?			

		Truth about the Pathology	
		Present	Absent
Test Result	+	True Positives (TP) *a*	False Positives (FP) *b*
	–	False Negatives (FN) *c*	True Negatives (TN) *d*

FIGURE 2 A 2 × 2 contingency table.

for each question, have been published, although a cumulative methodological score is not advocated.[39] Past studies[11,36,37] have used a score of 7 of 14 or greater "yeses" to indicate a high quality diagnostic accuracy study whereas scores below 7 were indicative of low quality. Based on our experience in the use of the QUADAS tool, the consensus is that higher quality articles are associated with 10 or greater unequivocal "yeses," whereas those articles with less than 10 unequivocal "yeses" are associated with poorly designed studies.[10,17–18]

Estimates of diagnostic accuracy are captured using various statistical terms. The simplest way to examine these statistical terms is via the 2 × 2 table (Figure 2). The 2 × 2 table is an epidemiologist's way of showing the results of the performance of the special test when that special test is compared to a "gold" standard, or a criterion standard. The criterion standard can be a laboratory test or an imaging test but, in the area of musculoskeletal practice, the criterion standard is often confirmation of the pathology via surgery.[7,8,13,28,29] Regardless of which criterion standard is chosen, the assumption in a 2 × 2 table is that the truth about the presence or absence of the pathology under investigation is known. Common information gleaned from the 2 × 2 table is as follows:

True positive (TP)—The special test is positive and the patient truly has the pathology. Traditionally represented by *a*.

False positive (FP)—The special test is positive but the patient does not have the pathology. Traditionally represented by *b*.

False negative (FN)—The special test is negative but the patient truly has the pathology. Traditionally represented by *c*.

True negative (TN)—The special test was negative and the patient truly does not have the pathology. Traditionally represented by *d*.

Sensitivity (SN)—The probability of a positive test result in someone with the pathology. Formula: $a/(a+c)$

Specificity (SP)—The probability of a negative test result in someone without the pathology. Formula: $d/(b+d)$

Positive Likelihood Ratio (LR+)—The ratio of a positive test result in people with the pathology to a positive test result in people without the pathology. The LR+ is a multiplier in Bayes' Theorem and is used to modify the posttest probability. Formula: $SN/(1-SP)$

Negative Likelihood Ratio (LR–)—The ratio of a negative test result in people with the pathology to a negative test result in people without the pathology. Formula: $(1-SN/SP)$

Bayes' Theorem—Pretest probability of a pathology × LR+ = Posttest probability of a pathology. Please see Fagan's nomogram[13] (Figure 3) for an example of the clinical application of likelihood ratios and Bayes' Theorem.

Positive Predictive Value (PPV)—The proportion of people with the disease of those with a positive test result. Formula: $a/(a+b)$

Baseline Probability | Odds Ratio | Post-exposure Probability

(A) 0.01, 0.02, 0.03, 0.05, 0.07, 0.1, 0.2, 0.3, 0.4, 0.5, 0.6, 0.7, 0.8, 0.9, 0.93, 0.95, 0.97, 0.98, 0.99

(B) 1000, 500, 100, 50, 10, 5, 1, 0.5, 0.1, 0.05, 0.01, 0.005, 0.001

(C) 0.99, 0.98, 0.97, 0.95, 0.93, 0.9, 0.8, 0.7, 0.6, 0.5, 0.4, 0.3, 0.2, 0.1, 0.07, 0.05, 0.03, 0.02, 0.01

FIGURE 3 Fagan's nomogram for using a likelihood ratio (LR) to modify pretest probability into an estimate of posttest probability accuracy.

TABLE 2 The Use of Likelihood Ratios (Adapted from Jaeschke et al.[19])

+ LR	Explanation	–LR
1 to 2	Alters posttest probability of a diagnosis to a very small degree	.5 to 1
2 to 5	Alters posttest probability of a diagnosis to a small degree	.2 to .5
5 to 10	Alters posttest probability of a diagnosis to a moderate degree	.1 to .2
More than 10	Alters posttest probability of a diagnosis to a moderate degree	Less than .1

Negative Predictive Value (NPV)—The proportion of people without the disease who had a negative test result. Formula: $d/(c+d)$

Accuracy—The proportion of subjects correctly identified by the test results. Formula: $(a+d)/(a+b+c+d)$

True positives, true negatives, false positives, and false negatives are terms to capture the raw data from a study examining the accuracy of special tests. All four of these measures contribute to sensitivity (SN) and specificity (SP). Tests with a high SN are valued as screening tests to rule out pathology when they are negative.[34,42] In studies that examine the diagnostic ability of a test, SN and SP are arguably the most popular measures of test performance. While SN and SP are popular, they are, nonetheless, incomplete measures of test performance. As SN increases, SP often decreases.[15] Further, paired indicators like SN/SP, PPV/NPV, and LR+/LR− cannot be used to easily rank special tests so that a clinician may easily pick the best test[15] despite the fact that, in 1994, Jaeschke et al.[20] attempted to make likelihood ratios more clinician-friendly by producing an outline of acceptable likelihood ratios (Table 2). Accuracy is a single, easily understood measure of test performance, but accuracy is greatly affected by the prevalence of a pathology.[15] The prevalence of a pathology can change from clinic to clinic. For example, a sports clinic is more likely to see patients with a torn anterior cruciate ligament than a primary care practice and thus, a special test that detects a torn anterior cruciate ligament is likely to appear to have greater accuracy when used in the sports clinic.

All of these measures, while capturing the performance of a special test in a research study, lack the ability to comment on the consistency/reliability with which the diagnostic test was performed and the overall quality of that study. If examiners are performing the same special test in a different fashion then they will have difficulty making valid decisions about patients.[2] Further, if the overall quality of a study is poor and full of bias, the accuracy of the special test will be over-estimated in that study and the measures from that study should be used with caution.[31,41]

How to Use This TEXT

The purposes of this text are to: (1) produce a comprehensive current list of Physical Examination Tests and, when possible, their original descriptions and (2) aid the musculoskeletal practitioner in the choosing of the best available Physical Examination Tests for his or her practice. With these goals in mind, we have attempted to make this text as clinician-friendly as possible. The text covers a broad anatomical area and is then subdivided into Physical Examination Tests that detect pathologies within that anatomical area. Further, within each pathoanatomic category, the studies are ordered so that the clinician will find the best tests first and the tests with little or no research to back them last. We do realize that this will cause some consternation when some clinical favorite Physical Examination Tests are not listed first. A detailed description (original if possible) and photograph will accompany each Physical Examination Test. All relevant literature studying the test's descriminatory ability and reliability will be summarized in a table format along with the epidemiological statistics gathered from that material (Figure 4). Finally, the number of "yeses" on the QUADAS tool will be recorded for each article and we will give the test a summary "Utility Score" which is our opinion of the clinical use of that special test after gathering and critically evaluating all of the literature. Please see Figure 4 for an example of the text's format. We feel it is important for the reader to know that, because the quality of research literature in the area of special tests is mediocre, some would say that providing a quality score for Physical Examination Tests is unwise.[39] Be that as it may, our goal is to create text that is as clinician-friendly as possible and the "Utility Score" is our expert opinion, as clinicians, teachers, and researchers, as to the clinical import of each special test. Our scale for the "Utility Score" is as follows:

- **1** Evidence strongly supports the use of this test
- **2** Evidence moderately supports the use of this test
- **3** Evidence minimally supports or does not support the use of this test
- **?** The test has not been researched sufficiently so we are unsure of its value

We hope that you find this text of use and that we contribute, in some small way, to the value of your clinical practice.

FIGURE 4 **Example of Textbook format.**

ANTERIOR DRAWER TEST [Anterior Cruciate Ligament (ACL) Tear]

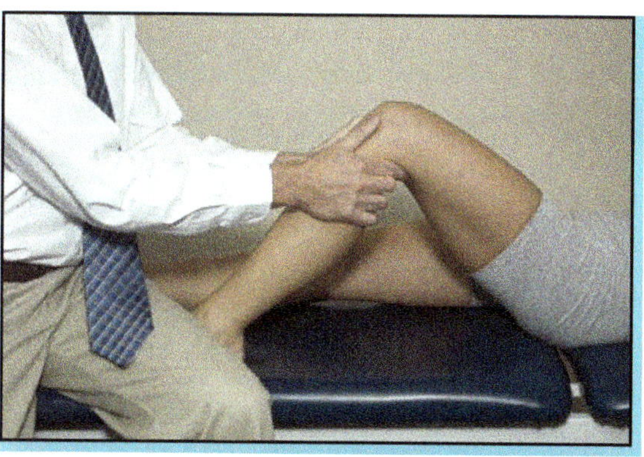

1) The patient is supine with the knee flexed to 90 degrees so that the foot is flat.

2) The examiner sits on the patient's foot and grasps behind the proximal tibia with thumbs palpating the tibial plateau and index fingers palpating the tendons of the hamstring muscle group medially and laterally.

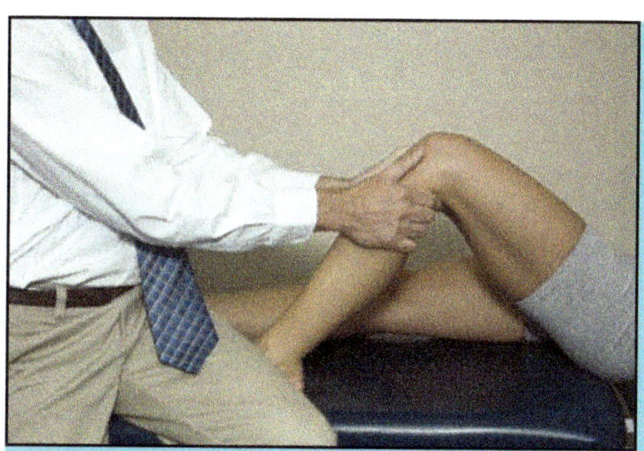

3) An anterior tibial force is applied by the examiner.

4) A positive test for a torn ACL is indicated by greater anterior tibial displacement on the affected side when compared to the unaffected side.

UTILITY SCORE 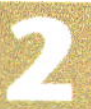

Study		Reliability	Sensitivity	Specificity	LR+	LR–	QUADAS Score (0–14)
Hardaker[16]		NT	18	NT	NA	NA	8
Bomberg[4]		NT	41	100	NA	NA	9
Jonsson[21]	Acute (A)	NT	33	NT	NA	NA	8
	Chronic (C)	NT	95	NT	NA	NA	8

Comments: The Anterior Drawer Test appears to be a specific test helpful at ruling in a torn ACL when the test is positive. The Anterior Drawer Test may become more sensitive in non-acute patients.
NT = Not Tested. This designation is used when the statistic was not reported in the study for whatever reason. Also, if a study reported only one of either sensitivity or specificity, then the rest of the statistics for that study are reported as NA.
NA = Not Applicable. This designation, in addition to being used when only one of either sensitivity or specificity are reported, is used for the likelihood ratios (LR+/LR–) when either sensitivity or specificity is reported as perfect (100) for a study. Also, if the study was not one of diagnostic accuracy then NA was used to indicate that QUADAS cannot be used to critique study quality.
Inf = Infinity, a value that cannot be truly calculated because the sensitivity or specificity is 100%.

References

1. Guide to Physical Therapist Practice. 2d ed. American Physical Therapy Association. *Phys Ther.* 2001;81:9–746.
2. Bartko JJ, Carpenter WT, Jr. On the methods and theory of reliability. *J Nerv Ment Dis.* 1976;163:307–317.
3. Benbassat J, Baumal R, Heyman SN, Brezis M. Viewpoint: suggestions for a shift in teaching clinical skills to medical students: the reflective clinical examination. *Acad Med.* 2005;80:1121–1126.
4. Bomberg BC, McGinty JB. Acute hemarthrosis of the knee: indications for diagnostic arthroscopy. *Arthroscopy.* 1990;6:221–225.
5. Bossuyt PM, Reitsma JB, Bruns DE, et al. Towards complete and accurate reporting of studies of diagnostic accuracy: The STARD Initiative. *Ann Intern Med.* 2003;138:40–44.
6. Bossuyt PM, Reitsma JB, Bruns DE, et al. The STARD statement for reporting studies of diagnostic accuracy: explanation and elaboration. *Ann Intern Med.* 2003;138:W1–12.
7. Chan YS, Lien LC, Hsu HL, et al. Evaluating hip labral tears using magnetic resonance arthrography: a prospective study comparing hip arthroscopy and magnetic resonance arthrography diagnosis. *Arthroscopy.* 2005;21:1250.
8. Charnley J. Orthopaedic signs in the diagnosis of disc protrusion. With special reference to the straight-leg-raising test. *Lancet.* 1951;1:186–192.
9. Cleland J. *Orthopaedic Clinical Examination: An Evidence-Based Approach for Physical Therapists.* 1st ed. Carlstadt, NJ: Icon Learning Systems; 2005.
10. Cook C, Hegedus E. Diagnostic utility of clinical tests for spinal dysfunction. *Man Ther.* 2011;16:21–25.
11. de Graaf I, Prak A, Bierma-Zeinstra S, Thomas S, Peul W, Koes B. Diagnosis of lumbar spinal stenosis: a systematic review of the accuracy of diagnostic tests. *Spine.* 2006;31:1168–1176.
12. Deeks JJ. Systematic reviews in health care: Systematic reviews of evaluations of diagnostic and screening tests. *BMJ.* 2001;323:157–162.
13. Eren OT. The accuracy of joint line tenderness by physical examination in the diagnosis of meniscal tears. *Arthroscopy.* 2003;19:850–854.
14. Fagan TJ. Letter: Nomogram for Bayes theorem. *N Engl J Med.* 1975;293:257.
15. Glas AS, Lijmer JG, Prins MH, Bonsel GJ, Bossuyt PM. The diagnostic odds ratio: a single indicator of test performance. *J Clin Epidemiol.* 2003;56:1129–1135.
16. Hardaker WT, Jr., Garrett WE, Jr., Bassett FH, 3rd. Evaluation of acute traumatic hemarthrosis of the knee joint. *South Med J.* 1990;83:640–644.
17. Hegedus EJ, Cook C, Hasselblad V, Goode A, McCrory DC. Physical examination tests for assessing a torn meniscus in the knee: a systematic review with meta-analysis. *J Orthop Sports Phys Ther.* 2007;37:541–550.
18. Hegedus EJ, Goode A, Campbell S, Morin A, Tamaddoni M, Moorman CT 3rd, Cook C. Physical examination tests of the shoulder: a systematic review with meta-analysis of individual tests. *Br J Sports Med.* 2008;42:80–92.
19. Jaeschke R, Guyatt G, Lijmer JG. *User's Guide to the Medical Literature: Essentials of Evidence-Based Practice.* Chicago, IL: AMA Press; 2002.
20. Jaeschke R, Guyatt GH, Sackett DL. Users' guides to the medical literature. III. How to use an article about a diagnostic test. B. What are the results and will they help me in caring for my patients? The Evidence-Based Medicine Working Group. *JAMA.* 1994;271:703–707.
21. Jonsson T, Althoff B, Peterson L, Renstrom P. Clinical diagnosis of ruptures of the anterior cruciate ligament: a comparative study of the Lachman test and the anterior drawer sign. *Am J Sports Med.* 1982;10:100–102.
22. Kassirer JP. Teaching clinical medicine by iterative hypothesis testing. Let's preach what we practice. *N Engl J Med.* 1983;309:921–923.
23. Knottnerus JA, van Weel C, Muris JW. Evaluation of diagnostic procedures. *BMJ.* 2002;324:477–480.
24. Landis JR, Koch GG. The measurement of observer agreement for categorical data. *Biometrics.* 1977;33:159–174.
25. Lijmer JG, Mol BW, Heisterkamp S, et al. Empirical evidence of design-related bias in studies of diagnostic tests. *JAMA.* 1999;282:1061–1066.
26. Magee DJ. *Orthopedic Physical Assessment.* Third ed. Philadelphia, PA: W.B. Saunders Company; 1997.
27. Mulrow CD, Linn WD, Gaul MK, Pugh JA. Assessing quality of a diagnostic test evaluation. *J Gen Intern Med.* 1989;4:288–295.
28. Murrell GA, Walton JR. Diagnosis of rotator cuff tears. *Lancet.* 2001;357:769–770.
29. Park HB, Yokota A, Gill HS, El Rassi G, McFarland EG. Diagnostic accuracy of clinical tests for the different degrees of subacromial impingement syndrome. *J Bone Joint Surg Am.* 2005;87:1446–1455.
30. Pauker SG, Kassirer JP. The threshold approach to clinical decision making. *N Engl J Med.* 1980;302:1109–1117.
31. Pewsner D, Battaglia M, Minder C, Marx A, Bucher HC, Egger M. Ruling a diagnosis in or out with "SpPIn" and "SnNOut": a note of caution. *BMJ.* 2004;329:209–213.
32. Reid MC, Lachs MS, Feinstein AR. Use of methodological standards in diagnostic test research. Getting better but still not good. *JAMA.* 1995;274:645–651.
33. Richardson J, Iglarsh Z. *Clinical Orthopaedic Physical Therapy.* Philadelphia: W.B. Saunders Company; 1994.
34. Sackett D, Strauss S, Richardson W, Rosenberg W, Haynes R. *Evidence-Based Medicine: How to Practice and Teach EBM.* 2d ed. Churchill Livingstone; 2000.
35. Schmitt BP, Kushner MS, Wiener SL. The diagnostic usefulness of the history of the patient with dyspnea. *J Gen Intern Med.* 1986;1:386–393.

36. Sehgal N, Shah RV, McKenzie-Brown AM, Everett CR. Diagnostic utility of facet (zygapophysial) joint injections in chronic spinal pain: a systematic review of evidence. *Pain Physician.* 2005;8:211–224.

37. Shah RV, Everett CR, McKenzie-Brown AM, Sehgal N. Discography as a diagnostic test for spinal pain: a systematic and narrative review. *Pain Physician.* 2005;8:187–209.

38. Sim J, Wright CC. The kappa statistic in reliability studies: use, interpretation, and sample size requirements. *Phys Ther.* 2005;85:257–268.

39. Whiting P, Harbord R, Kleijnen J. No role for quality scores in systematic reviews of diagnostic accuracy studies. *BMC Med Res Methodol.* 2005;5:19.

40. Whiting P, Rutjes AW, Dinnes J, Reitsma J, Bossuyt PM, Kleijnen J. Development and validation of methods for assessing the quality of diagnostic accuracy studies. *Health Technol Assess.* 2004;8:iii, 1–234.

41. Whiting P, Rutjes AW, Reitsma JB, Glas AS, Bossuyt PM, Kleijnen J. Sources of variation and bias in studies of diagnostic accuracy: a systematic review. *Ann Intern Med.* 2004;140:189–202.

42. Woolf AD. How to assess musculoskeletal conditions. History and physical examination. *Best Pract Res Clin Rheumatol.* 2003;17:381–402.

Physical Examination Tests for Medical Screening

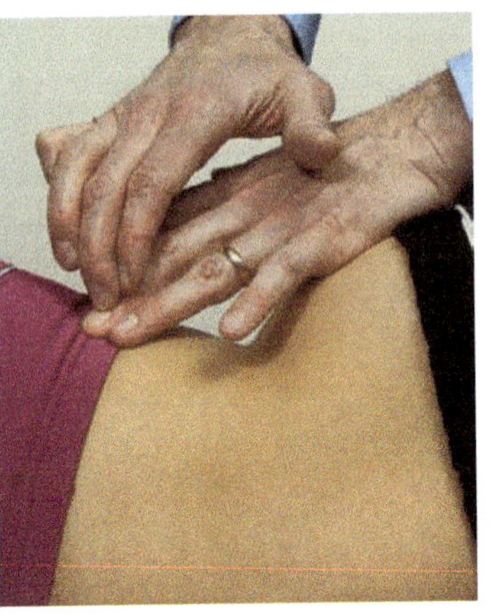

Physical Examination Tests for Medical Screening

Ken Learman

Please refer to the chapter "Introduction to Diagnostic Accuracy" before reading this chapter.

Index of Tests

Test for Cardiopulmonary, Vascular Disease, and Abdominal Aortic Aneurysm

Palpation of Abdominal Aorta

Tests for Deep Vein Thrombosis

Wells Criteria for Deep Vein Thrombosis

Tests for Upper Extremity Deep Vein Thrombosis

Tests for Pulmonary Embolism

Wells Criteria for Pulmonary Embolism

Geneva Criteria

Tests to Predict Future Cardiopulmonary Events

San Francisco Syncope Rule for Predicting Serious Short-term Outcome

Framingham Criteria for Heart Failure

Thrombolysis in Myocardial Infarction (TIMI) Score for Acute Coronary Syndromes

Risk Score for Acute Coronary Syndromes

Duke Treadmill Score for Identifying Risk of Ischaemic Heart Disease

Clinical Prediction Rule to Identify Individuals with Low Risk of Stroke from Atrial Fibrillation while Taking Aspirin

Ankle-Brachial Index for Predicting Coronary Artery Disease

Ankle Brachial Index for Predicting Stroke

Ankle-Brachial Index for Predicting any Cardiovascular Event

Ankle-Brachial Index for Predicting Peripheral Artery Disease

Ankle-Brachial Index for Predicting Cardiovascular Mortality

Ankle-Brachial Index for Predicting Total Mortality

Ankle-Brachial Index for Predicting Functional Deficits

Tests to Determine Need for Bone Mineral Densitometry

Male Osteoporosis Risk Estimation Score (MORES) Criteria for Bone Densitometry in Men

Osteoporosis Self-Assessment Tool (OST) Criteria for Bone Densitometry in Women

Osteoporosis Risk Assessment Instrument (ORAI) Criteria for Bone Densitometry

Simple Calculated Osteoporosis Risk Estimation (SCORE) for Bone Densitometry

National Osteoporosis Foundation (NOF) Criteria for Bone Densitometry

Age, Body Size, No Estrogen (ABONE) for Osteoporosis Prediction

Weight Criterion for Osteoporosis Prediction

Osteoporosis Index of Risk (OSIRIS)

Study of Osteoporotic Fractures Risk Index (SOFSURE)

Tests for Fracture Assessment

Barford Test for Fracture Assessment

Tuning Fork Test for Fracture Assessment

VISCERAL SCREENING

TESTS FOR SPLENOMEGALY

Nixon's Percussion

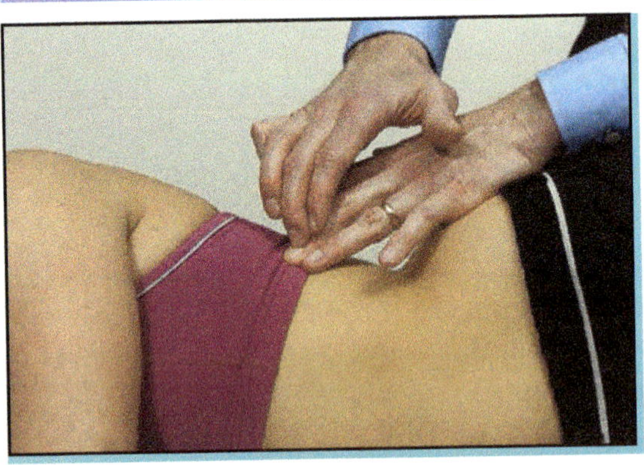

1) Patient is placed on right side lying with arms resting at shoulder level to allow full access of the spleen.

2) The distal end of lung resonance is found at the posterior axillary line.

3) Percussion is begun at the point found in step 2 and is continued in an anterior and inferior direction toward the midanterior costal margin.

4) A positive test is indicated when dullness extends over 8cm above the costal margin (normal is considered 6–8cm).

UTILITY SCORE 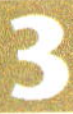

Study	Reliability	Sensitivity	Specificity	LR+	LR−	QUADAS Score (0–14)
Nixon[56]	NT	NT	NT	NT	NT	NA
Sullivan & Williams[76]	NT	59	94	9.83	0.44	8
Tamayo et al.[77]	0.31	37	79	1.76	0.80	11

Comments: Nixon[56] used successful splenic aspiration biopsies of 60 cases as the reference standard of splenomegaly confirmation; however, the study is not a true diagnostic accuracy study as very little description of methods and results were provided, making QUADAS assessment inappropriate. Sullivan & Williams[76] studied 65 subjects with suspected enlarged spleens who were scheduled to undergo ^{99m}Tc-sulfur colloid scans. Tamayo et al. calculated an overall reliability coefficient for 8 examiners with a Kendall's W (coefficient of concordance). Tamayo et al.'s[77] sensitivity and specificity values are data pooled for the 8 examiners and the likelihood ratios differ slightly from the Mantel-Haenszel estimates provided in the article.

TESTS FOR SPLENOMEGALY

Castell's Percussion

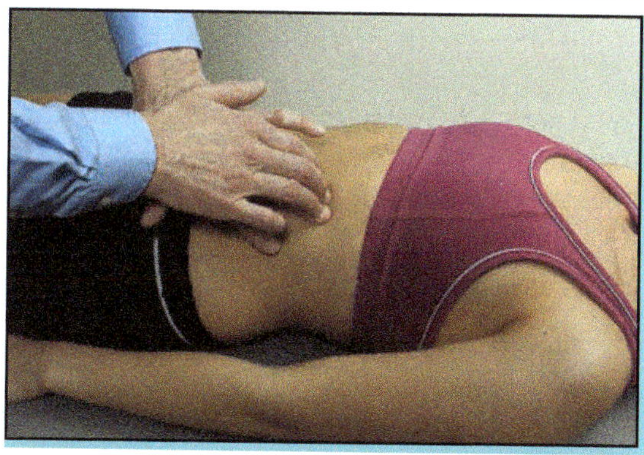

1) The patient is placed in supine with the examiner placing his or her fingers over the lowest intercostal space in line with the anterior axillary line (usually the 8th or 9th space).

2) Using a dummy finger technique, the examiner percusses the space at rest and with full inspiration.

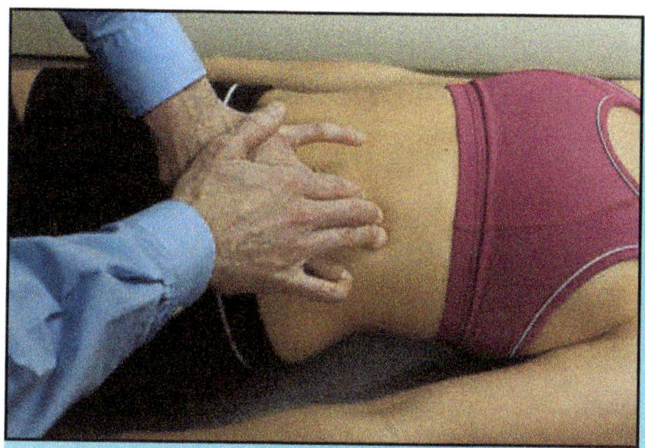

3) A positive test is perceived dullness of sound during percussion on full inspiration because the spleen descends during this condition. However, a grossly enlarged spleen could produce dullness in sound in both conditions, obfuscating the typical resonant sound at rest.

UTILITY SCORE 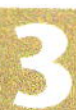 3

Study	Reliability	Sensitivity	Specificity	LR+	LR−	QUADAS Score (0–14)
Castell[12]	NT	NA	NA	NA	NA	8
Sullivan & Williams[76]	NT	82	83	4.82	0.22	8
Tamayo et al.[77]	0.31	39	80	1.95	0.76	11
Barkun et al.[5]	NT	79	46	1.46	0.46	9

Comments: Castell's[12] study included 10 subjects with a positive test and 10 subjects that were not expected to have splenomegaly. It is not a true diagnostic accuracy study; therefore, the results are not presented. Tamayo et al.[77] calculated an overall reliability coefficient for 8 examiners with a Kendall's W. Tamayo et al.'s[77] sensitivity and specificity values are data pooled for the 8 examiners and the likelihood ratios differ from the Mantel-Haenszel estimates provided in the article. Barkun et al.[5] called this test the splenic percussion sign. They performed the Castell maneuver but used the following grading criteria: 1) definitely tympanitic, 2) probably tympanitic, 3) uncertain, 4) probably dull, and 5) definitely dull. If the grade of the resonant sound progresses at least one level closer to definitely dull on full inspiration, it was considered positive. This criteria operationally defines a positive test more objectively than Castell's original description.

TESTS FOR SPLENOMEGALY

Percussion Test in Traube's Space

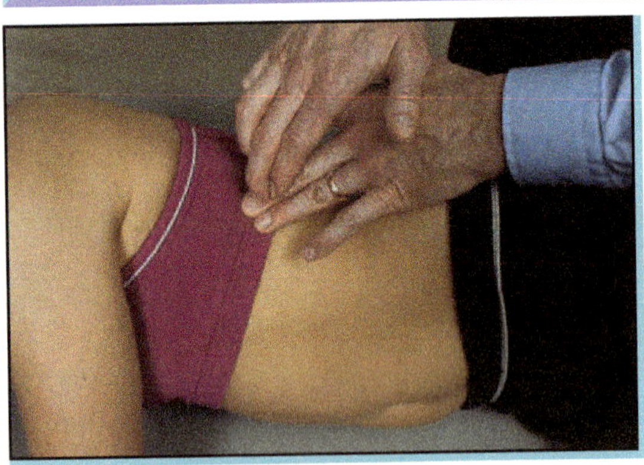

1) The patient is instructed to lie on right side.

2) Traube's space, defined by the 6th rib superiorly, the midaxillary line laterally, and the costal margin anteriorly, is percussed at one or more levels from lateral to medial margin while the subject breathes normally.

3) The quality of sound is graded on a five-point scale including 1) definitely tympanitic, 2) probably tympanitic, 3) uncertain, 4) probably dull, and 5) definitely dull.

4) A positive test is determined by the responses 3) uncertain, 4) probably dull, and 5) definitely dull.

UTILITY SCORE 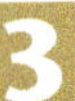

Study	Reliability	Sensitivity	Specificity	LR+	LR−	QUADAS Score (0–14)
Barkun et al.[6]	0.41, 0.22, 0.19	62	72	2.21	0.53	11
Barkun et al.[5]	NT	62	72	2.21	0.53	9
Tamayo et al.[77]	0.31	22	87	1.69	0.90	11

Comments: Barkun et al.[6] had 3 physicians clinically examine each patient resulting in 3 sets of paired reliability (kappa) coefficients. Barkun et al.[6] compared subjects known to have splenomegaly by ultrasonography with control subjects. Barkun et al.[5] used the same data set as Barkun 1989[6]. Tamayo et al.[77] calculated an overall reliability coefficient for 8 examiners with a Kendall's W. Tamayo et al.'s[77] sensitivity and specificity values are data pooled for the 8 examiners and the likelihood ratios differ from the Mantel-Haenszel estimates provided in the article.

Bimanual Palpation of Spleen

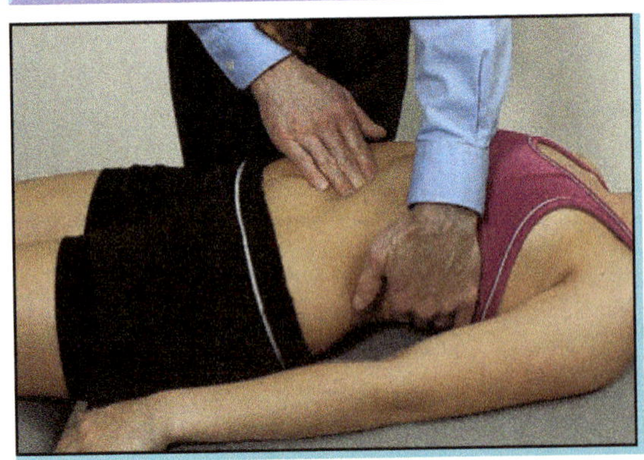

1) Patient is instructed to lie supine and breathe normally.

2) Standing at the patient's right side, the examiner reaches across the patient's body and, with the left hand, elevates the left rib cage and simultaneously creates skin slack on the costal margin.

3) With the right hand, the examiner palpates at the costal margin allowing the fingers to probe underneath the ribs attempting to feel the spleen's decent during inspiration. This palpation is performed along the whole costal margin. If needed, the patient can roll part way to the right allowing greater access to the lateral aspect of the costal margin.

4) A positive test is the ability to palpate the enlarged spleen.

TESTS FOR SPLENOMEGALY

UTILITY SCORE 3

Study	Reliability	Sensitivity	Specificity	LR+	LR−	QUADAS Score (0–14)
Tamayo et al.[77]	0.31	31	82	1.72	0.84	11
Barkun et al.[5]	0.7, 0.56, 0.57	56	93	8.00	0.57	9
Holzbach et al.[30]	NT	63	100	NA	0.37	6
Zhang & Lewis[91]	NT	56	69	1.81	0.64	7
Halpern et al.[28]	NT	28	98	14.0	0.73	6
Blendis et al.[7]	88%	79	100	NA	0.21	6
Sullivan & Williams[76]	NT	71	90	7.1	0.32	7

Comments: Tamayo et al.'s[77] sensitivity and specificity values are data pooled for 8 examiners and the likelihood ratios differ from the Mantel-Haenszel estimates provided in the article. Barkun et al.[5] combined the Bimanual and Middleton's maneuver techniques statistically and called the combination "Palpation." Holzbach et al.[30] do not describe which palpation technique was implemented in their study. In addition, the data set described in their narrative does not appear to match the sample size identified in the appropriate figure in the article. Zhang & Lewis[91] did not report which palpation technique was performed in the study. Blendis et al.[7] used a relatively small sample size and the methodology had many potential flaws, but did report that there was 88% agreement for all 4 clinical examiners and 97% agreement for 3 of 4 examiners. Halpern et al.[28] performed a retrospective chart review that may have verification bias since clinical vs. reference standards testing occurred up to 2 months apart. Sullivan & Williams[76] did not report which palpation technique was incorporated in the study resulting in a lower QUADAS score than in the percussion techniques study.

Ballottement of Spleen

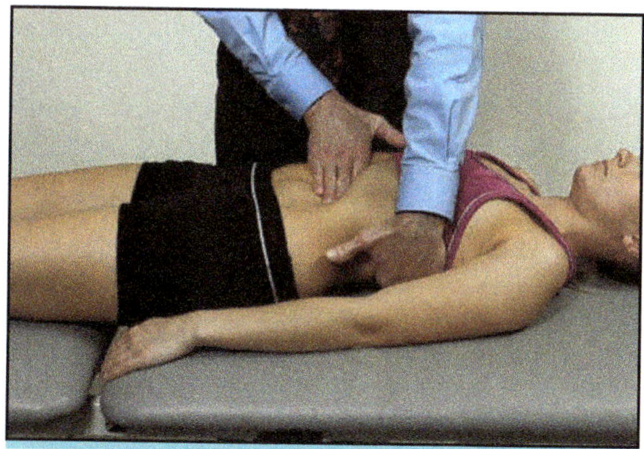

1. Patient is instructed to lie supine and breathe normally.
2. Standing at the patient's right side, the examiner reaches across the patient's body and, with the left hand, elevates the left rib cage and simultaneously creates skin slack on the costal margin.
3. With the right hand, the examiner palpates at the costal margin allowing the fingers to probe underneath the ribs.
4. A positive test is the ability to feel impulses from the spleen indicating an enlargement.

UTILITY SCORE 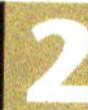

Study	Reliability	Sensitivity	Specificity	LR+	LR−	QUADAS Score (0–14)
Tamayo et al.[77]	0.31	38	83	2.24	0.75	11

Comments: Tamayo et al.'s[77] sensitivity and specificity values are data pooled for 8 examiners and the likelihood ratios differ from the Mantel-Haenszel estimates provided in the article.

TESTS FOR SPLENOMEGALY

Middleton's Maneuver for Splenomegaly (Palpation from above the Patient)

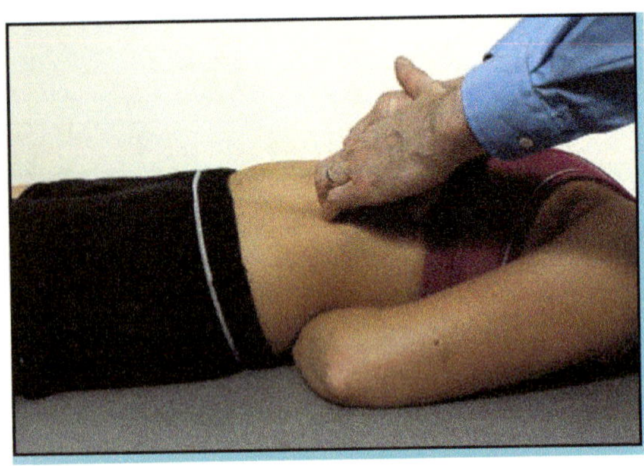

1) Patient is instructed to lie supine, place his or her own left fist under the left lower rib cage and breathe normally.

2) The examiner stands above the patient at their left shoulder and with both hands, curls the fingertips over the left costal margin and palpates for the spleen while the patient takes deep breaths.

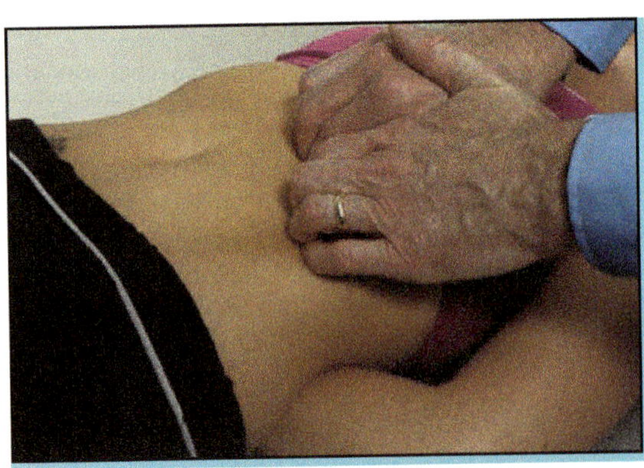

3) A positive test is a palpable spleen at any point during the examination.

UTILITY SCORE 

Study	Reliability	Sensitivity	Specificity	LR+	LR−	QUADAS Score (0–14)
Tamayo et al.[77]	0.31	35	87	2.69	0.75	11
Barkun et al.[5]	0.7, 0.56, 0.57	56	93	8.00	0.57	9
Comments: Tamayo et al.'s[77] sensitivity and specificity values are data pooled for 8 examiners and the likelihood ratios differ from the Mantel-Haenszel estimates provided in the article. Barkun et al.[5] combined the Bimanual and Middleton's maneuver techniques statistically and called the combination "Palpation."						

Percussion and Palpation of the Spleen

1) Perform either bimanual or Middleton's palpation as described above.

2) Perform a splenic percussion as described by Castell, Nixon, or in Traube's space.

3) A positive test is indicated when either the percussion test or the palpation test is positive.

UTILITY SCORE 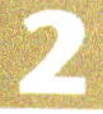

Study	Reliability	Sensitivity	Specificity	LR+	LR−	QUADAS Score (0–14)
Sullivan & Williams[76]	NT	88	83	5.18	0.14	7
Barkun et al.[5] [both tests concurrently (+)]	NT	46	97	15.33	0.56	9
Barkun et al.[5] [either test (+) or both tests (−)]	NT	72	68	2.25	0.41	9

Comments: Sullivan & Williams[76] did not make it clear whether or not both percussion techniques were combined with palpation in the combined condition nor did they describe which palpation maneuver was employed. Barkun et al.[5] used a combination of bimanual palpation and Middleton's maneuver for palpation and Traube's space percussion test.

TESTS FOR HEPATOMEGALY

Palpation of the Liver

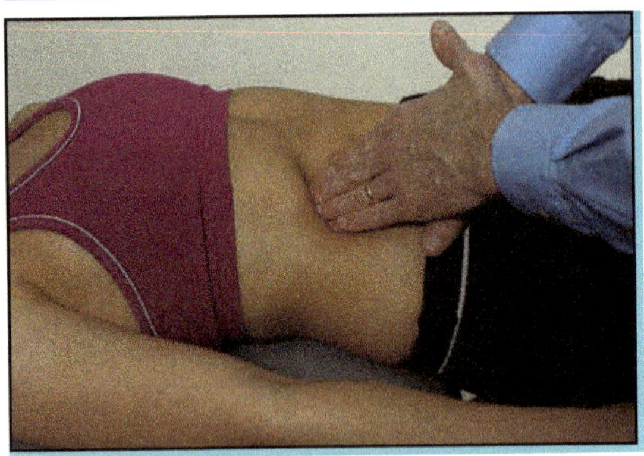

1. Patient lies supine and is asked to fully relax the abdomen.
2. The examiner's left hand is placed under the patient's inferior costovertebral region with the hand parallel to the lower ribs.
3. The examiner places one hand over the patient's right upper quadrant of the abdomen in line with the midclavicular line.
4. The examiner then palpates deeply in a posterior and superior direction while the patient takes a deep breath that causes the liver to descend toward the fingers.
5. A positive test is a readily palpable liver that may be painful. Please note, in certain circumstances, COPD and young children, the liver is more readily palpable, up to 3cm below the costal margin.

UTILITY SCORE 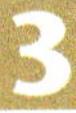

Study	Reliability	Sensitivity	Specificity	LR+	LR−	QUADAS Score (0–14)
Halpern et al.[28]	NT	71	62	1.87	0.47	6
Joshi et al.[32]	0.44, 0.49, 0.53	39–42	82–86	2.17–3.0	0.68–0.74	9
Blendis et al.[7]	54%	50	47	0.94	1.06	6
Ralphs et al.[64]	NT	36	83	2.18	0.76	10

Comments: Neither Halpern et al.[28] nor Joshi et al.[32] described the exact technique used to palpate the liver; therefore, a common technique for liver palpation was provided above. Joshi et al.[32] described the diagnostic accuracy of 3 independent examiners but did not provide sufficient data to pool; therefore, ranges were provided for all values. Blendis et al.[7] did not provide diagnostic accuracy information for the entire sample of subjects tested nor was the reference standard used to diagnose hepatomegaly consistent with other reports, bringing into question the validity of the reported values. Ralphs et al.[64] examined normal subjects only and compared investigator's ability to determine the liver that extends below the costal margin and performed the palpation and percussion exams together.

Percussion of the Liver

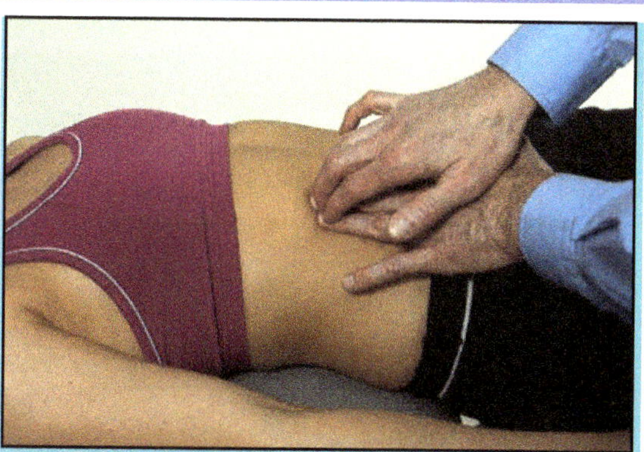

1) Patient lies supine and is asked to fully relax the abdomen.

2) The examiner locates the right midclavicular region and mentally draws a line down from this point through the right lower quadrant.

3) The examiner places the non-dominant third digit on the midclavicular line well below the expected point of liver dullness (in line with the umbilicus should be far enough in most cases).

4) The examiner then percusses the non-dominant finger with the dominant hand to create a sound of tympani or dullness. This procedure is continued every couple of centimeters in a proximal direction until the tympanitic sound of the abdomen gives way to a dull sound at the liver's border. This point is marked.

5) This technique is repeated from a point on the midclavicular line well proximal to the expected superior border of the liver in a distal direction until the superior border of the liver is perceived. This point is also marked and the distance between the marks is measured.

6) A positive test is a superior to inferior liver span of > 10cm. This may indicate hepatomegaly.

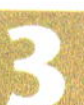

UTILITY SCORE 3

Study	Reliability	Sensitivity	Specificity	LR+	LR−	QUADAS Score (0–14)
Joshi et al.[32]	0.33, 0.31, 0.17	39–61	43–64	1.07–1.15	0.89–0.96	9
Ralphs et al.[64]	NT	36	83	2.18	0.76	10

Comments: Joshi et al.[32] did not describe the procedure used in liver percussion. Joshi et al.[32] described the diagnostic accuracy of 3 independent examiners but did not provide sufficient data to pool; therefore, ranges were provided for all values. Ralphs et al.[64] examined normal subjects only and compared investigator's ability to determine the liver that extends below the costal margin and performed the palpation and percussion exams together.

TEST FOR CHOLECYSTITIS

Murphy's Sign

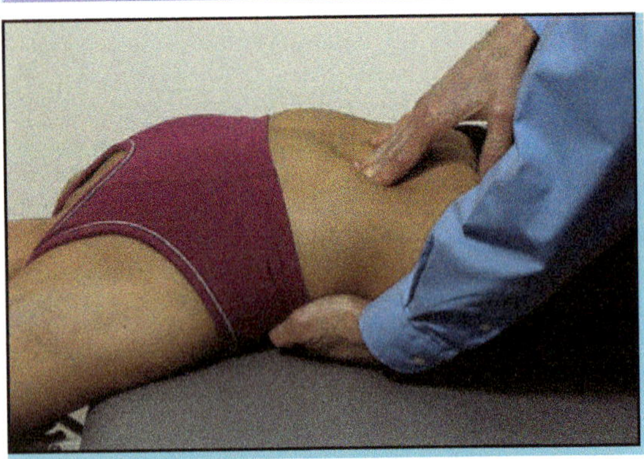

1. The patient is directed to lie supine and relax the abdomen.
2. The examiner places one hand on the right, posterior inferior costal margin.
3. The examiner places the other hand on the right upper quarter subcostal region.
4. The patient then draws in a deep breath while the examiner simultaneously palpates the subcostal region deeply.
5. A positive test is pain during inspiration and/or an associated inspiratory arrest.

UTILITY SCORE 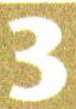

Study	Reliability	Sensitivity	Specificity	LR+	LR−	QUADAS Score (0–14)
Bree[8]	NT	86	35	1.32	0.40	9
Ralls et al.[63]	NT	63	94	9.84	0.40	9
Singer et al.[74]	NT	97	48	1.88	0.06	10

Comments: Bree[8] used a sonogram assisted Murphy's sign to ensure that the point of maximal tenderness was directly over the gallbladder which may increase the diagnostic accuracy of the test. Singer et al.[74] performed a retrospective chart analysis of subjects presenting to an emergency room with abdominal pain.

TESTS FOR KIDNEY SIZE

Palpation of Kidney

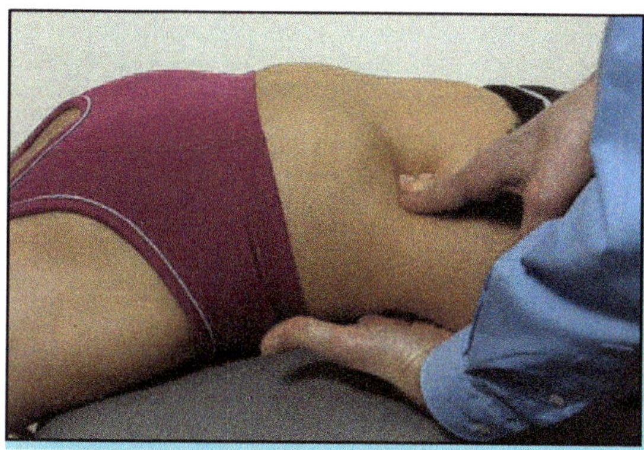

1) The patient lies supine and relaxes the abdomen.
2) The examiner places one hand on the posterior inferior costal margin.
3) The examiner places the other hand on the abdomen lateral to the rectus abdominus, proximal to the umbilicus, and distal to the ribs.
4) The examiner then draws the trunk anteriorly with the posterior hand while palpating deeply into the abdomen.
5) A positive test is pain during palpation or an appreciable difference in the size or texture of the kidneys.

UTILITY SCORE 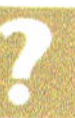

Study	Reliability	Sensitivity	Specificity	LR+	LR−	QUADAS Score (0–14)
NT	NT	NT	NT	NT	NT	NT
Comments: The diagnostic accuracy of kidney palpation does not appear to have been studied.						

Percussion of the Kidney (Murphy's Percussion Test or Test for Costovertebral Tenderness)

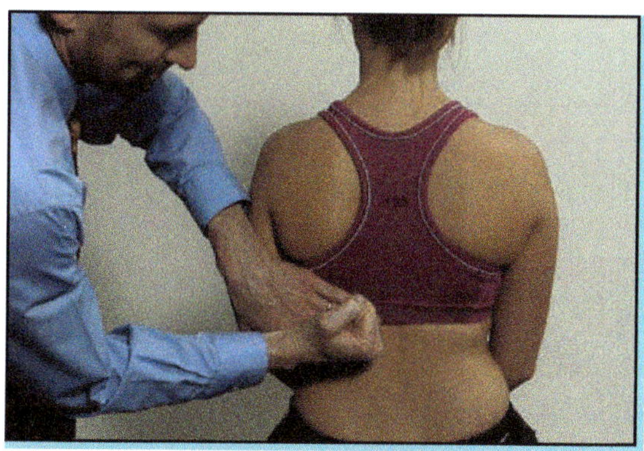

1) The patient lies prone or assumes a seated position without a chair back.
2) The examiner places one hand over the 12th rib at the costovertebral angle.
3) The examiner then raps the back of the palpatory hand with the other fist.
4) The normal patient will feel a firm thud but should feel no pain from the test. A positive test is pain in the back (subcostal region) and/or into the flank and lateral abdomen.

UTILITY SCORE 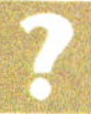

Study	Reliability	Sensitivity	Specificity	LR+	LR−	QUADAS Score (0–14)
NT	NT	NT	NT	NT	NT	NT
Comments: The diagnostic accuracy of kidney percussion does not appear to have been studied.						

TESTS FOR ACUTE APPENDICITIS

Palpation of McBurney's Point

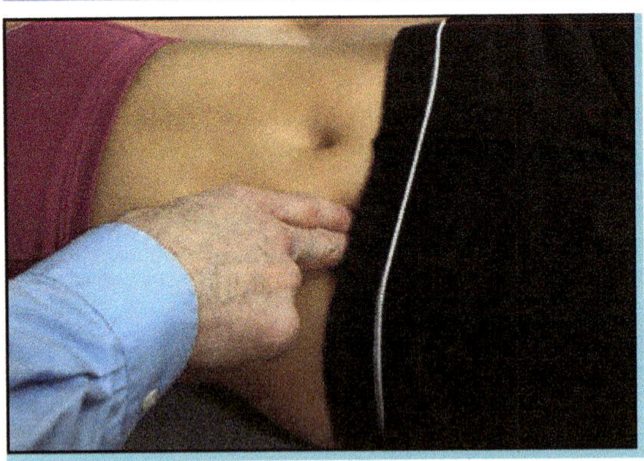

1. The patient lies supine and is asked to fully relax the abdomen.
2. The examiner gently and deeply palpates the right lower quadrant of the abdomen (midway between the umbilicus and the ASIS) looking for tenderness.
3. The examiner then palpates the tenderness deeply and releases the palpation quickly to see if rebound tenderness is present.
4. A positive test is greater tenderness with the rebound technique (Blumberg's sign) over McBurney's point.

UTILITY SCORE 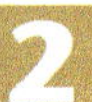 2

Study	Reliability	Sensitivity	Specificity	LR+	LR−	QUADAS Score (0–14)
Campbell & McPhail[11]	NT	76	NT	NT	NT	8
Alvarado[1] (tenderness)	NT	100	12	1.14	0.00	8
Alvarado[1] (Blumberg's sign)	NT	55	78	2.5	0.58	8
Tzanakis et al.[79] (tenderness)	NT	90	59	2.19	0.17	9
Tzanakis et al.[79] (Blumberg's sign)	NT	66	75	2.61	0.45	9
Soda et al.[75]	NT	87	90	8.42	0.15	9
Comments: Campbell & McPhail[11] only reported on cases confirmed as having appendicitis. Both Alvarado[1] and Tzanakis et al.[79] found tenderness to be more sensitive and Blumberg's sign (rebound pain) to be more specific.						

TESTS FOR ACUTE APPENDICITIS

Alvarado's Score to Predict Acute Appendicitis

1) The patient reports that pain migrated from epigastric region to right lower quadrant.
2) The patient reports anorexia.
3) The patient reports nausea and vomiting.
4) The patient has tenderness in the right lower quadrant.
5) Positive Blumberg's sign (rebound tenderness) over McBurney's point.
6) Fever.
7) Leucocytosis.
8) Shift to left (white count shifts to left).

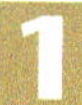

UTILITY SCORE 1

Study	Reliability	Sensitivity	Specificity	LR+	LR−	QUADAS Score (0–14)
Alvarado[1]	NT	97 81	38 74	1.56 3.12	0.09 0.26	8
Tzanakis et al.[79]	NT	90 66	59 75	2.19 2.61	0.17 0.45	9
Memon et al.[49] (cutoff < 5 rule out AA)	NT	100	44	1.80	0.00	7
Memon et al.[49] (cutoff > 6 rule in AA)	NT	58	89	5.24	0.47	7
Memon et al.[49] (cutoff > 7 rule in AA)	NT	45	100	NA	0.55	7

Comments: Alvarado[1] assessed components of a physical examination for acute appendicitis. The study concluded that scoring the probability of having acute appendicitis (AA) based on 6 clinical examinations and 2 laboratory tests was helpful in determining who could be conservatively managed and who required immediate surgery. Alvarado[1] developed the Alvarado score and discussed the use of stratification of score for diagnostic purposes. Scores < 5 were less likely to be acute appendicitis (AA) and scores > 6 were more likely. Tzanakis et al.[79] suggested a cutoff of > 7 for diagnostic purposes in identifying a high probability of AA. Memon et al.[49] examined two diagnostic cutoffs of > 6, as recommended by Alvarado, and > 7 as recommended by the author.

TEST FOR BLADDER SIZE

Palpation of Bladder Volume

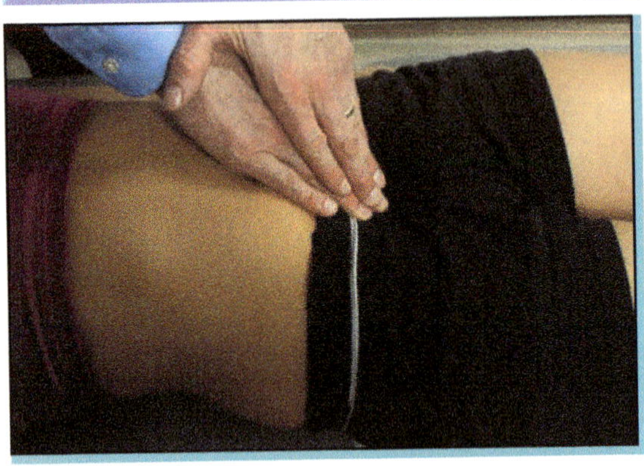

1) The patient lies supine.
2) The examiner places both hands on the patient's abdomen just distal to the umbilicus.

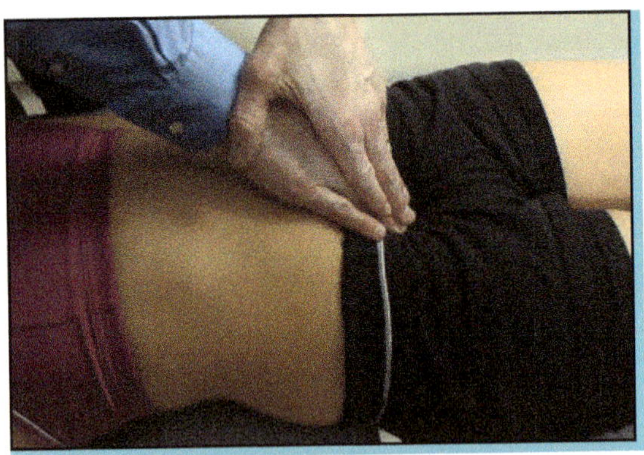

3) The examiner then palpates into the abdomen and proceeds to move distally until just proximal to the pubic symphysis.
4) The examiner assesses for a palpable bladder (sign of distention) and attempts to determine the size of the bladder.
5) A positive test is a palpable bladder that is either painful or difficult for the patient to empty appropriately.

UTILITY SCORE 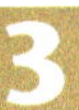

Study	Reliability	Sensitivity	Specificity	LR+	LR−	QUADAS Score (0–14)
Weatherall & Harwood[81]	NT	200cc: 72 400cc: 82 600cc: 81 800cc: 63 Pooled: 76	200cc: 65 400cc: 56 600cc: 50 800cc: 45 Pooled: 53	2.06 1.86 1.62 1.15 1.62	.43 .32 .38 .82 .45	10
Nygaard[57]	NT	14	68	0.44	1.27	10

Comments: Weatherall & Harwood's[81] study was performed on 16 healthy subjects by 8 examiners. The application of the technique to specific patient populations is unknown. Nygaard[57] found anecdotal evidence that BMI may alter results secondary to difficulty estimating bladder volume size in obese subjects.

TEST FOR CARDIOPULMONARY, VASCULAR DISEASE, AND ABDOMINAL AORTIC ANEURYSM

Palpation of Abdominal Aorta

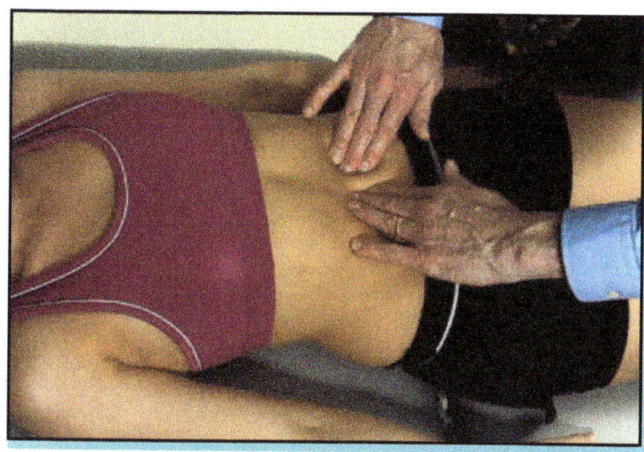

1) The patient lies supine with legs and abdomen relaxed.

2) The examiner places the fingertips over the epigastrium to determine if an epigastric pulse is present.

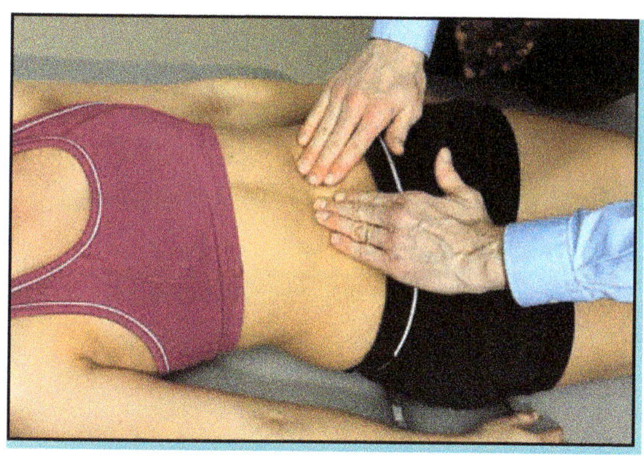

3) Both hands are placed on the abdomen with palms down and the index fingers placed on either side of the aorta to determine the width of the aortic pulse and thereby estimate the width of the aorta.

4) A positive test is the determination that the abdominal aorta is greater than 3cm in width (although some investigators feel 4cm is a better cutoff point for AAA).

(*continued*)

TESTS FOR CARDIOPULMONARY, VASCULAR DISEASE, AND ABDOMINAL AORTIC ANEURYSM

UTILITY SCORE 3

Study	Reliability	Sensitivity	Specificity	LR+	LR−	QUADAS Score (0–14)
Fink et al.[23]	0.66	68	75	2.70	0.43	9
Lederle et al.[38]	NT	50	NT	NT	NT	
Chervu et al.[15]	NT	38 77	NT NT	NT NT	NT NT	7
Collin et al.[16]	NT	44	91	5.00	0.62	8
Karkos et al.[33]	NT	48	NT	NT	NT	4
Kiev et al.[34]	NT	31	NT	NT	NT	7
Lederle & Simel[37]	NT	39	96	12.0	0.72	NA

Comments: Fink et al.[23] designed their study using 99 subjects with known AAA and 101 subjects known to be without AAA. The investigators also found that the sensitivity of the palpation examination increased with increasing size of the known aneurysm. Lederle et al.[38] found that the sensitivity increased to 100% in subjects with waist size < 100cm. Chervu et al.[15] examined diagnostic accuracy retrospectively. The first sensitivity value refers to the identification of the AAA by physical examination in the year leading up to radiographic confirmation. The second value refers to a physical examination performed by a physician just prior to AAA repair. Chervu et al.[15], Karkos et al.[33], and Kiev et al.[34]only provided accuracy values for subjects with known AAA. Lederle & Simel[37] is a meta-analysis of pooled data from several studies (N = 2955) with minor data adjustments to avoid dividing by 0 making a QUADAS score inappropriate for this type of article.

TESTS FOR DEEP VEIN THROMBOSIS

Wells Criteria for Deep Vein Thrombosis

The following clinical information is obtained from the patient, chart, or clinical examination and is scored as follows:

	Criterion	Score
1	Active cancer (within 6 months of Dx or palliative care)	1
2	Paralysis, paresis, or recent plaster immobilization of the lower extremity	1
3	Recently bedridden for > 3 days or major surgery within 4 weeks	1
4	Localized tenderness along the distribution of the deep venous system	1
5	Entire leg is swollen	1
6	Calf swelling of > 3 cm when compared with asymptomatic leg	1
7	Pitting edema that is worse in the symptomatic leg	1
8	Collateral superficial veins (nonvaricose)	1
9	Alternative diagnosis that is likely or more probable than DVT	– 2

Scoring risk on a scale of – 2 to 8 is the original Wells rule.
It has since been categorized into three groups: score ≤ 0 = low probability; score between 1 and 2 = intermediate probability; and score ≥ 3 = high probability.

TESTS FOR DEEP VEIN THROMBOSIS

UTILITY SCORE 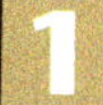

Study	Reliability	Sensitivity	Specificity	LR+	LR−	QUADAS Score (0–14)
Wells et al.[87]	0.85	91 61 67 78	100 99 98 98	NA 61 33.5 39	0.09 0.39 0.34 0.22	11
Wells et al.[83]	0.75	90 56	64 96	2.49 15.5	0.16 0.46	11
Wells et al.[82]	NT	86 54	41 94	1.46 8.39	0.35 0.49	9
Wells et al.[84] (Wells score alone)	NT	90	64	2.49	0.16	8
Wells et al.[84] (Wells score with D-dimer testing)	NT	98	46	1.79	0.05	8
Kraaijenhagen et al.[36] (Wells score alone)	NT	83	63	2.23	0.27	10
Kraaijenhagen et al.[36] (Wells score with D-dimer testing)	NT	98	42	1.68	0.06	10
Oudega et al.[59] (Score ≤ 0)	NT	79	44	1.42	0.48	13
Oudega et al.[59](score ≤ 0 with – D-dimer test)	NT	98	22	1.25	0.08	13
Oudega et al.[59](score ≤ 1 with – D-dimer test)	NT	97	26	1.32	0.11	13
Riddle et al.[67]	NT	71 48	71 92	2.49 6.17	0.40 0.57	11
Shields et al.[73]	NT	94	47	1.78	0.13	10
Anderson et al.[2]	NT	90	49	1.75	0.21	8
Miron et al.[50]	0.32	93 60	57 94	2.18 9.93	0.12 0.43	10
Cornuz et al.[20]	0.31	83 39	48 92	1.61 4.76	0.35 0.66	13
Dryjski et al.[22]	NT	100	50	2.00	0.00	11

Comments: Wells et al.[87] provided diagnostic accuracy values for subjects clinically considered at high, moderate, low, and combined risk values. Wells et al.[87] used a version of criteria that stratifies predictor variables as major and minor risks and served as a starting point for the currently used Wells criteria of later studies. Wells et al.[83] stratified data into low, medium, and high probability of DVT and the first set of numbers is calculated at low probability to rule out DVT and the second set is based on high probability to rule in DVT. Wells et al.[82] used a diagnostic algorithm to determine risk of DVT. This clinically more relevant procedure reduces the QUADAS score as there was variability in the implementation of reference standards. Oudega et al.[59] used the Wells rule in primary care rather than secondary care as historically tested. Diagnostic accuracy values were based on the ability to discriminate the low risk category. The article went on to add D-dimer testing to enhance diagnostic accuracy of the Wells rule. For Riddle et al.[67] the first values identify the low-risk patient and serve to rule out the condition. The second values identify the high-risk patient and serve to rule in the pathology. Miron et al.[50] was a comparative study assessing the Wells rule against an empirical clinical assessment. The values provided here were extrapolated from data tables in the manuscript with the first values representing low risk to rule out DVT and the second values high risk to rule in DVT. The kappa statistic reported was the reliability of both tools used to classify the subjects in the same category. Cornuz et al.[20] measured a kappa statistic for agreement between the Wells criteria and the physician's assessment. Cornuz et al.[20] allowed subjects with a previous history of DVT to be included in the study which differs from most other studies examining the Wells criteria. Dryjski et al.[22] combined the Wells criteria with D-dimer results in a particularly small sample of subjects (N = 66); therefore, generalizability of these results may be questionable.

Tests for Upper Extremity Deep Vein Thrombosis

The following criteria are taken from the history or clinical examination:

1)	The presence of venous material (catheter, venous access, or pacemaker)	1
2)	Upper extremity, unilateral pitting edema	1
3)	Localized upper extremity pain	1
4)	Another diagnosis is reasonably plausible	–1

Scoring is as follows: score ≤ 0 low risk for DVT; score = 1 intermediate risk; and score ≥ 2 = higher risk for UEDVT

UTILITY SCORE 2

Study	Reliability	Sensitivity	Specificity	LR+	LR–	QUADAS Score (0–14)
Constans et al.[18]	NT	79	64	2.21	0.33	9
Constans et al.[18]	NT	96	37	1.51	0.12	10
Comments: The sensitivity, specificity, and likelihood ratios were calculated from the data provided by the authors using ≤ 0 as the cutoff score for ruling out UEDVT. Both internal and external validation samples were reported on in the same article with minor differences in methodology accounting for the QUADAS score differences.						

TESTS FOR PULMONARY EMBOLISM

Wells Criteria for Pulmonary Embolism

1) Clinical signs and symptoms of DVT (pain with palpation of the deep veins and leg swelling at a minimum) +3.0
2) Pulmonary embolism is as likely or more likely than an alternative diagnosis +3.0
3) Pulse greater than 100 +1.5
4) Previous history of DVT or PE +1.5
5) Immobilization or major surgery in the past 4 weeks +1.5
6) Hemoptysis +1
7) Active cancer with ongoing treatment or within the past 6 months +1

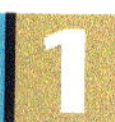

Wells criteria for pulmonary embolism scoring: Score < 2 = low probability; score between 2 and 6 = moderate probability; and score > 4 = high probability

Dichotomized Wells criteria: score ≤ 4 = PE unlikely; score > 4 PE likely

UTILITY SCORE 1

Study	Reliability	Sensitivity	Specificity	LR+	LR−	QUADAS Score (0–14)
Penaloza et al.[60] (low pretest probability to rule out)	0.66	93	65	2.62	0.11	12
Penaloza et al.[60] (high pretest probability to rule in)	0.66	66	87	5.13	0.39	12
Wells et al.[86]	NT	89 37	69 98	2.89 16.77	0.17 0.65	10
Wells et al.[85]	NT	92	57	2.12	0.14	10
Wolf et al.[90]	0.54 0.72	94 81	49 72	1.85 2.90	0.13 0.26	10
Moores et al.[53]	NT	83 19	40 91	1.38 2.1	0.43 0.89	8
Chagnon et al.[13]	0.43	73 14	69 99.5	2.39 28.2	0.39 0.86	7

Comment: Penaloza et al.[60] provided a kappa statistic comparing reliability between physicians in training with supervising physicians. Wolf et al.[90] provided kappa statistics for trichotomized and dichotomized Wells criteria scoring respectively. The Moores et al.[53] study was based on a retrospective chart analysis and provides two sets of numbers to rule out PE and to rule in PE respectively. Chagnon et al.[13] provided a kappa reliability statistic for a Geneva score vs. Wells criteria.

TESTS FOR PULMONARY EMBOLISM

Geneva Criteria

1) Previous pulmonary embolism or deep vein thrombosis	+2.0
2) Pulse greater than 100	+1.0
3) Recent surgery	+3.0
4) Age (years)	
60–79	+1.0
≥ 80	+2.0
5) P_aCO_2	
<4.8 kPa (36 mmHg)	+2.0
4.8–5.19 kPa (36–38.9 mmHg)	+1.0
6) P_aO_2	
<6.5 kPa (48.7 mmHg)	+4.0
6.5–7.99 kPa (48.7–59.9 mmHg)	+3.0
8–9.49 kPa (60–71.2 mmHg)	+2.0
9.5–10.99 kPa (71.3–82.4 mmHg)	+1.0
7) Atelactasis	+1.0
8) Elevated hemidiaphragm	+1.0

Geneva criteria for pulmonary embolism scoring: Score ≤ 4 = low probability; score between 5 and 8 = moderate probability; and score ≥ 9 = high probability.

UTILITY SCORE 2

Study	Reliability	Sensitivity	Specificity	LR+	LR−	QUADAS Score (0–14)
Moores et al.[53]	NT	70 26	36 93	1.08 3.68	.85 .80	8
Chagnon et al.[13]	0.43	72 11	64 98	2.00 5.95	.44 .90	7

Comment: Moores et al.[53] study was based on a retrospective chart analysis and provided two sets of diagnostic accuracy numbers to rule out PE and to rule in PE respectively. Chagnon et al.[13] provided a kappa reliability statistic for a Geneva score vs. Wells criteria.

TESTS TO PREDICT FUTURE CARDIOPULMONARY EVENTS

San Francisco Syncope Rule for Predicting Serious Short-term Outcome

Presence of any of the following after a syncope episode:

1) Abnormal ECG
2) Shortness of breath
3) Systolic blood pressure < 90 mmHg
4) Hematocrit < 30%
5) History of congestive heart failure

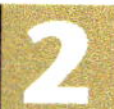

UTILITY SCORE 2

Study	Reliability	Sensitivity	Specificity	LR+	LR−	QUADAS Score (0–14)
Quinn et al.[62]	NT	96	62	2.53	0.06	10
Quinn et al.[61] (syncope related mortality 6 months)	NT	100	52	2.08	0.00	10
Quinn et al.[61] (syncope related mortality 12 months)	NT	93	53	1.98	0.13	10
Quinn et al.[61] (any mortality 6 months)	NT	89	53	1.89	0.21	10
Quinn et al.[61] (any mortality 12 months)	NT	83	54	1.80	0.31	10

Comments: In the derivation study by Quinn et al.[62], multiple variables were examined for reliability; however, the clinical criteria in its entirety were not analyzed for reliability.

TESTS TO PREDICT FUTURE CARDIOPULMONARY EVENTS

Framingham Criteria for Heart Failure

Major Criteria

1) Paroxysmal nocturnal dyspnea or orthopnea
2) Neck vein distention
3) Rales
4) Cardiomegaly
5) Acute pulmonary edema
6) S3 gallop
7) Hepatojugular reflex

Minor Criteria

1) Ankle edema
2) Nocturnal cough
3) Dyspnea on exertion
4) Hepatomegaly
5) Pleural effusion
6) Tachycardia (>120 bpm)

Diagnosis of heart failure is made by the presence of 2 major criteria or 1 major criteria with 2 minor criteria. The minor criteria should not be able to be explained by an alternative diagnosis.

UTILITY SCORE 2

Study	Reliability	Sensitivity	Specificity	LR+	LR−	QUADAS Score (0–14)
Maestre et al.[41] (overall heart failure)	0.76	92	79	4.35	0.1	10
Maestre et al.[41] (systolic heart failure)	0.76	97	79	4.57	0.04	10
Maestre et al.[41] (diastolic heart failure)	0.76	89	79	4.21	0.13	10
Comments: In Maestre et al.[41] the kappa value stated represents the mean value for all diagnostic criteria.						

Thrombolysis in Myocardial Infarction (TIMI) Score for Acute Coronary Syndromes

1) Age: > 65 +1
2) Known CAD with stenosis ≥ 50% +1
3) ASA use in past week +1
4) Severe angina with ≥ 2 episodes in 24 hours +1
5) ST changes ≥ 0.5mm +1
6) Have cardiac marker +1
7) ≥ 3 known cardiac risk factors +1

TIMI score is based on a 0–7 scale and can be risk stratified as 0–2 low risk, 3–4 intermediate risk, and 5–7 high risk.

TESTS TO PREDICT FUTURE CARDIOPULMONARY EVENTS

UTILITY SCORE 1

Study	Reliability	Sensitivity	Specificity	LR+	LR−	QUADAS Score (0–14)
Antman et al.[3] (outcome of all CV events)	NT	69 15	47 95	1.31 2.83	0.66 0.90	10
Antman et al.[3] (outcome of mortality)	NT	85 33	32 88	1.25 2.78	0.48 0.76	10
Antman et al.[3] (outcome of acute MI)	NT	84 29	33 88	1.25 2.47	0.48 0.81	10
Antman et al.[3] (outcome of revascularization)	NT	85 21	34 88	1.27 1.78	0.46 0.90	10
Antman et al.[3] (outcome of mortality & MI combined)	NT	83 29	33 89	1.24 2.49	0.50 0.81	10
Garcia et al.[25]	NT	76 27	71 99	2.62 30.0	0.33 0.74	10
Morrow et al.[54]	NT	94 46	16 72	1.12 1.65	0.36 0.75	9
Scirica et al.[70] (6 week outcomes)	NT	69 23	44 90	1.23 2.31	0.70 0.85	8
Scirica et al.[70] (1 year outcomes)	NT	71 24	45 91	1.29 2.67	0.64 0.84	8
Chase et al.[14] (outcome is death)	NT	43 0	77 97	1.89 0.00	0.74 1.03	11
Chase et al.[14] (outcome is total serious event)	NT	54 12	80 98	2.76 5.90	0.57 0.90	11
Chase et al.[14] (outcome is MI)	NT	49 2	79 97	2.29 0.67	0.65 1.01	11
Conway et al.[19] (modified TIMI)	NT	55 15	73 97	2.02 5.21	0.62 0.88	10
Conway et al.[19] (standard TIMI)	NT	72 26	72 97	2.58 7.97	0.39 0.77	10
Tong et al.[78] (modified TIMI)	NT	62 6	63 95	1.67 1.30	0.61 0.99	12
Tong et al.[78] (standard TIMI)	NT	83 37	61 92	2.14 4.74	0.29 0.69	12

Comments: Antman et al.[3] provided data on two sets of subjects and they are combined in this table. The rows correspond to 14 day outcomes and, within each cell, calculations based on low-risk to rule-out and high-risk to rule-in events are provided respectively.Garcia et al.[25] stratified results by low, intermediate, and high risk categories and diagnostic accuracy values listed are for low risk (ruling out) and high risk (ruling in) the conditions in question. Morrow et al.[54] included the TIMI risk stratification to a group of subjects receiving tirofiban and heparin therapy to reduce the risk of future coronary events. The first set of numbers are based on the low risk category for ruling out potential future events and the second set are based on the high risk category for ruling in future coronary events. Scirica et al.[70] data are for low risk (0–2) for ruling out CV events and high risk (5–7) for ruling in CV events respectively. Scirica et al.[70] did not provide raw data but these diagnostic accuracy values are estimates constructed from data on bar charts in the text. Within each cell, Chase et al.[14] based calculations on low-risk to rule-out and high-risk to rule-in events respectively. Both Conway et al.[19] and Tong et al.[78] used two versions of the TIMI score including a modified version (mTIMI) that did not include the cardiac marker (Troponin I: because it takes time to get back the lab results). Within each cell, calculations based on low-risk to rule-out and high-risk to rule-in events are provided respectively.

TESTS TO PREDICT FUTURE CARDIOPULMONARY EVENTS

Risk Score for Acute Coronary Syndromes

1) Age: > 67 +1

2) IDDM +2

3) Chest pain score ≥ 10 points +1

4) ≥ 2 chest pain episodes in past 24 hours +1

5) Prior PTCA +1

Risk Score is based on a 0–6 scale and can be risk stratified as very low risk 0, low risk 1, intermediate risk 2, high risk 3, and very high risk ≥ 4.

UTILITY SCORE 2

Study	Reliability	Sensitivity	Specificity	LR+	LR−	QUADAS Score (0–14)
Sanchis et al.[69] (risk score ≤ 1 to rule out)	NT	86	50	1.72	0.28	8
Sanchis et al.[69] (risk score ≥ 3 to rule in)	NT	19	97	5.64	0.84	8
Sanchis et al.[69] (risk score ≥ 4 to rule in)	NT	61	83	3.48	0.48	8
Comments: Sanchis et al.[69] provided data on risk of death and MI at 12 month follow-up for each risk level. It can be seen that diagnostic accuracy has a higher LR+ for ruling in at the higher risk cutoff.						

Duke Treadmill Score for Identifying Risk of Ischaemic Heart Disease

1) Treadmill exercise protocol involves minute recordings of heart rate and blood pressure. ST depression during exercise was recorded to the nearest 25 mm. Angina was recorded as 0 = none, 1 = nonlimiting, and 2 = exercise limiting.

2) Exercise is stopped if exertional hypotension, malignant ventricular arrhythmias, ST depression of ≥ 3mm, or exercise limiting chest pain is present.

3) Exercise time (min) – (5 × ST segment deviation) – (4 × exercise angina)

4) Scores of ≥ 5 are considered low risk, +4 to –10 are moderate risk, and ≤ –11 are high risk. The usual range is between –25 to +15.

TESTS TO PREDICT FUTURE CARDIOPULMONARY EVENTS

UTILITY SCORE 2

Study	Reliability	Sensitivity	Specificity	LR+	LR−	QUADAS Score (0–14)
Shaw et al.[71] outcome = death	NT	88 34	39 93	1.44 5.11	0.30 0.71	12
Shaw et al.[71] [severe CAD (3 vessels ≥ 75% blockage)]	NT	87 25	45 97	1.57 7.35	0.29 0.78	12
Shaw et al.[71] [significant CAD (at least 1 vessel ≥ 75% blockage)]	NT	67 7	38 90	1.08 0.68	0.87 1.04	12
Shaw et al.[71] [no significant CAD(no vessel ≥ 75% blocked)]	NT	76 15	55 99.9	1.67 152.0	0.44 0.85	12
Mark et al.[42]	NT	89 32	45 94	1.61 5.44	0.24 0.72	10
Marwick et al.[44]	NT	64 5	62 98	1.67 2.94	0.58 0.97	10

Comments: Shaw et al.'s[71] results are presented as ruling out the condition with low risk and ruling in the condition with high risk scores respectively. Mark et al.[42] measured mortality at 4 years post treadmill testing. Marwick et al.[44] reported total mortality at 5 years post treadmill testing. The authors acknowledge that increasing age alters relative risk of death (they should be credited for this); however, they do no not report how many subjects in the study were elderly, making independent assessment of the possible effects on the results impossible.

Clinical Prediction Rule to Identify Individuals with Low Risk of Stroke from Atrial Fibrillation while Taking Aspirin

1) If the patient has nonvalvular atrial fibrillation and:
2) Has no previous history of stroke or transient ischemic attack,
3) Has no history of treated hypertension or systolic blood pressure ≥ 140 mmHg,
4) Has no history of myocardial infarction or angina,
5) Does not have Diabetes;
6) If all conditions are met, the patient can use daily aspirin rather than oral anticoagulants to minimize potential cerebral events.

UTILITY SCORE 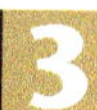

Study	Reliability	Sensitivity	Specificity	LR+	LR−	QUADAS Score (0–14)
van Walraven et al.[80]	NT	91	NT	NT	NT	NT

Comments: van Walraven et al.[80] did not provide sufficient detail to determine all diagnostic accuracy values. The authors did report that in the low risk group, observed event rate was 1.1 per 100 patient years vs. 4.2 per 100 patient years for the moderate to high risk groups.

TESTS TO PREDICT FUTURE CARDIOPULMONARY EVENTS

Ankle-Brachial Index for Predicting Coronary Artery Disease

1) The patient lies supine for at least 5–10 minutes to achieve a resting state.

2) The systolic blood pressure is taken in each arm and each leg. The lower extremity pressures may be taken at either the dorsalispedis or posterior tibial arteries.

3) The patient should have no history of treated hypertension or systolic blood pressure ≥ 140 mmHg.

4) The ABI calculation is the ratio of the lower extremity systolic pressure divided by the brachial systolic pressure.

5) The method of determining the systolic pressures used has some variability depending on the source referenced. Some use the higher value of each arm and each leg, others have used the mean values of the arms and legs. Others have calculated the ratio of one side compared with the other to determine if asymmetrical disease processes may exist.

6) An ABI cutoff value may be used to predict future cardiovascular event including mortality, or stratified values may be employed to determine the severity of the disease process. The most frequent value cited is ≥ 0.90 for predictive purposes. Values between ≥ 1.2 and ≥ 1.5 have been used to exclude patients from a diagnostic accuracy study based on the belief that these are non-compressible veins due to atherosclerotic disease and represent false negatives. This strategy has been inconsistently done and may alter the values calculated.

UTILITY SCORE 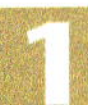

Study	Reliability	Sensitivity	Specificity	LR+	LR−	QUADAS Score (0–14)
Doobay & Anand[21]	NT	17	93	2.26	0.90	NA
Resnick et al.[65]	NT	18	96	4.21	0.86	10
Leng et al.[39]	NT	27	82	1.51	0.89	9
Otah et al.[58] (no CAD)	NT	62	94	10.28	0.41	12
Otah et al.[58] (significant CAD)	NT	86	81	4.39	0.18	12

Comments: Doobay & Anand[21] is a systematic review of diagnostic accuracy studies; therefore, the QUADAS assessment is not applicable to this study. Otah et al.[58] studied African-Americans exclusively, limiting generalizability of results to other populations.

Ankle-Brachial Index for Predicting Stroke

1) The patient lies supine for at least 5–10 minutes to achieve a resting state.

2) The systolic blood pressure is taken in each arm and each leg. The lower extremity pressures may be taken at either the dorsalispedis or posterior tibial arteries.

3) The patient should have no history of treated hypertension or systolic blood pressure ≥ 140 mmHg.

4) The ABI calculation is the ratio of the lower extremity systolic pressure divided by the brachial systolic pressure.

5) The method of determining the systolic pressures used has some variability depending on the source referenced. Some use the higher value of each arm and each leg, others have used the mean values of the arms and legs. Others have calculated the ratio of one side compared with the other to determine if asymmetrical disease processes may exist.

6) An ABI cutoff value may be used to predict future cardiovascular event including mortality, or stratified values may be employed to determine the severity of the disease process. The most frequent value cited is ≥ 0.90 for predictive purposes. Values between ≥ 1.2 and ≥ 1.5 have been used to exclude patients from a diagnostic accuracy study based on the belief that these are non-compressible veins due to atherosclerotic disease and represent false negatives. This strategy has been inconsistently done and may alter the values calculated.

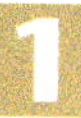

UTILITY SCORE 1

Study	Reliability	Sensitivity	Specificity	LR+	LR−	QUADAS Score (0–14)
Doobay & Anand[21]	NT	16	92	2.05	0.91	NA
Leng et al.[39]	NT	29	82	1.59	0.87	9
Koh et al.[35]	NT	10	97	3.64	0.92	9
Newman et al.[55] (history of CAD)	NT	29	76	1.19	0.94	8
Newman et al.[55] (no history of CAD)	NT	17	91	1.85	0.91	8
Newman et al.[55] (all subjects combined)	NT	21	87	1.63	0.91	8

Comments: Doobay & Anand[21] is a systematic review of diagnostic accuracy studies; therefore, the QUADAS assessment is not applicable to this study.

TESTS TO PREDICT FUTURE CARDIOPULMONARY EVENTS

Ankle-Brachial Index for Predicting any Cardiovascular Event

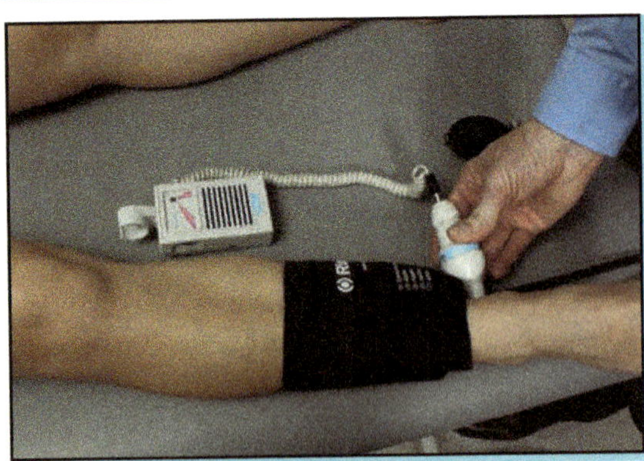

1. The patient lies supine for at least 5–10 minutes to achieve a resting state.
2. The systolic blood pressure is taken in each arm and each leg. The lower extremity pressures may be taken at either the dorsalispedis or posterior tibial arteries.
3. The patient should have no history of treated hypertension or systolic blood pressure ≥ 140 mmHg.
4. The ABI calculation is the ratio of the lower extremity systolic pressure divided by the brachial systolic pressure.
5. The method of determining the systolic pressures used has some variability depending on the source referenced. Some use the higher value of each arm and each leg, others have used the mean values of the arms and legs. Others have calculated the ratio of one side compared with the other to determine if asymmetrical disease processes may exist.
6. An ABI cutoff value may be used to predict future cardiovascular event including mortality, or stratified values may be employed to determine the severity of the disease process. The most frequent value cited is ≥ 0.90 for predictive purposes. Values between ≥ 1.2 and ≥ 1.5 have been used to exclude patients from a diagnostic accuracy study based on the belief that these are non-compressible veins due to atherosclerotic disease and represent false negatives. This strategy has been inconsistently done and may alter the values calculated.

UTILITY SCORE 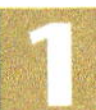

Study	Reliability	Sensitivity	Specificity	LR+	LR−	QUADAS Score (0–14)
Doobay et al.[21]	NT	17	93	2.26	0.90	NA
Wild et al.[88]	NT	24	88	1.89	0.81	9
Leng et al.[39]	NT	32	84	1.99	0.81	9
Newman et al.[55] (history of CAD)	NT	35	88	2.88	0.74	9
Newman et al.[55] (no history of CAD)	NT	15	93	2.23	0.91	9
Newman et al.[55] (all subjects combined)	NT	21	92	2.83	0.85	9
Hooi et al.[31]	NT	24	91	2.53	0.84	9

Comments: Doobay et al.[21] is a systematic review of diagnostic accuracy studies; therefore, the QUADAS assessment is not applicable to this study.

Ankle-Brachial Index for Predicting Peripheral Artery Disease

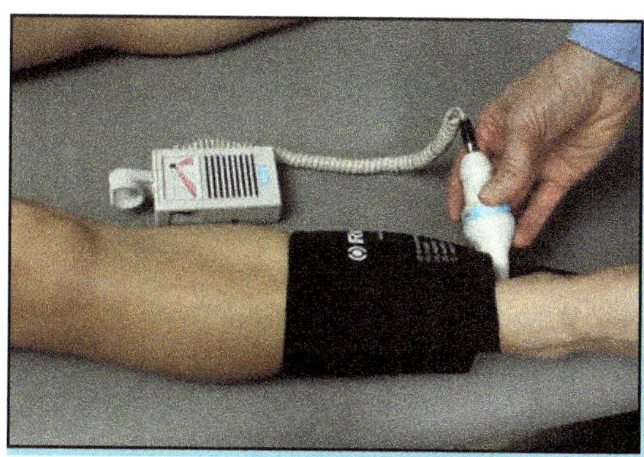

1) The patient lies supine for at least 5–10 minutes to achieve a resting state.

2) The systolic blood pressure is taken in each arm and each leg. The lower extremity pressures may be taken at either the dorsalispedis or posterior tibial arteries.

3) The patient should have no history of treated hypertension or systolic blood pressure ≥ 140 mmHg.

4) The ABI calculation is the ratio of the lower extremity systolic pressure divided by the brachial systolic pressure.

5) The method of determining the systolic pressures used has some variability depending on the source referenced. Some use the higher value of each arm and each leg, others have used the mean values of the arms and legs. Others have calculated the ratio of one side compared with the other to determine if asymmetrical disease processes may exist.

6) An ABI cutoff value may be used to predict future cardiovascular event including mortality, or stratified values may be employed to determine the severity of the disease process. The most frequent value cited is ≥ 0.90 for predictive purposes. Values between ≥ 1.2 and ≥ 1.5 have been used to exclude patients from a diagnostic accuracy study based on the belief that these are non-compressible veins due to atherosclerotic disease and represent false negatives. This strategy has been inconsistently done and may alter the values calculated.

(*continued*)

TESTS TO PREDICT FUTURE CARDIOPULMONARY EVENTS

UTILITY SCORE 1

Study	Reliability	Sensitivity	Specificity	LR+	LR−	QUADAS Score (0–14)
Newman et al.[55](history of CAD)	NT	56	76	2.39	0.57	9
Newman et al.[55](no history of CAD)	NT	43	91	4.71	0.63	9
Newman et al.[55](all subjects combined)	NT	49	87	3.87	0.58	9
Hooi et al.[31]	NT	52	89	4.53	0.55	9
Guo et al.[27] (ABI cutoff = 1.12)	NT	100	40	1.67	0.0	12
Guo et al.[27] (ABI cutoff = 0.95)	NT	91	86	6.50	0.1	12
Guo et al.[27] (ABI cutoff = 0.90)	NT	76	90	7.60	0.27	12
Guo et al.[27] (ABI cutoff = 0.53)	NT	14	100	0.14	0.86	12
Holland-Letz et al.[29]	0.42	NT	NT	NT	NT	NA
Mätzke et al.[45]	0.02 16% > 0.15	NT	NT	NT	NT	NA

Comments: Guo et al.[27] excluded patients with non-compressible vessels (ABI ≥ 1.40). Holland-Letz et al.[29] calculated a total variance intraclass correlation coefficient (ICC) based on measurements taken by vascular experts, family physicians, and nurses. Mätzke et al.[45] only examined the reproducibility of ABI and found a median difference of 0.02 when two experienced vascular nurses performed ABI testing. They also found that overall 16% of ABI measurements differed by > 0.15 (accepted critical value of measurement error).

Ankle-Brachial Index for Predicting Cardiovascular Mortality

1) The patient lies supine for at least 5–10 minutes to achieve a resting state.

2) The systolic blood pressure is taken in each arm and each leg. The lower extremity pressures may be taken at either the dorsalispedis or posterior tibial arteries.

3) The patient should have no history of treated hypertension or systolic blood pressure ≥ 140 mmHg.

4) The ABI calculation is the ratio of the lower extremity systolic pressure divided by the brachial systolic pressure.

5) The method of determining the systolic pressures used has some variability depending on the source referenced. Some use the higher value of each arm and each leg, others have used the mean values of the arms and legs. Others have calculated the ratio of one side compared with the other to determine if asymmetrical disease processes may exist.

6) An ABI cutoff value may be used to predict future cardiovascular event including mortality, or stratified values may be employed to determine the severity of the disease process. The most frequent value cited is ≥ 0.90 for predictive purposes. Values between ≥ 1.2 and ≥ 1.5 have been used to exclude patients from a diagnostic accuracy study based on the belief that these are non-compressible veins due to atherosclerotic disease and represent false negatives. This strategy has been inconsistently performed and may alter the values calculated.

TESTS TO PREDICT FUTURE CARDIOPULMONARY EVENTS

UTILITY SCORE 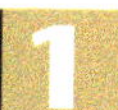

Study	Reliability	Sensitivity	Specificity	LR+	LR−	QUADAS Score (0–14)
Doobay & Anand[21]	NT	41	88	3.39	0.67	NA
Leng et al.[39]	NT	38	83	2.25	0.74	9
Wild et al.[88]	NT	31	85	2.08	0.81	9
Newman et al.[55] (history of CAD)	NT	64	77	2.78	0.47	9
Newman et al.[55] (no history of CAD)	NT	30	91	3.24	0.78	9
Newman et al.[55] (all subjects combined)	NT	36	88	3.00	0.73	9
Hooi et al.[31]	NT	32	89	2.79	0.77	9
Resnick et al.[65] (ABI cutoff < 0.90)	NT	18	96	4.21	0.86	10
Resnick et al.[65] (ABI cutoff < 0.90 or >1.40)	NT	34	87	2.62	0.76	10

Comments: Doobay & Anand[21] is a systematic review of diagnostic accuracy studies; therefore, the QUADAS assessment is not applicable to this study. Hooi et al.[31] used an ABI value of ≤ 0.95 as their cutoff for measuring disease. Most studies exclude subjects with ABI > 1.40 but Resnick et al.[65] included them for analysis.

Ankle-Brachial Index for Predicting Total Mortality

1) The patient lies supine for at least 5–10 minutes to achieve a resting state.

2) The systolic blood pressure is taken in each arm and each leg. The lower extremity pressures may be taken at either the dorsalispedis or posterior tibial arteries.

3) The patient should have no history of treated hypertension or systolic blood pressure ≥ 140 mmHg.

4) The ABI calculation is the ratio of the lower extremity systolic pressure divided by the brachial systolic pressure.

5) The method of determining the systolic pressures used has some variability depending on the source referenced. Some use the higher value of each arm and each leg, others have used the mean values of the arms and legs. Others have calculated the ratio of one side compared with the other to determine if asymmetrical disease processes may exist.

6) An ABI cutoff value may be used to predict future cardiovascular event including mortality, or stratified values may be employed to determine the severity of the disease process. The most frequent value cited is ≥ 0.90 for predictive purposes. Values between ≥ 1.2 and ≥ 1.5 have been used to exclude patients from a diagnostic accuracy study based on the belief that these are non-compressible veins due to atherosclerotic disease and represent false negatives. This strategy has been inconsistently done and may alter the values calculated.

(continued)

TESTS TO PREDICT FUTURE CARDIOPULMONARY EVENTS

UTILITY SCORE 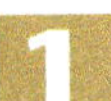

Study	Reliability	Sensitivity	Specificity	LR+	LR−	QUADAS Score (0–14)
Doobay & Anand[21]	NT	31	89	2.81	0.77	NA
Leng et al.[39]	NT	31	84	1.92	0.82	9
Wild et al.[88]	NT	26	87	2.05	0.85	9
Newman et al.[55] (history of CAD)	NT	44	77	1.91	0.73	9
Newman et al.[55] (no history of CAD)	NT	24	92	3.00	0.83	9
Newman et al.[55] (all subjects combined)	NT	28	89	2.52	0.81	9
Hooi et al.[31]	NT	27	90	2.52	0.82	9
Resnick et al.[65] (ABI cutoff < 0.90)	NT	26	97	7.37	0.77	10
Resnick et al.[65] (ABI cutoff < 0.90 or >1.40)	NT	51	91	5.60	0.54	10

Comments: Doobay & Anand[21] is a systematic review of diagnostic accuracy studies; therefore, the QUADAS assessment is not applicable to this study. Hooi et al.[31] used an ABI value of ≤ 0.95 as their cutoff for measuring disease. Most studies exclude subjects with ABI > 1.40 but Resnick et al.[65] included them for analysis.

Ankle-Brachial Index for Predicting Functional Deficits

1) The patient lies supine for at least 5–10 minutes to achieve a resting state.

2) The systolic blood pressure is taken in each arm and each leg. The lower extremity pressures may be taken at either the dorsalispedis or posterior tibial arteries.

3) The patient should have no history of treated hypertension or systolic blood pressure ≥ 140 mmHg.

4) The ABI calculation is the ratio of the lower extremity systolic pressure divided by the brachial systolic pressure.

5) The method of determining the systolic pressures used has some variability depending on the source referenced. Some use the higher value of each arm and each leg, others have used the mean values of the arms and legs. Others have calculated the ratio of one side compared with the other to determine if asymmetrical disease processes may exist.

6) An ABI cutoff value may be used to predict future cardiovascular event including mortality, or stratified values may be employed to determine the severity of the disease process. The most frequent value cited is ≥ 0.90 for predictive purposes. Values between ≥ 1.2 and ≥ 1.5 have been used to exclude patients from a diagnostic accuracy study based on the belief that these are non-compressible veins due to atherosclerotic disease and represent false negatives. This strategy has been inconsistently done and may alter the values calculated.

TESTS TO PREDICT FUTURE CARDIOPULMONARY EVENTS

UTILITY SCORE 2

Study	Reliability	Sensitivity	Specificity	LR+	LR−	QUADAS Score (0–14)
McDermott et al.[47] (exertional leg pain)	NT	36	66	1.04	0.98	9
McDermott et al.[47] (difficulty walking ¼ mile)	NT	35	83	2.00	0.79	9
McDermott et al.[47] (difficulty climbing 10 steps)	NT	35	75	1.37	0.87	9
McDermott et al.[48]	NT	29	92	3.49	0.77	9

Comments: The diagnostic accuracy values found by McDermott et al.[47] suggest that the ABI does not predict functional deficits particularly well, indicating that other co-morbidities may play a role in this relationship as confounder variables. McDermott et al.[48] provided a bar chart, which served as estimates for the calculations presented.

Key Points

1. Screening tools used for identifying cardiopulmonary disease processes have variable levels of diagnostic accuracy. Depending on the study, most of the values calculated would provide small to moderate shifts in posttest probability.
2. It would appear that most of the tools have cutoff scores that can be adjusted to enhance ruling out or ruling in potential disease.
3. Confounding variables (such as age) may reduce the diagnostic accuracy of some of the screening tools.
4. Physical examination techniques, such as the ABI, may have diagnostic accuracy compromised by variability of experience of the examiner.

TESTS TO DETERMINE NEED FOR BONE MINERAL DENSITOMETRY

Male Osteoporosis Risk Estimation Score (MORES) Criteria for Bone Densitometry in Men

1) Age:

≥ 75	+4
56–74	+3
≤ 55	+0

2) Weight:

> 80 kg	+0
70–80 kg	+4
≤ 70 kg	+6

3) Chronic obstructive pulmonary disease +3

MORES scoring: score ≥ 6, DEXA scanning is recommended.

UTILITY SCORE 3

Study	Reliability	Sensitivity	Specificity	LR+	LR−	QUADAS Score (0–14)
Shepherd et al.[72]	NT	91 95 93	58 61 59	2.17 2.44 2.27	0.16 0.08 0.12	10
Comments: Shepherd et al.[72] used National Health and Nutrition Examination Survey III data and separated these data (as reported above) into developmental, validation, and overall data sets respectively.						

TESTS TO DETERMINE NEED FOR BONE MINERAL DENSITOMETRY

Osteoporosis Self-Assessment Tool (OST) Criteria for Bone Densitometry in Women

1) (Weight in kg – age in years) x 0.2.

2) Truncate value from 1st step to yield an integer. This integer is the risk score.

OST ≤ – 1. bone densitometry is recommended.

UTILITY SCORE 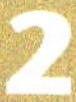

Study	Reliability	Sensitivity	Specificity	LR+	LR−	QUADAS Score (0–14)
Koh et al.[35]	NT	90	29	2.44	0.08	11
Rud et al.[68]	NT	92	71	3.17	0.11	9
Geusens et al.[26]	NT	88	52	1.83	0.30	9
Fujiwara et al.[24]	NT	87	43	1.53	0.23	9
Martinez-Aguila et al.[43]	NT	69	59	1.68	0.52	9
Richy et al.[66]	NT	97	34	1.47	0.09	10
Comments: Rud et al.[68], Geusens et al.[26], and Richy et al.[66] used ≤ 2 as their cut-off score. Fujiwara et al.[24] refers to this test as FOSTA.						

Osteoporosis Risk Assessment Instrument (ORAI) Criteria for Bone Densitometry

1) Age:

≥ 75	+15
65–74	+9
55–64	+5

2) Weight:

< 60 kg	+9
60–69.9 kg	+3

3) If not currently taking estrogen +2

ORAI scoring: score ≥ 9 suggests recommendation for DEXA scanning.

(continued)

TESTS TO DETERMINE NEED FOR BONE MINERAL DENSITOMETRY

UTILITY SCORE 1

Study	Reliability	Sensitivity	Specificity	LR+	LR−	QUADAS Score (0–14)
Mauck et al.[46]	NT	99 91 100	36 69 0	1.5 2.9 1.0	0.0 0.1 0.0	10
Cadarette et al.[10] (T score <−1.0 SD)	NT	83	44	1.48	0.38	9
Cadarette et al.[10] (T score <−2.0 SD)	NT	94	32	1.38	0.18	9
Cadarette et al.[10] (T score <−2.5 SD)	NT	97	28	1.35	0.09	9
*Cadarette et al.[9]	NT	77 90 97	57 45 41	1.78 1.64 1.65	0.40 0.22 0.07	9
**Cadarette et al.[9]	NT	77 93 94	58 46 41	1.85 1.74 1.61	0.39 0.14 0.14	9
Rud et al.[68]	NT	50	75	2.00	0.67	8
Geusens et al.[26]	NT	90	52	1.88	0.19	9
Richy et al.[66]	NT	90	43	1.58	0.23	10
Martinez-Aguila et al.[43]	NT	64	59	1.56	0.61	10
Fujiwara et al.[24]	NT	89	39	1.46	0.28	9

Comments: Mauck et al.[46] calculated diagnostic accuracy under three separate conditions in the order presented above: overall, ages 45–64 years, and ages 65 years and older. Cadarette et al.[9] calculated diagnostic accuracy off two separate samples including: * a developmental cohort of 924 women and ** a validation cohort of 450 women. Fujiwara et al.[24] used <15 as their cut-off score.

Simple Calculated Osteoporosis Risk Estimation (SCORE) for Bone Densitometry

1) Patient is not black. +5

2) Patient has rheumatoid arthritis. +4

3) Patient has a history of fracture from minimal trauma after age 45 years. Scored +4 for each fracture of the wrist, ribs, or hip to a maximum of +12.

4) Age: take first digit of age, multiply by 3.

5) Estrogen therapy has never been taken. +1

6) Weight in pounds, divided by 10 and truncated to an integer –integer

SCORE scoring: score is ≥ 6, DEXA scanning is recommended.

UTILITY SCORE 2

Study	Reliability	Sensitivity	Specificity	LR+	LR−	QUADAS Score (0–14)
Cadarette et al.[10] (T score < − 1.0 SD)	NT	91	31	1.31	0.31	9
Cadarette et al.[10] (T score < − 2.0 SD)	NT	98	21	1.23	0.12	9
Cadarette et al.[10] (T score < − 2.5 SD)	NT	100	18	1.21	0.02	9
Mauck et al.[46] (overall)	NT	100	25	1.3	0.0	10
Mauck et al.[46] (ages 45–64)	NT	100	41	1.7	0.0	10
Mauck et al.[46] (age ≥ 65)	NT	100	8	1.1	0.0	10
Geusens et al.[26]	NT	89	58	2.12	0.19	9
Richy et al.[66]	NT	94	37	1.49	0.16	10
Fujiwara et al.[24]	NT	90	42	1.55	0.24	9
Rud et al.[68]	NT	61	68	1.91	0.57	9
Comments: Useful screening tool.						

National Osteoporosis Foundation (NOF) Criteria for Bone Densitometry

1) Age ≥ 65 +1
2) Weight < 57.6 kg +1
3) Personal history of fracture from minimal trauma after age 40 +1
4) Parental history of hip, spine, or wrist fracture after age 50 +1
5) Currently smoking cigarettes +1

NOF scoring: score ≥ 1, requires DEXA scanning.

UTILITY SCORE 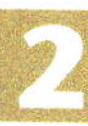

Study	Reliability	Sensitivity	Specificity	LR+	LR−	QUADAS Score (0–14)
Cadarette et al.[10] (T score < − 1.0 SD)	NT	88	26	1.18	0.47	9
Cadarette et al.[10] (T score < − 2.0 SD)	NT	94	20	1.17	0.32	9
Cadarette et al.[10] (T score < −2.5 SD)	NT	96	18	1.17	0.21	9
Mauck et al.[46] (Overall)	NT	100	10	1.1	0.0	10
Mauck et al.[46] (ages 45–64)	NT	100	19	1.2	0.0	10
Mauck et al.[46] (age ≥ 65)	NT	100	0	1.0	0.0	10
Comments: Cadarette et al.[10] calculated diagnostic accuracy under three separate conditions in the order presented above: BMD T score <−1.0 SD, BMD T score <−2.0 SD, and BMD T score <−2.5 SD.						

TESTS TO DETERMINE NEED FOR BONE MINERAL DENSITOMETRY

Age, Body Size, No Estrogen (ABONE) for Osteoporosis Prediction

1) Age > 65 +1

2) Patient weight is < 63.5 kg +1

3) Patient has not used oral contraception or estrogen therapy for ≥ 6 months +1

ABONE scoring: score ≥ 6, DEXA scanning is recommended.

UTILITY SCORE 3

Study	Reliability	Sensitivity	Specificity	LR+	LR−	QUADAS Score (0–14)
Cadarette et al.[10] (T score < − 1.0 SD)	NT	64	64	1.80	0.55	9
Cadarette et al.[10] (T score < − 2.0 SD)	NT	79	53	1.67	0.40	9
Cadarette et al.[10] (T score < − 2.5 SD)	NT	83	48	1.59	0.35	9
Comments:						

TESTS TO DETERMINE NEED FOR BONE MINERAL DENSITOMETRY

Weight Criterion for Osteoporosis Prediction

1) Weight < 70 kg

UTILITY SCORE 3

Study	Reliability	Sensitivity	Specificity	LR+	LR−	QUADAS Score (0–14)
Cadarette et al.[10] (T score < − 1.0 SD)	NT	64	62	1.68	0.58	9
Cadarette et al.[10] (T score < − 2.0 SD)	NT	80	52	1.67	0.39	9
Cadarette et al.[10] (T score < − 2.5 SD)	NT	87	48	1.66	0.27	9
Martinez-Aguila et al.[43]	NT	70	84	1.26	0.49	10
Comments: Lesser value as a screening tool.						

Osteoporosis Index of Risk (OSIRIS)

1) Age: age × −0.2

2) Weight: bodyweight in kg x +0.2

3) History of estrogen therapy +2.0

4) History of low impact fracture +2.0

Threshold for BMD testing is < 1.

UTILITY SCORE 3

Study	Reliability	Sensitivity	Specificity	LR+	LR−	QUADAS Score (0–14)
Richy et al.[66]	NT	84	63	2.27	0.25	10
Martinez-Aguila et al.[43]	NT	58	68	1.81	0.62	10
Comments:						

TESTS TO DETERMINE NEED FOR BONE MINERAL DENSITOMETRY

Study of Osteoporotic Fractures Risk Index (SOFSURE)

1)	Age: for every year over 65	+0.2
	for every year under 65	−0.2
2)	Weight: between 59 and 68 kg	+1
	< 59 kg	+3
3)	Current smoker	+1
4)	History of fracture after menopause	+1

Threshold for BMD testing is ≥ 1.

UTILITY SCORE 3

Study	Reliability	Sensitivity	Specificity	LR+	LR−	QUADAS Score (0–14)
Fujiwara et al.[24]	NT	89	38	1.44	0.29	9
Geusens et al.[26]	NT	92	37	1.46	0.22	9
Comments: Useful screening tool.						

Key Points

1. There are a number of clinical decision making rules available for predicting the need for DEXA scanning in individuals with suspected low bone mineral density.
2. Several decisions are well studied and have been found to have sufficient sensitivity to make them good screening tools for subjects with suspected low bone mineral density.
3. Other decision rules have not been studied adequately to suggest recommendation for clinical use even though they are simpler to implement.

TESTS FOR FRACTURE ASSESSMENT

Barford Test for Fracture Assessment

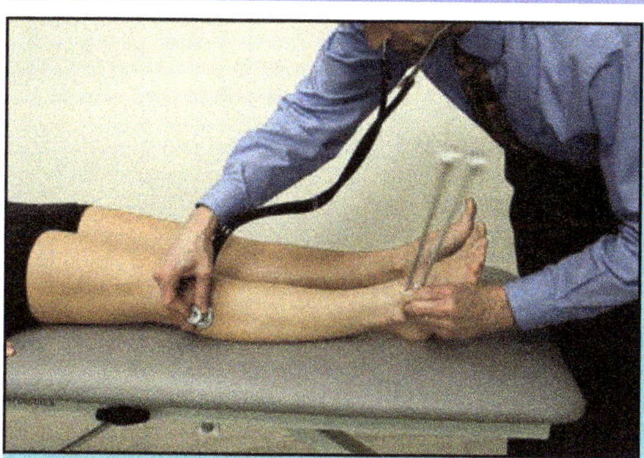

1) The examiner places a stethoscope on the pubic symphysis of the supine lying patient or at one end of the bone suspected of being fractured.

2) The examiner then strikes a tuning fork and places it on the patella of the lower extremity (or at the opposite end of the bone suspected of being fractured) listening to the quality of the sound propagated through the bony structures.

3) A positive test is determined when the sound transmitted through the involved lower extremity is muffled by comparison with the uninvolved.

UTILITY SCORE 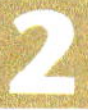

Study	Reliability	Sensitivity	Specificity	LR+	LR−	QUADAS Score (0–14)
Bache & Cross[4]	NT	91	82	5.01	0.11	7
Lesho[40]	NT	75	67	2.27	0.37	9
Misurya et al.[51] (all fractures combined)	NT	94	NT	NA	NA	7
Misurya et al.[51] (femoral neck fractures)	NT	89	NT	NA	NA	7
Misurya et al.[51] (femoral shaft fractures)	NT	95	NT	NA	NA	7
Misurya et al.[51] (tibial shaft fractures)	NT	100	NT	NA	NA	7
Colwill & Berg[17]	NT	88	100	NA	0.12	8
Moore[52]	NT	83	80	4.17	0.21	10

Comments: Misurya et al.[51] separated fractures by location within the femur, which is clinically impractical to attempt. Colwill & Berg[17] substituted percussion with a finger rather than a tuning fork for vibration. Moore[52] used a 128 Hz tuning fork and tested many different bones of the extremity exploring the generalizability of the technique to other bones beyond the femur.

TESTS FOR FRACTURE ASSESSMENT

Tuning Fork Test for Fracture Assessment

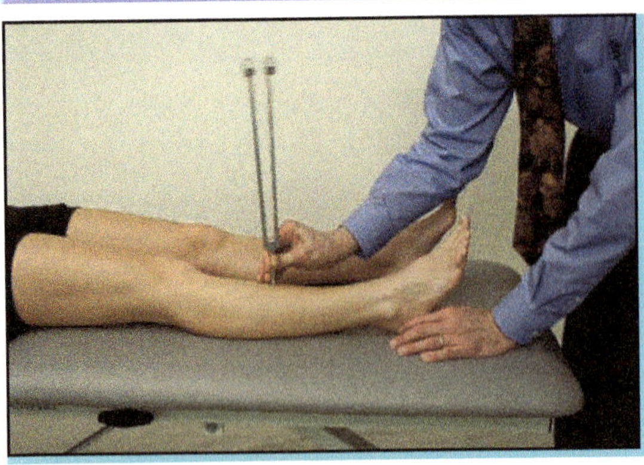

1) The examiner places a vibrating tuning fork over the portion of the bone with the greatest tenderness from the physical examination.

2) The examiner then queries the patient for change in perceived pain level.

3) A positive test is determined when the perceived pain level increases from application of the tuning fork.

UTILITY SCORE 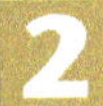

Study	Reliability	Sensitivity	Specificity	LR+	LR−	QUADAS Score (0–14)
Wilder et al.[89] (radiograph reference)	NT	83 80 71	38 50 60	1.33 1.60 1.76	0.45 0.40 0.49	8
Wilder et al.[89] (MRI reference)	NT	92 90 78	19 20 25	1.14 1.13 1.04	0.40 0.50 0.89	8
Wilder et al.[89] (bone scan reference)	NT	77 50 35	65 83 40	2.17 2.99 0.59	0.36 0.60 1.62	8

Comments: Each row within each cell for Wilder et al.[89] corresponds to 128 Hz, 256 Hz, and 512 Hz tuning forks respectively. The frequency of tuning fork used affected the diagnostic accuracy of the test. The entire sample did not receive each imaging technique which may introduce sampling bias into the findings for the MRI and bone scan as the sample sizes were smaller and a higher percentage of those subjects had already experienced a negative radiograph. The authors report that rating pain from the test as severe increased the likelihood of identifying a fracture with the odds ratio being 5.91 for pain level of severe rather than any pain level less than severe.

Key Points

1. Many of the abdominal palpation techniques frequently used in the clinical assessment of abdominal pain lack sufficient sensitivity to be considered excellent screening tools.
2. Many of the studies available are fairly old and are not well designed (or at least lack the description necessary to evaluate them as being well done).
3. Reliability of these techniques and variation in their description (or a lack of sufficient description) make it difficult to strongly recommend their use. The pretest probability of visceral involvement should be high based on other clinical features in order to enhance the posttest probability of visceral diagnosis.
4. The use of the tuning fork to assist in clinical assessment of potential fractures has not been well studied to date.
5. The available studies found in the literature lack sufficient power to make strong recommendations based on their results; however, these data seem promising for the use of the tuning fork either with a stethoscope or with direct placement of the tuning fork over the fracture site.
6. When the tuning fork has failed to classify a fracture appropriately, diagnostic imaging appears to support that the fracture was impacted sufficiently to ensure strong cortical bone contact preserving bony conduction.

References

1. Alvarado A. A practical score for the early diagnosis of acute appendicitis. *Ann Emerg Med.* 1986;15:557–564.
2. Anderson DR, Kovacs MJ, Kovacs G, et al. Combined use of clinical assessment and D-dimer to improve the management of patients presenting to the emergency department with suspected deep vein thrombosis (the edited study). *J Thromb Haemost.* 2003;1:645–651.
3. Antman EM, Cohen M, Bernink PJ, et al. The TIMI risk score for unstable angina/non-st elevation M I: A method for prognostication and therapeutic decision making. *JAMA.* 2000;284:835–842.
4. Bache JB, Cross AB. The Barford test. A useful diagnostic sign in fractures of the femoral neck. *Practitioner.* 1984;228:305–308.
5. Barkun AN, Camus M, Green L, et al. The bedside assessment of splenic enlargement. *Am J Med.* 1991;91:512–518.
6. Barkun AN, Camus M, Meagher T, et al. Splenic enlargement and Traube's space: How useful is percussion? *Am J Med.* 1989;87:562–566.
7. Blendis LM, McNeilly WJ, Sheppard L, et al. Observer variation in the clinical and radiological assessment of hepatosplenomegaly. *Br Med J.* 1970;1:727–730.
8. Bree RL. Further observations on the usefulness of the sonographic Murphy Sign in the evaluation of suspected acute cholecystitis. *J Clin Ultrasound.* 1995;23:169–172.
9. Cadarette SM, Jaglal SB, Kreiger N, et al. Development and validation of the osteoporosis risk assessment instrument to facilitate selection of women for bone densitometry. *CMAJ.* 2000;162:1289–1294.
10. Cadarette SM, Jaglal SB, Murray TM, et al. Evaluation of decision rules for referring women for bone densitometry by dual-energy x-ray absorptiometry. *JAMA.* 2001;286:57–63.
11. Campbell JA, McPhail DC. Acute appendicitis. *Br Med J.* 1958;1:852–855.
12. Castell DO. The spleen percussion sign. A useful diagnostic technique. *Ann Intern Med.* 1967;67:1265–1267.
13. Chagnon I, Bounameaux H, Aujesky D, et al. Comparison of two clinical prediction rules and implicit assessment among patients with suspected pulmonary embolism. *Am J Med.* 2002;113:269–275.
14. Chase M, Robey JL, Zogby KE, et al. Prospective validation of the thrombolysis in myocardial infarction risk score in the emergency department chest pain population. *Ann Emerg Med.* 2006;48:252–259.
15. Chervu A, Clagett GP, Valentine RJ, et al. Role of physical examination in detection of abdominal aortic aneurysms. *Surgery.* 1995;117:454–457.
16. Collin J, Araujo L, Walton J, et al. Oxford screening programme for abdominal aortic aneurysm in men aged 65 to 74 years. *Lancet.* 1988;2:613–615.
17. Colwill JC, Berg EH. Auscultation as an important aid to the diagnosis of fractures. *Surg Gynecol Obstet.* 1958;106:713–714.
18. Constans J, Salmi LR, Sevestre-Pietri MA, et al. A clinical prediction score for upper extremity deep venous thrombosis. *Thromb Haemost.* 2008;99:202–207.
19. Conway Morris A, Caesar D, Gray S, et al. TIMI risk score accurately risk stratifies patients with undifferentiated chest pain presenting to an emergency department. *Heart.* 2006;92:1333–1334.
20. Cornuz J, Ghali WA, Hayoz D, et al. Clinical prediction of deep venous thrombosis using two risk assessment methods in combination with rapid quantitative D-dimer testing. *Am J Med.* 2002;112:198–203.
21. Doobay AV, Anand SS. Sensitivity and specificity of the ankle-brachial index to predict future cardiovascular outcomes: A systematic review. *Arterioscler Thromb Vasc Biol.* 2005;25:1463–1469.

22. Dryjski M, O'Brien-Irr MS, Harris LM, et al. Evaluation of a screening protocol to exclude the diagnosis of deep venous thrombosis among emergency department patients. *J Vasc Surg.* 2001;34:1010–1015.

23. Fink HA, Lederle FA, Roth CS, et al. The accuracy of physical examination to detect abdominal aortic aneurysm. *Arch Intern Med.* 2000;160:833–836.

24. Fujiwara S, Masunari N, Suzuki G, et al. Performance of osteoporosis risk indices in a japanese population. *Curr Ther Res Clin Exp.* 2001;62:586–594.

25. Garcia S, Canoniero M, Peter A, et al. Correlation of TIMI risk score with angiographic severity and extent of coronary artery disease in patients with non-st-elevation acute coronary syndromes. *Am J Cardiol.* 2004;93:813–816.

26. Geusens P, Hochberg MC, van der Voort DJ, et al. Performance of risk indices for identifying low bone density in postmenopausal women. *Mayo Clin Proc.* 2002;77:629–637.

27. Guo X, Li J, Pang W, et al. Sensitivity and specificity of ankle-brachial index for detecting angiographic stenosis of peripheral arteries. *Circ J.* 2008;72:605–610.

28. Halpern S, Coel M, Ashburn W, et al. Correlation of liver and spleen size. Determinations by nuclear medicine studies and physical examination. *Arch Intern Med.* 1974;134:123–124.

29. Holland-Letz T, Endres HG, Biedermann S, et al. Reproducibility and reliability of the ankle-brachial index as assessed by vascular experts, family physicians and nurses. *Vasc Med.* 2007;12:105–112.

30. Holzbach RT, Clark RE, Shipley RA, et al. Evaluation of spleen size by radioactive scanning. *J Lab Clin Med.* 1962;60:902–913.

31. Hooi JD, Stoffers HE, Kester AD, et al. Peripheral arterial occlusive disease: Prognostic value of signs, symptoms, and the ankle-brachial pressure index. *Med Decis Making.* 2002;22:99–107.

32. Joshi R, Singh A, Jajoo N, et al. Accuracy and reliability of palpation and percussion for detecting hepatomegaly: A rural hospital-based study. *Indian J Gastroenterol.* 2004;23:171–174.

33. Karkos CD, Mukhopadhyay U, Papakostas I, et al. Abdominal aortic aneurysm: The role of clinical examination and opportunistic detection. *Eur J Vasc Endovasc Surg.* 2000;19:299–303.

34. Kiev J, Eckhardt A, Kerstein MD. Reliability and accuracy of physical examination in detection of abdominal aortic aneurysms. *Vasc Endovascular Surg.* 1997;31:143–146.

35. Koh LK, Sedrine WB, Torralba TP, et al. A simple tool to identify Asian women at increased risk of osteoporosis. *Osteoporos Int.* 2001;12:699–705.

36. Kraaijenhagen RA, Piovella F, Bernardi E, et al. Simplification of the diagnostic management of suspected deep vein thrombosis. *Arch Intern Med.* 2002;162:907–911.

37. Lederle FA, Simel DL. The rational clinical examination. Does this patient have abdominal aortic aneurysm? *JAMA.* 1999;281:77–82.

38. Lederle FA, Walker JM, Reinke DB. Selective screening for abdominal aortic aneurysms with physical examination and ultrasound. *Arch Intern Med.* 1988;148:1753–1756.

39. Leng GC, Fowkes FG, Lee AJ, et al. Use of ankle brachial pressure index to predict cardiovascular events and death: A cohort study. *BMJ.* 1996;313:1440–1444.

40. Lesho EP. Can tuning forks replace bone scans for identification of tibial stress fractures? *Mil Med.* 1997;162:802–803.

41. Maestre A, Gil V, Gallego J, et al. Diagnostic accuracy of clinical criteria for identifying systolic and diastolic heart failure: Cross-sectional study. *J Eval Clin Pract.* 2009;15:55–61.

42. Mark DB, Shaw L, Harrell FE, Jr., et al. Prognostic value of a treadmill exercise score in outpatients with suspected coronary artery disease. *N Engl J Med.* 1991;325:849–853.

43. Martinez-Aguila D, Gomez-Vaquero C, Rozadilla A, et al. Decision rules for selecting women for bone mineral density testing: Application in postmenopausal women referred to a bone densitometry unit. *J Rheumatol.* 2007;34:1307–1312.

44. Marwick TH, Case C, Vasey C, et al. Prediction of mortality by exercise echocardiography: A strategy for combination with the Duke treadmill score. *Circulation.* 2001;103:2566–2571.

45. Mätzke S, Franckena M, Alback A, et al. Ankle brachial index measurements in critical leg ischaemia—the influence of experience on reproducibility. *Scand J Surg.* 2003;92:144–147.

46. Mauck KF, Cuddihy MT, Atkinson EJ, et al. Use of clinical prediction rules in detecting osteoporosis in a population-based sample of postmenopausal women. *Arch Intern Med.* 2005;165:530–536.

47. McDermott MM, Fried L, Simonsick E, et al. Asymptomatic peripheral arterial disease is independently associated with impaired lower extremity functioning: The women's health and aging study. *Circulation.* 2000;101:1007–1012.

48. McDermott MM, Greenland P, Liu K, et al. The ankle brachial index is associated with leg function and physical activity: The walking and leg circulation study. *Ann Intern Med.* 2002;136:873–883.

49. Memon AA, Vohra LM, Khaliq T, et al. Diagnostic accuracy of Alvarado score in the diagnosis of acute appendicitis. *Pak J Med Sci.* 2009;25:118–121.

50. Miron MJ, Perrier A, Bounameaux H. Clinical assessment of suspected deep vein thrombosis: Comparison between a score and empirical assessment. *J Intern Med.* 2000;247:249–254.

51. Misurya RK, Khare A, Mallick A, et al. Use of tuning fork in diagnostic auscultation of fractures. *Injury.* 1987;18:63–64.

52. Moore MB. The use of a tuning fork and stethoscope to identify fractures. *J Athl Train.* 2009;44:272–274.

53. Moores LK, Collen JF, Woods KM, et al. Practical utility of clinical prediction rules for suspected acute pulmonary embolism in a large academic institution. *Thromb Res.* 2004;113:1–6.

54. Morrow DA, Antman EM, Snapinn SM, et al. An integrated clinical approach to predicting the benefit of tirofiban in non-st elevation acute coronary syndromes. Application of the TIMI risk score for ua/nstemi in prism-plus. *Eur Heart J.* 2002;23:223–229.

55. Newman AB, Shemanski L, Manolio TA, et al. Ankle-arm index as a predictor of cardiovascular disease and mortality in the cardiovascular health study. The cardiovascular health study group. *Arterioscler Thromb Vasc Biol.* 1999;19:538–545.

56. Nixon RK, Jr. The detection of splenomegaly by percussion. *N Engl J Med.* 1954;250:166–167.

57. Nygaard IE. Postvoid residual volume cannot be accurately estimated by bimanual examination. *Int Urogynecol J Pelvic Floor Dysfunct.* 1996;7:74–76.

58. Otah KE, Madan A, Otah E, et al. Usefulness of an abnormal ankle-brachial index to predict presence of coronary artery disease in African-Americans. *Am J Cardiol.* 2004;93:481–483.

59. Oudega R, Hoes AW, Moons KG. The Wells rule does not adequately rule out deep venous thrombosis in primary care patients. *Ann Intern Med.* 2005;143:100–107.

60. Penaloza A, Melot C, Dochy E, et al. Assessment of pretest probability of pulmonary embolism in the emergency department by physicians in training using the Wells model. *Thromb Res.* 2007;120:173–179.

61. Quinn J, McDermott D, Kramer N, et al. Death after emergency department visits for syncope: How common and can it be predicted? *Ann Emerg Med.* 2008;51:585–590.

62. Quinn JV, Stiell IG, McDermott DA, et al. Derivation of the San Francisco syncope rule to predict patients with short-term serious outcomes. *Ann Emerg Med.* 2004;43:224–232.

63. Ralls PW, Halls J, Lapin SA, et al. Prospective evaluation of the sonographic Murphy Sign in suspected acute cholecystitis. *J Clin Ultrasound.* 1982;10:113–115.

64. Ralphs DN, Venn G, Khan O, et al. Is the undeniably palpable liver ever 'normal'? *Ann R Coll Surg Engl.* 1983;65:159–160.

65. Resnick HE, Lindsay RS, McDermott MM, et al. Relationship of high and low ankle brachial index to all-cause and cardiovascular disease mortality: The strong heart study. *Circulation.* 2004;109:733–739.

66. Richy F, Gourlay M, Ross PD, et al. Validation and comparative evaluation of the osteoporosis self-assessment tool (OST) in a Caucasian population from Belgium. *QJM.* 2004;97:39–46.

67. Riddle DL, Hoppener MR, Kraaijenhagen RA, et al. Preliminary validation of clinical assessment for deep vein thrombosis in orthopaedic outpatients. *Clin Orthop Relat Res.* 2005:252–257.

68. Rud B, Jensen JE, Mosekilde L, et al. Performance of four clinical screening tools to select peri- and early postmenopausal women for dual x-ray absorptiometry. *Osteoporos Int.* 2005;16:764–772.

69. Sanchis J, Bodi V, Nunez J, et al. New risk score for patients with acute chest pain, non-st-segment deviation, and normal troponin concentrations: A comparison with the TIMI risk score. *J Am Coll Cardiol.* 2005;46:443–449.

70. Scirica BM, Cannon CP, Antman EM, et al. Validation of the thrombolysis in myocardial infarction (TIMI) risk score for unstable angina pectoris and non-ST-elevation myocardial infarction in the TIMIiii registry. *Am J Cardiol.* 2002;90:303–305.

71. Shaw LJ, Peterson ED, Shaw LK, et al. Use of a prognostic treadmill score in identifying diagnostic coronary disease subgroups. *Circulation.* 1998;98:1622–1630.

72. Shepherd AJ, Cass AR, Carlson CA, et al. Development and internal validation of the male osteoporosis risk estimation score. *Ann Fam Med.* 2007;5:540–546.

73. Shields GP, Turnipseed S, Panacek EA, et al. Validation of the Canadian clinical probability model for acute venous thrombosis. *Acad Emerg Med.* 2002;9:561–566.

74. Singer AJ, McCracken G, Henry MC, et al. Correlation among clinical, laboratory, and hepatobiliary scanning findings in patients with suspected acute cholecystitis. *Ann Emerg Med.* 1996;28:267–272.

75. Soda K, Nemoto K, Yoshizawa S, et al. Detection of pinpoint tenderness on the appendix under ultrasonography is useful to confirm acute appendicitis. *Arch Surg.* 2001;136:1136–1140.

76. Sullivan S, Williams R. Reliability of clinical techniques for detecting splenic enlargement. *Br Med J.* 1976;2:1043–1044.

77. Tamayo SG, Rickman LS, Mathews WC, et al. Examiner dependence on physical diagnostic tests for the detection of splenomegaly: A prospective study with multiple observers. *J Gen Intern Med.* 1993;8:69–75.

78. Tong KL, Kaul S, Wang XQ, et al. Myocardial contrast echocardiography versus thrombolysis in myocardial infarction score in patients presenting to the emergency department with chest pain and a nondiagnostic electrocardiogram. *J Am Coll Cardiol.* 2005;46:920–927.

79. Tzanakis NE, Efstathiou SP, Danulidis K, et al. A new approach to accurate diagnosis of acute appendicitis. *World J Surg.* 2005;29:1151–1156, discussion 1157.

80. van Walraven C, Hart RG, Wells GA, et al. A clinical prediction rule to identify patients with atrial fibrillation and a low risk for stroke while taking aspirin. *Arch Intern Med.* 2003;163:936–943.

81. Weatherall M, Harwood M. The accuracy of clinical assessment of bladder volume. *Arch Phys Med Rehabil.* 2002;83:1300–1302.

82. Wells PS, Anderson DR, Bormanis J, et al. Application of a diagnostic clinical model for the management of hospitalized patients with suspected deep-vein thrombosis. *Thromb Haemost.* 1999;81:493–497.

83. Wells PS, Anderson DR, Bormanis J, et al. Value of assessment of pretest probability of deep-vein thrombosis in clinical management. *Lancet.* 1997;350:1795–1798.

84. Wells PS, Anderson DR, Rodger M, et al. Evaluation of D-dimer in the diagnosis of suspected deep-vein thrombosis. *N Engl J Med.* 2003;349:1227–1235.

85. Wells PS, Anderson DR, Rodger M, et al. Excluding pulmonary embolism at the bedside without diagnostic imaging: Management of patients with suspected pulmonary embolism presenting to the emergency department by using a simple clinical model and D-dimer. *Ann Intern Med.* 2001;135:98–107.

86. Wells PS, Ginsberg JS, Anderson DR, et al. Use of a clinical model for safe management of patients with suspected pulmonary embolism. *Ann Intern Med.* 1998;129:997–1005.

87. Wells PS, Hirsh J, Anderson DR, et al. Accuracy of clinical assessment of deep-vein thrombosis. *Lancet.* 1995;345:1326–1330.

88. Wild SH, Byrne CD, Smith FB, et al. Low ankle-brachial pressure index predicts increased risk of cardiovascular disease independent of the metabolic syndrome and conventional cardiovascular risk factors in the Edinburgh artery study. *Diabetes Care.* 2006;29:637–642.

89. Wilder RP, Vincent HK, Stewart J, et al. Clinical use of tuning forks to identify running-related stress fractures. *Ath Train Sport Health Care.* 2009;1:12–18.

90. Wolf SJ, McCubbin TR, Feldhaus KM, et al. Prospective validation of Wells Criteria in the evaluation of patients with suspected pulmonary embolism. *Ann Emerg Med.* 2004;44:503–510.

91. Zhang B, Lewis SM. A study of the reliability of clinical palpation of the spleen. *Clin Lab Haematol.* 1989;11:7–10.

PEARSON myhealthprofessionskit™

Use this address to access the Companion Website created for this textbook. Simply select "Physical Therapy" from the choice of disciplines. Find this book and log in using your username and password to access video clips of selected tests.

Physical Examination Tests for Neurological Testing and Screening

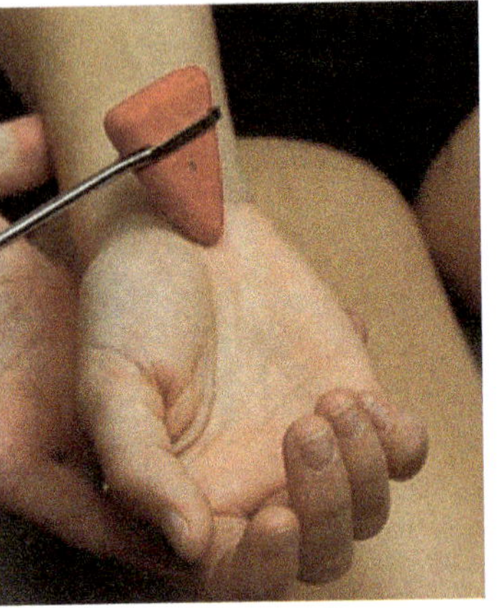

Physical Examination Tests for Neurological Testing and Screening

Chad E. Cook and Mark Wilhelm

Please refer to the chapter "Introduction to Diagnostic Accuracy" before reading this chapter.

Index of Tests

Tests for Focal or Monohemispheric Brain Tumors/Lesions

- Digit Quinti Sign
- Pronator Drift Test
- Finger Rolling Test
- Forearm Rolling Test
- Finger Tap
- Modified Mingazzini's Maneuver
- Rapid Alternating Movements of the Hands
- Barre Test
- Teitelbaum's Clinical Prediction Rule for Unilateral Cerebral Lesions

Tests for Peripheral Neuropathy

- Superficial Pain
- Vibration Testing
- Monofilament Testing
- Position Sense of the Great Toe
- Achilles Reflex
- Phalen's Test
- Tinel's Sign
- Richardson's Clinical Prediction Rule for Peripheral Neuropathy Criteria

Tests for Peripheral Nerve Pathology

- Long Thoracic Nerve Injury
- Pronator Teres Syndrome Test
- Common Fibular Nerve Injury
- Pencil Test

Test for Facioscapulohumeral Dystrophy

- Beevor's Sign

Tests for Cervical Radiculopathy

- Biceps Deep Tendon Reflex
- Triceps Deep Tendon Reflex
- Brachioradialis Deep Tendon Reflex
- Muscle Power Testing
- Sensibility Testing
- Combined Tests Upper Extremity

Tests for Lumbar Radiculopathy

- Quadriceps Deep Tendon Reflex
- Achilles Deep Tendon Reflex
- Extensor Digitorum Brevis Deep Tendon Reflex Test
- Muscle Power Testing
- Sensibility Testing
- Combined Tests Lower Extremity
- Brudzinski's Sign
- Bowstring Test

TESTS FOR CRANIAL NERVE ASSESSMENT

Cranial Nerve I: Olfactory Nerve

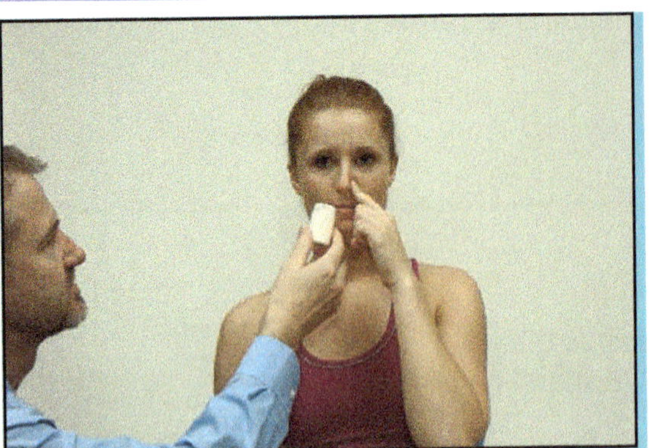

1) The patient is placed in a sitting or standing position.
2) Can the patient recognize common scents, such as coffee or vanilla?
3) Test each nostril separately.

UTILITY SCORE 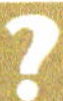

Study	Reliability	Sensitivity	Specificity	LR+	LR−	QUADAS Score (0–14)
Cameron & Klein[7]	NT	NT	NT	NA	NA	NA
Comments: Choose commonly used scents that are accessible at the clinic.						

Cranial Nerve II: Optic Nerve

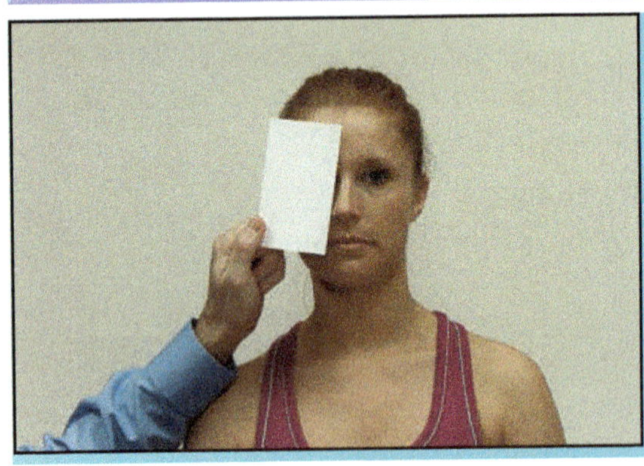

1) The patient is placed in a sitting or standing position.
2) Patient may have history of vision loss.
3) Test visual acuity using an eye chart.
4) Test each eye separately.

UTILITY SCORE 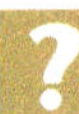

Study	Reliability	Sensitivity	Specificity	LR+	LR−	QUADAS Score (0–14)
Cameron & Klein[7]	NT	NT	NT	NA	NA	NA
Comments: A standard Snellen chart is useful for testing the optic nerve.						

TESTS FOR CRANIAL NERVE ASSESSMENT

Cranial Nerve III: Oculomotor Nerve

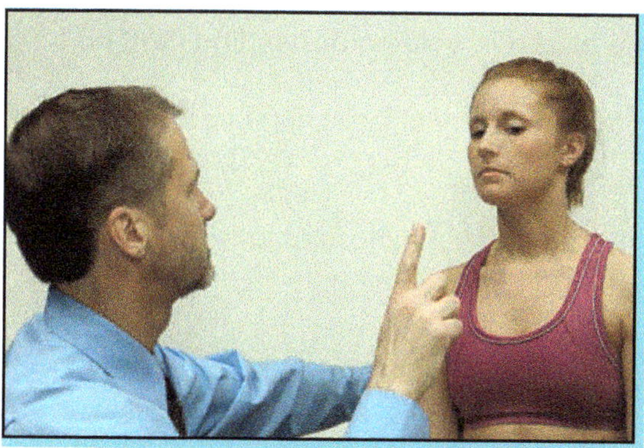

1) The patient is placed in a sitting or standing position.
2) Patient may have a history of double or blurred vision.
3) Ask the patient to follow the clinician's finger in the vertical and horizontal directions with the eyes without moving the head.
4) Look for the ability of the patient to follow movements without report of double vision.

UTILITY SCORE 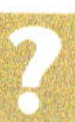

Study	Reliability	Sensitivity	Specificity	LR+	LR−	QUADAS Score (0–14)
Cameron & Klein[7]	NT	NT	NT	NA	NA	NA
Comments: Look for asymmetry of movement or lagging during eye movements.						

Cranial Nerve IV: Trochlear Nerve

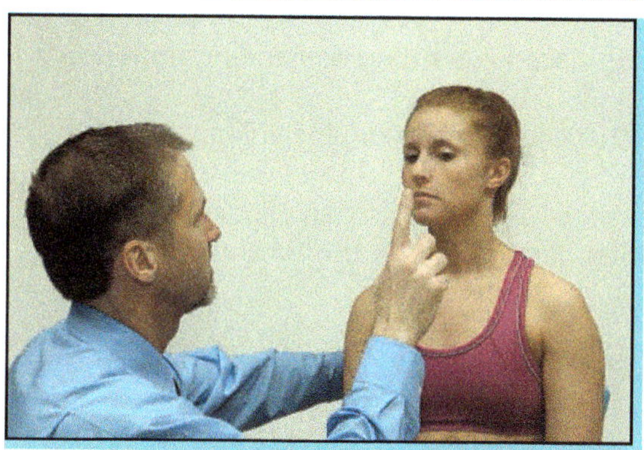

1) The patient is placed in a sitting or standing position.
2) Patient may have a history of double vision.
3) Ask the patient to follow the clinician's finger in the vertical and horizontal directions with the eyes without moving the head.
4) A positive sign is the inability of the eye to move down and in. The eye may also be held up and out when impaired.

UTILITY SCORE 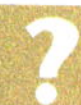

Study	Reliability	Sensitivity	Specificity	LR+	LR−	QUADAS Score (0–14)
Cameron & Klein[7]	NT	NT	NT	NA	NA	NA
Comments: Look for asymmetry of movement or lagging during eye movements.						

TESTS FOR CRANIAL NERVE ASSESSMENT

Cranial Nerve V: Trigeminal Nerve

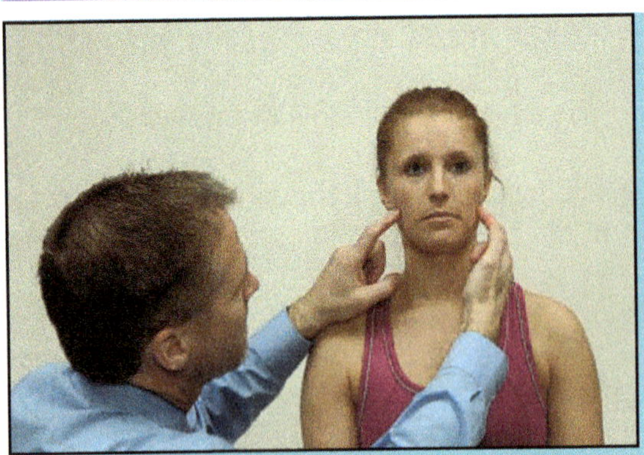

1) The patient is placed in a sitting or standing position.
2) Patient may have a history of facial numbness or difficulty chewing.
3) Lightly touch the upper, middle, and lower face on each side.
4) Check strength of jaw clenching and the masseter muscles.

UTILITY SCORE 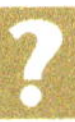

Study	Reliability	Sensitivity	Specificity	LR+	LR−	QUADAS Score (0–14)
Cameron & Klein[7]	NT	NT	NT	NA	NA	NA
Comments: Test both sides. Look for atrophy of the masseter muscles as well.						

Cranial Nerve VI: Abducens Nerve

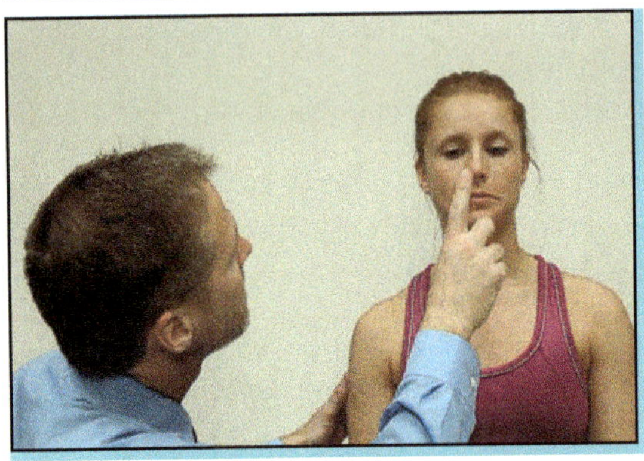

1) The patient is placed in a sitting or standing position.
2) Patient may have a history of double vision.
3) Ask the patient to follow the clinician's finger in the vertical and horizontal directions with the eyes without moving the head.
4) A positive sign is the inability of the eye to move laterally. The eye may also be medially deviated.

UTILITY SCORE 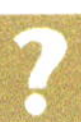

Study	Reliability	Sensitivity	Specificity	LR+	LR−	QUADAS Score (0–14)
Cameron & Klein[7]	NT	NT	NT	NA	NA	NA
Comments: Look for asymmetry of movement or lagging during eye movements.						

TESTS FOR CRANIAL NERVE ASSESSMENT

Cranial Nerve VII: Facial Nerve

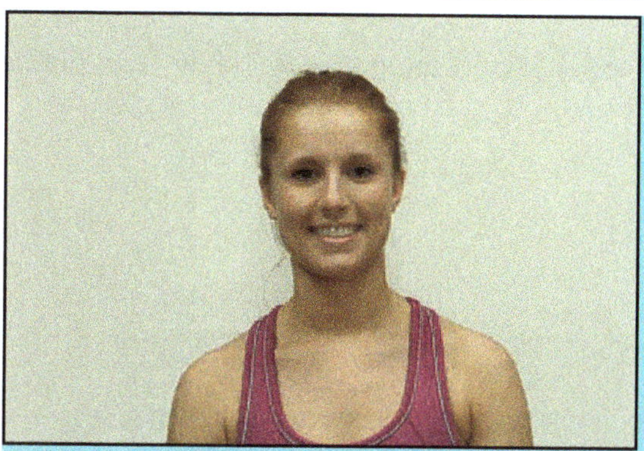

1) The patient is placed in a sitting or standing position.

2) The patient may have a history of facial droop.

3) The examiner asks the patient to smile.

UTILITY SCORE 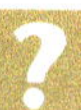

Study	Reliability	Sensitivity	Specificity	LR+	LR−	QUADAS Score (0–14)
Cameron & Klein[7]	NT	NT	NT	NA	NA	NA
Comments: Look for symmetry of facial structures during face muscle movements.						

Cranial Nerve VIII: Vestibulocochlear Nerve

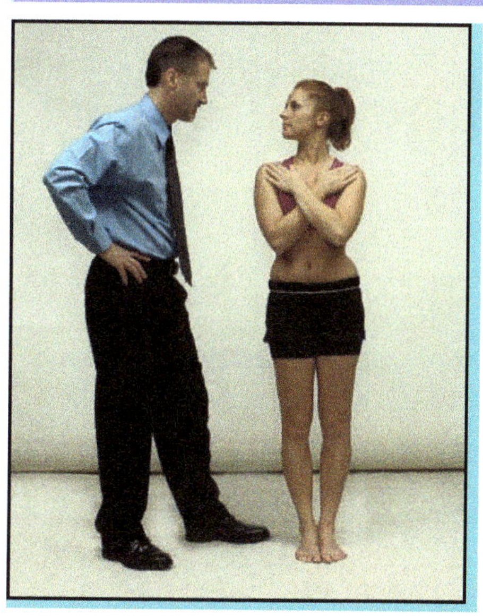

1) The patient is placed in a sitting or standing position.

2) The patient may have a history of dizziness, imbalance, and hearing loss.

3) To test vestibular portion, the examiner asks the patient to look as far as possible in each direction without moving his or her head.

4) The examiner observes the patient's eyes.

(continued)

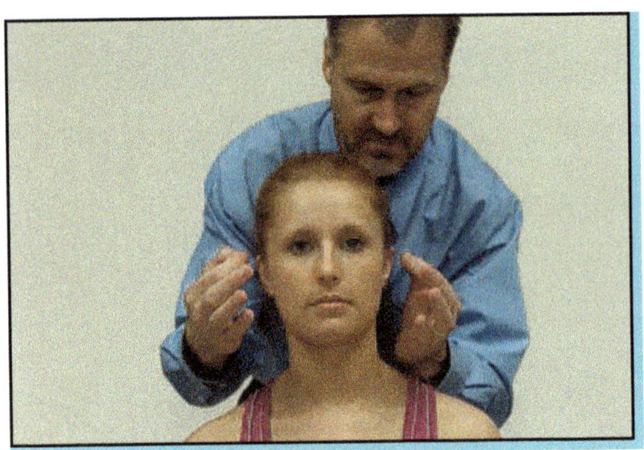

5) A positive sign for the vestibular portion is nystagmus when the patient looks in each direction.

6) To test the cochlear portion, the examiner will rub his fingers together next to each of the patient's ears.

UTILITY SCORE 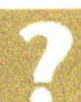

Study	Reliability	Sensitivity	Specificity	LR+	LR−	QUADAS Score (0–14)
Cameron & Klein[7]	NT	NT	NT	NA	NA	NA
Comments: Nystagmus involves involuntary eye movements.						

Cranial Nerve IX: Glossopharyngeal Nerve

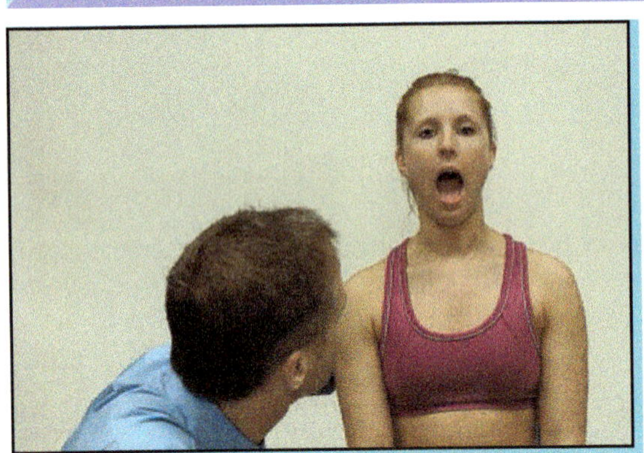

1) The patient is placed in a sitting or standing position.

2) The patient may have a history of difficulty swallowing.

3) Check that the patient can elevate the palate when saying "ahh."

UTILITY SCORE 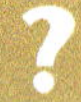

Study	Reliability	Sensitivity	Specificity	LR+	LR−	QUADAS Score (0–14)
Cameron & Klein[7]	NT	NT	NT	NA	NA	NA
Comments: Look at the uvula during mouth opening and saying "ahh" to see if it elevates symmetrically.						

Cranial Nerve X: Vagus Nerve

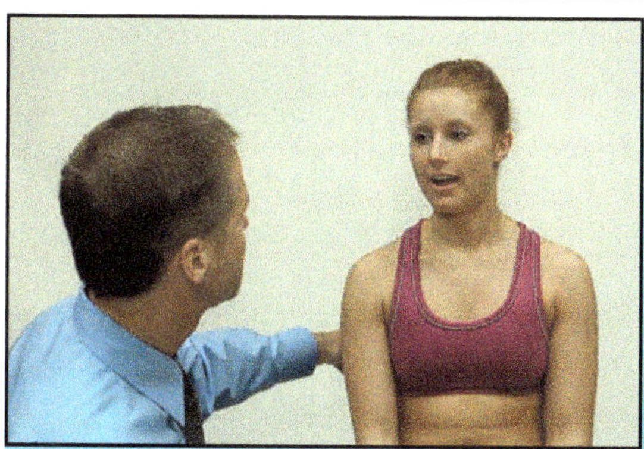

1) The patient is placed in a sitting or standing position.
2) The patient may have a history of a hoarse voice or difficulty swallowing.
3) The examiner will listen to the patient's speech.
4) Check that the patient gags when a cotton swab touches the soft palate.

UTILITY SCORE 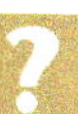

Study	Reliability	Sensitivity	Specificity	LR+	LR−	QUADAS Score (0–14)
Cameron & Klein[7]	NT	NT	NT	NA	NA	NA
Comments: Explain to the patient the procedure you are using.						

Cranial Nerve XI: Spinal Accessory Nerve

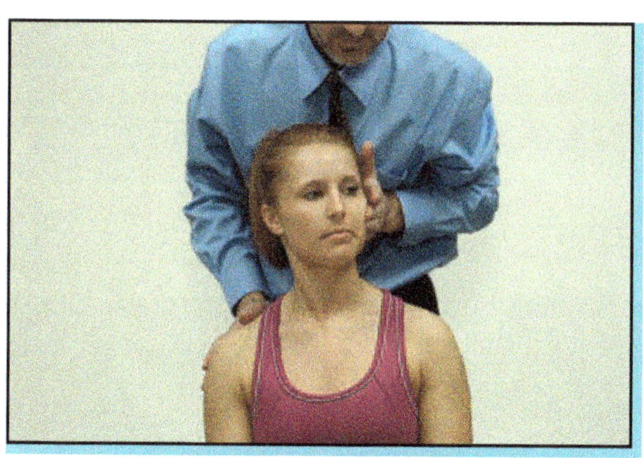

1) The patient is placed in a sitting or standing position.
2) The patient may have a history of neck weakness.
3) Ask the patient to rotate his or her neck against the resistance of the examiner's hand.

UTILITY SCORE 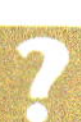

Study	Reliability	Sensitivity	Specificity	LR+	LR−	QUADAS Score (0–14)
Cameron & Klein[7]	NT	NT	NT	NA	NA	NA
Comments: Typically, the patient (unless very acute) will also demonstrate significant atrophy of the neck muscles if the spinal accessory nerve is affected.						

TESTS FOR CRANIAL NERVE ASSESSMENT

Cranial Nerve XII: Hypoglossal Nerve

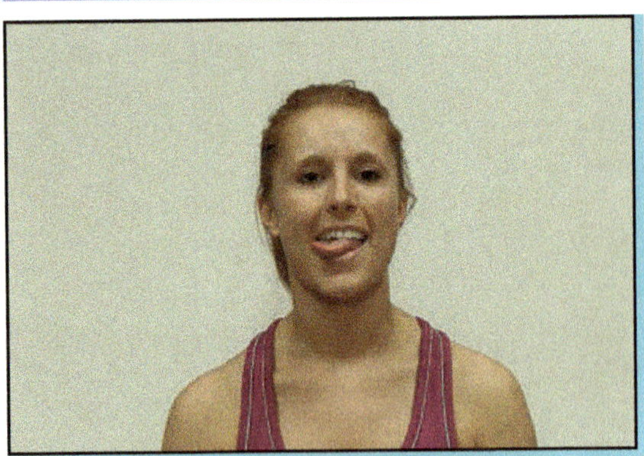

1) The patient is placed in a sitting or standing position.
2) The patient may have a history of tongue weakness (rarely complains of this).
3) Ask the patient to stick out his or her tongue and observe for deviation to either side.

UTILITY SCORE 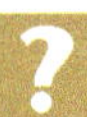

Study	Reliability	Sensitivity	Specificity	LR+	LR−	QUADAS Score (0–14)
Cameron & Klein[7]	NT	NT	NT	NA	NA	NA
Comments: Another method one can use is having the patient poke their tongue in the side of their cheek on both sides.						

TEST FOR CONCUSSION OR POSTCONCUSSION SYNDROME

Single Limb Stance

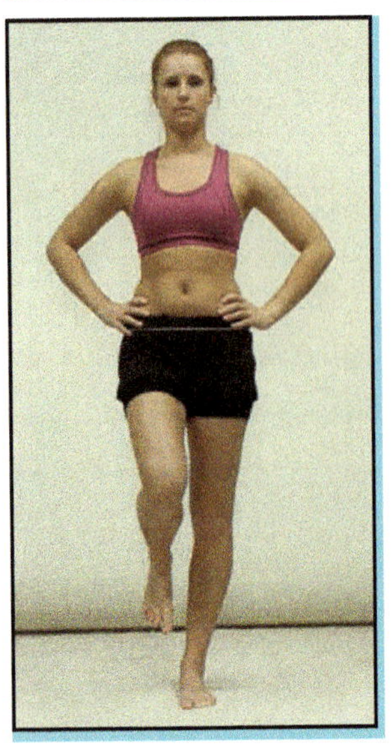

1) The patient is placed in a standing position.
2) Instruct the patient to place his or her hands on his or her hips (pictured). Once the patient has exhibited stability request that they close both eyes.
3) The patient then stands on one foot.
4) A positive test is the inability of the patient to maintain standing balance without opening his or her eyes; touching the floor with the non-test leg, breaking contact with the floor and the standing limb; or removal of the hands from the hips.

TEST FOR CONCUSSION OR POSTCONCUSSION SYNDROME

UTILITY SCORE ?

Study	Reliability	Sensitivity	Specificity	LR+	LR−	QUADAS Score (0–14)
Schneiders et al.[45]	NT	NT	NT	NT	NT	NA

Comments: Some studies have shown an age-related deterioration in balance starting in the 4th decade of life. With multiple trials, there may be a slight learning effect which may increase performance on subsequent trials.

Tandem Walk Test

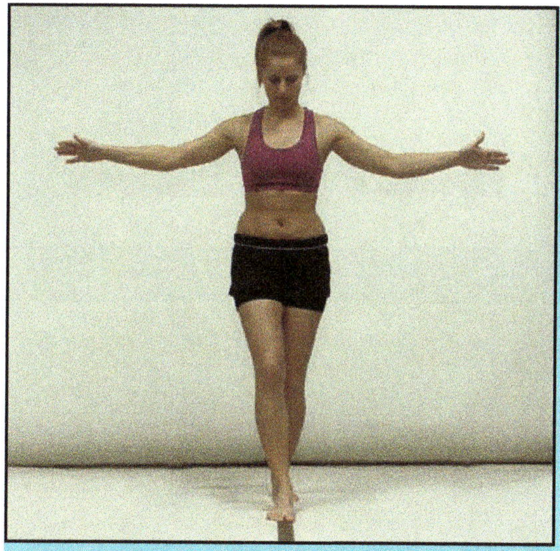

1) Prior to testing the patient, the clinician should set up a line that is approximately 38 mm wide and 3 meters long.
2) The patient is placed in a standing position.
3) Instruct the patient to walk from one end of the line to the other using a tandem gait maintaining approximation of the heel and toes.
4) Once the patient reaches the end, he or she should turn 180° and return to the starting point.
5) A positive test is the inability of the patient to maintain approximation between his or her heel and toes or deviation from the track.

UTILITY SCORE 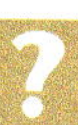

Study	Reliability	Sensitivity	Specificity	LR+	LR−	QUADAS Score (0–14)
Schneiders et al.[45]	NT	NT	NT	NT	NT	NA

Comments: The utilization of tandem gait for assessment of sports related concussion is relatively new despite the fact that it has a long history of being used for neuromotor function. Schneiders et al.[45] described normative values for tandem gait and did not study the utility of the test. With multiple trials, there may be a slight learning effect which may increase performance on subsequent trials.

TEST FOR CONCUSSION OR POSTCONCUSSION SYNDROME

Finger to Nose Test

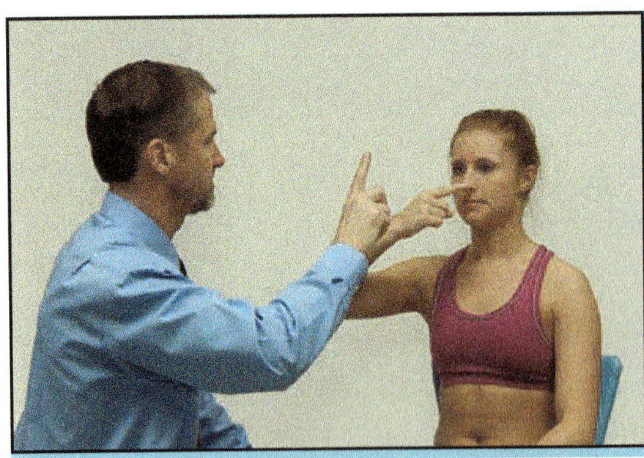

1) The patient is placed in a seated position in a chair with a back rest.

2) Instruct the patient to flex the shoulder to 90° with the test arm outstretched and the elbow and index finger extended.

3) The patient's head is to remain stationary and eyes should be open.

4) The patient is instructed to touch his or her nose with the tip of the index finger and return to starting position five times.

5) A positive sign is the inability of the patient to repetitively touch the tip of his or her nose using a smooth motion.

UTILITY SCORE 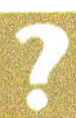

Study	Reliability	Sensitivity	Specificity	LR+	LR−	QUADAS Score (0–14)
Schneiders et al.[45]	NT	NT	NT	NT	NT	NA
Scifers[46]	NT	NT	NT	NT	NT	NA
Comments: Finger to nose assesses upper limb coordination and speed. To increase the difficulty of the test, instruct the patient to increase the speed. With multiple trials, there may be a slight learning effect which may increase performance on subsequent trials.						

ICD-10 Criteria

Criteria consisted of the following 9 self report symptoms:

1) Headaches
2) Dizziness/Vertigo
3) Fatiguing quickly/Getting tired quickly
4) Irritability
5) Poor concentration for extended periods of time
6) Being forgetful/Difficulty remembering things
7) Sleep disturbances
8) Depression
9) Anxiety/Tension

TEST FOR CONCUSSION OR POSTCONCUSSION SYNDROME

UTILITY SCORE 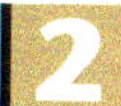

Study	Reliability	Sensitivity	Specificity	LR+	LR−	QUADAS Score (0–14)
Kashluba et al.[25]	NT	See Below	See Below	See Below	See Below	6
Number of symptoms present						
9	NT	21.8	96.6	6.4	0.81	6
8	NT	30.0	94.9	5.88	0.74	6
7	NT	46.4	83.9	2.88	0.64	6
6	NT	57.3	78.0	2.60	0.55	6
5	NT	72.7	61.0	1.86	0.45	6
4	NT	9.1	86.4	0.67	1.05	6
3	NT	10.9	85.6	0.76	1.04	6
2	NT	3.6	85.6	0.25	1.13	6
1	NT	2.7	86.4	0.2	1.13	6
0	NT	0.9	94.9	0.18	1.04	6
Comments: Assessment of symptoms was performed at 1 month and again at 3 months post MTBI. This data was taken from the assessment 1 month post mild traumatic brain injury.						

TESTS FOR PATHOLOGICAL UPPER MOTOR NEURON REFLEX OR SPINAL CORD COMPRESSION (MYELOPATHY)

Hoffmann's Reflex

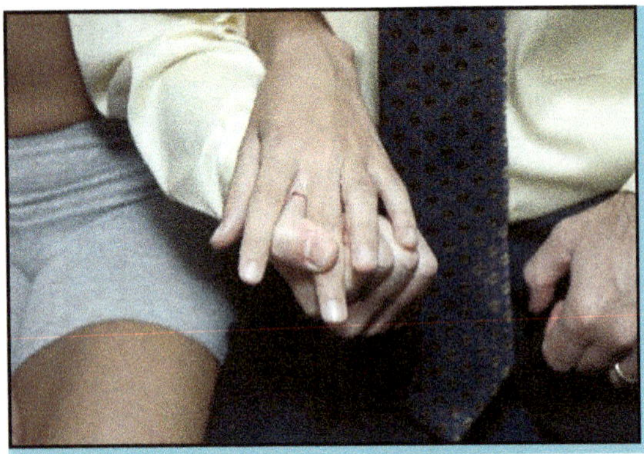

1) The patient is placed in sitting or standing.

2) The examiner stabilizes the middle finger proximally to the distal interphalangeal joint and cradles the hand of the patient.

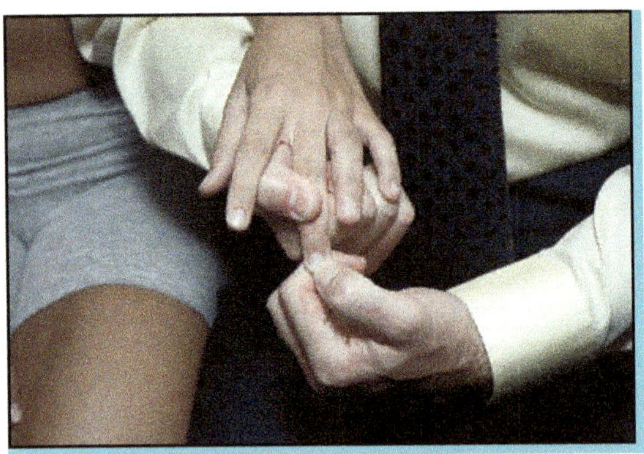

3) The examiner applies a stimulus to the middle finger by nipping the fingernail of the patient between his or her thumb and index finger or by flicking the middle finger with the examiner's fingernail.

4) A positive test is adduction and opposition of thumb and slight flexion of the fingers.

UTILITY SCORE 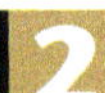

Study	Reliability	Sensitivity	Specificity	LR+	LR−	QUADAS Score (0–14)
Denno & Meadows[13] (sample was biased, negative Hoffmann's was selected)	NT	0	0	0	0	6
Sung & Wang[49] (sample consisted of those with positive tests only)	NT	94	NT	NA	NA	7
Wong et al.[55] (sample consisted of patients with cervical myelopathy)	NT	82	NT	NA	NA	3
Glaser et al.[17] (unblinded tester)	NT	58	74	2.23	0.57	8
Glaser et al.[17] (blinded tester)	NT	28	71	0.96	1.01	8
Cook et al.[10]	89% agreement	44	75	1.8	0.7	11
Rhee et al.[42]	NT	59	84	3.69	0.49	4

TESTS FOR PATHOLOGICAL UPPER MOTOR NEURON REFLEX OR SPINAL CORD COMPRESSION (MYELOPATHY)

Study	Reliability	Sensitivity	Specificity	LR+	LR−	QUADAS Score (0–14)
Cook et al.[9]	NT	31	73	4.9	0.74	7
Kiely et al.[27] (sample consisted of asymptomatic patients)	NT	NT	90	NA	NA	2
Houten & Noce[22] (bilateral or unilateral)	NT	68	NT	NA	NA	7
Chikuda et al.[8]	NT	81	NT	NA	NA	6
Comments: Positive findings are typically very subtle. False positives may occur in patients with a history of head injury or concussion. Note that the only blinded reference involves the Glaser et al.[17] study. The values associated with blinding and unblinding are significantly affected. We feel that the Hoffmann's is not a good screening test.						

Babinski Sign

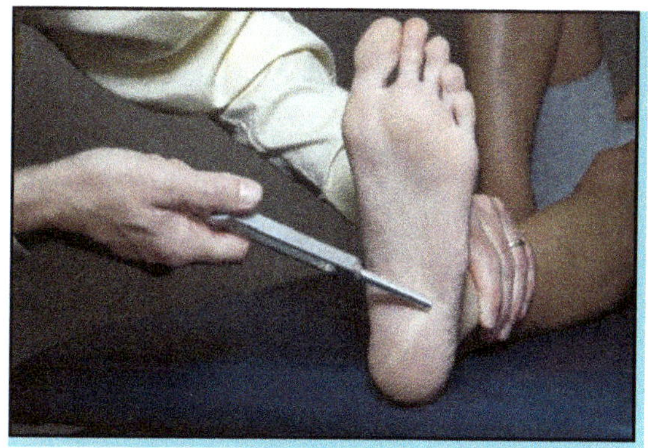

1) The patient is placed in supine. The foot is held in relative neutral by the examiner.

2) The examiner applies stimulation with the blunt end of a reflex hammer to the plantar aspect of the foot (typically laterally to medial from heel to metatarsal).

3) A negative finding is slight toe flexion, smaller digits greater than great toe.

UTILITY SCORE 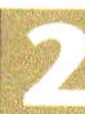

Study	Reliability	Sensitivity	Specificity	LR+	LR−	QUADAS Score (0–14)
Bertilson et al.[6]	98% agreement	NT	NT	NA	NA	NA
De Freitas & Andre[12] (tested to determine brain death)	NT	0	NT	NA	NA	6
Berger et al.[4] (tested concurrently with sock off and sheet removal)	NT	80	90	8	0.05	7
Ghosh[16]	NT	76	NT	NA	NA	11
Hindfelt et al.[21]	NT	18	NT	NA	NA	6
Miller & Johnston[35]	.73 kappa	35	77	1.5	0.8	9
Cook et al.[10]	89% agreement	33	92	4.0	0.7	11
Rhee et al.[42]	NT	13	100	Inf	0.87	4
Cook et al.[9]	NT	7	100	Inf	0.93	7

(continued)

TESTS FOR PATHOLOGICAL UPPER MOTOR NEURON REFLEX OR SPINAL CORD COMPRESSION (MYELOPATHY)

Study	Reliability	Sensitivity	Specificity	LR+	LR−	QUADAS Score (0–14)
Kiely et al.[27] (sample consisted of asymptomatic patients)	NT	NT	100	NA	NA	2
Houten & Noce[22]	NT	33	NT	NA	NA	7
Chikuda et al.[8]	NT	53	NT	NA	NA	6

Comments: A positive finding is generally associated with a pyramidal defect. Response changes after 1 year of birth. There are a number of ways to perform the stroking of the foot, and it is doubtful if technique or location affects findings.

Lhermitte's Sign

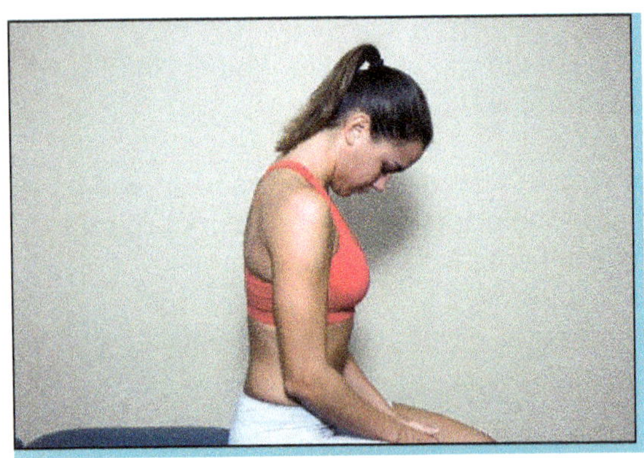

1) The patient is placed in standing or supine.

2) The patient is instructed to flex the neck with emphasis on lower cervical flexion.

3) Some examiners have advocated use of hyperextension to produce a Lhermitte's response.

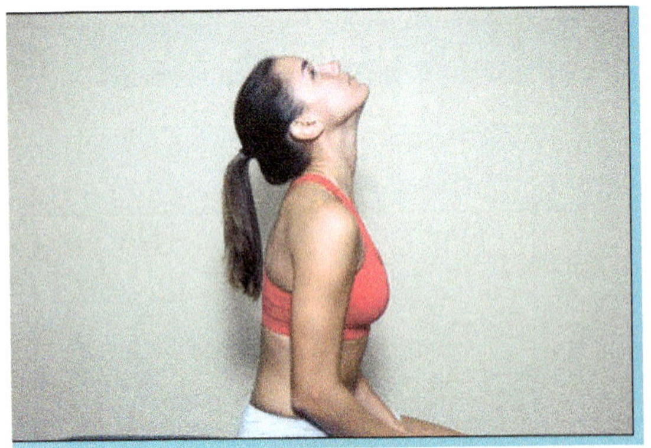

4) The patient is queried for "electrical-type" responses during the flexion or if used, extension. A positive test is an "electrical-type" sensation in the midline and occasionally to the extremities during flexion.

UTILITY SCORE 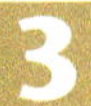

Study	Reliability	Sensitivity	Specificity	LR+	LR−	QUADAS Score (0–14)
Uchihara et al.[52]	NT	3	97	1	1	8

Comments: A positive finding is associated with focal lesions of the spinal cord, multiple sclerosis, or other degenerative processes causing stenosis (cord compression).

TESTS FOR PATHOLOGICAL UPPER MOTOR NEURON REFLEX OR SPINAL CORD COMPRESSION (MYELOPATHY)

Gonda-Allen Sign

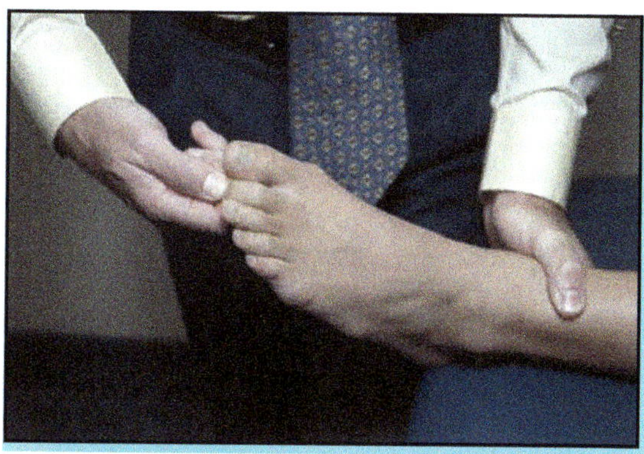

1) The patient is placed in a supine position.

2) The examiner provides a forceful downward stretch or snaps the distal phalanx of the 2nd or 4th toe. The examiner may also press on the toe nail, twist the toe, and hold for a few seconds.

3) A positive response is the extensor toe sign (great toe extension), a similar response to a positive Babinski sign.

UTILITY SCORE 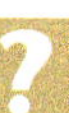

Study	Reliability	Sensitivity	Specificity	LR+	LR−	QUADAS Score (0–14)
Denno & Meadows[13]	NT	90	NT	NA	NA	11
Comments: The sample was biased because only patients with a negative Hoffmann's were selected.						

Allen-Cleckley Sign

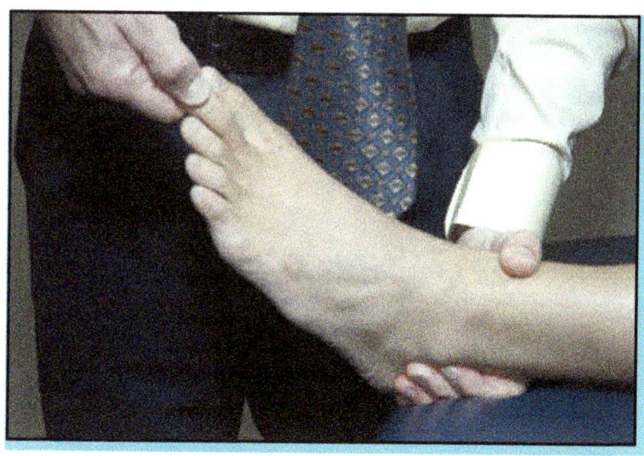

1) The patient is placed in a supine position.

2) The examiner provides a sharp upward flick of the 2nd toe or pressure over the distal aspect or ball of the toe.

3) A positive response is the extensor toe sign.

UTILITY SCORE 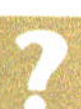

Study	Reliability	Sensitivity	Specificity	LR+	LR−	QUADAS Score (0–14)
Denno & Meadows[13]	NT	82	NT	NA	NA	11
Comments: The diagnostic value of this test suggests high sensitivity but caution must be taken. The sample was biased, only patients with a negative Hoffmann's were selected.						

TESTS FOR PATHOLOGICAL UPPER MOTOR NEURON REFLEX OR SPINAL CORD COMPRESSION (MYELOPATHY)

Inverted Supinator Sign

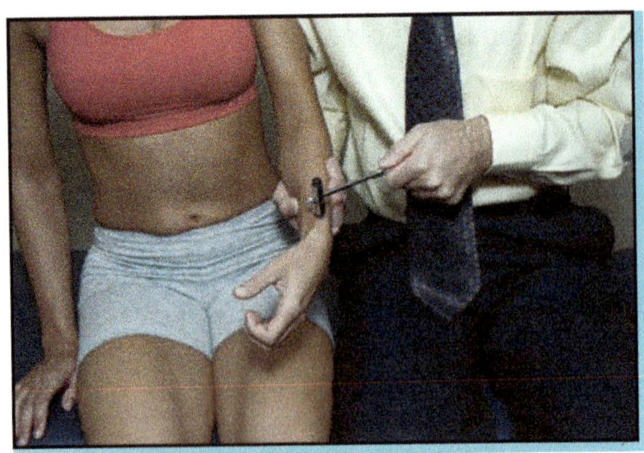

1) The patient assumes a sitting position.

2) The examiner places the patient's forearm on his or her forearm to ensure relaxation. The patient's forearm is held in slight pronation.

3) The examiner applies a series of quick strikes near the styloid process of the radius at the attachment of the brachioradialis and the tendon.

4) A positive test is finger flexion or slight elbow extension.

UTILITY SCORE 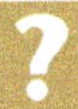

Study	Reliability	Sensitivity	Specificity	LR+	LR−	QUADAS Score (0–14)
Estanol & Marin[15]	NT	NT	NT	NA	NA	NA
Cook et al.[10]	78% agreement	61	78	2.8	0.5	11
Rhee et al.[42]	NT	51	81	2.68	0.60	4
Cook et al.[9]	NT	18	99	29.1	0.82	7
Kiely et al.[27] (sample consisted of asymptomatic patients)	NT	NT	72.4	NA	NA	2
Wong et al.[55] (sample consisted of patients with cervical myelopathy)	NT	53	NT	NA	NA	3
Comments: A positive finding is likely related to increased alpha motor neurons below the level of the lesion.						

Finger Escape Sign

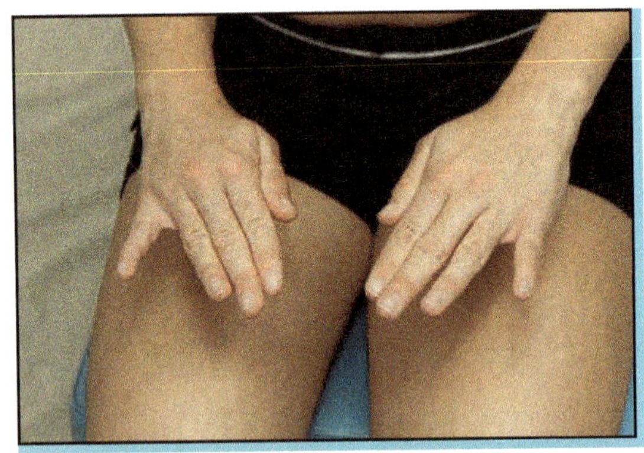

1) The patient is placed in a seated position.

2) The patient is asked to flex both elbows to 90° and keep them at his or her side.

3) The forearms are then pronated and all fingers are adducted.

4) A positive sign is the inability of the patient to maintain adduction of the 5th digit. The 5th digit will start to drift in an ulnar and volar direction.

TESTS FOR PATHOLOGICAL UPPER MOTOR NEURON REFLEX OR SPINAL CORD COMPRESSION (MYELOPATHY)

UTILITY SCORE ?

Study	Reliability	Sensitivity	Specificity	LR+	LR−	QUADAS Score (0–14)
Kiely et al.[27] (sample consisted of asymptomatic patients)	NT	NT	100	NA	NA	2
Wong et al.[55] (sample consisted of patients with cervical myelopathy)	NT	55	NT	NA	NA	3
Comments: The studies are so poorly performed that it is difficult to extract a value from this test.						

Crossed Upgoing Toe Sign (Cut)

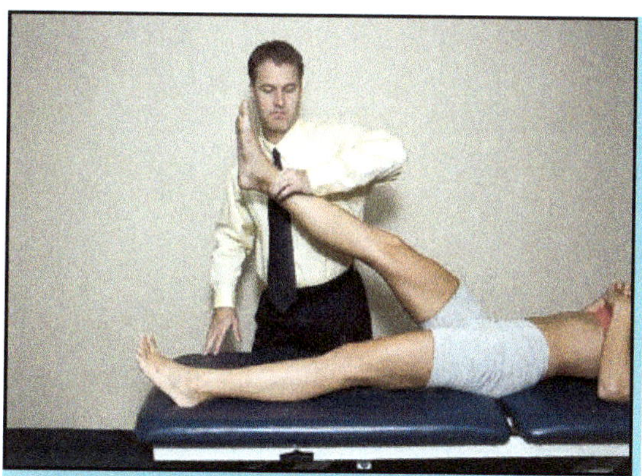

1) The patient is placed in a supine position.
2) The examiner passively raises the opposite limb into hip flexion. The examiner then instructs the patient to hold the leg in flexion.
3) The examiner applies a downward force against the leg.
4) Visual inspection of the opposite great toe is required to observe great toe extension.
5) A positive test is associated with great toe extension of the opposite leg during resistance of hip flexion.

UTILITY SCORE 

Study	Reliability	Sensitivity	Specificity	LR+	LR−	QUADAS Score (0–14)
Hindfelt et al.[21]	NT	31	96	7.8	0.72	6
Comments: Bias limits the true assessment of diagnostic value.						

Mendel-Bechterew Sign

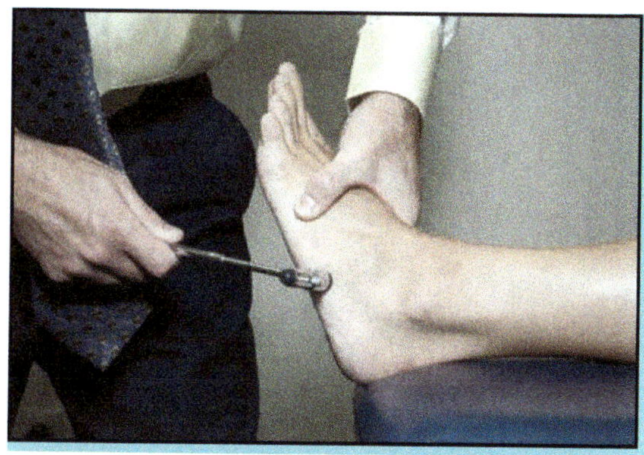

1) The patient is placed in a supine or sitting position.
2) The examiner taps on the cuboid bone (on the dorsal aspect) using the sharp end of the reflex hammer.
3) A positive response is flexion of the four lateral toes.

(*continued*)

TESTS FOR PATHOLOGICAL UPPER MOTOR NEURON REFLEX OR SPINAL CORD COMPRESSION (MYELOPATHY)

UTILITY SCORE

Study	Reliability	Sensitivity	Specificity	LR+	LR−	QUADAS Score (0–14)
Kumar & Ramasubramanian[29]	NT	NT	NT	NA	NA	NT
Comments: The diagnostic value of this test is unknown.						

Schaefer's Sign

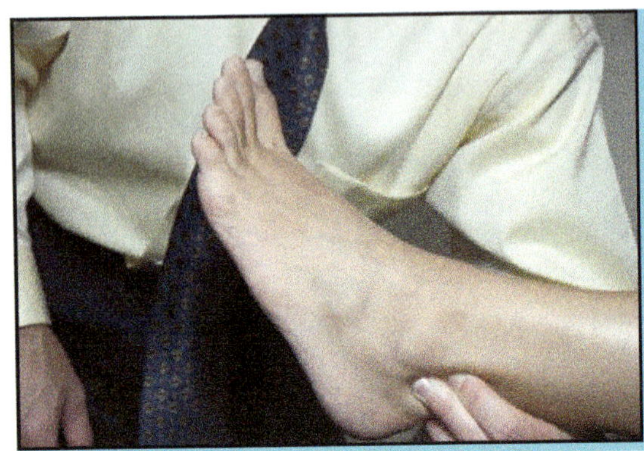

1) The patient is placed in a supine or sitting position.
2) The examiner provides a sharp, quick squeeze of the Achilles tendon.
3) A positive response is the extensor toe sign.

UTILITY SCORE 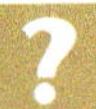

Study	Reliability	Sensitivity	Specificity	LR+	LR−	QUADAS Score (0–14)
Kumar & Ramasubramanian[29]	NT	NT	NT	NA	NA	NT
Comments: The diagnostic value of this test is unknown.						

Oppenheim Sign

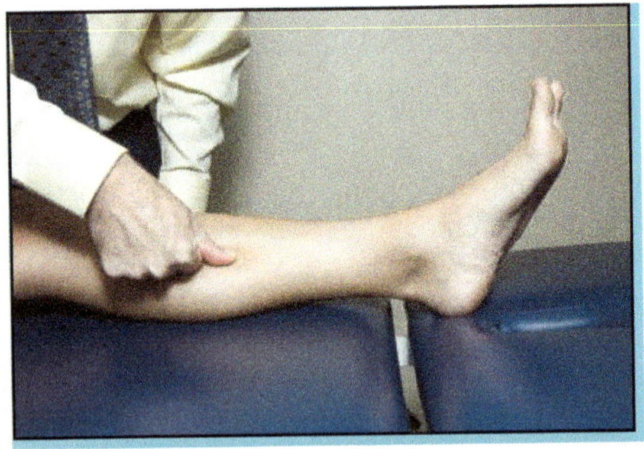

1) The patient is placed in a supine or sitting position.
2) The examiner provides pressure along the shin of the tibia, while sliding downward toward the foot.
3) A positive response is the extensor toe sign.

TESTS FOR PATHOLOGICAL UPPER MOTOR NEURON REFLEX OR SPINAL CORD COMPRESSION (MYELOPATHY)

UTILITY SCORE 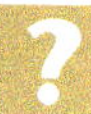

Study	Reliability	Sensitivity	Specificity	LR+	LR−	QUADAS Score (0–14)
Kumar & Ramasubramanian[29]	NT	NT	NT	NA	NA	NT
Comments: The diagnostic value of this test is unknown.						

Chaddock's Sign

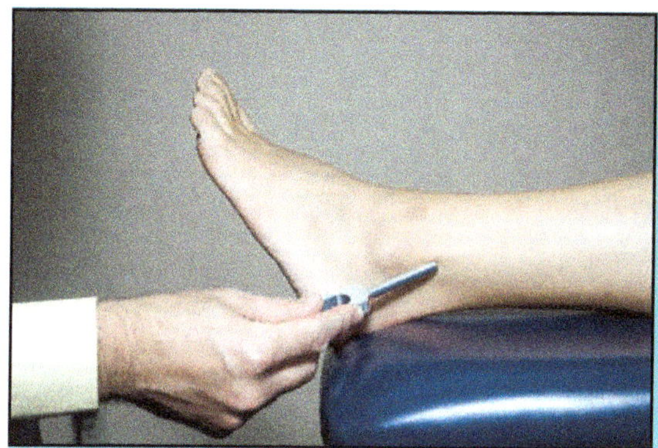

1) The patient is placed in a supine or sitting position.
2) The examiner strokes the lateral malleolus from proximal to distal with a solid, relatively sharp object.
3) A positive response is the extensor toe sign.

UTILITY SCORE 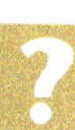

Study	Reliability	Sensitivity	Specificity	LR+	LR−	QUADAS Score (0–14)
Kumar & Ramasubramanian[29]	NT	NT	NT	NA	NA	NT
Comments: The diagnostic value of this test is unknown.						

Clonus

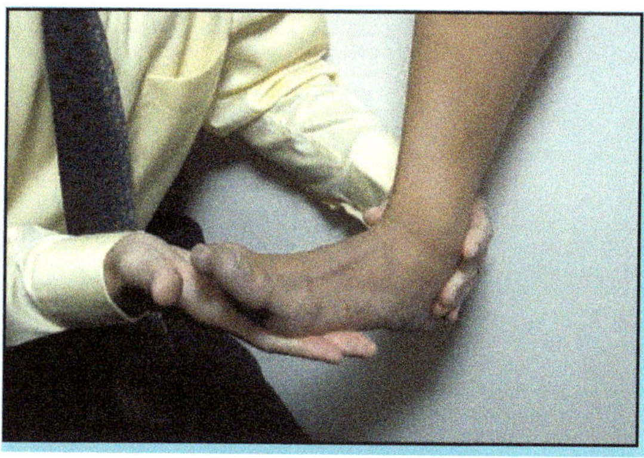

1) The patient is placed in a supine or sitting position.
2) The technique can be applied to the wrist or to the ankle.
3) The examiner takes up the slack of the wrist (into extension; not pictured). The examiner then applies a quick overpressure with maintained pressure to the wrist.
4) The examiner takes up the slack of the ankle (into dorsiflexion; pictured). The examiner then applies a quick overpressure with maintained pressure to the ankle.
5) A positive response is more than three involuntary beats of the ankle or wrist.

(*continued*)

TESTS FOR PATHOLOGICAL UPPER MOTOR NEURON REFLEX OR SPINAL CORD COMPRESSION (MYELOPATHY)

UTILITY SCORE 2

Study	Reliability	Sensitivity	Specificity	LR+	LR−	QUADAS Score (0–14)
Rhee et al.[42]	NT	13	100	Inf	0.87	4
Cook et al.[10]	98% agreement	11	96	2.7	0.9	11
Cook et al.[9]	NT	7	99	5.4	0.94	7
Chikuda et al.[8] (sustained ankle clonus)	NT	35	NT	NA	NA	6
Comments: One or two beats is relatively normal and is not indicative of pathology. Three beats or more is considered abnormal. One may see a positive for patients with a history of concussion.						

Deep Tendon Reflex Tests

Biceps Tendon

1) In biceps tendon testing, the patient is positioned in sitting.
2) The clinician slightly supinates the patient's forearm and places it on his own forearm assuring relaxation.
3) The clinician's thumb is placed on the patient's biceps tendon and he strikes his own thumb with quick strikes of a reflex hammer.
4) A positive test is indicated by hyperreflexia of the biceps deep tendon reflex.

Triceps Tendon

1) In triceps tendon testing, the patient is positioned in sitting.
2) The patient's shoulder is elevated to 90° with the elbow passively flexed to 90°.
3) The clinician places his thumb over the distal aspect of the patient's triceps tendon and applies a series of quick strikes with the reflex hammer to the back of his thumb.
4) A positive test is indicated by hyperreflexia of the triceps deep tendon reflex.

UTILITY SCORE 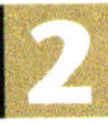

Study	Reliability	Sensitivity	Specificity	LR+	LR−	QUADAS Score (0–14)
Cook et al.[10]	89% agreement	44	71	1.5	0.8	11
Cook et al.[9]	NT	18	96	4.8	0.85	7
Comments: Cook et al.[9] tested only for biceps tendon hyperreflexia. Reflex testing is commonly scored as 0+ = absent (no visible or palpable muscle contraction with reinforcement), 1+ = tone change (slight, transitory impulse, with no movement of the extremities), 2+ = normal (visual, brief movement of the extremity), 3+ = exaggerated (full movement of the extremities), 4+ = abnormal (compulsory and sustained movement, lasting for more than 30 seconds). The test is frequently performed as a component of the upper quarter screen. The biceps reflex test is purported to target C6, and the triceps reflex test is purported to target C7.						

TESTS FOR PATHOLOGICAL UPPER MOTOR NEURON REFLEX OR SPINAL CORD COMPRESSION (MYELOPATHY)

Suprapatellar Quadriceps Test

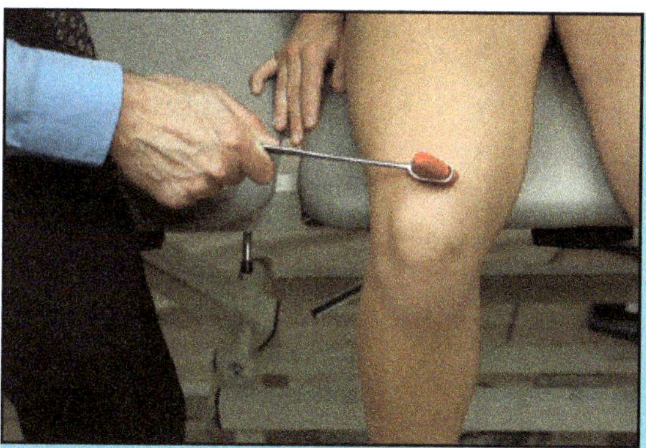

1) The patient is positioned in seated with his or her feet off the ground.

2) The clinician applies quick strikes of the reflex hammer to the suprapatellar tendon.

3) A positive test is indicated by hyperreflexive knee extension.

UTILITY SCORE 3

Study	Reliability	Sensitivity	Specificity	LR+	LR−	QUADAS Score (0–14)
Cook et al.[10]	84% agreement	56	33	0.8	1.3	11
Cook et al.[9]	NT	22	97	6.9	0.81	7
Comments: Reflex testing is commonly scored as 0+ = absent (no visible or palpable muscle contraction with reinforcement), 1+ = tone change (slight, transitory impulse, with no movement of the extremities), 2+ = normal (visual, brief movement of the extremity), 3+ = exaggerated (full movement of the extremities), 4+ = abnormal (compulsory and sustained movement, lasting for more than 30 seconds). The test is frequently performed as a component of the upper quarter screen.						

Achilles Tendon Reflex Test

1) The patient is placed in with the foot to be tested not touching the ground.

2) Using a reflex hammer, either strike the tendon itself or use the plantar strike technique to elicit a reflex.

3) If the reflex is absent, ask the patient to gently plantarflex the foot, tightly close the eyes, and pull their clasped hands apart just prior to striking.

4) A positive test is indicated by hyperreflexia of the Achilles tendon reflex.

UTILITY SCORE 2

Study	Reliability	Sensitivity	Specificity	LR+	LR−	QUADAS Score (0–14)
Cook et al.[9]	NT	15	98	7.8	0.87	7
Rhee et al.[42]	NT	26	81	1.37	0.91	4
Comments: Reflex testing is commonly scored as 0+ = absent (no visible or palpable muscle contraction with reinforcement), 1+ = tone change (slight, transitory impulse, with no movement of the extremities), 2+ = normal (visual, brief movement of the extremity), 3+ = exaggerated (full movement of the extremities), 4+ = abnormal (compulsory and sustained movement, lasting for more than 30 seconds).						

TESTS FOR PATHOLOGICAL UPPER MOTOR NEURON REFLEX OR SPINAL CORD COMPRESSION (MYELOPATHY)

Infrapatellar Tendon Reflex

1) The patient is positioned in sitting with the leg to be tested not touching the ground.

2) Using a reflex hammer, strike the patellar tendon inferior to the patella.

3) A positive test is indicated by hyperreflexia of the patellar tendon reflex.

UTILITY SCORE 3

Study	Reliability	Sensitivity	Specificity	LR+	LR−	QUADAS Score (0–14)
Chikuda et al.[8]	NT	94	NT	NA	NA	6
Rhee et al.[42]	NT	33	76	1.37	0.88	4
Comments: Reflex testing is commonly scored as 0+ = absent (no visible or palpable muscle contraction with reinforcement), 1+ = tone change (slight, transitory impulse, with no movement of the extremities), 2+ = normal (visual, brief movement of the extremity), 3+ = exaggerated (full movement of the extremities), 4+ = abnormal (compulsory and sustained movement, lasting for more than 30 seconds).						

Hand Withdrawal Reflex

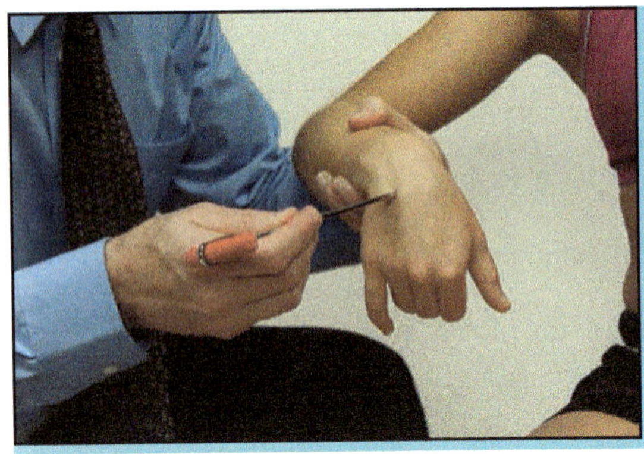

1) The patient is positioned in either sitting or standing.

2) The clinician grasps the patient's palm and strikes the dorsum of the patient's hand with a reflex hammer.

3) A positive test is indicated by an abnormal flexor response.

UTILITY SCORE 3

Study	Reliability	Sensitivity	Specificity	LR+	LR−	QUADAS Score (0–14)
Cook et al.[10]	80% agreement	41	63	1.1	0.9	11
Comments: This test has questionable value.						

TESTS FOR PATHOLOGICAL UPPER MOTOR NEURON REFLEX OR SPINAL CORD COMPRESSION (MYELOPATHY)

Static and Dynamic Romberg's Sign

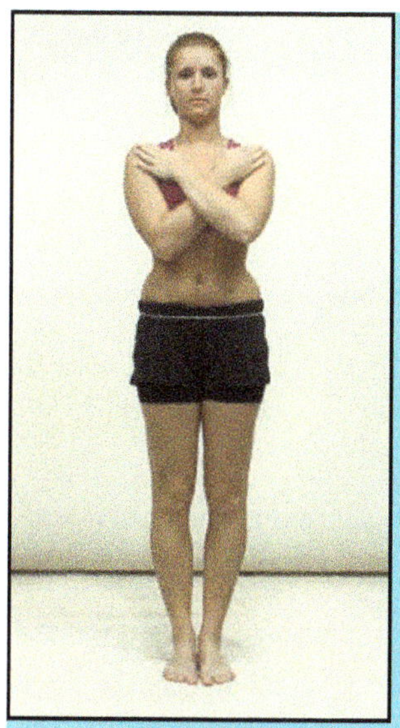

1) The patient is in a standing position.
2) The patient's feet are together, eyes are closed after the patient demonstrates stability, and hands are by his or her side.
3) A positive sign is obvious swaying or falling.
4) The Dynamic Romberg sign is performed similarly to the static test; however, a light external moment is applied to the patient.
5) A positive sign is still indicated by obvious swaying or falling.

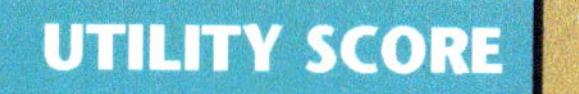

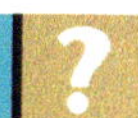

Study	Reliability	Sensitivity	Specificity	LR+	LR−	QUADAS Score (0–14)
Kiely et al.[27] (sample consisted of asymptomatic patients)	NT	NT	100	NA	NA	2
Comments: The use of this test for assessment of myelopathic symptoms requires additional investigation.						

Gait Deviation

1) The patient is asked to ambulate as the clinician observes the patient's gait.
2) A positive sign is the presence of abnormally wide based gait, ataxia, or spastic gait.

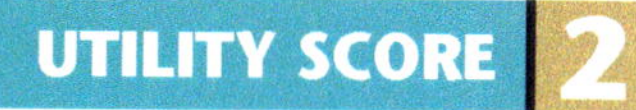

Study	Reliability	Sensitivity	Specificity	LR+	LR−	QUADAS Score (0–14)
Cook et al.[9]	NT	19	94	3.4	0.85	7
Comments: Promising finding but requires a better operational definition than the one described in the study.						

TESTS FOR PATHOLOGICAL UPPER MOTOR NEURON REFLEX OR SPINAL CORD COMPRESSION (MYELOPATHY)

Cook's Clinical Prediction Rule for Myelopathy Tests Included in Clinical Prediction Rule

1) Gait Deviation
2) Positive Hoffmann's Test
3) Inverted Supinator Sign
4) Positive Babinski Test
5) Patient age >45 years old

UTILITY SCORE 2

Study	Reliability	Sensitivity	Specificity	LR+	LR−	QUADAS Score (0–14)
Cook et al.[9] 1 of 5 Positive Tests	NT	94	31	1.4	0.18	7
Cook et al.[9] 2 of 5 Positive Tests	NT	39	88	3.3	0.63	7
Cook et al.[9] 3 of 5 Positive Tests	NT	19	99	30.9	0.81	7
Cook et al.[9] 4 of 5 Positive Tests	NT	9	100	Inf	0.91	7
Comments: This is the first study which is known to show a high sensitivity rather than just high specificity for cervical myelopathy.						

TEST FOR PATHOLOGICAL UPPER MOTOR NEURON REFLEX

Palmomental Reflex

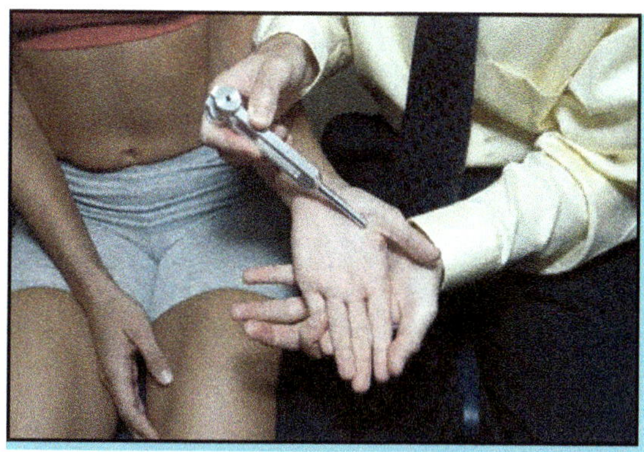

1) The patient is positioned in sitting or supine.

2) A number of methods to elicit this reflex have been advocated. The examiner may stroke the thenar eminence of the hand in a proximal to distal direction with a reflex hammer or may stroke the hypothenar eminence in a similar fashion.

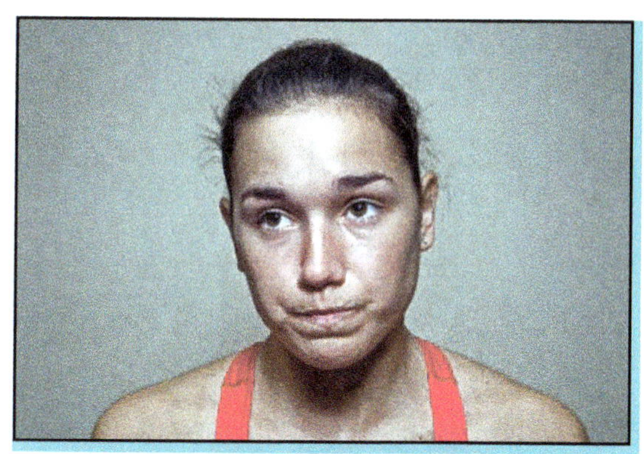

3) The process can be repeated up to five times to detect a continuous response. If the response diminishes the test is considered negative.

4) A positive test is contraction of the mentalis and orbicularis oris muscles causing wrinkling of the skin of the chin and slight retraction (and occasionally elevation of the mouth).

UTILITY SCORE 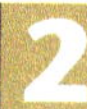 2

Study	Reliability	Sensitivity	Specificity	LR+	LR−	QUADAS Score (0–14)
Gotkine et al.[18]	98.9% agreement	24	NT	NA	NA	9
August & Miller[2]	NT	95	98	38	.21	4
Isakov et al.[23]	NT	78	58	1.8	.22	11
Comments: This test is associated with a high degree of false positives. There is a higher prevalence of positive findings in Parkinson's and other neurological diseases.						

TESTS FOR FOCAL OR MONOHEMISPHERIC BRAIN TUMORS/LESIONS

Digit Quinti Sign

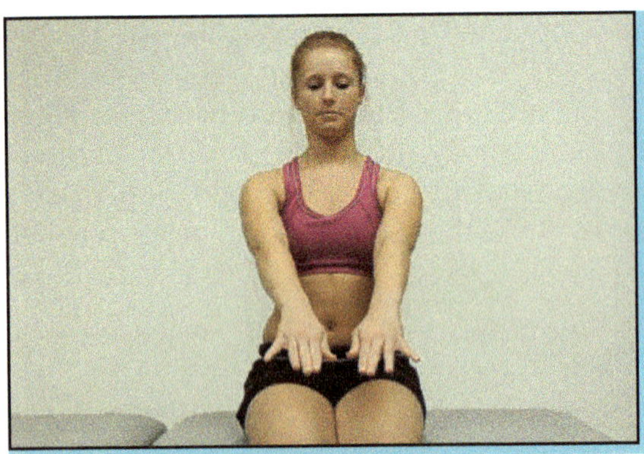

1) The patient is instructed to horizontally extend the arms and fingers forward with palms down.

2) If the fifth finger adducts on one side, that side is considered to test positive. If the fifth digit on both sides is abducted symmetrically, there is no clinical significance.

UTILITY SCORE 3

Study	Reliability	Sensitivity	Specificity	LR+	LR−	QUADAS Score (0–14)
Maranhao et al.[31]	NT	51	70	1.7	0.7	11
Comments: Well done study but less than promising results.						

Pronator Drift Test

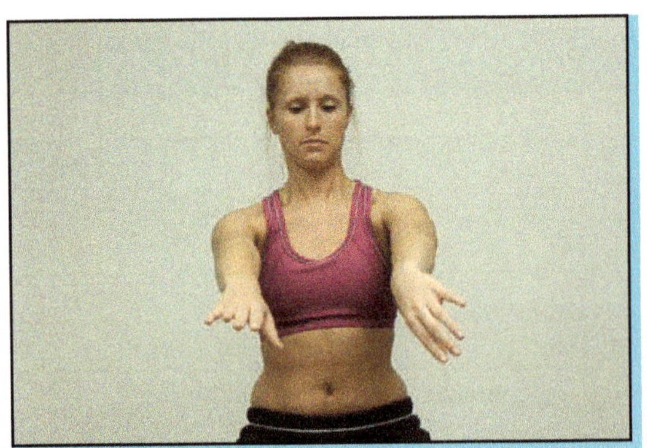

1) The patient is asked to hold the upper extremities outstretched in front with 90° of shoulder flexion, palms up and elbows and wrists extended.

2) Positive test is indicated by the inability of the patient to maintain this position for 20–30 seconds and asymmetric pronation or downward drifting of the arm.

TESTS FOR FOCAL OR MONOHEMISPHERIC BRAIN TUMORS/LESIONS

UTILITY SCORE 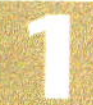

Study	Reliability	Sensitivity	Specificity	LR+	LR–	QUADAS Score (0–14)
Maranhao et al.[31]	NT	41	96	10.25	0.61	11
Anderson et al.[1]	NT	22	100	Inf	0.78	8
Teitelbaum et al.[50]	81.6	92.2	90	9.2	0.09	9
Comments: Anderson et al.[1] only required the patients to hold their arms supinated for 10 seconds instead of 20–30 seconds.						

Finger Rolling Test

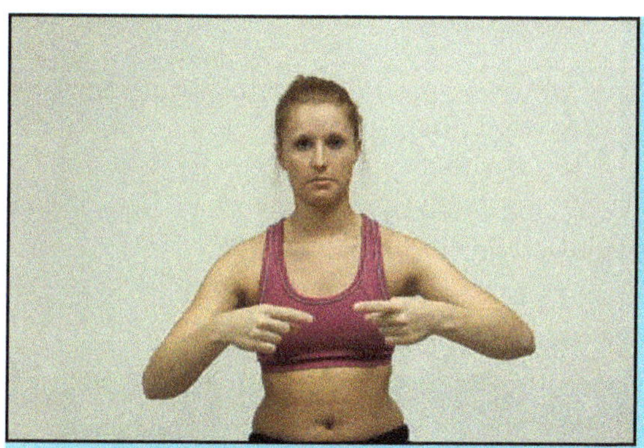

1) Patient is instructed to extend both index fingers and point them towards each other in front of the torso approximately 1 finger length apart with each index finger pointing at the metacarpophalangeal joint of the flexed fingers on the opposite hand.

2) The patient is instructed to roll the fingers around each other.

3) A positive sign is one finger orbiting around the other (the affected side moves less than the unaffected side).

UTILITY SCORE 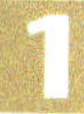

Study	Reliability	Sensitivity	Specificity	LR+	LR–	QUADAS Score (0–14)
Maranhao et al.[31]	NT	41	93	5.86	0.63	11
Anderson et al.[1]	NT	33	100	Inf	0.67	8
Comments: This is a modified version of the forearm rolling test.						

TESTS FOR FOCAL OR MONOHEMISPHERIC BRAIN TUMORS/LESIONS

Forearm Rolling Test

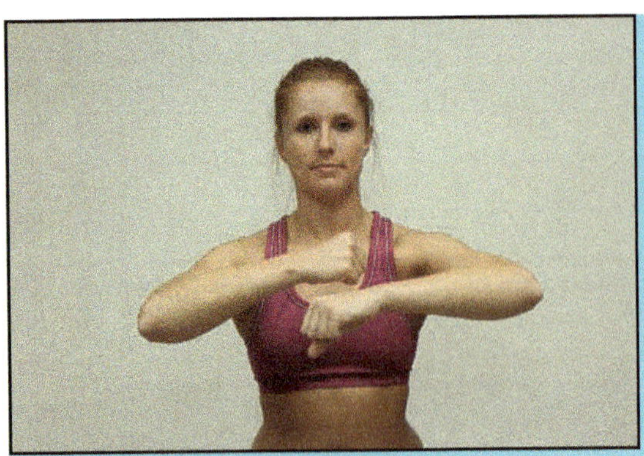

1) The patient is placed in either sitting or standing position.

2) Patient is instructed to make a fist with both hands.

3) Patient then flexes both shoulders and both elbows to approximately 90° so that the fists and forearms overlap by approximately 15 cm in front of the patient and horizontal to the ground.

4) The patient is then instructed to rotate both fists around each other in this position for 5 to 10 seconds in each direction of rotation.

5) The examiner observes the movement of both forearms for symmetry of movement.

6) A positive sign is indicated by one side orbiting around the other (the involved side will move less than the uninvolved side).

UTILITY SCORE 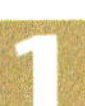

Study	Reliability	Sensitivity	Specificity	LR+	LR−	QUADAS Score (0–14)
Maranhao et al.[31]	NT	16	100	Inf	0.84	11
Anderson et al.[1]	NT	24	100	Inf	0.76	8
Teitelbaum et al.[50]	77.6	45.6	97.5	18.2	0.56	9
Comments: The forearm rolling test demonstrates very promising results.						

Finger Tap

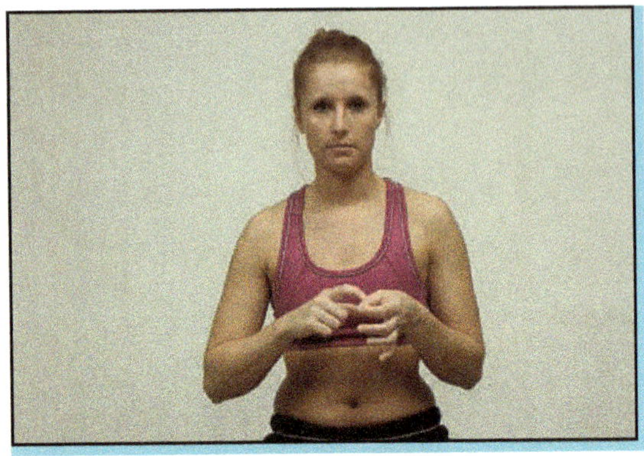

1) The patient is placed in sitting or standing.

2) The patient is instructed to tap the tip of the index finger to the interphalangeal joint of the thumb as many times as possible in 10 seconds.

3) A positive sign is a difference of 5 or more taps between the right and left index fingers. The movement will be slower on the affected side.

TESTS FOR FOCAL OR MONOHEMISPHERIC BRAIN TUMORS/LESIONS

UTILITY SCORE 2

Study	Reliability	Sensitivity	Specificity	LR+	LR−	QUADAS Score (0–14)
Maranhao et al.[31]	NT	18	90	1.8	0.91	11
Anderson et al.[1]	NT	15	100	Inf	0.85	8
Teitelbaum et al.[50]	80.6	73.3	87.5	5.9	0.31	9

Comments: It is unknown whether both fingers should be tested at the same time or one after the other. Interpretation of this test can be difficult due to the fact that the non-dominant hand may have a slower performance of the test.

Modified Mingazzini's Maneuver

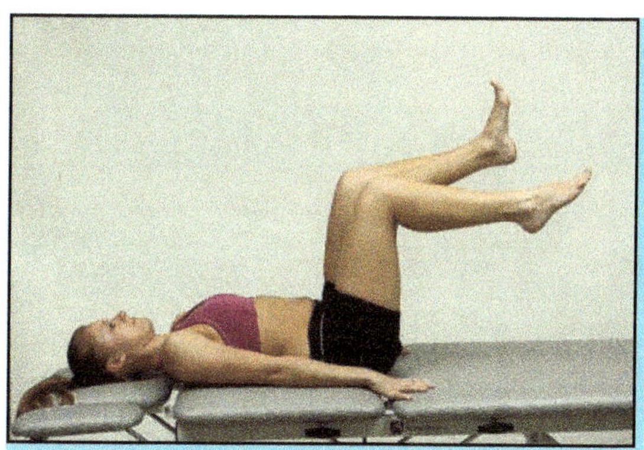

1) The patient is placed in supine.

2) Patient is instructed to flex both hips to 75–80° with the knees flexed to approximately 100° so the lower legs are parallel to the bed.

3) The ankles are dorsiflexed to 90°.

4) The patient is then instructed to hold this position for as long as possible up to 30 seconds.

5) A positive sign occurs if the leg or hip begins to fall or if the foot begins to lose dorsiflexion.

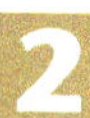

UTILITY SCORE 2

Study	Reliability	Sensitivity	Specificity	LR+	LR−	QUADAS Score (0–14)
Teitelbaum et al.[50]	NT	55.3	91	6.1	0.49	9

Comments: Originally this test was performed with the knees in full extension with the hips flexed only to 45°. This was then changed by Barre to 90° of flexion at the knees and hips. Teitelbaum et al.[51] performed a variant of this version.

TESTS FOR FOCAL OR MONOHEMISPHERIC BRAIN TUMORS/LESIONS

Rapid Alternating Movements of the Hands

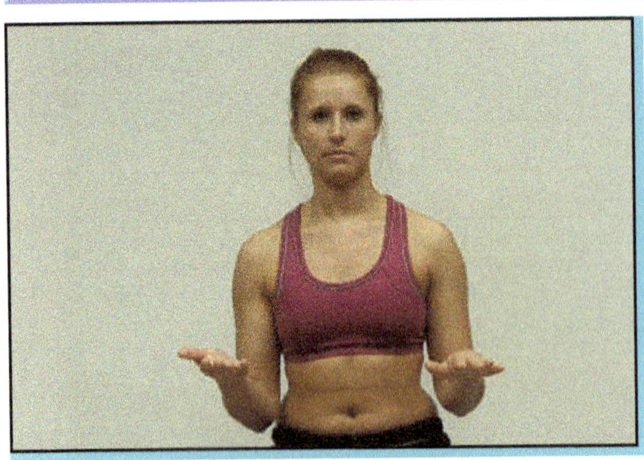

1) The patient is placed in a seated position.
2) Patient is instructed to place his or her hands on his or her thighs.
3) The patient is then instructed to pat the thighs alternately with the dorsum or palm of his or her hands for 10 seconds.
4) This test can also be performed using rapidly extending and flexing the fingers of each hand for 10 seconds.
5) A positive test is indicated by an asymmetry of movement between the two upper extremities.

UTILITY SCORE 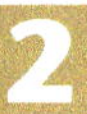

Study	Reliability	Sensitivity	Specificity	LR+	LR−	QUADAS Score (0–14)
Anderson et al.[1]	NT	15	100	Inf	0.85	8
Comments: Somewhat flawed study but the test results appear promising.						

Barre Test

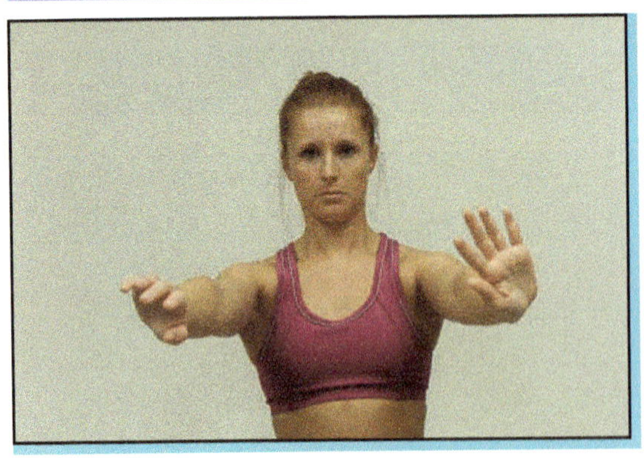

1) The patient is placed in a seated position.
2) The patient's arms are held at 90° of shoulder flexion with elbows fully extended, forearms pronated, wrists in full extension, and finger extended and abducted. If the patient is not able to sit, this can be done in supine with shoulders flexed to 45° instead of 90°.
3) The patient is instructed to hold this position for as long as possible up to 1 minute.
4) A test is considered positive if the patient's fingers, wrist, or arm start to fall, or if the fingers are not able to maintain abduction. If the problem is due to an upper motor neuron lesion, the fingers will adduct or the fingers and wrist will begin to drop before the arms drop.

UTILITY SCORE 2

Study	Reliability	Sensitivity	Specificity	LR+	LR−	QUADAS Score (0–14)
Teitelbaum et al.[50]	79.6	86.7	90.0	8.7	0.15	9
Comments: When the Barre Test was originally described the wrist was positioned in flexion, but Teitelbaum et al.[50] tested with the wrist in dorsiflexion.						

Teitelbaum's Clinical Prediction Rule for Unilateral Cerebral Lesions

1) This CPR is a combination of three maneuvers.
2) Pronator Drift
3) Finger Tap
4) Deep Tendon Reflexes

UTILITY SCORE 1

Study	Reliability	Sensitivity	Specificity	LR+	LR−	QUADAS Score (0–14)
Teitelbaum et al.[50] + = all 3 pos − = >1 neg	NT	75.5	97.5	30.2	0.25	9
Teitelbaum et al.[50] + = >1 pos − = all three neg	NT	97.8	86.3	7.25	0.03	9
Comments: Deep tendon reflexes tested were biceps, triceps, brachioradialis, infrapatellar, Achilles and plantar. Positive reflex test included abnormal increase of two or more reflexes on the same side or the presence of a positive Babinski's sign.						

TESTS FOR PERIPHERAL NEUROPATHY

Superficial Pain

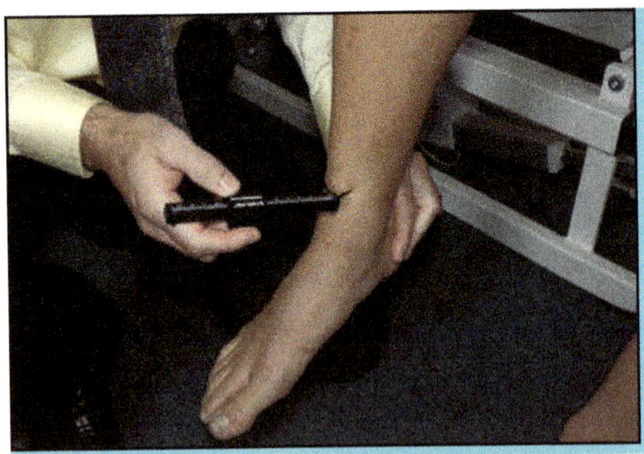

1) The patient is placed in sitting or standing.
2) The examiner applies a superficial painful stimuli and queries the patient regarding pain level. The patient's eyes are closed during the testing.
3) A positive response is a lack of report of pain during application of painful stimuli.

UTILITY SCORE 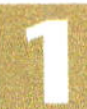

Study	Reliability	Sensitivity	Specificity	LR+	LR−	QUADAS Score (0–14)
Olaleye et al.[37] (2 correct responses)	NT	47	89	4.27	0.59	7
Olaleye et al.[37] (3 correct responses)	NT	42	90	4.2	0.64	7
Olaleye et al.[37] (4 correct responses)	NT	25	97	8.33	0.77	7
Olaleye et al.[37] (5 correct responses)	NT	23	98	11.5	0.78	7
Perkins et al.[40] (>5 out of 8 attempts)	NT	59	97	19.7	0.42	9
Comments: To stimulate superficial pain, a sharp–dull response was used. Anesthesia is considered a positive finding.						

Vibration Testing

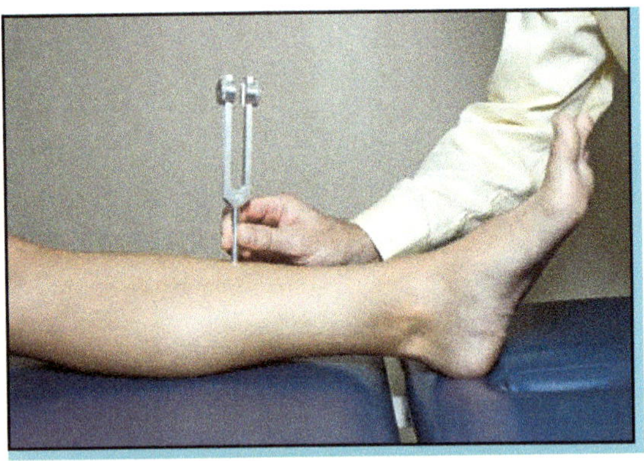

1) The patient is placed in sitting or supine position.
2) The examiner applies the tuning fork over the selected bony prominence. The patient is instructed to close his or her eyes and to indicate when the vibration begins and when the vibration is complete.
3) The examiner applies a series of five trials to determine the cumulative ability of correct responses.
4) A positive test is decreased ability to report when the vibration was applied and when the vibration dampened while still applied.

TESTS FOR PERIPHERAL NEUROPATHY

UTILITY SCORE 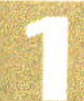

Study	Reliability	Sensitivity	Specificity	LR+	LR−	QUADAS Score (0–14)
Olaleye et al.[37] (2 correct responses)	NT	46	94	7.66	0.57	7
Olaleye et al.[37] (3 correct responses)	NT	42	97	14	0.59	7
Olaleye et al.[37] (4 correct responses)	NT	25	99	25	0.75	7
Olaleye et al.[37] (5 correct responses)	NT	22	99	22	0.78	7
Perkins et al.[40] (>5 out of 8 attempts) (On–Off method)	NT	53	99	53	0.47	9
Perkins et al.[40] (>5 out of 8 attempts) (Timed Method)	NT	80	98	40	0.20	9
Jepsen et al.[24] (Median Nerve)	.70 kappa	NT	NT	NA	NA	NA
Jepsen et al.[24] (Ulnar Nerve)	.45 kappa	NT	NT	NA	NA	NA
Comments: Although primarily tested in this population, the test is not specific for peripheral neuropathy.						

Monofilament Testing

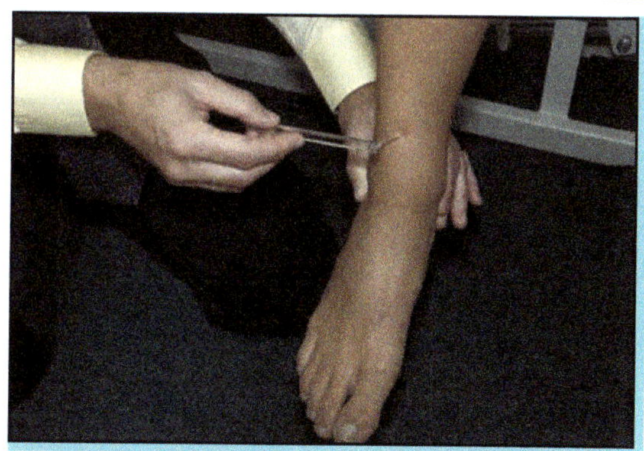

1) The patient is placed in sitting.

2) The examiner applies a Semmes-Weinstein 10-g monofilament to the selected noncalloused areas of the foot. With eyes closed, the patient is queried as to whether he or she feels the application.

3) A positive response is the inability to feel the applied stimulus. If no stimulus is felt at the palmar aspect of the foot, this reflects the lack of a protective sensation from the patient.

(continued)

TESTS FOR PERIPHERAL NEUROPATHY

UTILITY SCORE 1

Study	Reliability	Sensitivity	Specificity	LR+	LR−	QUADAS Score (0–14)
Olaleye et al.[37] (2 correct responses)	NT	70	75	2.8	0.4	7
Olaleye et al.[37] (3 correct responses)	NT	63	82	3.5	0.45	7
Olaleye et al.[37] (4 correct responses)	NT	39	96	9.8	0.63	7
Olaleye et al.[37] (5 correct responses)	NT	31	97	10.3	0.71	7
Perkins et al.[40] (>5 out of 8 attempts)	NT	77	96	19.3	0.24	9
Mythili et al.[36] (> or = 1 incorrect out of 6 attempts)	NT	98.5	55	2.19	0.027	7

Comments: The articles addressed the protective sensation secondary to peripheral neuropathy of the diabetic foot. Each article used a 10-g monofilament to test protective sensation. This procedure is different from a standard assessment of monofilament testing, which has not undergone diagnostic accuracy analysis. The test is frequently performed as a component of the upper quarter screen. Mythili et al.[36] performed six trials using a 10-g monofilament with enough pressure to buckle the monofilament. Test sites were the plantar surface of the hallux and centrally on the plantar surface of the heel.

Position Sense of the Great Toe

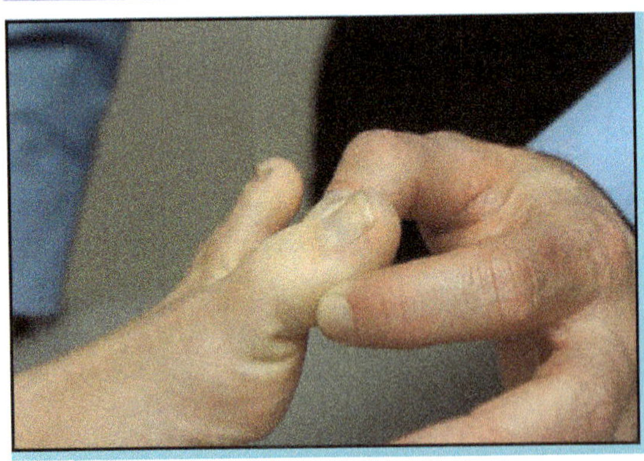

1. Position sense is tested with the patient in supine.
2. The dominant toe is grasped on the medial and lateral sides by the examiner's thumb and index finger.
3. Up and down movements are first performed with the subject's eyes open. Then with the subjects eyes closed, a series of 10 small amplitude movements are performed. The amplitude should be approximately 1 cm over a time of 1 second each and the movement should be performed smoothly.
4. The patient is asked to identify if there was any movement as well as the direction if it was sensed.
5. A positive test is the inability of the patient to give correct responses on 8 or fewer of the 10 movements.

TESTS FOR PERIPHERAL NEUROPATHY

UTILILTY SCORE 2

Study	Reliability	Sensitivity	Specificity	LR+	LR−	QUADAS Score (0–14)
Richardson[43]	NT	88.2	68.8	2.83	0.17	9
Comments: No verbal cues were given to the patient, so an incorrect response was marked if the patient failed to recognize movement and respond (no response) as well as incorrect identification of the direction of movement.						

Achilles Reflex

1) The patient is placed in sitting with the foot to be tested not touching the ground.
2) Using a reflex hammer, either strike the tendon itself or use the plantar strike technique to elicit a reflex.
3) If the reflex is absent, ask the patient to gently plantarflex the foot, tightly close the eyes, and pull their clasped hands apart just prior to striking.
4) A positive test is the inability to elicit a reflex even with facilitation.

UTILILTY SCORE 2

Study	Reliability	Sensitivity	Specificity	LR+	LR−	QUADAS Score (0–14)
Richardson[43]	NT	72.1	90.6	7.67	0.31	9
Comments: Some studies show that the Achilles reflex decreases normally with aging.						

Phalen's Test

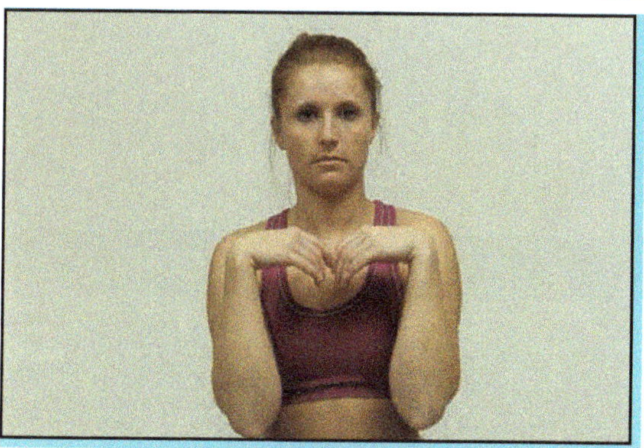

1) The patient is placed in sitting or standing position.
2) The patient is asked to hold the forearms vertically and maximally flex both wrists for a period of 60 seconds.
3) A positive test is indicated by the reproduction of symptoms along the distribution of the median nerve's cutaneous distribution.

UTILILTY SCORE 

Study	Reliability	Sensitivity	Specificity	LR+	LR−	QUADAS Score (0–14)
Onde et al.[38]	NT	85.7	50	1.71	0.29	6
Comments: Carpal tunnel syndrome is the most common entrapment neuropathy in diabetes.						

TESTS FOR PERIPHERAL NEUROPATHY

Tinel's Sign

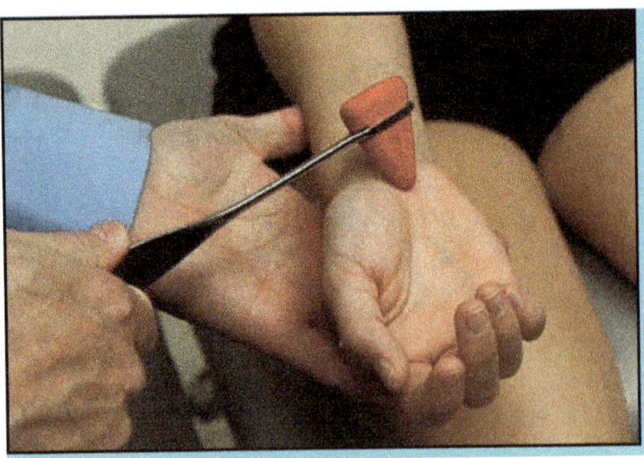

1. The patient is placed in a sitting position.
2. The patient's wrist is placed in a neutral position.
3. The examiner uses his or her finger or a reflex hammer to tap on the median nerve where it enters the carpal tunnel.
4. A positive sign is the presence of pain or parasthesia radiating into the hand.

UTILILTY SCORE 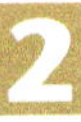

Study	Reliability	Sensitivity	Specificity	LR+	LR−	QUADAS Score (0–14)
Onde et al.[38]	NT	72.7	83.3	4.35	0.33	6
Comments: Carpal tunnel syndrome is the most common entrapment neuropathy in diabetes. A positive Tinel's sign indicates axonal regeneration.						

Richardson's Clinical Prediction Rule for Peripheral Neuropathy Criteria

1. Absence of the Achilles reflex even with facilitation.
2. Vibration Sense using a 128-Hz tuning fork. A positive test is the ability of the patient to detect vibration for less than 8 seconds at a site proximal to the nail bed of the first digit of the lower extremities.
3. Position Sense of the dominant side great toe.
4. Positive CPR is presence of 2 or 3 positive tests.

UTILITY SCORE 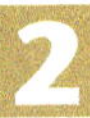

Study	Reliability	Sensitivity	Specificity	LR+	LR−	QUADAS Score (0–14)
Richardson[43]	.83 kappa	94.1	84.4	6.03	0.07	9
Comments: In patients with known diabetes, the sensitivity increased to 97.2 and specificity increased to 90. This changes the LR+ to 9.72 and the LR− to 0.03.						

TESTS FOR PERIPHERAL NERVE PATHOLOGY

Long Thoracic Nerve Injury

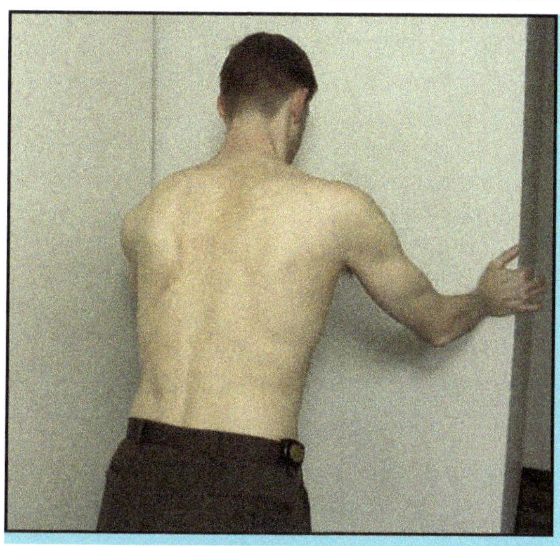

1) The patient is positioned in standing facing a wall.
2) Instruct the patient to complete a wall push-up.
3) Observe the patient's scapula for signs of winging.
4) A positive test is indicated by scapular winging on the involved side.

UTILITY SCORE 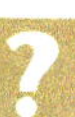

Study	Reliability	Sensitivity	Specificity	LR+	LR−	QUADAS Score (0–14)
Scifers[46]	NT	NT	NT	NT	NT	NA
Comments: Patient may also have difficulty performing active glenohumeral flexion or abduction due to altered scapulohumeral rhythm.						

Pronator Teres Syndrome Test

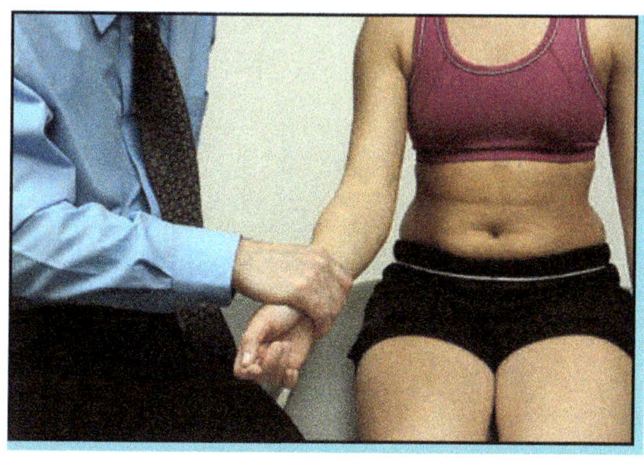

1) The patient is positioned in sitting.
2) Instruct the patient to flex his or her elbows to 90° with the forearm in supination.
3) The clinician resists pronation of the patient's forearm while allowing active elbow extension.
4) A positive test is indicated by parasthesia in the median nerve distribution of the involved hand.

UTILITY SCORE 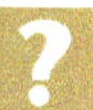

Study	Reliability	Sensitivity	Specificity	LR+	LR−	QUADAS Score (0–14)
Scifers[46]	NT	NT	NT	NT	NT	NA
Comments: This test indicates compression of the median nerve by the pronator teres.						

TESTS FOR PERIPHERAL NERVE PATHOLOGY

Common Fibular Nerve Injury

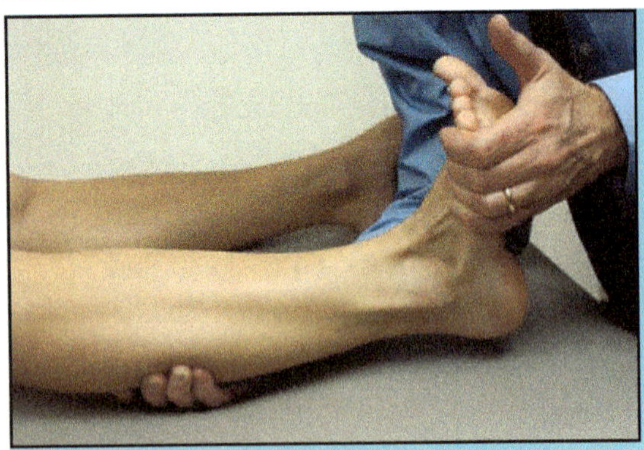

1) The patient is positioned in sitting or supine.
2) Instruct the patient to provide maximal resistance as the examiner performs manual muscle tests for ankle dorsiflexion and eversion.
3) A positive test is indicated by significantly decreased ability to resist the examiner's force.

UTILITY SCORE 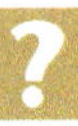

Study	Reliability	Sensitivity	Specificity	LR+	LR−	QUADAS Score (0–14)
Scifers[46]	NT	NT	NT	NT	NT	NA
Comments: The patient may also have a loss of sensation in the common fibular nerve distribution.						

Pencil Test

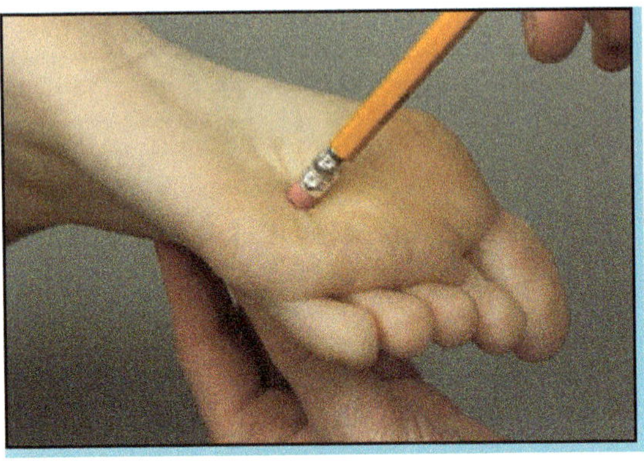

1) The patient is positioned in supine, long sitting, or sitting.
2) Using the blunt end of a pen or the eraser end of a pencil, the clinician applies a compressive force to the intermetatarsal space between the third and fourth metatarsals.
3) A positive sign is indicated by pain or reproduction of the patient's concordant sign indicating a Morton's Neuroma.

UTILITY SCORE 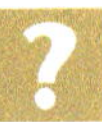

Study	Reliability	Sensitivity	Specificity	LR+	LR−	QUADAS Score (0–14)
Scifers[46]	NT	NT	NT	NT	NT	NA
Comments: In most cases Morton's Neuromas are present between the 3rd and 4th metatarsals, but can also occur between the 2nd and 3rd metatarsals as well.						

TEST FOR FACIOSCAPULOHUMERAL DYSTROPHY

Beevor's Sign

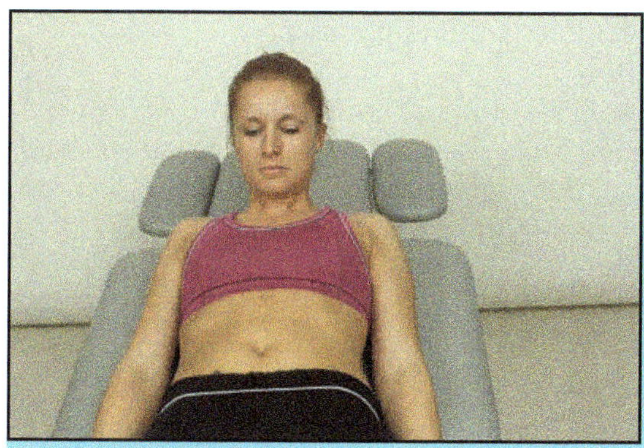

1) The patient lies supine.

2) The examiner directs the patient to actively move their head into flexion.

3) The examiner watches for upward movement of the umbilicus during neck flexion.

4) The test is considered positive if there is marked upward movement of the umbilicus following neck flexion.

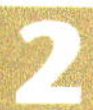

UTILITY SCORE 2

Study	Reliability	Sensitivity	Specificity	LR+	LR−	QUADAS Score (0–14)
Eger et al.[14]	NT	46.4	96.9	15.1	0.55	6
Shahrizaila & Wills[47]	NT	95	96	23.8	0.05	5
Awerbuch et al.[3]	NT	90	100	Inf	0.1	5
Comments: The test is similar to the Hyperabduction Test but adds rotation away from the affected side.						

TESTS FOR CERVICAL RADICULOPATHY

Biceps Deep Tendon Reflex

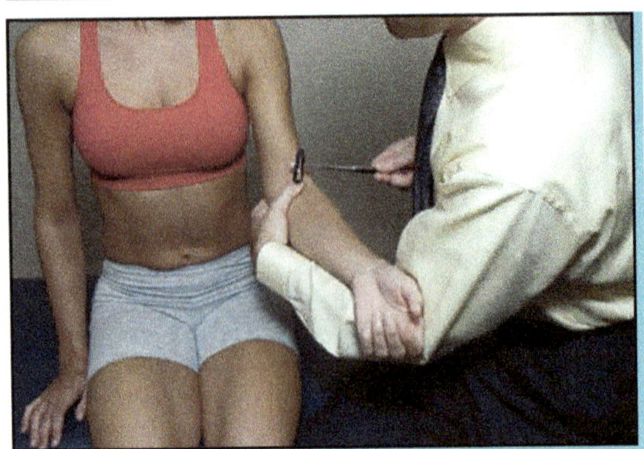

1) The patient assumes a sitting position.

2) The examiner places the patient's forearm on his or her forearm to ensure relaxation. The patient's forearm is held in slight supination. The examiner's thumb is placed on the biceps tendon of the patient.

3) The examiner applies a series of quick strikes to his or her own thumb. The quick strikes should elicit a reflex response of elbow flexion.

4) A positive test is a depression of reflex when compared to the opposite side or "normal."

5) The patient may be instructed to perform the lower extremity Jendrassik's maneuver to improve the response of the reflex.

UTILITY SCORE 2

Study	Reliability	Sensitivity	Specificity	LR+	LR−	QUADAS Score (0–14)
Bertilson et al.[6]	94% agreement	NT	NT	NA	NA	NA
Wainner et al.[54]	.73 kappa	24	95	4.8	0.8	10
Matsumoto et al.[33] (C4–5)	NT	65	95	13	0.37	6
Matsumoto et al.[33] (C5–6)	NT	65	94	10.8	0.37	6
Lauder et al.[30] (C5–6)	NT	14	90	1.4	0.95	9

Comments: Reflex testing is commonly scored as 0+ = absent (no visible or palpable muscle contraction with reinforcement), 1+ = tone change (slight, transitory impulse, with no movement of the extremities), 2+ = normal (visual, brief movement of the extremity), 3+ = exaggerated (full movement of the extremities), 4+ = abnormal (compulsory and sustained movement, lasting for more than 30 seconds). The test is frequently performed as a component of the upper quarter screen. The test is purported to target C6.

TESTS FOR CERVICAL RADICULOPATHY

Triceps Deep Tendon Reflex

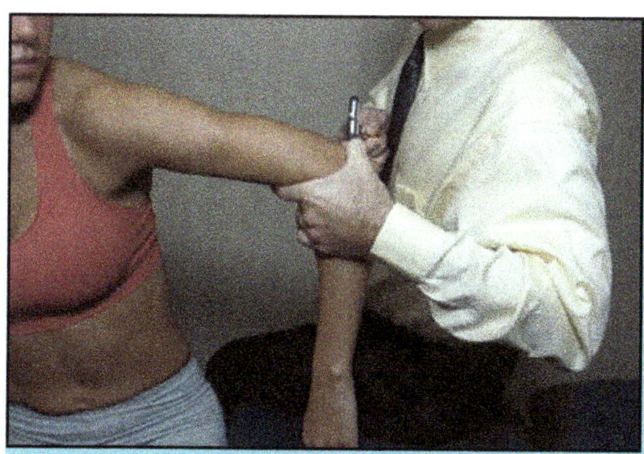

1) The patient assumes a sitting position.

2) The examiner flexes the patient's elbow and lifts the shoulder to 90 degrees. The examiner places his or her thumb over the distal aspect of the triceps tendon.

3) The examiner applies a series of strikes to his or her thumb. The strikes should elicit a reflex response of elbow extension.

4) A positive test is a depression of reflex when compared to the opposite side or "normal."

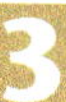

UTILITY SCORE 3

Study	Reliability	Sensitivity	Specificity	LR+	LR−	QUADAS Score (0–14)
Bertilson et al.[6]	88% agreement	NT	NT	NA	NA	NA
Wainner et al.[54]	NT	3	93	0.42	1.04	10
Matsumoto et al.[33]	NT	38	98	19	0.63	6
Lauder et al.[30] (C7)	NT	14	92	1.75	0.93	9

Comments: Reflex testing is commonly scored as 0+ = absent (no visible or palpable muscle contraction with reinforcement), 1+ = tone change (slight, transitory impulse, with no movement of the extremities), 2+ = normal (visual, brief movement of the extremity), 3+ = exaggerated (full movement of the extremities), 4+ = abnormal (compulsory and sustained movement, lasting for more than 30 seconds). The test is frequently performed as a component of the upper quarter screen. The test is purported to target C7.

Brachioradialis Deep Tendon Reflex

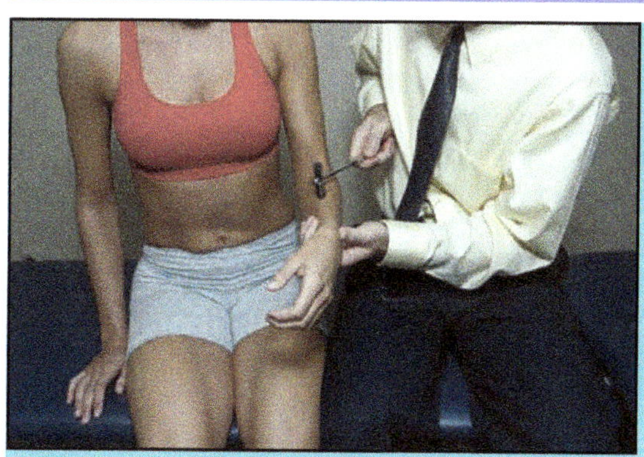

1) The patient assumes a sitting position.

2) The examiner places the patient's forearm on his or her forearm to ensure relaxation. The patient's forearm is held in slight pronation.

3) The examiner applies a series of quick strikes to the intersection point of the brachioradialis and the tendon. The quick strikes should elicit a reflex response of pronation and elbow flexion.

4) A positive test is a depression of reflex when compared to the opposite side or "normal."

(continued)

TESTS FOR CERVICAL RADICULOPATHY

UTILITY SCORE 3

Study	Reliability	Sensitivity	Specificity	LR+	LR−	QUADAS Score (0–14)
Bertilson et al.[6]	92% agreement	NT	NT	NA	NA	NA
Wainner et al.[54]	NT	6	95	1.2	0.98	10
Lauder et al.[30] (C6–7)	NT	17	94	2.8	0.88	9

Comments: Reflex testing is commonly scored as 0+ = absent (no visible or palpable muscle contraction with reinforcement), 1+ = tone change (slight, transitory impulse, with no movement of the extremities), 2+ = normal (visual, brief movement of the extremity), 3+ = exaggerated (full movement of the extremities), 4+ = abnormal (compulsory and sustained movement, lasting for more than 30 seconds). The test is frequently performed as a component of the upper quarter screen. The test is purported to target C6.

Muscle Power Testing

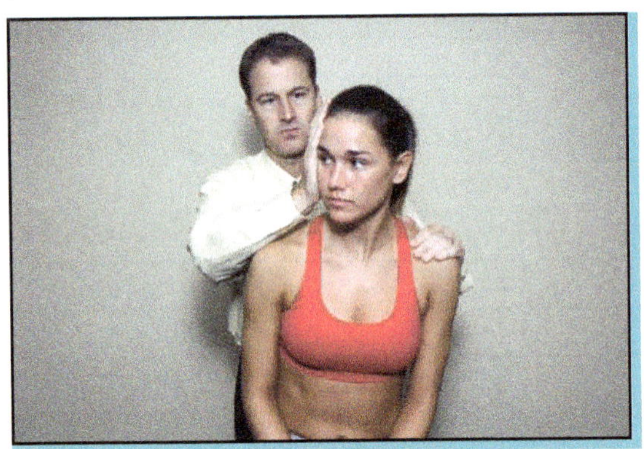

1) The patient is placed in sitting.

2) To test C1–3, cervical rotation is resisted.

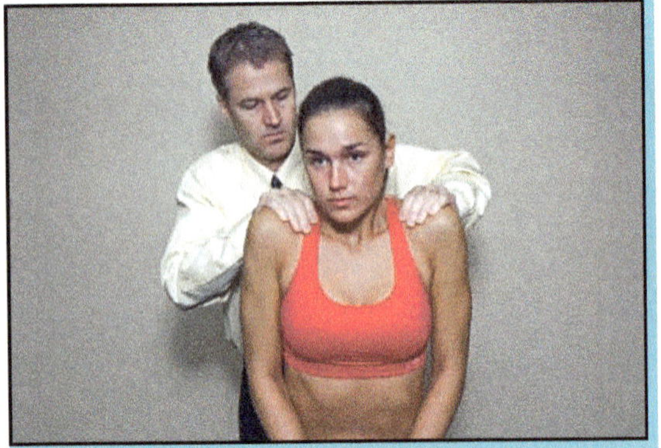

3) The patient is placed in sitting.

4) To test C4, shoulder shrug is resisted.

TESTS FOR CERVICAL RADICULOPATHY

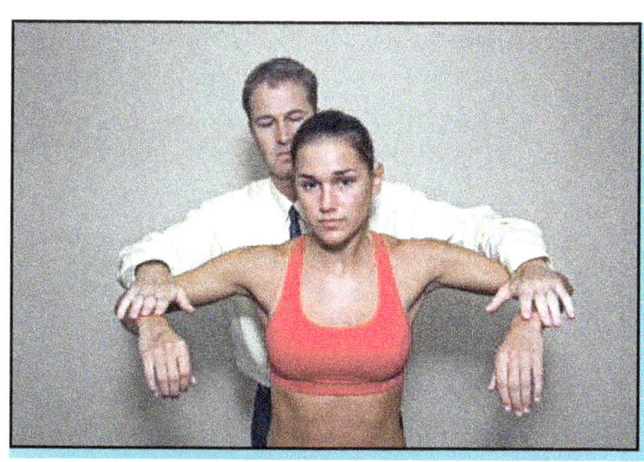

5) The patient is placed in sitting.

6) To test C5, shoulder abduction is resisted.

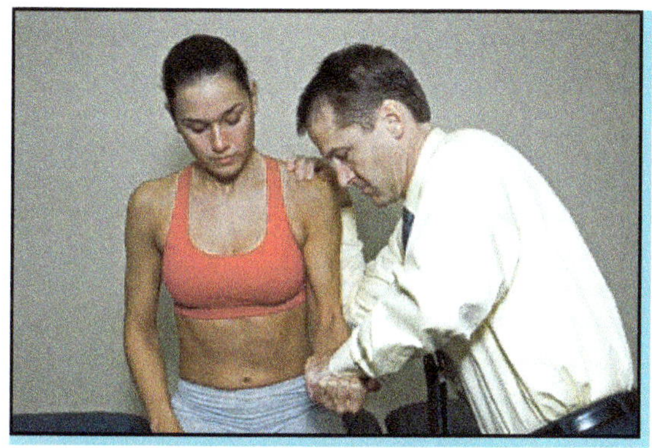

7) The patient is placed in sitting.

8) To test C6, the biceps are resisted.

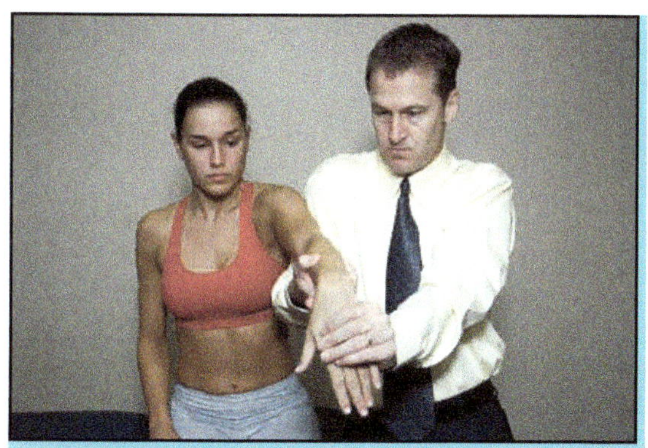

9) The patient is placed in sitting.

10) To test C7, wrist flexion is resisted.

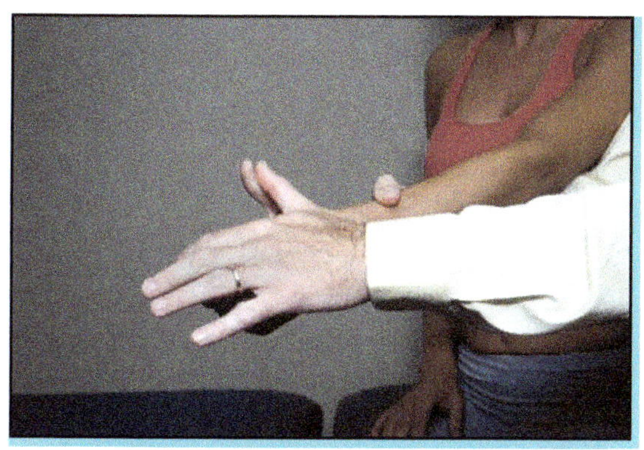

11) The patient is placed in sitting.

12) To test C8, thumb extension is resisted.

(continued)

TESTS FOR CERVICAL RADICULOPATHY

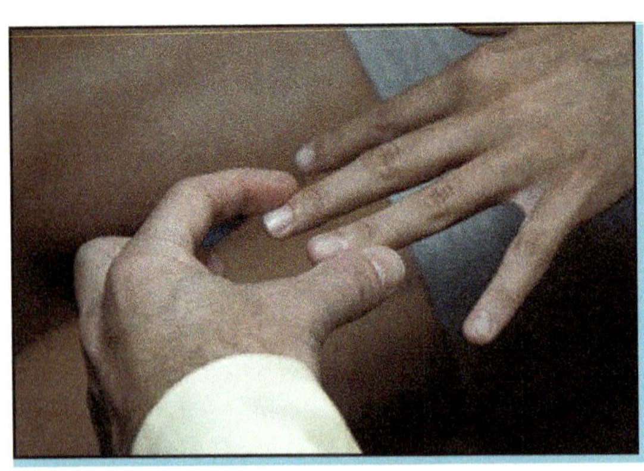

13) The patient is placed in sitting.

14) To test T1, finger abduction is resisted.

15) With all areas, a positive test is noticeable weakness when compared to the opposite side or versus expectations if bilateral symptoms are present.

UTILITY SCORE 2

Study	Reliability	Sensitivity	Specificity	LR+	LR−	QUADAS Score (0–14)
Wainner et al.[54] (Deltoid)	.62 kappa	24	89	2.18	0.85	10
Wainner et al.[54] (Biceps)	.69 kappa	24	94	4	0.8	10
Wainner et al.[54] (Extensor Carpi Radialis)	.63 kappa	12	90	1.2	0.97	10
Wainner et al.[54] (Triceps Brachii)	.29 kappa	12	94	2	0.93	10
Wainner et al.[54] (Flexor Carpi Radialis)	.23 kappa	6	89	0.54	1.05	10
Wainner et al.[54] (Abductor Pollicis Brevis)	.39 kappa	6	84	0.37	1.12	10
Wainner et al.[54] (First Dorsal Interosseus)	.37 kappa	3	93	0.42	1.04	10
Matsumoto et al.[33] (C4–5) (Deltoid Weakness)	NT	35	98	17.5	0.66	6
Matsumoto et al.[33] (C7 or below) (Wrist Extensor Weakness)	NT	28	74	1.07	0.97	6
Comments: Note that the test tends to exhibit strong specificity and low sensitivity, suggesting it may lack practicality as a screen. The test is frequently performed as a component of the upper quarter screen.						

TESTS FOR CERVICAL RADICULOPATHY

Sensibility Testing

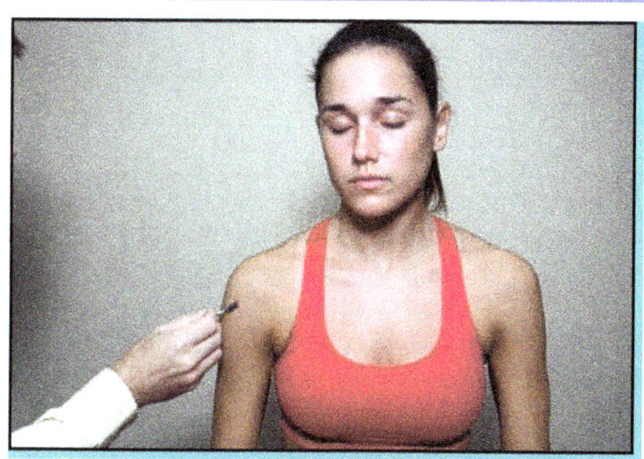

1. The patient is placed in sitting or supine.
2. The examiner applies a series of concurrent sensibility tests to both sides (light touch, sharp/dull). The examiner makes careful effort to apply sensation testing along known dermatomes.
3. Sharp/dull is assessed using pin prick.
4. A positive test is considered impaired sensation when tested against the opposite side.

UTILITY SCORE 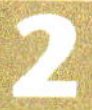

Study	Reliability	Sensitivity	Specificity	LR+	LR−	QUADAS Score (0–14)
Jepsen et al.[24] (Axillary Nerve) (Light Touch)	.69 kappa	NT	NT	NA	NA	NA
Jepsen et al.[24] (Medial Cutaneous of Arm) (Light Touch)	.90 kappa	NT	NT	NA	NA	NA
Jepsen et al.[24] (Medial Cutaneous of Forearm) (Light Touch)	.75 kappa	NT	NT	NA	NA	NA
Jepsen et al.[24] (Musculocutaneous) (Light Touch)	.67 kappa	NT	NT	NA	NA	NA
Jepsen et al.[24] (Radial Nerve) (Light Touch)	.31 kappa	NT	NT	NA	NA	NA
Jepsen et al.[24] (Median Nerve) (Light Touch)	.73 kappa	NT	NT	NA	NA	NA
Jepsen et al.[24] (Ulnar Nerve) (Light Touch)	.59 kappa	NT	NT	NA	NA	NA
Jepsen et al.[24] (Axillary Nerve) (Pain)	.54 kappa	NT	NT	NA	NA	NA
Jepsen et al.[24] (Medial Cutaneous of Arm) (Pain)	.42 kappa	NT	NT	NA	NA	NA
Jepsen et al.[24] (Medial Cutaneous of Forearm) (Pain)	.69 kappa	NT	NT	NA	NA	NA
Jepsen et al.[24] (Musculocutaneous) (Pain)	.48 kappa	NT	NT	NA	NA	NA
Jepsen et al.[24] (Radial Nerve) (Pain)	.48 kappa	NT	NT	NA	NA	NA
Jepsen et al.[24] (Median Nerve) (Pain)	.43 kappa	NT	NT	NA	NA	NA
Jepsen et al.[24] (Ulnar Nerve) (Pain)	.48 kappa	NT	NT	NA	NA	NA
Wainner et al.[54] (C5) (Pin Prick)	.67 kappa	29	86	2.07	0.82	10
Wainner et al.[54] (C6) (Pin Prick)	.28 kappa	24	66	0.70	1.15	10
Wainner et al.[54] (C7) (Pin Prick)	.40 kappa	28	77	1.21	0.93	10
Wainner et al.[54] (C8) (Pin Prick)	.16 kappa	12	81	0.63	1.08	10

(continued)

TESTS FOR CERVICAL RADICULOPATHY

Study	Reliability	Sensitivity	Specificity	LR+	LR−	QUADAS Score (0–14)
Wainner et al.[54] (T1) (Pin Prick)	.46 kappa	18	79	0.85	1.03	10
Matsumoto et al.[33] (C3, 4, 5)	NT	56	82	3.11	0.53	6
Matsumoto et al.[33] (6 and below)	NT	45	81	2.36	0.68	6
Comments: Results suggest that bilateral stimulus with the patient's eyes closed generates the most valid findings. Unless indicated, results were associated with light touch sensibility testing. The test is frequently performed as a component of the upper quarter screen.						

Combined Tests Upper Extremity

UTILITY SCORE 3

Study	Reliability	Sensitivity	Specificity	LR+	LR−	QUADAS Score (0–14)
Matsumoto et al.[34] (All Deep Tendon Reflexes)	63% agreement	52	NT	NA	NA	7
Matsumoto et al.[34] (All Muscle Weakness)	63% agreement	23	NT	NA	NA	7
Matsumoto et al.[34] (All Dermatomes)	63% agreement	62	NT	NA	NA	7
Lauder et al.[30] (Weakness Any Muscle)	NT	73	61	1.87	0.44	9
Lauder et al.[30] (Sensory and Reflexes)	NT	9	97	3	0.93	9
Lauder et al.[30] (Sensory and Weakness)	NT	27	74	1.04	0.98	9
Lauder et al.[30] (Weakness and Reflexes)	NT	18	98	9	0.83	9
Lauder et al.[30] (Weakness, Sensory, and Reflex Abnormalities)	NT	7	98	3.5	0.94	9
Lauder et al.[30] (Any Component-Weakness or Sensory or Reflex Abnormalities)	NT	84	31	1.2	0.51	9
Lauder et al.[30] (Sensation Loss-Vibration or Pin Prick)	NT	38	46	0.70	1.35	9
Davidson et al.[11] (Loss or Depression of Reflexes)	NT	50	NT	NA	NA	8
Davidson et al.[11] (Any Muscle Strength Loss)	NT	91	NT	NA	NA	8
Spurling & Scoville[48] (Any Muscle Strength Loss)	NT	58	NT	NA	NA	4
Spurling & Scoville[48] (Any Loss or Depression of Reflexes)	NT	33	NT	NA	NA	4
Comments: For diagnostic purposes, combined values exceeded the findings of single neurological screening testing.						

TESTS FOR LUMBAR RADICULOPATHY

Quadriceps Deep Tendon Reflex

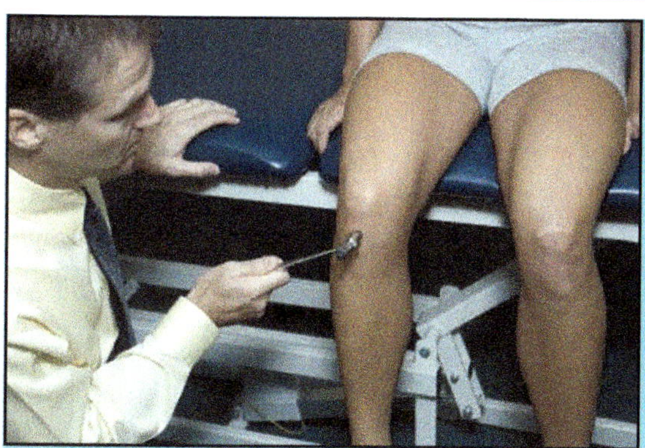

1) The patient assumes a sitting position.

2) The examiner strikes the infrapatellar tendon just above the tibial tuberosity. Three to five strikes are necessary to examine fatigue.

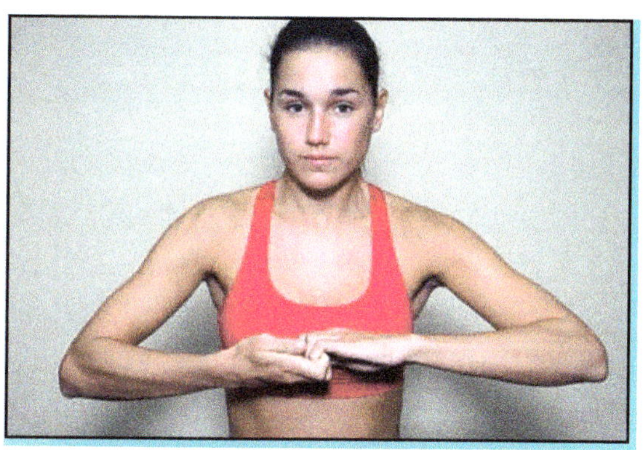

3) A positive test is a depression of knee extension directly after the tendon strike in comparison to the opposite side.

4) The Jendrassik's maneuver is often used to improve reflex response.

UTILITY SCORE 

Study	Reliability	Sensitivity	Specificity	LR+	LR−	QUADAS Score (0–14)
Knuttson[28] (L3–L4)	NT	100	65	2.86	0	3
Knuttson[28] (L5–S1)	NT	14	65	0.41	1.32	3
Knuttson[28] (L4–L5)	NT	12	65	0.34	1.36	3
Hakelius & Hindmarsh[20] (All Levels Included)	NT	75	NT	NA	NA	3
Lauder et al.[30] (All Levels Included)	NT	12	96	3	0.92	6

Comments: Reflex testing is commonly scored as 0+ = absent (no visible or palpable muscle contraction with reinforcement), 1+ = tone change (slight, transitory impulse, with no movement of the extremities), 2+ = normal (visual, brief movement of the extremity), 3+ = exaggerated (full movement of the extremities), 4+ = abnormal (compulsory and sustained movement, lasting for more than 30 seconds). Please note that the majority of the studies were very poorly performed and this predicament likely biases findings. The test is frequently performed as a component of the lower quarter screen. The test is purported to target L2–3.

TESTS FOR LUMBAR RADICULOPATHY

Achilles Deep Tendon Reflex (Lumbar Radiculopathy Secondary to Disk Herniation or Protrusion)

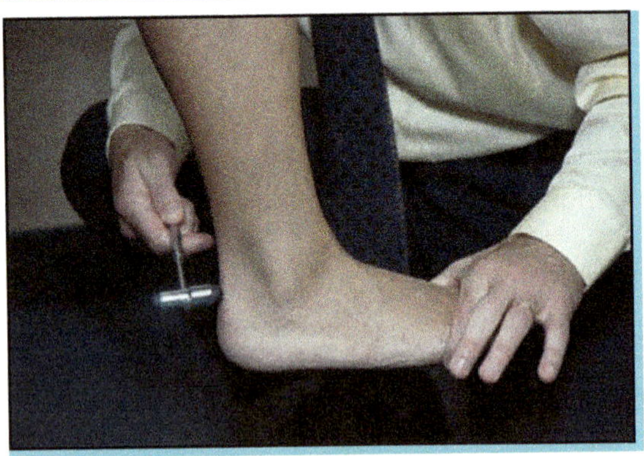

1. The patient assumes a sitting or supine position.
2. The examiner places the ankle in slight dorsiflexion by pulling the palmar aspect of the forefoot into dorsiflexion.
3. The examiner applies 3 to 5 quick strikes to the Achilles tendon. The examiner observes plantarflexion immediately after each strike.
4. A positive test is depression of the reflex in comparison to the opposite side.

UTILITY SCORE 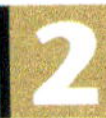

Study	Reliability	Sensitivity	Specificity	LR+	LR−	QUADAS Score (0–14)
Knuttson[28] (L5–S1)	NT	80	76	3.36	0.26	3
Knuttson[28] (L4–L5)	NT	36.5	76	1.53	0.83	3
Kerr et al.[26] (L5–S1)	NT	87	89	7.91	0.15	7
Kerr et al.[26] (L4–L5)	NT	12	89	1.1	0.99	7
Hakelius & Hindmarsh[20] (All Levels Included)	NT	80	NT	NA	NA	3
Lauder et al.[30] (All Levels Included)	NT	15	92	1.88	0.9	6
Rico & Jonkman[44] (S1)	NT	85	89	7.9	0.2	6

Comments: Reflex testing is commonly scored as 0+ = absent (no visible or palpable muscle contraction with reinforcement), 1+ = tone change (slight, transitory impulse, with no movement of the extremities), 2+ = normal (visual, brief movement of the extremity), 3+ = exaggerated (full movement of the extremities), 4+ = abnormal (compulsory and sustained movement, lasting for more than 30 seconds). Studies were poorly done. The test is frequently performed as a component of the lower quarter screen. The test is purported to target L5–S1.

TESTS FOR LUMBAR RADICULOPATHY

Extensor Digitorum Brevis Deep Tendon Reflex Test (Radiculopathy of L5–S1)

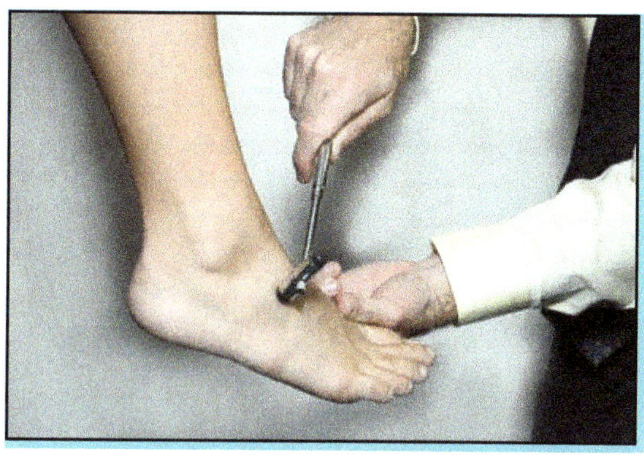

1) The patient assumes a sitting position.
2) The examiner prepositions the foot into slight inversion and plantarflexion. The great toe is placed in plantarflexion.
3) The examiner taps the EDB tendons distal to the muscle belly near the metatarsalphalangeal joints.
4) The examiner repeats the process six times in an effort to elicit a reflex response.
5) A positive test is absence of a reflex (L5 with small contribution of S1) and is indicative of radiculopathy.

UTILITY SCORE 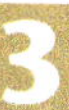

Study	Reliability	Sensitivity	Specificity	LR+	LR−	QUADAS Score (0–14)
Marin et al.[32] (L5)	NT	18	91	2	.90	8
Marin et al.[32] (S1)	NT	11	91	1.22	.98	8
Marin et al.[32] (L5 and S1)	NT	14	91	1.56	.95	8
Comments: Although not acknowledged by Marin et al.[32], eliciting any reflex response with this test has shown to be very difficult. The test is purported to target L4–L5.						

Muscle Power Testing (Lumbar Radiculopathy Secondary to Disk Herniation or Protrusion)

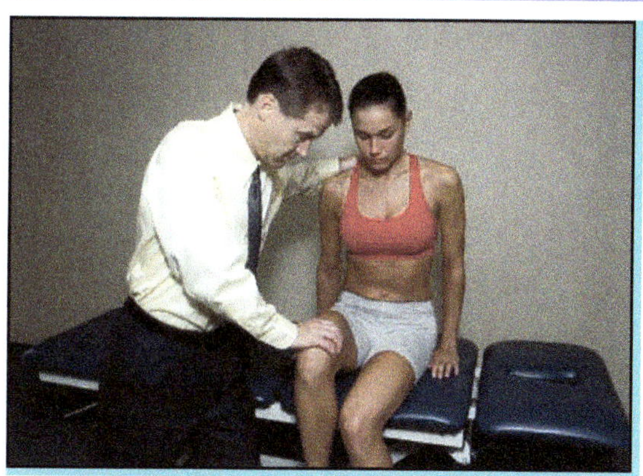

1) The patient is placed in sitting.
2) To test L1–L2, hip flexion is resisted.

(continued)

TESTS FOR LUMBAR RADICULOPATHY

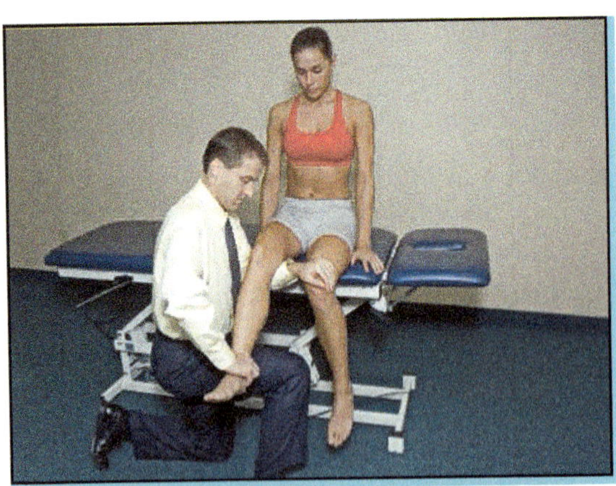

3) The patient is placed in sitting.

4) To test L3–L4, knee extension is resisted.

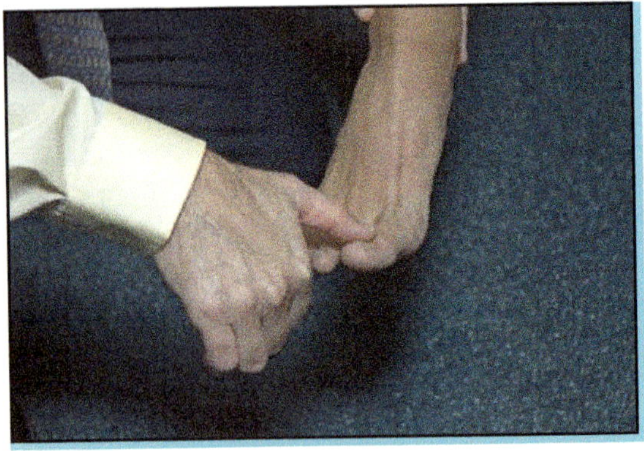

5) The patient is placed in sitting.

6) To test L5, great toe extension is resisted.

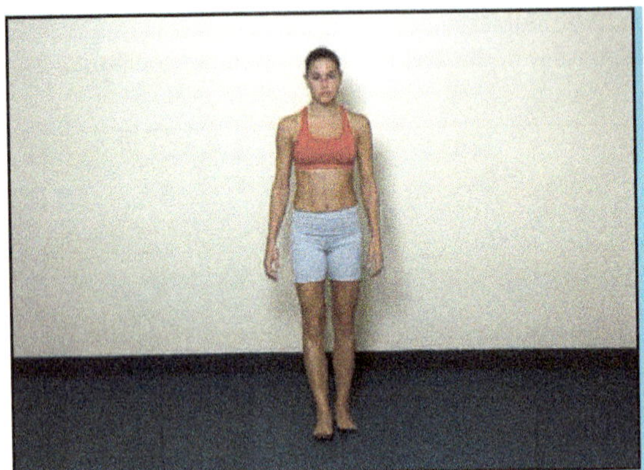

7) The patient is placed in standing.

8) To test L4–L5 (dorsiflexion), the patient is requested to walk on his or her heels.

TESTS FOR LUMBAR RADICULOPATHY

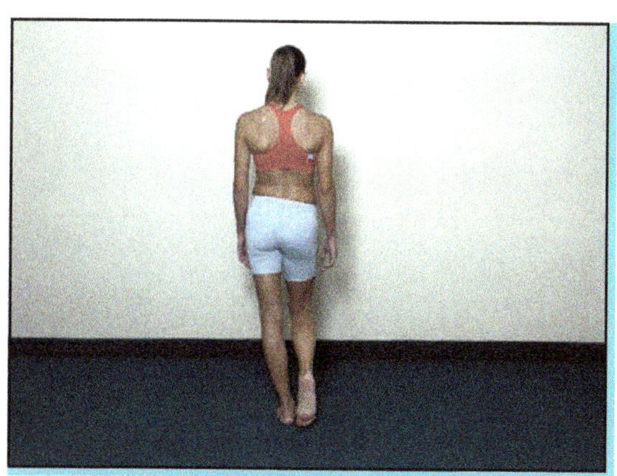

9) The patient is placed in standing.

10) To test L5–S1, the patient is requested to unilaterally stand.

11) The examiner observes pelvic drop on the opposite side for weakness in the hip abductors.

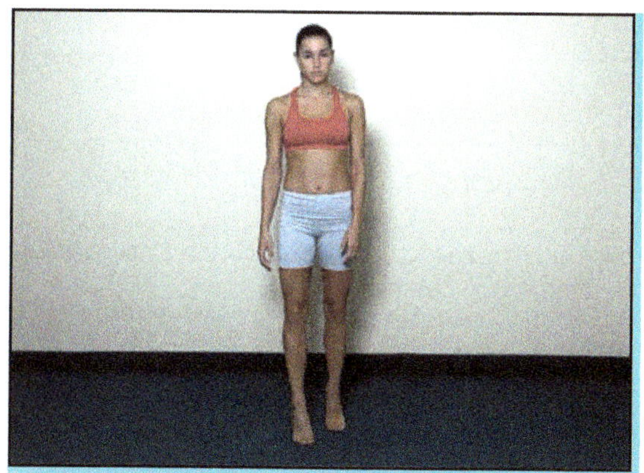

12) The patient is placed in standing.

13) To test S1, the patient is requested to walk on his or her toes.

14) With all areas, a positive test is noticeable weakness when compared to the opposite side or versus expectations if bilateral symptoms are present.

UTILITY SCORE 3

Study	Reliability	Sensitivity	Specificity	LR+	LR−	QUADAS Score (0–14)
Knuttson[28] (L5–S1) (Great Toe Weakness)	NT	48	50	0.95	1.1	3
Knuttson[28] (L4–L5) (Great Toe Weakness)	NT	74	50	1.5	0.52	3
Knuttson[28] (L3–L4) (Great Toe Weakness)	NT	100	50	NA	NA	3
Knuttson[28] (L4–L5) (Great Toe Weakness)	NT	36	50	0.72	1.3	3

(continued)

TESTS FOR LUMBAR RADICULOPATHY

Study	Reliability	Sensitivity	Specificity	LR+	LR−	QUADAS Score (0–14)
Gurdjian et al.[19] (Great Toe Weakness)	NT	16	50	0.32	1.7	4
Gurdjian et al.[19] (Foot Drop-Dorsiflexion)	NT	1	50	0.02	1.98	4
Kerr et al.[26] (L4–L5) (Hip Extension Weakness)	NT	12	96	3	0.92	7
Kerr et al.[26] (L5–S1) (Hip Extension Weakness)	NT	9	89	0.77	1.03	7
Kerr et al.[26] (L3–L4) (Ankle Dorsiflexion)	NT	33	89	3.03	0.75	7
Kerr et al.[26] (L4–L5) (Ankle Dorsiflexion)	NT	60	89	5.45	0.45	7
Kerr et al.[26] (L5–S1) (Ankle Dorsiflexion)	NT	49	89	4.45	0.6	7
Kerr et al.[26] (L3–L4) (Ankle Plantarflexion)	NT	0	100	NA	NA	7
Kerr et al.[26] (L4–L5) (Ankle Plantarflexion)	NT	0	100	NA	NA	7
Kerr et al.[26] (L5–S1) (Ankle Plantarflexion)	NT	28	100	NA	NA	7
Hakelius & Hindmarsh[20] (Great Toe Extension, All Levels)	NT	79	NT	NA	NA	3
Hakelius & Hindmarsh[20] (Dorsiflexion, All Levels)	NT	75	NT	NA	NA	3
Hakelius & Hindmarsh[20] (Quadriceps, All Levels)	NT	79	NT	NA	NA	3
Comments: Note that the study results are highly variable and depend on the population examined. In addition, positive findings are affected by the prevalence of conditions represented in the study. Most patients in the studies demonstrated L4–L5 or L5–S1 disorders, thus it's expected to see better diagnostic value with muscle groups that reflect this innervation pattern. The test is frequently performed as a component of the lower quarter screen.						

Sensibility Testing (Lumbar Radiculopathy from Disk Herniation or Protrusion)

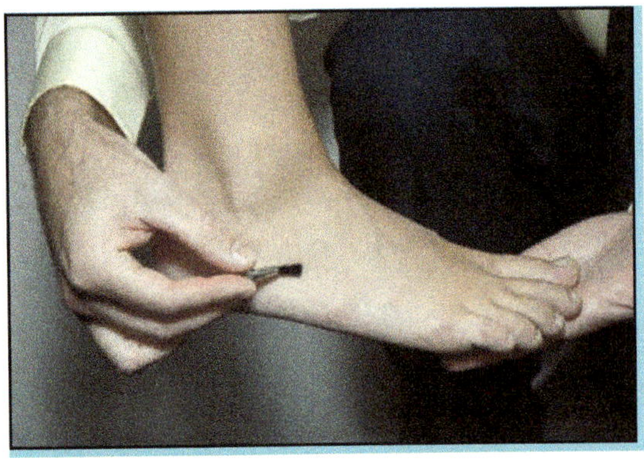

1) The patient is placed in sitting or supine.

2) The examiner applies a series of concurrent sensibility tests (light touch) to both sides. The examiner makes careful effort to apply sensation testing along known dermatomes.

3) Sharp/dull is assessed using pin prick.

4) A positive test is considered impaired sensation when tested against the opposite side.

TESTS FOR LUMBAR RADICULOPATHY

UTILITY SCORE 3

Study	Reliability	Sensitivity	Specificity	LR+	LR−	QUADAS Score (0–14)
Porchet et al.[41]	NT	57	NT	NA	NA	5
Kerr et al.[26] (L5 Dermatome)	NT	16	86	1.14	0.98	7
Kerr et al.[26] (S1 Dermatome)	NT	28	86	2	0.84	7
Lauder et al.[30] (Any Level, Vibration and Pinprick)	NT	55	77	2.4	0.6	6
Vroomen et al.[53] (Any Form, Any Level—Sensory Loss)	NT	45	50	0.9	1.1	10
Knuttson[28] (L3–L4)	NT	67	65	1.9	0.5	3
Knuttson[28] (L4–L5)	NT	30	65	0.87	1.1	3
Knuttson[28] (L5–S1)	NT	27	65	.8	1.1	3
Gurdjian et al.[19] (Hyperesthesia, Anesthesia, or Paresthesia)	NT	40	NT	NA	NA	4
Peeters et al.[39] (L4) (L3–L4 Disk Herniation)	NT	50	87.5	4	0.6	8
Peeters et al.[39] (L5) (L3–L4 Disk Herniation)	NT	50	100	NA	NA	8
Peeters et al.[39] (S1) (L3–L4 Disk Herniation)	NT	0	87.5	0	0	8
Peeters et al.[39] (L4) (L4–L5 Disk Herniation)	NT	59	87.5	4.7	0.5	8
Peeters et al.[39] (L5) (L4–L5 Disk Herniation)	NT	50	100	NA	NA	8
Peeters et al.[39] (S1) (L4–L5 Disk Herniation)	NT	23	87.5	1.8	0.9	8
Peeters et al.[39] (L4) (L5–S1 Disk Herniation)	NT	16	87.5	1.3	0.96	8
Peeters et al.[39] (L5) (L5–S1 Disk Herniation)	NT	42	100	NA	NA	8
Peeters et al.[39] (S1) (L5–S1 Disk Herniation)	NT	74	87.5	5.9	0.3	8
Tokuhashi et al.[51] (L4, L5, S1) (Light Touch)	NT	62	NT	NA	NA	4
Tokuhashi et al.[51] (L4, L5, S1) (Tuning Fork)	NT	53	NT	NA	NA	4
Tokuhashi et al.[51] (L4, L5, S1) (Pressure)	NT	52	NT	NA	NA	4
Bertilson et al.[5] (L4)	.50 kappa	NT	NT	NA	NA	NA
Bertilson et al.[5] (L5)	.71 kappa	NT	NT	NA	NA	NA
Bertilson et al.[5] (S1)	.68 kappa	NT	NT	NA	NA	NA

Comments: Results suggest that bilateral stimulus with the patient's eyes closed generates the most valid findings. Unless indicated, results were associated with light touch sensibility testing. The test is frequently performed as a component of the lower quarter screen.

TESTS FOR LUMBAR RADICULOPATHY

Combined Tests Lower Extremity

UTILITY SCORE 3

Study	Reliability	Sensitivity	Specificity	LR+	LR−	QUADAS Score (0–14)
Porchet et al.[41] (All LE Reflexes, Lateral Disk Herniation)	NT	82	NT	NA	NA	5
Porchet et al.[41] (Any Sensory Deficit, Lateral Disk Herniation)	NT	57	NT	NA	NA	5
Porchet et al.[41] (Any Strength Loss, Lateral Disk Herniation)	NT	79	NT	NT	NT	5
Lauder et al.[30] (Weakness, Any Muscle)	NT	69	61	1.77	0.51	6
Lauder et al.[30] (Sensory Loss and Weakness)	NT	41	88	3.41	0.67	6
Lauder et al.[30] (Sensory Loss and Reflexes)	NT	14	96	3.5	8.9	6
Lauder et al.[30] (Weakness and Reflexes)	NT	19	96	4.75	0.84	6
Lauder et al.[30] (Sensory, Reflexes, and Weakness)	NT	12	100	NA	NA	6
Vroomen et al.[53] (Ankle and Knee Loss)	NT	14	93	2.2	0.92	10
Comments: For diagnostic purposes, combined values exceed the findings of single neurological screening testing.						

Brudzinski's Sign

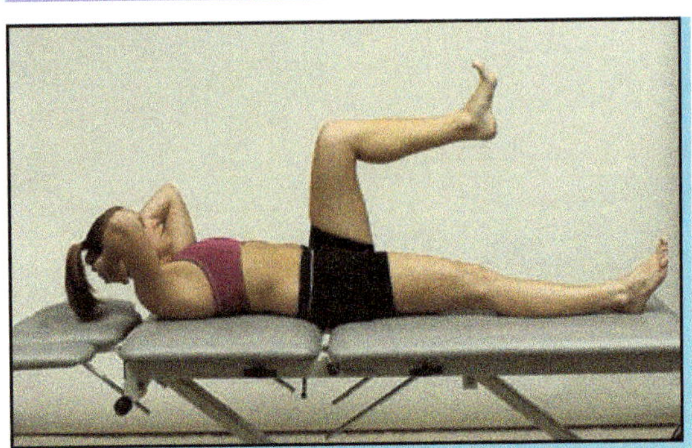

1) The patient is positioned in supine.

2) The patient is instructed to place his or her hands behind his or her head and passively flex his or her cervical spine.

3) The patient is instructed to then flex the hip on the tested side to end range or to the point of pain. The patient's knee should remain fully extended.

4) The patient should then be instructed to actively flex the knee to 90° on the tested side while maintaining full extension on the opposite side.

5) A positive test is indicated by spine pain or lower extremity symptoms which increase with neck and hip flexion but are relieved with knee flexion.

TESTS FOR LUMBAR RADICULOPATHY

UTILITY SCORE ?

Study	Reliability	Sensitivity	Specificity	LR+	LR−	QUADAS Score (0–14)
Scifers[46]	NT	NT	NT	NT	NT	NA

Comments: A positive test indicates a nerve root impingement, irritation of the dura, and meningeal irritation. This test is also used to test for bacterial or viral meningitis.

Bowstring Test

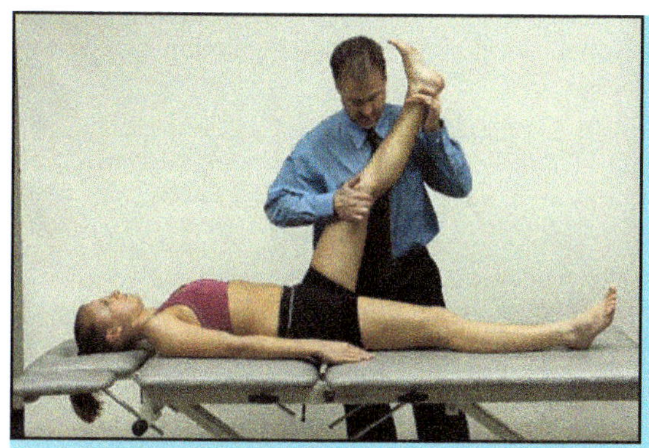

1) The patient is positioned in supine.
2) The clinician performs a passive straight leg raise of the involved side. If the patient reports radiating pain during the straight leg raise, the clinician should flex the patient's leg approximately 20° in order to relieve the patient's symptoms.
3) The clinician should then palpate the sciatic nerve in the popliteal fossa in an attempt to reproduce the patient's familiar symptoms.
4) A positive sign is the presence of radicular symptoms during straight leg raise which is relieved by flexion of the knee but exacerbated with palpation of the popliteal fossa.

UTILITY SCORE 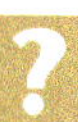

Study	Reliability	Sensitivity	Specificity	LR+	LR−	QUADAS Score (0–14)
Scifers[46]	NT	NT	NT	NT	NT	NA

Comments: The patient should maintain the same degree of hip flexion throughout the test.

Key Points

1. Nearly all of the neurological clinical special tests exhibit high levels of procedural bias.
2. Despite the fact that many of the neurological clinical special tests are purported to function as screens, the majority demonstrate poor sensitivity and fair to strong specificity, the opposite diagnostic values expected in a screening examination.
3. Hoffmann's test, a test for upper motor neuron assessment, is frequently included as a gold standard in most studies, but demonstrates only poor to fair diagnostic value when examined independently.
4. Those studies with higher QUADAS values routinely demonstrate that many of the neurological screen tests have less accuracy than studies with lower QUADAS scores.
5. The Babinski sign and offshoots of this test (Allen-Cleckley and Gonda-Allen) demonstrate good sensitivity for testing upper motor neuron disorders.
6. The sensibility tests for peripheral neuropathy demonstrate very good diagnostic value but the sensibility tests for radiculopathy demonstrate poor value for lower extremities and poor to moderate value for upper extremities.
7. Only the biceps reflex test demonstrates fair diagnostic value. The brachioradialis and triceps reflex tests demonstrate poor diagnostic value and do not function well as screens.

8. Nearly all the lower extremity reflex studies are riddled with bias.
9. As a whole, muscle power testing yields poor diagnostic value in lower and upper extremities.
10. Combining the test values only marginally improves the accuracy of the test. Specificity is improved by the sensitivity declines.

References

1. Anderson NE, Mason DF, Fink JN, Bergin PS, Charleston AJ, Gamble GD. Detection of focal cerebral hemisphere lesions using the neurological examination. *J Neurol Neurosurg Psychiatry.* 2005;76:545–549.
2. August B, Miller FB. Clinical value of the palmomental reflex. *J Am Med Assoc.* 1952;148(2):120–121.
3. Awerbuch GI, Nigro MA, Wishnow R. Beevor's sign and facioscapulohumeral dystrophy. *Arch Neurol.* 1990;47(11):1208–1209.
4. Berger JR, Fannin M. The "bedsheet" Babinski. *South Med J.* 2002;95(10):1178–1179.
5. Bertilson B, Bring J, Sjoblom A, Sundell K, Strender LE. Inter-examiner reliability in the assessment of low back pain (LBP) using the Kirkaldy-Willis classification (KWC). *Eur Spine J.* 2006;15(11):1695–1703.
6. Bertilson B, Grunnesjo M, Strender LE. Reliability of clinical tests in the assessment of patient with neck/shoulder problems—impact of history. *Spine.* 2003;19:2222–2231.
7. Cameron MH, Klein EL. Screening for medical disease—Nervous system disorders. *J Hand Ther.* 2010;23:158–172.
8. Chikuda H, Seichi A, Takeshita K, et al. Correlation between pyramidal signs and the severity of cervical myelopathy. *European Spine J.* 2010;19:1684–1689.
9. Cook C, Brown C, Isaacs R, Roman M, Davis S, Richardson W. Clustered clinical findings for diagnosis of cervical spine myelopathy. *J Man Manip Ther.* 2010;18(4):175–180.
10. Cook C, Roman M, Stewart KM, Gray Leithe L, Isaacs R. Reliability and diagnostic accuracy of clinical special tests for myelopathy in patients seen for cervical dysfunction. *J Orthop Sports Phys Ther.* 2009;39(3):172–178.
11. Davidson R, Dunn E, Metzmaker J. The shoulder abduction test in the diagnosis of radicular pain in cervical extradural compression monoradiculopathies. *Spine.* 1981;6:441–445.
12. De Freitas G, Andre C. Absence of the Babinski sign in brain death. *J Neurol.* 2005;252:106–107.
13. Denno JJ, Meadows GR. Early diagnosis of cervical spondylotic myelopathy. A useful clinical sign. *Spine.* 1991;16(12):1353–1355.
14. Eger K, Jordan B, Habermann S, Sierz S. Beevor's sign in facioscapulohumeral muscular dystrophy: an old sign with new implications. *J Neurol.* 2010;257:436–438.
15. Estanol BV, Marin OS. Mechanism of the inverted supinator reflex. A clinical and neurophysiological study. *J Neurol Neurosurg Psychiatry.* 1976;39:905–908.
16. Ghosh D, Pradhan S. Extensor toe sign: by various methods in spastic children with cerebral palsy. *J Child Neurol.* 1998;13:216–220.
17. Glaser J, Cure J, Bailey K, Morrow D. Cervical spinal cord compression and the Hoffmann sign. *Iowa Orthop J.* 2001;21:49–52.
18. Gotkine M, Haggiag S, Abramsky O, Biran I. Lack of hemispheric localizing value of the palmomental reflex. *Neurology.* 2005;64(9):1656.
19. Gurdjian E, Webster J, Ostrowski AZ, Hardy W, Lindner D, Thomas L. Herniated lumbar intervertebral discs: an analysis of 1176 operated cases. *J Trauma.* 1961;1:158–176.
20. Hakelius A, Hindmarsh J. The comparative reliability of preoperative diagnostic methods in lumbar disc surgery. *Acta Orthop Scand.* 1972;43:234–238.
21. Hindfelt B, Rosen I, Hanko J. The significance of a crossed extensor hallucis response in neurological disorders: a comparison with the Babinski sign. *Acta Neurol Scandinav.* 1976;53:241–250.
22. Houten JK, Noce LA. Clinical correlations of cervical myelopathy and the Hoffmann sign. *J Neurosurg Spine.* 2008;9(3):237–242.
23. Isakov E, Sazbon L, Costeff H, Luz Y, Najenson T. The diagnostic value of three common primitive reflexes. *Eur Neurol.* 1984;23(1):17–21.
24. Jepsen JR, Laursen LH, Hagert CG, Kreiner S, Larsen A. Diagnostic accuracy of the neurological upper limb examination I: inter-rater reproducibility of selected findings and patterns. *BMC Neurology.* 2006;6:8.
25. Kashluba S, Casey JE, Paniak C. Evaluating the utility of ICD-10 diagnostic criteria for postconcussion syndrome following mild traumatic brain injury. *J Int Neuropsychol Soc.* 2006;12:111–118.
26. Kerr RSC, Cadoux-Hudson TA, Adams CBT. The value of accurate clinical assessment in the surgical management of the lumbar disc protrusion. *J Neurol Neurosurg Psychiatr.* 1988;51:169–173.
27. Kiely P, Baker JF, O'hEireamhoin S, Butler JS, Ahmed M, Lui DF, Devitt B, Walsh A, Poynton AR, Synnot KA. The evaluation of the inverted supinator reflex in asymptomatic patients. *Spine.* 2010;35(9):955–957.
28. Knuttson B. Comparative value of electromyographic, myelographic, and clinical-neurological examinations in diagnosis of lumbar root compression syndrome. *Acta Ortho Scand.* 1961;(Suppl 49):19–49.
29. Kumar SP, Ramasubramanian D. The Babinski sign—a reappraisal. *Neurology India.* 2000;48:314–318.

30. Lauder T, Dillingham T, Andary M, Kumar S, Pezzin L, Stephens R. Predicting electrodiagnostic outcome in patients with upper limb symptoms: are the history and physical examination helpful? *Arch Phys Med Rehabil.* 2000;81:436–441.

31. Maranhao ET, Maranhao-Filho P, Lima MA, Vincent MB. Can clinical tests detect early signs of monohemispheric brain tumors? *J Neurologic Phys Ther.* 2010;34(3):145–149.

32. Marin R, Dillingham TR, Chang A, Belandres P. Extensor digitorum brevis reflex in normals and patients with radiculopathies. *Muscle Nerve.* 1995;18:52–59.

33. Matsumoto M, Fujimura Y, Toyama Y. Usefulness and reliability of neurological signs for level diagnosis in cervical myelopathy caused by soft disc herniation. *J Spinal Disord.* 1996;9(4):317–21.

34. Matsumoto M, Ishikawa M, Ishii K, Nishizawa T, Maruiwa H, Nakamura M, Chiba K, Toyama Y. Usefulness of neurological examination for diagnosis of the affected level in patients with cervical compressive myelopathy: prospective comparative study with radiological evaluation. *J Neurosurg Spine.* 2005;2(5):535–539.

35. Miller T, Johnston SC. Should the Babinski sign be part of the routine neurological examination? *Neurology.* 2005;65:1165–1168.

36. Mythili A, Dileep Kumar K, Subrahmanyam KAV, Venkateswarlu K, Butchi RG. A comparative study of examination scores and quantitative sensory testing in diagnosis of diabetic polyneuropathy. *Int J Diab Dev Ctries.* 2010;30(1):43–48.

37. Olaleye D, Perkins BA, Bril V. Evaluation of three screening tests and a risk assessment model for diagnosing peripheral neuropathy in the diabetes clinic. *Diabetes Res Clin Pract.* 2001;54(2):115–128.

38. Onde ME, Ozge A, Senol MG, Togrol E, Ozdag F, Saracoglu M, Misirli H. The sensitivity of clinical diagnostic methods in the diagnosis of diabetic neuropathy. *J International Med Res.* 2008;36:63–70.

39. Peeters GG, Aufdemkampe G, Oostendorp RA. Sensibility testing in patients with a lumbosacral radicular syndrome. *J Manipulative Physiol Ther.* 1998;21(2):81–88.

40. Perkins BA, Olaleye D, Zinman B, Bril V. Simple screening tests for peripheral neuropathy in the diabetes clinic. *Diabetes Care.* 2001;24(2):250–256.

41. Porchet F, Fankhauser H, de Tribolet N. Extreme lateral lumbar disc herniation: clinical presentation in 178 patients. *Acta Neurochir (Wien).* 1994;127(3-4):203–209.

42. Rhee JM, Heflin JA, Hamasaki T, Freedman B. Prevalence of physical signs in cervical myelopathy: a prospective, controlled study. *Spine.* 2009;34(9):890–895.

43. Richardson JK. The clinical identification of peripheral neuropathy among older persons. *Arch Phys Med Rehabil.* 2002;83:1553–1558.

44. Rico RE, Jonkman EJ. Measurement of the Achilles tendon reflex for the diagnosis of lumbosacral root compression syndromes. *J Neurol Neurosurg Psychiatry.* 1982;45(9):791–795.

45. Schneiders AG, Sullivan SJ, Gray AR, Hammond-Tooke GD, McCrory PR. Normative values for three clinical measures of motor performance used in the neurological assessment of sports concussion. *J Science Med Sport.* 2010;13:196–201.

46. Scifers JR. *Special tests for Neurologic Examination.* Thorofare, NJ: Slack Incorporated; 2008.

47. Shahrizaila N, Wills AJ. Significance of Beevor's sign in facioscapulohumeral dystrophy and other neuromuscular diseases. *J Neurol Neurosurg Psychiatry.* 2005;76:869–870.

48. Spurling RG, Scoville WB. Lateral rupture of the cervical intervertebral disc. *Surg Gynecol Obstet.* 1944;78:350–358.

49. Sung R, Wang J. Correlation between a positive Hoffmann's reflex and cervical pathology in asymptomatic individuals. *Spine.* 2001;26:67–70.

50. Teitelbaum JS, Eliasziw M, Garner M. Tests of motor function in patients suspected of having mild unilateral cerebral lesions. *Can J Neurol Sci.* 2002;29:337–344.

51. Tokuhashi Y, Satoh K, Funami S. A quantitative evaluation of sensory dysfunction in lumbosacral radiculopathy. *Spine.* 1991;16(11):1321–1328.

52. Uchihara T, Furukawa T, Tsukagoshi H. Compression of brachial plexus as a diagnostic test of cervical cord lesion. *Spine.* 1994;19(19):2170–2173.

53. Vroomen P, de Krom M, Wilmink J, Kester A, Knottnerus J. Diagnostic value of history and physical examination in patients suspected of lumbosacral nerve root compression. *J Neurol Neurosurg Psychiatry.* 2002;72:630–634.

54. Wainner R, Fritz J, Irrgang J, Boninger M, Delitto A, Allison S. Reliability and diagnostic accuracy of the clinical examination and patient self-report measures for cervical radiculopathy. *Spine.* 2003;28:52–62.

55. Wong TM, Leung HB, Wong WC. Correlation between magnetic resonance imaging and radiographic measurement of cervical spine in cervical myelopathic patients. *J Orthop Surg.* 2004;12:239–242.

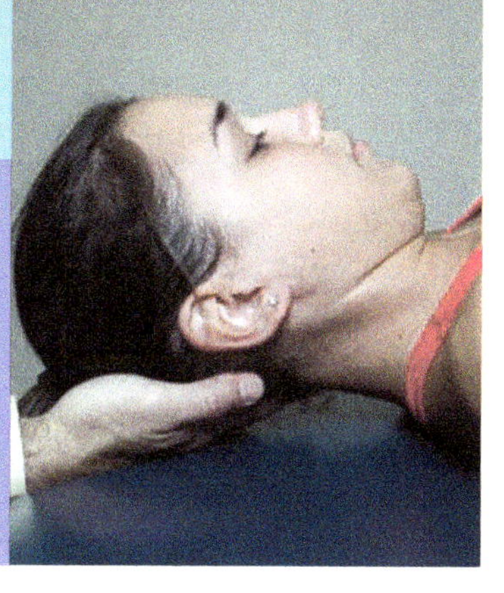

Physical Examination Tests for the Cervical Spine

Chad E. Cook

Please refer to the chapter "Introduction to Diagnostic Accuracy" before reading this chapter.

Index of Tests

Tests for Cervical Radiculopathy

Spurling's Compression Test
Valsalva Maneuver
Brachial Plexus Compression Test
Cervical Hyperflexion Test
Cervical Distraction Test
Upper Limb Tension Test (ULTT)
Cervical Hyperextension (Jackson's Test)
Shoulder Abduction Test
Quadrant Test
Cervical Compression Test
Wainner's Clinical Prediction Rule for Cervical Radiculopathy

Tests for Upper Cervical Instability

Modified Sharp Purser Test
Alar Ligament Stability Test
Upper Cervical Flexion Test
Original Sharp Purser Test
Anterior Stability Test of the Atlanto-Occipital Joint
Direct Anterior Translation Stress Test
Lateral Shear Test of the Atlanto-Axial Articulation
Tectorial Membrane Test
Posterior Atlanto-Occipital Membrane Test

Tests for Mid-Cervical Instability

AP and PA Stress Testing of the Mid-Cervical Spine
Lateral Stress Testing of the Mid-Cervical Spine

Tests for Potential Vertebral Artery Dysfunction

Vertebral Basilar Insufficiency (VBI) Test
Wallenberg's Position (Extension and Rotation)

Tests for Cervicogenic Headache

Cervical-Flexion Rotation Test
C0–1, C1–2, C2–3 Joint Mobility Assessment

Tests for Postural Dysfunction

Neck Flexor Muscle Endurance Test

Scapular Muscle Endurance Test

Posterior Extensors Endurance Test

Tests for Level of Dysfunction or Linear Stability

Posterior-Anterior Mobilization Test

Palpation of Physiological Movement

Tests to Identify Neck Pain from Asymptomatic Conditions

Manual Examination of Rotation

Combined Manual Rotation and a Visual Analog Scale

Tests to Determine if a Radiograph Is Required

Canadian C-Spine Rules

Nexus (National Emergency X-Radiography Utilization Study)

TESTS FOR CERVICAL RADICULOPATHY

Spurling's Compression Test

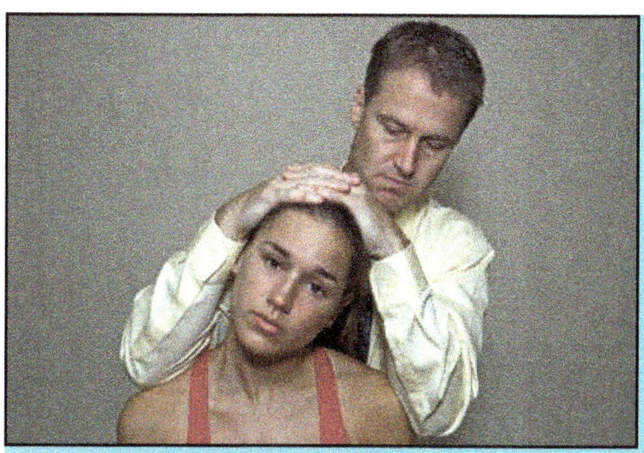

1) The patient assumes a neutral cervical posture while in sitting position. Assess resting symptoms.

2) The patient is instructed to side flex his or her head to the side of his or her referred symptoms. If radicular pain is present, the test is positive.

3) If no symptoms up to this point, the examiner then applies a combined compression and side flexion force in the direction of side flexion. If radicular pain is present, the test is positive.

UTILITY SCORE 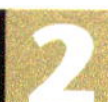

Study	Reliability	Sensitivity	Specificity	LR+	LR−	QUADAS Score (0–14)
Bertilson et al.[2]	.14 to .28 kappa	NT	NT	NA	NA	NA
Spurling & Scoville[25]	NT	100	NT	NA	NA	4
Uchihara et al.[29]	NT	11	100	NA	NA	8
Tong et al.[28]	NT	30	93	4.3	.75	9
Shah & Rajshekhar[22]	NT	93	95	18.6	0.07	9
Wainner et al.[33]	.60 kappa	50	86	3.57	0.58	10
Wainner et al.[33] (included side flexion toward the rotation and extension)	.62 kappa	50	74	1.92	0.67	10
Viikari-Juntura et al.[32] (right side)	NT	36	92	4.5	0.69	11
Viikari-Juntura et al.[32] (left side)	NT	39	92	4.87	0.66	11
Sandmark & Nisell[21] (not for radiculopathy)	NT	77	92	9.62	0.25	9
DeHertogh et al.[6]	NT	77.8	77.3	3.4	0.28	9

Comments: The Spurling's maneuver appears to be specific but not sensitive and would not function well as a screen. Some have described the test by including ipsilateral rotation with side flexion while others have included extension. DeHertogh et al. used a case control design to identify neck pain versus no neck pain. The description provided is the original description from Spurling & Scoville.[25]

TESTS FOR CERVICAL RADICULOPATHY

Valsalva Maneuver

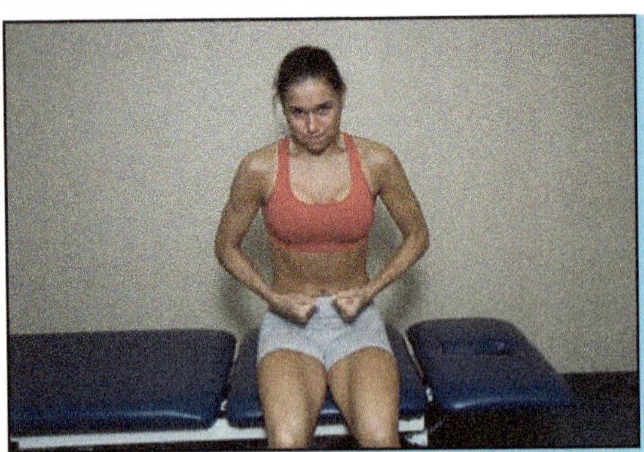

1. The patient assumes a sitting position.
2. The patient is instructed to hold his or her breath then "bear down" as in performing a toileting procedure.
3. Reproduction of concordant pain during bearing down is considered a positive response.

UTILITY SCORE 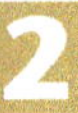

Study	Reliability	Sensitivity	Specificity	LR+	LR−	QUADAS Score (0–14)
Wainner et al.[33]	.69 kappa	22	94	3.67	0.82	10
Comments: The test appears to be moderately reliable and specific for patients with cervical radiculopathy. The test should not be used as a screen.						

Brachial Plexus Compression Test

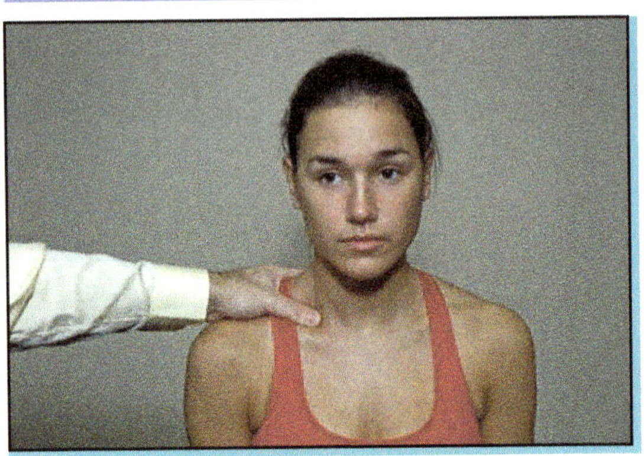

1. The patient assumes a sitting position.
2. The examiner applies a compressive force with his or her hand, just above the clavicle on the symptomatic side.
3. Special effort to apply compression lateral to the scalenes is made to apply traction to the nerve bundle.
4. A positive test is reproduction of radicular symptoms.

UTILITY SCORE 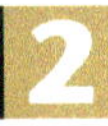

Study	Reliability	Sensitivity	Specificity	LR+	LR−	QUADAS Score (0–14)
Uchihara et al.[29]	NT	69	83	4.1	0.37	8
Comments: The test mimics those of thoracic outlet syndrome. It is doubtful that the test could discriminate between cervical radiculopathy and thoracic outlet syndrome, and may demonstrate false positives if localized pain only is queried.						

TESTS FOR CERVICAL RADICULOPATHY

Cervical Hyperflexion Test

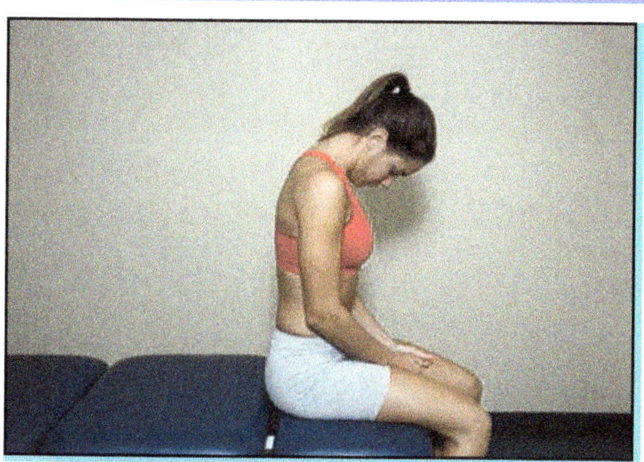

1) The patient assumes a sitting position.

2) The patient is instructed to flex his or her neck to the first point of pain. If no pain, the patient is instructed to flex toward end range.

3) Reproduction of radicular symptoms during hyperflexion is considered a positive response.

UTILITY SCORE 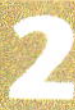

Study	Reliability	Sensitivity	Specificity	LR+	LR−	QUADAS Score (0–14)
Uchihara et al.[29]	NT	8	100	NA	NA	8
Wainner et al.[33] (limited < 55°)	.60 kappa	89	41	1.51	0.27	10

Comments: The dramatic differences in values are unexplained. Wainner et al.[33] provided better methodology for their study and the results are likely more transferable to a population with cervical radiculopathy.

Cervical Distraction Test

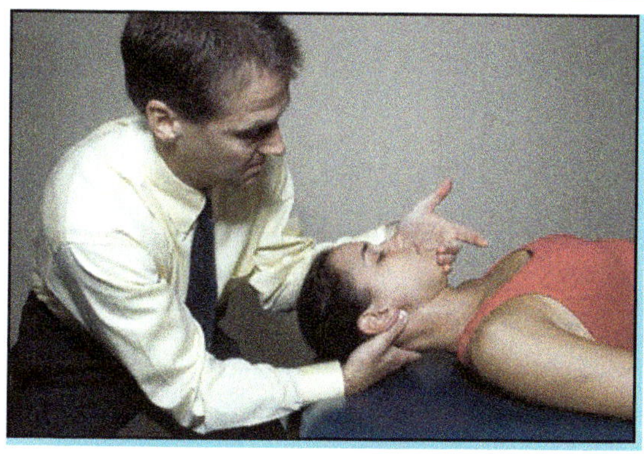

1) The patient assumes a supine position. The patient's symptoms require assessment prior to the examination.

2) The examiner uses a chin cradle grip around the head of the patient, specifically targeting the occipital shelf of the neck.

3) A traction force is applied and the patient's symptoms are reassessed. Pain is respected and the same pattern of movement to pain, movement beyond pain, and repeated movement should be implemented.

4) A positive test is reduction of symptoms during traction.

UTILITY SCORE 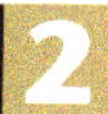

Study	Reliability	Sensitivity	Specificity	LR+	LR−	QUADAS Score (0–14)
Bertilson et al.[2]	.63 to .43 kappa	NT	NT	NA	NA	NA
Wainner et al.[33]	.88 kappa	44	90	4.4	0.62	10
Viikari-Juntura et al.[32]	NT	40	100	NA	NA	11

Comments: Though only moderate, this test provides one of the best diagnostic scores of the tests for cervical radiculopathy. The test is highly specific for cervical radiculopathy.

TESTS FOR CERVICAL RADICULOPATHY

Upper Limb Tension Test (ULTT)

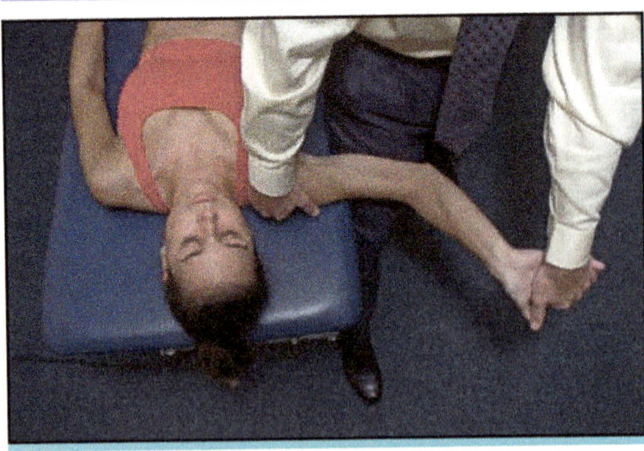

1) The patient assumes a supine position. The examiner assesses resting symptoms.

2) The examiner blocks the shoulder girdle to stabilize the scapulae. Symptoms are again assessed.

3) If no reproduction of symptoms has occurred, the glenohumeral joint is abducted to 110 degrees with slight coronal plane extension. Symptoms are again assessed.

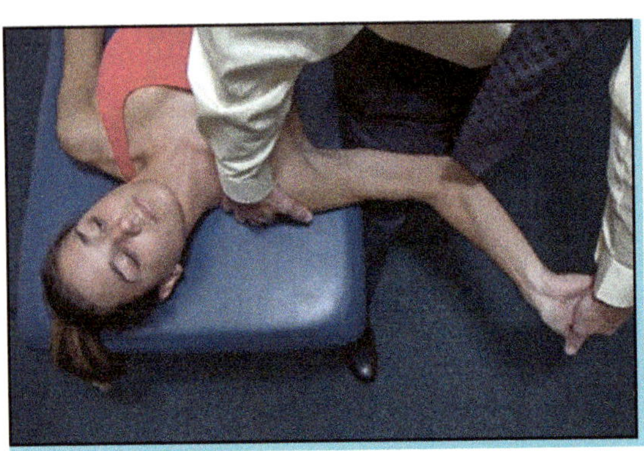

4) If no reproduction of symptoms has occurred, the forearm is supinated completely and the wrist and fingers are extended. Ulnar deviation is implemented. Symptoms are again assessed.

5) If no reproduction of symptoms has occurred, elbow extension is applied. Symptoms are again assessed. One may measure the degree of elbow extension if range of motion is an objective.

6) Lateral flexion of the neck is used to sensitize the procedure. A positive test is reproduction of symptoms during distal movement.

UTILITY SCORE 2

Study	Reliability	Sensitivity	Specificity	LR+	LR−	QUADAS Score (0–14)
Wainner et al.[33] (median nerve bias)	.76 kappa	97	22	1.24	.14	10
Wainner et al.[33] (radial nerve bias)	.83 kappa	72	33	1.07	.84	10
Bertilson et al.[2] (median nerve bias)	.03 kappa	NT	NT	NA	NA	NA
Bertilson et al.[2] (radial nerve bias)	.11 kappa	NT	NT	NA	NA	NA
Bertilson et al.[2] (ulnar nerve bias)	NT	NT	NT	NA	NA	NA
Sandmark & Nisell[21] (not for radiculopathy)	NT	77	94	12.8	.24	9

Comments: This sensitive test is most likely associated with a number of dysfunctions. Studies have supported that a positive ULTT is not specific to a selected disorder secondary to anatomical considerations. To increase the specificity of the test, one should look for concordant symptoms, sensitization, and asymmetry from side to side. The test should be considered an excellent screen for radiculopathy as a negative finding is compelling toward the lack of existence of radiculopathy.

TESTS FOR CERVICAL RADICULOPATHY

Cervical Hyperextension (Jackson's Test)

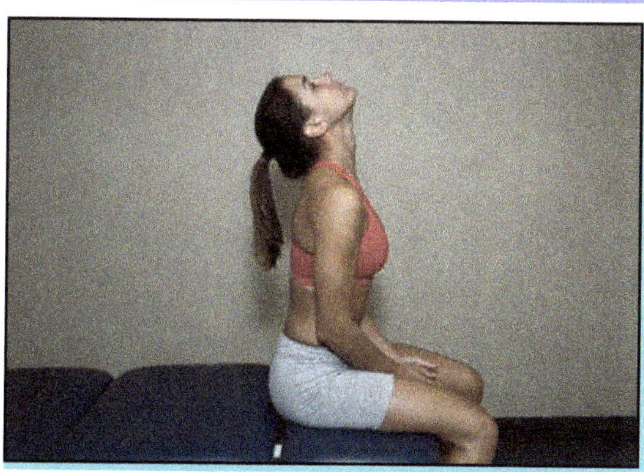

1) The patient assumes a sitting position.

2) The patient is instructed to extend his or her neck to the first point of pain. If no pain, the patient is instructed to extend toward end range.

3) Reproduction of symptoms is considered a positive response.

UTILITY SCORE 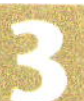

Study	Reliability	Sensitivity	Specificity	LR+	LR−	QUADAS Score (0–14)
Uchihara et al.[29]	NT	25	90	2.5	0.83	8
Sandmark & Nisell[21] (not for radiculopathy)	NT	27	90	2.7	0.81	9

Comments: Although the test is specific, the examiner would be best served to differentiate localized pain compared to radicular symptoms.

Shoulder Abduction Test

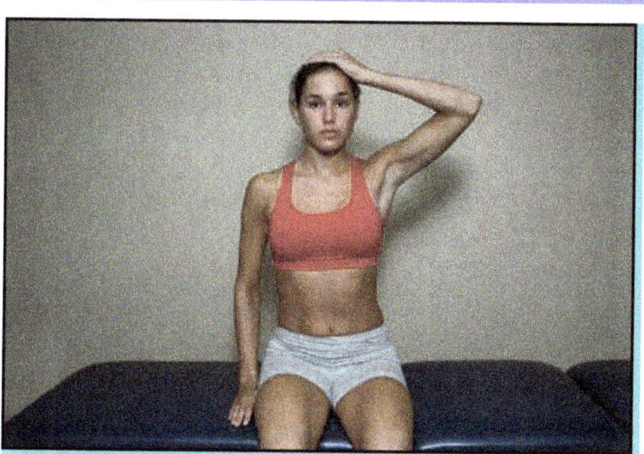

1) The patient assumes a sitting position. The examiner assesses resting symptoms.

2) The patient actively places his or her hand on top of his or her head. The examiner then determines the presence or absence of the symptoms. It is unlikely that causative level of the cervical radiculopathy can be discriminated with this test.

3) A positive test is identified by reduction of the patient's concordant pain.

UTILITY SCORE 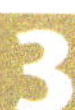

Study	Reliability	Sensitivity	Specificity	LR+	LR−	QUADAS Score (0–14)
Davidson et al.[5]	NT	68	NT	NA	NA	8
Wainner et al.[33]	.20 kappa	17	92	2.12	0.90	10
Viikari-Juntura et al.[32] (right side)	NT	38	80	1.9	0.77	11
Viikari-Juntura et al.[32] (left side)	NT	43	80	2.2	0.71	11

Comments: The test is not considered a good screen but is moderately specific. Overall, the diagnostic value is not compelling for diagnosis.

TESTS FOR CERVICAL RADICULOPATHY

Quadrant Test

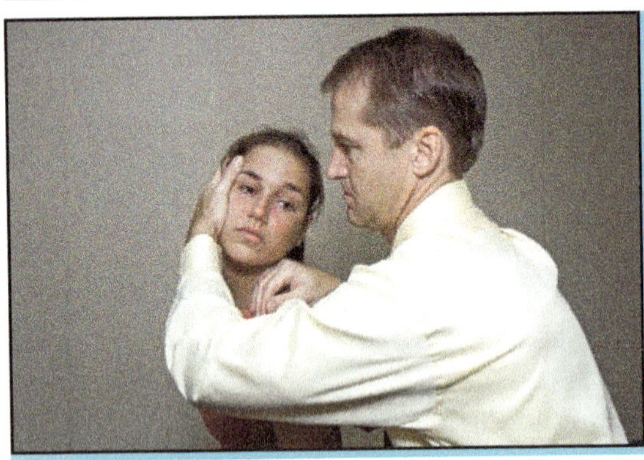

1) The patient assumes a sitting position.

2) The examiner instructs the patient to side flex, rotate, and extend his or her neck toward the side of pain.

3) The examiner gently provides overpressure to the zygomatic process toward side flexion, rotation, and extension.

4) Reproduction of arm symptoms is considered a positive finding.

UTILITY SCORE 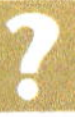

Study	Reliability	Sensitivity	Specificity	LR+	LR−	QUADAS Score (0–14)
Uchihara et al.[29]	NT	NT	NT	NA	NA	NT
Comments: This test is commonly used to "rule out" cervical dysfunction but at present is untested.						

Cervical Compression Test

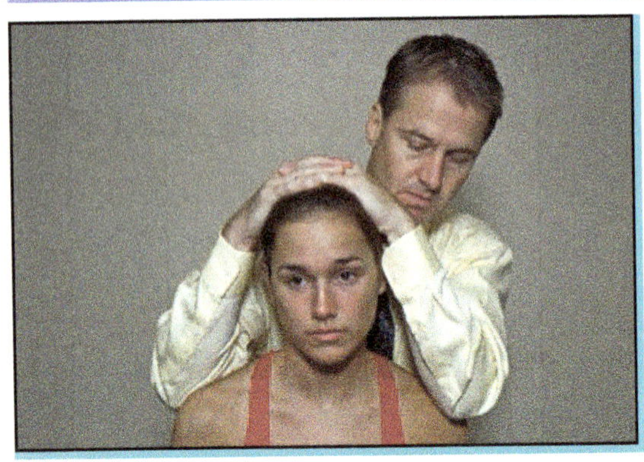

1) The patient assumes a sitting position.

2) The examiner stands behind the patient. With the elbows on each shoulder, the examiner applies a downward force to the head.

3) Reproduction of symptoms is considered a positive response.

UTILITY SCORE 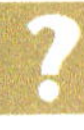

Study	Reliability	Sensitivity	Specificity	LR+	LR−	QUADAS Score (0–14)
Bertilson et al.[2]	.44 kappa	NT	NT	NA	NA	NA
Comments: The kappa value suggests the test has only fair agreement. The diagnostic value remains untested.						

TESTS FOR CERVICAL RADICULOPATHY

Wainner's Clinical Prediction Rule for Cervical Radiculopathy

The study includes four criteria: Cervical rotation less than 60 degrees, a positive Spurling's test, a positive distraction test, and a positive upper limb tension sign.

UTILITY SCORE 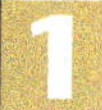

Study	Reliability	Sensitivity	Specificity	LR+	LR−	QUADAS Score (0–14)
Wainner et al.[33] (2 of 4 positive tests)	NT	39	56	0.88	1.08	10
Wainner et al.[33] (3 of 4 positive tests)	NT	39	94	6.1	0.64	10
Wainner et al.[33] (4 of 4 positive tests)	NT	24	99	30.3	0.76	10
Comments: A well done study that demonstrates a useful combination for diagnosis.						

TESTS FOR UPPER CERVICAL INSTABILITY

Modified Sharp Purser Test

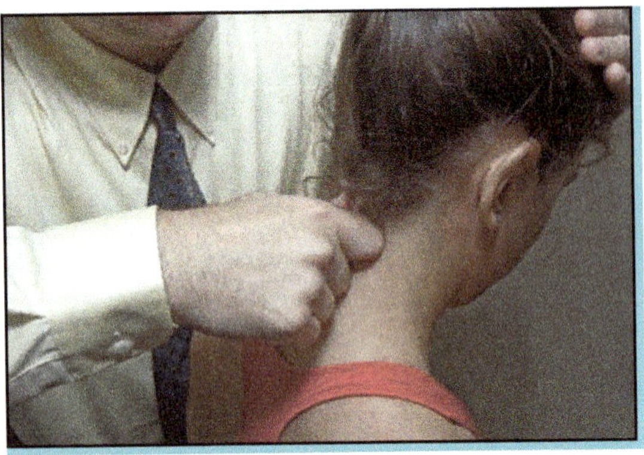

1) The patient assumes a sitting position. The patient's head should be slightly flexed. The examiner assesses resting symptoms.

2) The examiner stands to the side of the patient and stabilizes the C2 spinous process using a pincer grasp.

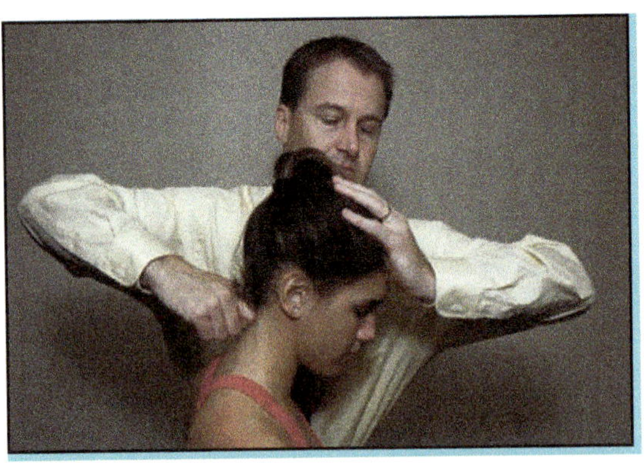

3) Gently at first, the examiner applies a posterior translation force from the palm of the hand on the patient's forehead toward a posterior direction.

4) Symptoms are assessed for both degree of linear displacement (palpated) or symptom provocation.

5) Collectively, a positive test is identified either by reproduction of myelopathic symptoms during forward flexion or decrease in symptoms during an anterior to posterior movement or excess displacement during the AP movement.

UTILITY SCORE 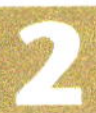

Study	Reliability	Sensitivity	Specificity	LR+	LR−	QUADAS Score (0–14)
Cattrysse et al.[3] (includes only those that were significantly related)	.67 kappa	NT	NT	NA	NA	NA
Uitvlugt & Indenbaum[30]	NT	69	96	17.3	0.32	8

Comments: Uitvlugt & Indenbaum[30] found high specificity with the Sharp Purser and described the test as "symptom reduction upon posterior force through the head." The test differs from the original Sharp Purser, which was poorly defined and only consisted of upper cervical flexion. Precautions should be taken prior to use on patients who may have a dens fracture.

TESTS FOR UPPER CERVICAL INSTABILITY

Alar Ligament Stability Test

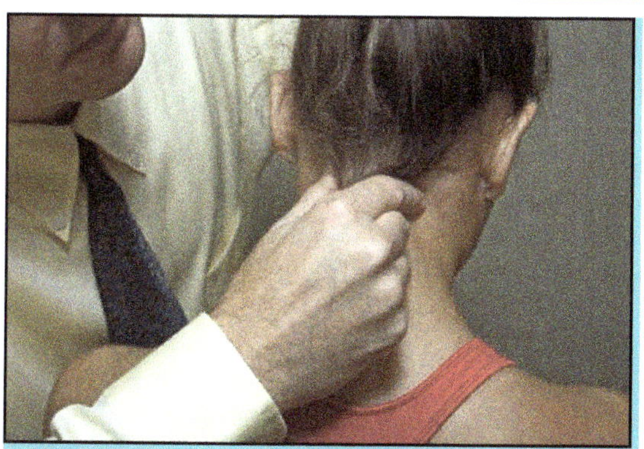

1) The patient assumes a sitting or supine position. The head is slightly flexed to further engage the Alar ligament. The examiner assesses resting symptoms.

2) The examiner stabilizes the C2 spinous process using a pincer grasp. A firm grip ensures appropriate assessment of movement.

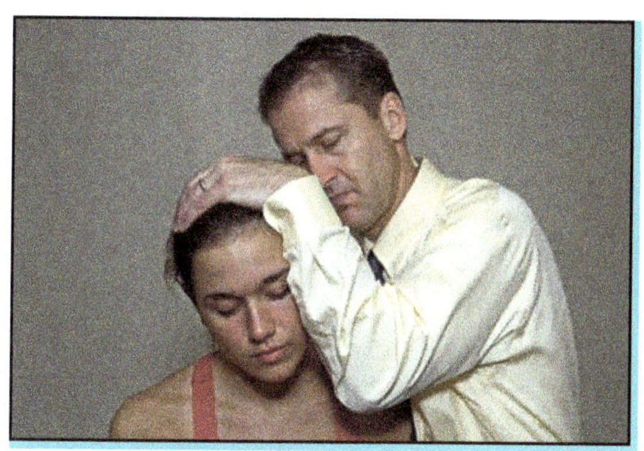

3) Either side flexion or rotation is passively initiated by the examiner. During these passive movements, the examiner attempts to feel movement of C2.

4) A positive test is the failure to "feel" movement of the C2 process during side flexion and rotation.

UTILITY SCORE 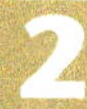

Study	Reliability	Sensitivity	Specificity	LR+	LR−	QUADAS Score (0–14)
Kaale et al. [16] (right)	0.71 kappa	69	100	Inf	0.31	7
Kaale et al. [16] (left)	0.69 kappa	72	96	18	0.29	7

Comments: Precautions should be taken prior to use on patients who may have a dens fracture. There are several considerations associated with the Alar ligament test. First, any movement of C2 during side flexion or rotation should be considered normal. Second, the patient may experience some discomfort during the procedure, specifically post-trauma, and this finding should be considered a "red flag" for high-velocity techniques. Finally, some individuals have recommended using the coupling pattern of C0–1 or C1–2 to identify pathology; however, because the coupling pattern is inconsistent, this is not advised. Others suggest that selected range of motion loss is indicative of capsular restrictions or hypermobility but this line of thought has not been tested. Kaale et al.[16] used a slight variation of the traditional Alar ligament test which involved palpation of the C1 transverse process to feel for movement between C1 and C2.

TESTS FOR UPPER CERVICAL INSTABILITY

Upper Cervical Flexion Test

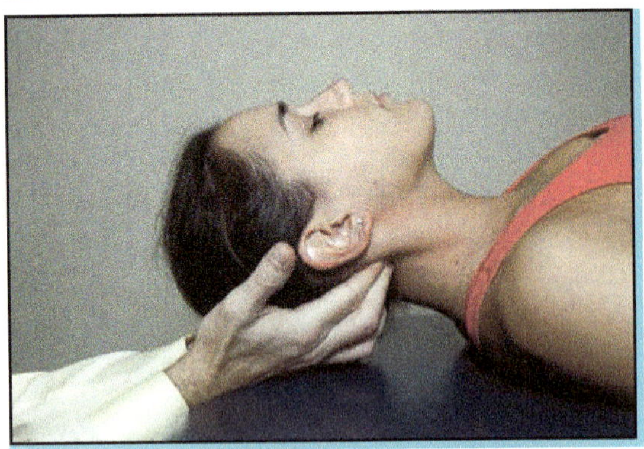

1) The patient assumes a supine position. The examiner assesses resting symptoms.

2) Using a friction massage grip (digits 2 and 3 are held tightly together) the examiner contacts the posterior aspect of the bilateral C1 transverse processes. The palms of the examiner are placed under the occiput of the patient.

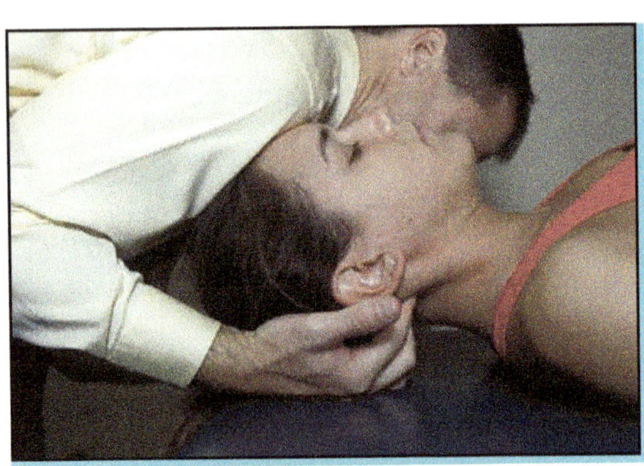

3) The examiner then applies an anterior force to the C1 transverse processes, lifting the head as the force is applied. This position is held for 15 to 20 seconds.

4) If no symptoms occur, the examiner can apply a downward force on the patient's forehead using the anterior aspect of the shoulder. This position is held for 15 to 20 seconds.

5) A positive test is identified by excessive translation or reproduction of instability-related symptoms.

UTILITY SCORE 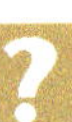

Study	Reliability	Sensitivity	Specificity	LR+	LR−	QUADAS Score (0–14)
Cattrysse et al.[3] (includes only those that were significantly related among raters)	.64 to 1.00 kappa	NT	NT	NA	NA	NA
Comments: This test exhibits moderate to strong reliability but has not been tested for validity. The test is similar in construct to the Sharp Purser test. Precautions should be taken prior to use on patients who may have a dens fracture.						

TESTS FOR UPPER CERVICAL INSTABILITY

Original Sharp Purser Test

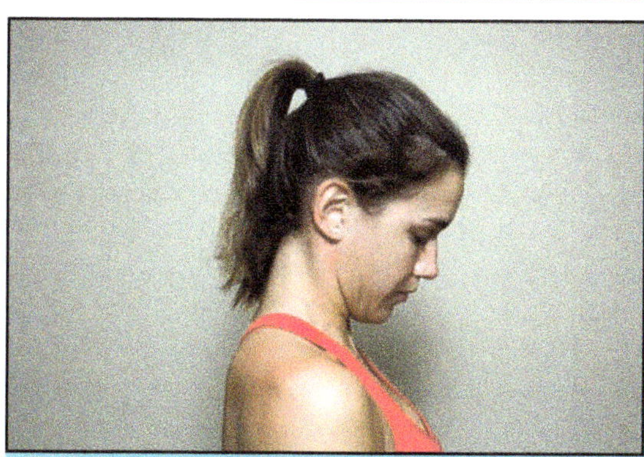

1) The patient assumes a sitting position.

2) The patient is instructed to nod the head into flexion. Reproduction of myelopathic symptoms is considered a positive test.

3) If no symptoms are encountered, the examiner can apply very gentle flexion to the forehead of the patient.

4) A positive test is identified by reproduction of myelopathic symptoms during flexion movements.

UTILITY SCORE 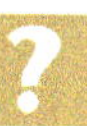

Study	Reliability	Sensitivity	Specificity	LR+	LR−	QUADAS Score (0–14)
Sharp et al.[23]	NT	NT	NT	NA	NA	NA
Comments: Sharp et al.[23] provided a very poor description of the procedure in the seminal paper. The manner in which this test is commonly taught is not the description provided by the original authors.						

Anterior Stability Test of the Atlanto-Occipital Joint

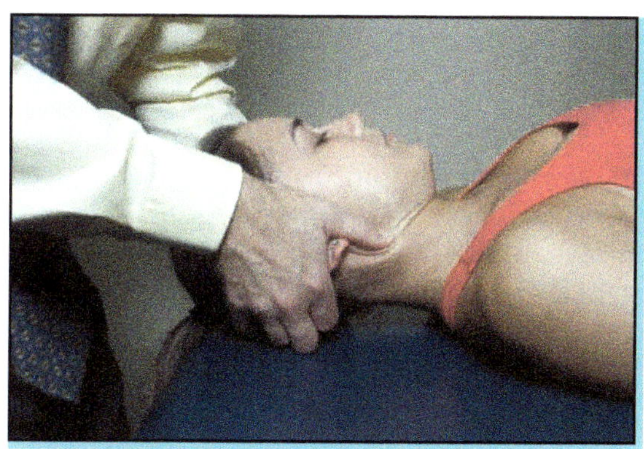

1) The patient assumes a supine position.

2) The cranium of the patient is supported with the examiner's finger under the occiput. The thumbs of the examiner are placed medially on the anterior aspect of the patient's C1–2 transverse processes.

3) The examiner lifts the occiput while simultaneously applying pressure to the anterior aspect of C1–2 transverse processes.

4) A positive test is identified either by reproduction of myelopathic symptoms during anterior translation or excess displacement during the PA movement.

UTILITY SCORE 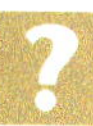

Study	Reliability	Sensitivity	Specificity	LR+	LR−	QUADAS Score (0–14)
Kaale et al.[16]	0.69 kappa	65	99	65	0.35	7
Comments: Precautions should be taken prior to use on patients who may have a dens fracture. This is another of the many cervical spine instability tests that remain uninvestigated.						

TESTS FOR UPPER CERVICAL INSTABILITY

Direct Anterior Translation Stress Test

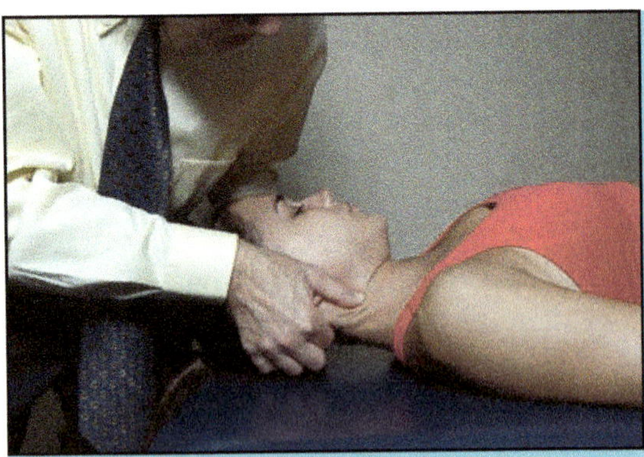

1. The patient assumes a supine position.
2. The examiner's thumbs are placed medially and anteriorly over the anterolateral aspect of the axis. The examiner's fingers are placed posteriorly over the posterior arch of the atlas.
3. The examiner applies a stress between the fingers and the thumbs.
4. A positive test is identified either by reproduction of myelopathic symptoms during translation or excess displacement during the movement.

UTILITY SCORE 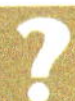

Study	Reliability	Sensitivity	Specificity	LR+	LR−	QUADAS Score (0–14)
Dobbs[8]	NT	NT	NT	NA	NA	NA
Comments: This is another poorly investigated cervical spine instability test. Precautions should be taken prior to use on patients who may have a dens fracture. This technique is difficult to perform and may not provide information beyond the modified Sharp Purser test.						

Lateral Shear Test of the Atlanto-Axial Articulation

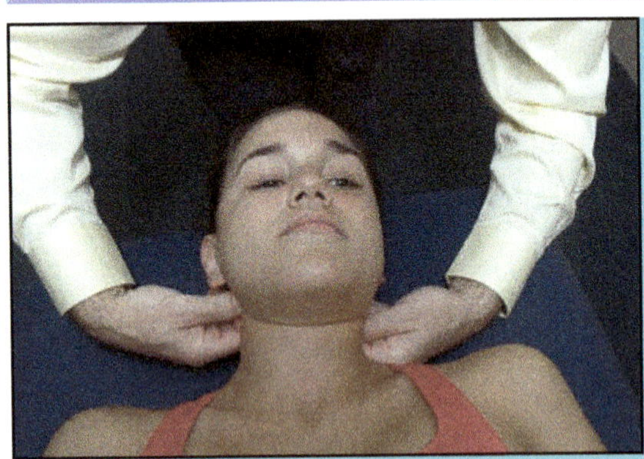

1. The patient assumes a supine position.
2. The examiner uses a "key fob" grip and stabilizes/contacts the C1 transverse process on one side. Using a key fob grip, the examiner applies the same form of grip on the opposite side of the neck at the transverse aspect of C2.
3. The examiner applies a stress between the two grips incorporating a transverse shear force.
4. A positive test is identified either by reproduction of myelopathic symptoms during translation or excess displacement during the movement.

UTILITY SCORE 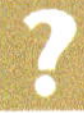

Study	Reliability	Sensitivity	Specificity	LR+	LR−	QUADAS Score (0–14)
Dobbs[8]	NT	NT	NT	NA	NA	NA
Comments: Precautions should be taken prior to use on patients who may have a dens or a Jefferson's fracture. This is another poorly studied cervical spine instability test.						

TESTS FOR UPPER CERVICAL INSTABILITY

Tectorial Membrane Test

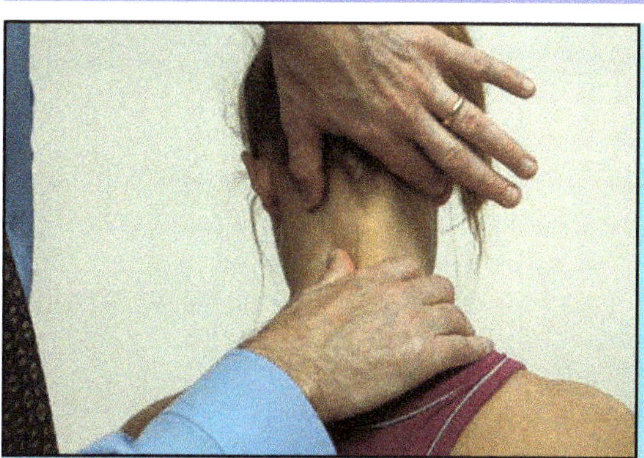

1) The patient assumes a sitting position.

2) The examiner places one hand in the suboccipital region using the thumb and the first finger against the lower aspect of the occiput. The bottom three fingers (while flexed) are placed against the spinous processes of the cervical spine and block the spine.

3) Using the other hand the examiner provides a posterior and upward force on the mastoid processes of the patient, to translate the head posteriorly. The thumb and first finger of the first hand provide a traction force.

4) A positive test is identified as excessive translation between the occiput and C1and C2.

UTILITY SCORE 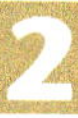

Study	Reliability	Sensitivity	Specificity	LR+	LR−	QUADAS Score (0–14)
Kaale et al.[16]	0.93 kappa	94	99	94	0.06	7
Comments: This is a difficult technique to master. The study comparative group was MRI findings in patients with whiplash associated disorders.						

Posterior Atlanto-Occipital Membrane Test

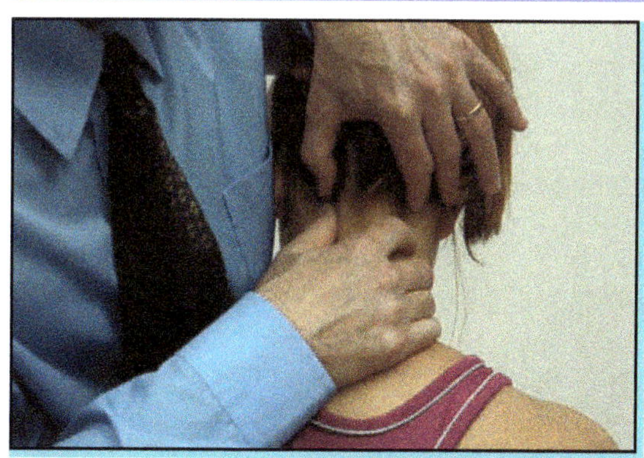

1) The patient assumes a sitting position.

2) The examiner uses one hand to pull downward on the lateral aspects of C1.

3) The examiner uses the other hand to pull upward on the occiput.

4) A positive test is identified as excessive motion during the traction assessment.

UTILITY SCORE 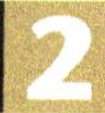

Study	Reliability	Sensitivity	Specificity	LR+	LR−	QUADAS Score (0–14)
Kaale et al.[16]	0.97 kappa	96	100	Inf	0.04	7
Comments: Precautions should be taken prior to use on patients who may have a dens or a Jefferson's fracture. This is another poorly studied cervical spine instability test.						

TESTS FOR MID-CERVICAL INSTABILITY

AP and PA Stress Testing of the Mid-Cervical Spine

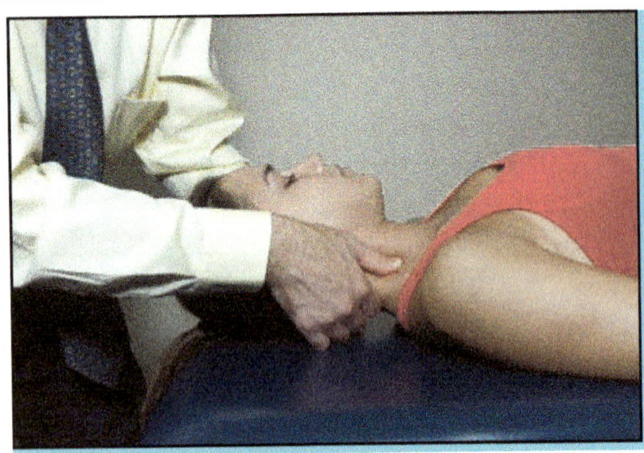

1) The patient assumes a supine position.
2) The examiner's thumbs are placed medially and anteriorly over the anterolateral aspect of the mid-cervical segments. The examiner's fingers are placed posteriorly over the posterior arch of segment above or below the tested mid-cervical segment.
3) The examiner applies a stress between the fingers and the thumbs.
4) A positive test is identified either by reproduction of myelopathic symptoms during translation or excess displacement during the movement.

UTILITY SCORE 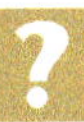

Study	Reliability	Sensitivity	Specificity	LR+	LR−	QUADAS Score (0–14)
Dobbs[8]	NT	NT	NT	NA	NA	NA
Comments: This is an untested stress test of the mid-cervical spine.						

Lateral Stress Testing of the Mid-Cervical Spine

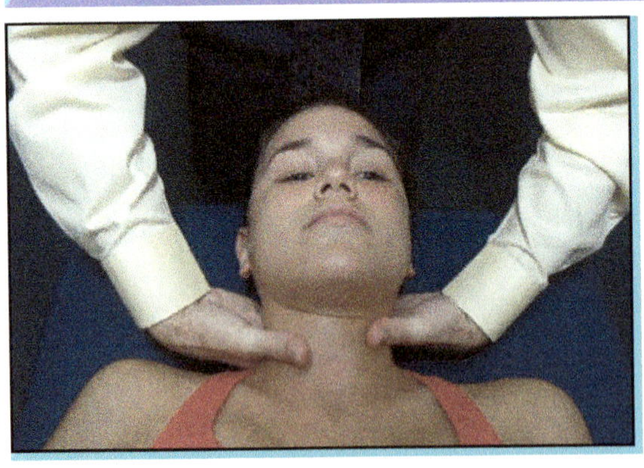

1) The patient assumes a supine position.
2) The examiner's lateral border of his or her metacarpalphalangeal joint is placed against the transverse process of a selected mid-cervical level. On the opposite side of the cervical spine, the opposite hand of the examiner provides a similar MCP grip on a mid-cervical level above or below the previous level.
3) The examiner applies a medial force to the patient's neck with each hand.
4) A positive test is identified either by reproduction of myelopathic symptoms during translation or excess displacement during the movement.

UTILITY SCORE 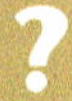

Study	Reliability	Sensitivity	Specificity	LR+	LR−	QUADAS Score (0–14)
Dobbs[8]	NT	NT	NT	NA	NA	NA
Comments: This is an untested stress test of the mid-cervical spine.						

TESTS FOR POTENTIAL VERTEBRAL ARTERY DYSFUNCTION

Vertebral Basilar Insufficiency (VBI) Test

1) The patient is interviewed to extract signs and symptoms of VBI. If remarkable, the patient is referred out for appropriate medical consult.

2) Prior to a comprehensive clinical examination, the examiner performs end-range cervical rotation tests on the patient in a sitting or supine position. The position is held for 10 seconds with observation for signs and symptoms of VBI.

3) The head is returned to a neutral position and held for a minimum of 10 seconds.

4) Rotation is repeated to the opposite side and the position is held for 10 seconds. The examiner observes for signs and symptoms of VBI. If remarkable, the patient is referred for appropriate medical consult.

5) A positive test is identified by initiation of symptoms such as dizziness, diplopia, dysphasia, dysarthria, drop attacks, nausea, and nystagmus.

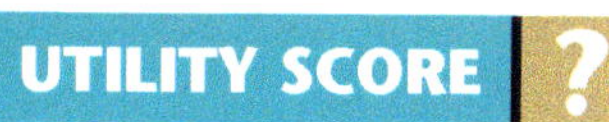

Study	Reliability	Sensitivity	Specificity	LR+	LR−	QUADAS Score (0–14)
Not tested	NT	NT	NT	NA	NA	NA

Comments: Much debate exists on the safety and applicability of the VBI tests. We recommend that it is inappropriate to perform the VBI if significant signs are present during the patient history. The test may reproduce symptoms and can be dangerous if applied injudiciously. In addition to the patient complaints listed above, numbness around the mouth, anxiety, and other neurological sensations should be investigated. The protocol selected is associated with literature that promotes end-range rotation. Others have described tests that include extension, rotation and extension, and traction. All are likely beneficial. Although VBI testing has been associated with measured reductions in blood flow, patients rarely demonstrate clinical symptoms, leading to potential finding of false positives.

TESTS FOR POTENTIAL VERTEBRAL ARTERY DYSFUNCTION

Wallenberg's Position (Extension and Rotation)

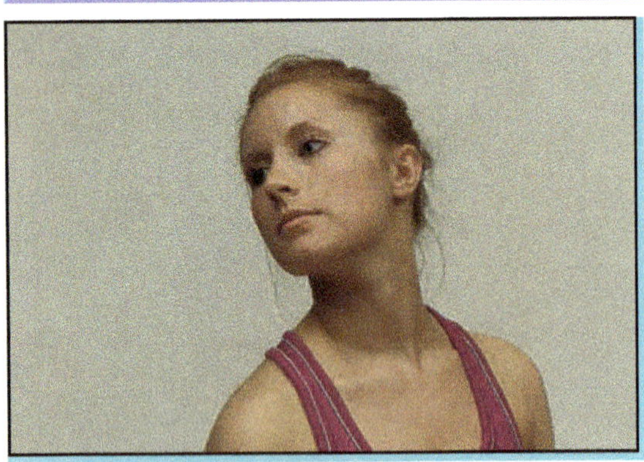

1) The patient is placed in a sitting position.

2) The head is rotated to one side and extension is added. This position is held for 30 seconds.

3) The process is repeated on the opposite side.

4) A positive test is identified by initiation of symptoms such as dizziness, diplopia, dysphasia, dysarthria, drop attacks, nausea, and nystagmus.

UTILITY SCORE 3

Study	Reliability	Sensitivity	Specificity	LR+	LR−	QUADAS Score (0–14)
Cote et al.[4] (left side 2.78 velocity)	NT	0	67	0	1.5	5
Cote et al.[4] (left side 3.49 velocity)	NT	0	71	0	1.4	5
Cote et al.[4] (right side 2.78 velocity)	NT	0	86	0	1.2	5
Cote et al.[4] (right side 3.49 velocity)	NT	0	90	0	1.1	5

Comments: Cote et al.'s[4] study used blood velocity measures (upper confidence intervals) when determining symptoms. It is unlikely that this could be replicated in the clinic. Not a well done study.

TESTS FOR CERVICOGENIC HEADACHE

Cervical-Flexion Rotation Test

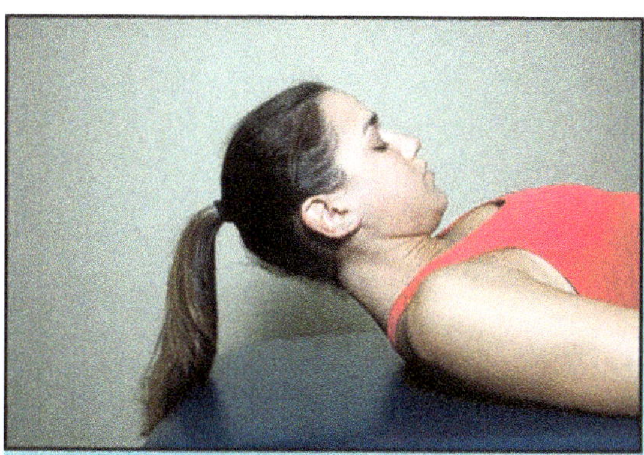

1) The patient assumes a supine position. The examiner stands at the head of the patient. Resting symptoms are assessed.

2) The patient actively moves his or her neck into maximum flexion.

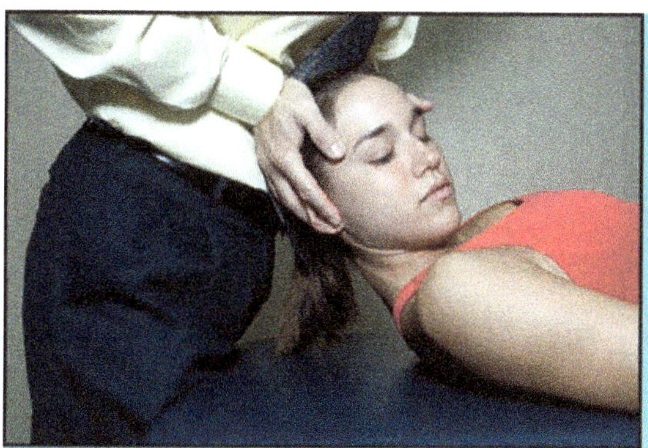

3) The examiner then applies a full rotational force to both sides. Symptoms are queried to determine if concordant.

4) The test is both a pain provocation test and a test for range of motion loss. If a loss of 10 degrees or greater is noted, the test is considered positive.

UTILITY SCORE 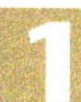

Study	Reliability	Sensitivity	Specificity	LR+	LR−	QUADAS Score (0–14)
Hall & Robinson[10]	NT	86	100	NA	NA	12
Ogince et al.[18]	0.81 kappa	91	90	9.1	0.10	10
Hall et al.[11]	0.93 kappa	90	88	7.5	0.11	8
Comments: The test likely isolates C1–C2, and most likely does not assess the presence of cervicogenic headache at other levels. All studies used a case control or a modified case control design, thus there is a risk for bias.						

TESTS FOR CERVICOGENIC HEADACHE

C0–1, C1–2, C2–3 Joint Mobility Assessment

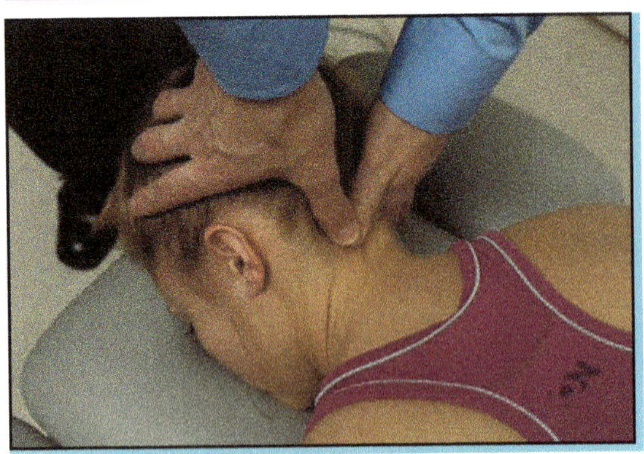

1) The patient assumes a prone position. The examiner stands at the head of the patient. Resting symptoms are assessed.

2) The examiner applies a downward force with his or her thumbs on the C1 transverse process (right and left), the C2–3 facet (right and left) (pictured) and the C2–3 facet with the head rotated toward the targeted side (right and left).

3) The test is both a pain provocation test and a test for hypomobility.

UTILITY SCORE 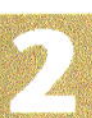

Study	Reliability	Sensitivity	Specificity	LR+	LR−	QUADAS Score (0–14)
Zito et al.[34] (C0–C1)	NT	59	82	3.3	0.49	10
Zito et al.[34] (C1–C2)	NT	62	87	4.9	0.43	10
Zito et al.[34] (C2–C3)	NT	65	78	2.9	0.44	10
Comments: This "test" is often used during normal spine differentiation. Some of the subjects were asymptomatic, which can amplify the diagnostic accuracy. Seems to be especially beneficial for C1–2.						

TESTS FOR POSTURAL DYSFUNCTION

Neck Flexor Muscle Endurance Test

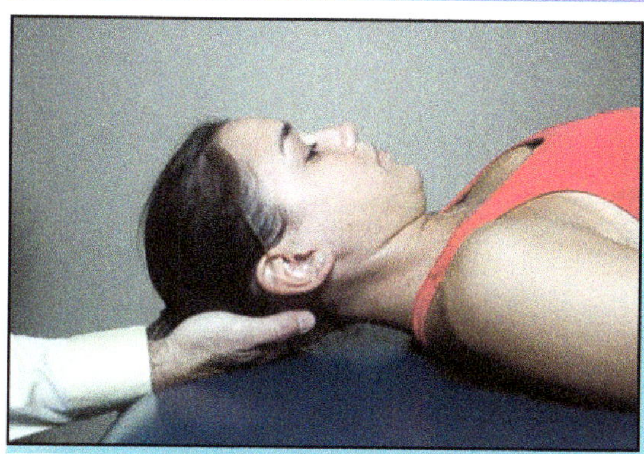

1) The patient lies in a supine position.

2) The examiner positions the patient so that the head is actively retracted and held approximately 2.5 cm off the plinth (the examiner places his or her hand under the head for knowledge of position). Visually a skin fold is present in the anterior lateral neck. A line is drawn on this skin fold.

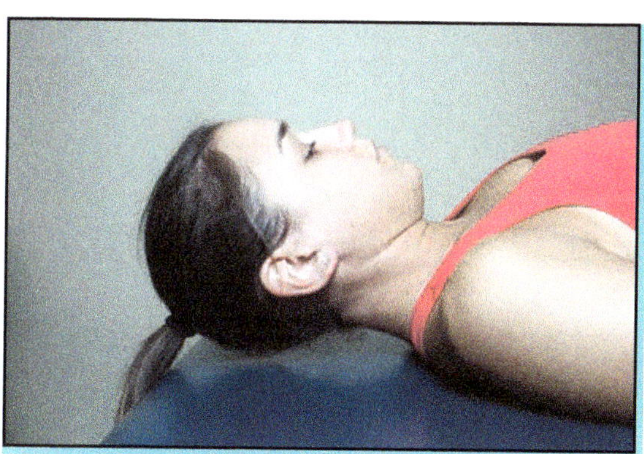

3) The patient is instructed to hold this position. If the patient's head touches the examiner's hand or he or she loses the skin folds, he or she is instructed to hold the head or tuck the chin.

4) A positive test is undefined but the test is terminated if the patient cannot hold the lines of the skin fold or cannot hold his or her head up for over a second.

UTILITY SCORE

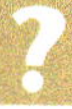

Study	Reliability	Sensitivity	Specificity	LR+	LR−	QUADAS Score (0–14)
Harris et al.[12] (without neck pain)	.82 – 91 ICC	NT	NT	NA	NA	NA
Harris et al.[12] (with neck pain)	.67 ICC	NT	NT	NA	NA	NA
Olsen et al.[19] (with neck pain)	.83, .85, .88 ICC	NT	NT	NA	NA	NA
Edmondston et al.[9]	0.93	NT	NT	NA	NA	NA

Comments: This test would benefit from a validity investigation for patients with cervicogenic headaches. It is likely that this test reflects lower cervical flexor strength, not upper cervical. The test is also used for assessment of postural dysfunction.

TESTS FOR POSTURAL DYSFUNCTION

Scapular Muscle Endurance Test

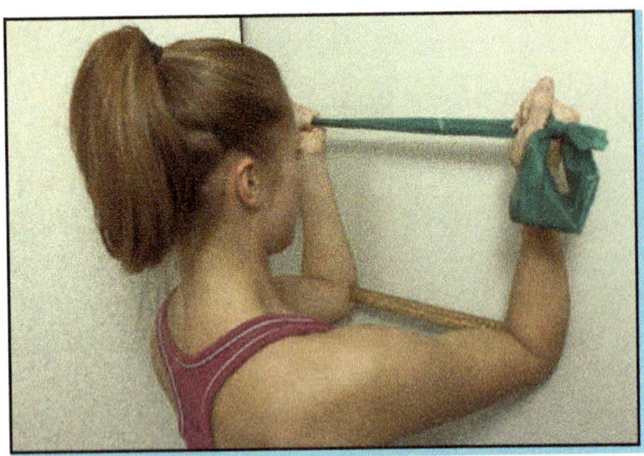

1) The patient stands near a wall and places their shoulders in 90 degrees of flexion and the elbows in 90° of flexion.

2) A ruler is placed between the elbows and the patient is requested to externally rotate their shoulders with a 1 kg force between the hands.

3) The end of the test occurs when the patient is unable to maintain the set resistance of 1 kg, or drops the ruler-spacer, or drops their shoulder below 90 degrees.

UTILITY SCORE 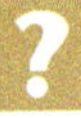

Study	Reliability	Sensitivity	Specificity	LR+	LR−	QUADAS Score (0–14)
Edmondston et al.[9]	0.67	NT	NT	NA	NA	NA
Comments: Also used as an outcome measure.						

Posterior Extensors Endurance Test

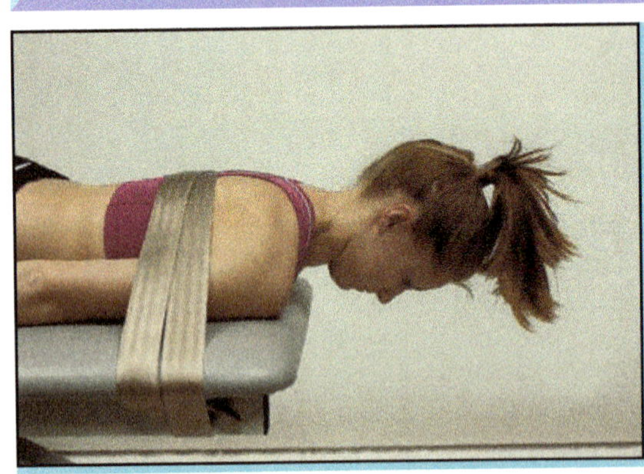

1) The patient lies in a prone position, with the head off the end of the plinth.

2) A belt is placed around the thoracic spine to reduce the chance of thoracic extension. A 2 kg weight can be placed on the patients head for loading.

3) The patient is instructed to chin retract and hold this position as long as possible.

4) A positive test when the patients head moves 5 degrees from the horizontal.

UTILITY SCORE 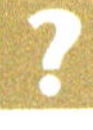

Study	Reliability	Sensitivity	Specificity	LR+	LR−	QUADAS Score (0–14)
Edmondston et al.[9]	0.88	NT	NT	NA	NA	NA
Comments: Also used as an outcome measure.						

TESTS FOR LEVEL OF DYSFUNCTION OR LINEAR STABILITY

Posterior-Anterior Mobilization Test

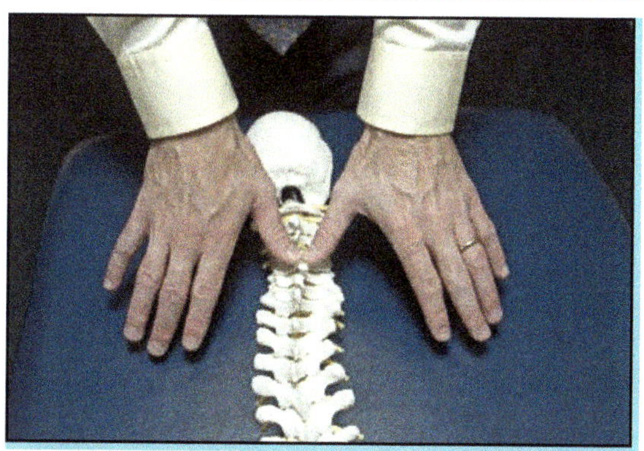

1) The patient may lie in prone or side lying. The neck is positioned in neutral and resting symptoms are assessed.

2) The examiner palpates the C2 spinous process using the tips of the thumb. Using a thumb-to-thumb application, the examiner applies a gentle downward force up to the first point of the patient's complaint of pain and the pain response is assessed.

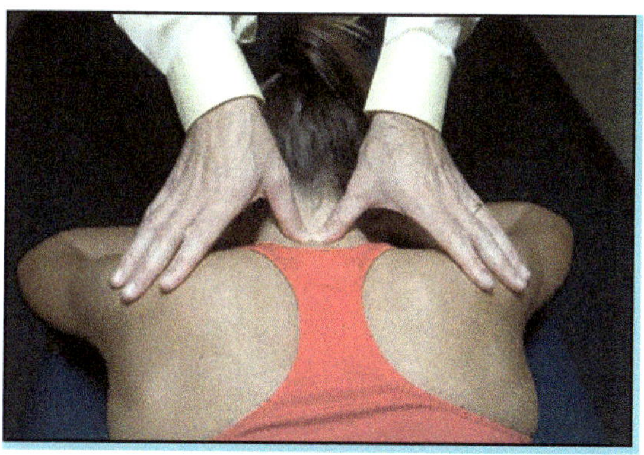

3) The examiner then pushes beyond the first point of pain, toward end range, and reassesses pain and quality of movement. Additionally, splinting or muscle spasm should be assessed. The clinician should assess if pain is concordant.

4) The examiner repeats the movements toward end range while assessing pain. One should use caution if the patient reports significant pain that is unrelenting.

5) The process is repeated on each spinous process to T4 to identify the concordant segment.

6) A positive test is identified by reproduction of the patient's concordant pain.

UTILITY SCORE 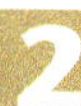

Study	Reliability	Sensitivity	Specificity	LR+	LR−	QUADAS Score (0–14)
Jull, et al.[15]	NT	100	100	NA	NA	9
Van Suijlekom et al.[31] (upper cervical tenderness)	.14 kappa	NT	NT	NA	NA	8
Van Suijlekom et al.[31] (mid-cervical tenderness)	.37 kappa	NT	NT	NA	NA	8
Van Suijlekom et al.[31] (lower cervical tenderness)	.31 kappa	NT	NT	NA	NA	8
King et al.[17] (C2–C3)	NT	88	39	1.4	0.30	5
King et al.[17] (C5–C6)	NT	89	50	1.8	0.22	5

Comments: The test results may vary based on application force, determination of what is considered a positive finding, and the examiner's conception of stiffness. It is likely that this test is highly sensitive at implicating the level of a disorder, but is not specific for a pathological process.

TESTS FOR LEVEL OF DYSFUNCTION OR LINEAR STABILITY

Palpation of Physiological Movement

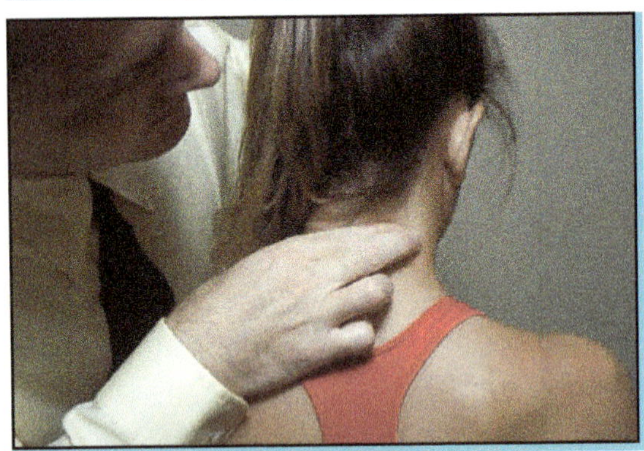

1) The patient is placed in a sitting position.

2) The examiner palpates the lateral aspect of C2–3 (articular pillars) with his or her fingers. The opposite hand stabilizes the head in order to apply a lateral/extension movement.

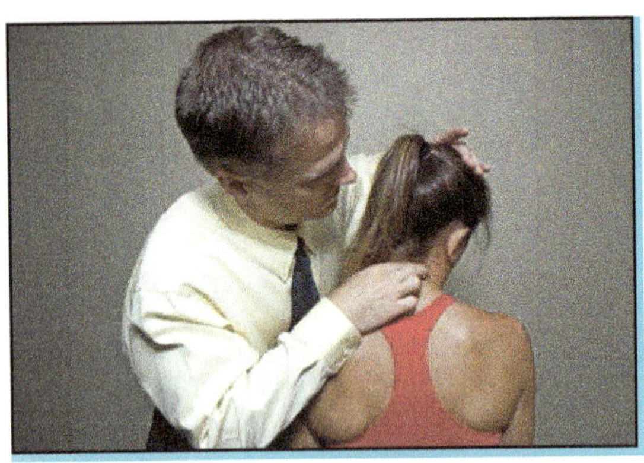

3) The examiner applies a series of lateral/extension movements to feel the amount of motion at that segment. The same procedure can be used for lower segments.

4) Increased movement at one level versus another is considered positive.

UTILITY SCORE 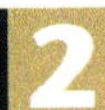

Study	Reliability	Sensitivity	Specificity	LR+	LR−	QUADAS Score (0–14)
Smedmark et al.[24] (C1–2 rotation)	.28 kappa	NT	NT	NA	NA	NA
Smedmark et al.[24] (C2–3 rotation)	.43 kappa	NT	NT	NA	NA	NA
Smedmark et al.[24] (C7 flex-extension)	.36 kappa	NT	NT	NA	NA	NA
Humphreys et al.[14] (C2–3 block)	.76 kappa	98	91	10.9	0.02	11
Humphreys et al.[14] (C5–6 block)	.46 kappa	78	55	1.7	0.4	11
Sandmark & Nisell[21] (not for radiculopathy)	NT	82	79	3.9	0.23	9
Rey-Einz et al.[20] (C3–C4)	0.75 kappa	83.3	76.3	3.5	0.21	11
Rey-Einz et al.[20] (C4–C5)	0.65	100	79.5	4.9	0.00	11
Rey-Einz et al.[20] (C5–C6)	0.60	100	34.8	1.5	0.00	11
Comments: The testing procedure appears to be sensitive in identifying fused joint levels or degenerative levels identified during a radiograph. Sensitivity may decline in lower joints.						

TESTS TO IDENTIFY NECK PAIN FROM ASYMPTOMATIC CONDITIONS

Manual Examination of Rotation

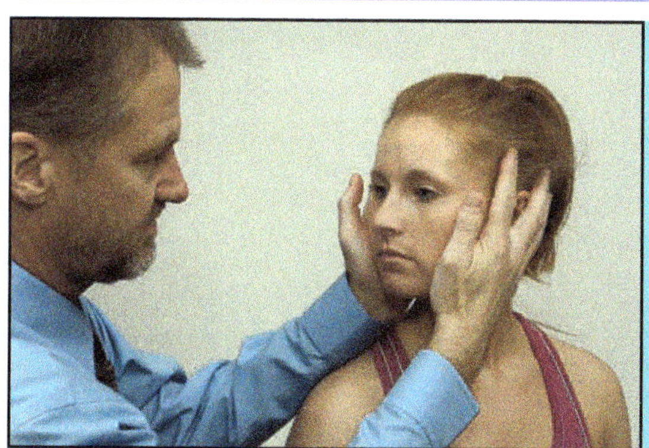

1) The patient is placed in a sitting position.

2) The examiner palpates the spinous processes of C0, C2, and C7 and uses these locations as landmarks.

3) The examiner applies a passive rotation to the neck (left and right) and scores the passive movement as hypermobile, normal, and hypomobile).

4) A positive finding is hyper/hypomobility and/or a hard or empty end feel.

UTILITY SCORE 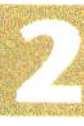

Study	Reliability	Sensitivity	Specificity	LR+	LR−	QUADAS Score (0–14)
DeHertogh et al.[6]	NT	77.2	90.0	7.7	025	9
Comments: It was a nicely done study but there were patients with no symptoms (case control design).						

Combined Manual Rotation and a Visual Analog Scale

The clustered findings included a standard 100 mm visual analog scale (using 20 mm or greater as a positive finding) and the manual rotation described above.

UTILITY SCORE 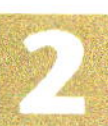

Study	Reliability	Sensitivity	Specificity	LR+	LR−	QUADAS Score (0–14)
DeHertogh et al.[6]	NT	88.9	86.5	6.6	0.21	9
Comments: It was a nicely done study but there were patients with no symptoms (case control design). It's very likely that one can tell who has neck pain versus who doesn't and that's probably why the results are pretty high.						

TESTS TO DETERMINE IF A RADIOGRAPH IS REQUIRED

Canadian C-Spine Rules

1) Patients who are cognitively intact and have no neurological symptoms; or
2) Patients who are under the age of 65; or
3) Patients who are not fearful of moving the head upon command; or
4) Patients who were not involved in a distraction-based injury; or
5) Patients who demonstrate no midline pain do not need a radiograph.
6) Any positive finding in any of the above five categories should result in a radiographic test.

UTILITY SCORE 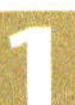

Study	Reliability	Sensitivity	Specificity	LR+	LR−	QUADAS Score (0–14)
Stiell et al.[26] (not including indeterminate cases)	NT	99	45	1.81	0.01	12
Stiell et al.[26] (not including indeterminate cases)	NT	99	45	1.81	0.01	12
Stiell et al.[26] (including indeterminant cases)	NT	99	91	10.7	0.01	12
Stiell et al.[27]	.6 kappa	100	43	NT	NT	12
Bandiera et al.[1]	.6 kappa	100	43	NT	NT	9

Comments: Because the test is designed as a screen it is imperative that the findings exhibit high sensitivity. In order to rule out the need for an x-ray, all five categories should be negative. The decision rules are designed to be used in the acute stage of the injury.

NEXUS (National Emergency X-Radiography Utilization Study)

1) Patients who do not have tenderness at posterior midline of the cervical spine.
2) Patients who have no focal neurological deficit.
3) Patients who have a normal level of alertness.
4) Patients who have no evidence of intoxication.
5) Patients who do not have a clinically apparent, painful injury that may distract them from a cervical injury.
6) Any positive finding in any of the above five categories should result in a radiographic test.

TESTS TO DETERMINE IF A RADIOGRAPH IS REQUIRED

UTILITY SCORE 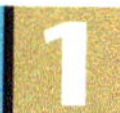

Study	Reliability	Sensitivity	Specificity	LR+	LR–	QUADAS Score (0–14)
Stiell et al.[26]	.52 to .72 kappa	91	37	1.43	0.25	12
Dickinson et al.[7]	.23 to .78 kappa	93	38	1.49	0.19	9
Hoffman et al.[13]	NT	99	13	1.14	0.08	11
Comments: Note the lower sensitivity values, suggesting this "screen" is less effective than the Canadian C-Spine rules. Nonetheless, the test still demonstrates value. The rules are designed to be used in the acute stage of the injury.						

Key Points

1. The majority of clinical special tests for cervical radiculopathy have been investigated within the literature.
2. Many of the clinical special tests for cervical instability have not been investigated for diagnostic accuracy. Those that have been studied may be influenced by bias.
3. Tests such as the ULTT and Brachial Plexus Compression have high sensitivity for detection of cervical radiculopathy.
4. The Spurling's compression test demonstrates variable findings, depending on the studies cited.
5. Although untested for diagnostic accuracy, the vertebral basilar insufficiency test is likely not sensitive but a specific test, albeit of high risk if findings are noted.
6. Prior to administration of cervical spine instability tests, specifically after trauma, one should perform the Canadian C-Spine rules.
7. The Canadian C-Spine rules, used to detect who would benefit from a radiograph, are highly sensitive and function very well as a screen in the acutely injured patient.
8. The flexion-rotation test for cervicogenic headaches detection is likely diagnostic because the criteria included for patients with cervicogenic headaches was very specific.

References

1. Bandiera G, Stiell IG, Wells GA, Clement C, De Maio V, Vandemheen KL, Greenberg GH, Lesiuk H, Brison R, Cass D, Dreyer J, Eisenhauer MA, Macphail I, McKnight RD, Morrison L, Reardon M, Schull M, Worthington J; Canadian C-Spine and CT Head Study Group. The Canadian C-spine rule performs better than unstructured physician judgment. *Ann Emerg Med.* 2003;42(3):395–402.
2. Bertilson B, Grunnesjo M, Strender LE. Reliability of clinical tests in the assessment of patient with neck/shoulder problems—impact of history. *Spine.* 2003;19:2222–2231.
3. Cattrysse E, Swinkels RA, Oostendorp RA, Duquet W. Upper cervical instability: Are clinical tests reliable? *Man Ther.* 1997;2(2):91–97.
4. Cote P, Krietz BG, Cassidy JD, Thiel H. The validity of the extension-rotation test as a clinical screening procedure before neck manipulation: A secondary analysis. *J Manip Physiol Therapeutics.* 1996;19:159–164.
5. Davidson R, Dunn E, Metzmaker J. The shoulder abduction test in the diagnosis of radicular pain in cervical extradural compression monoradiculopathies. *Spine.* 1981;6:441–445.

6. DeHertogh WJ, Vaes PH, Vijverman V, DeCordt A, Duquet W. The clinical examination of neck pain patients: The validity of a group of tests. *Man Ther.* 2007;12:50–55.

7. Dickinson G, Stiell IG, Schull M, Brison R, Clement CM, Vandemheen KL, Cass D, McKnight D, Greenberg G, Worthington JR, Reardon M, Morrison L, Eisenhauer MA, Dreyer J, Wells GA. Retrospective application of the NEXUS low-risk criteria for cervical spine radiography in Canadian emergency departments. *Ann Emerg Med.* 2004;43(4):507–514.

8. Dobbs A. Manual therapy assessment of cervical instability. *Orthopaedic Physical Therapy Clinics of North America.* 2001;10:431–454.

9. Edmondston SJ, Wallumrod M, MacLeid F, Kvamme L, Joebges S, Brabham GC. Reliability of isometric muscle endurance tests in subjects with postural neck pain. *J Manipulative Physiol Ther.* 2008;31:348–354.

10. Hall T, Robinson K. The flexion-rotation test and active cervical mobility—a comparative measurement study in cervicogenic headache. *Man Ther.* 2004;9(4): 197–202.

11. Hall T, Robinson K, Fujinawa O, Alkaska K, Pyne E. Interester reliability and diagnostic validity of the cervical flexion-rotation test. *J Manipulative Physiol Ther.* 2008;31:293–300.

12. Harris KD, Heer DM, Roy TC, Santos DM, Whitman JM, Wainner RS. Reliability of a measurement of neck flexor muscle endurance. *Phys Ther.* 2005;85(12): 1349–1355.

13. Hoffman JR, Mower WR, Wolfson AB, Todd KH, Zucker MI. Validity of a set of clinical criteria to rule out injury to the cervical spine in patients with blunt trauma. National Emergency X-Radiography Utilization Study Group. *N Engl J Med.* 2000;343(2):94–99.

14. Humphreys BK, Delahaye M, Peterson CK. An investigation into the validity of cervical spine motion palpation using patients with congenital block vertebrae as a "gold standard." *BMC Musculoskelet Disord.* 2004;5:19.

15. Jull G, Bogduk N, Marsland A. The accuracy of manual diagnosis for cervical zygapophyseal joint pain syndromes. *Med J Aust.* 1988;148(5):233–236.

16. Kaale BR, Krakenes J, Albrektsen G, Wester K. Clinical assessment techniques for detecting ligament and membrane injuries in the upper cervical spine region—A comparison with MRI results. *Man Ther.* 2008;13: 397–403.

17. King W, Lau P, Lees R, Bogduk N. The validity of manual examination in assessing patients with neck pain. *Spine J.* 2005;7:22–26.

18. Ogince M, Hall T, Robinson K, Blackmore AM. The diagnostic validity of the cervical flexion-rotation test in C1–2 related cervicogenic headache. *Man Ther.* 2007;12:256–262.

19. Olsen L, Millar L, Dunker J, Hicks J, Glanz D. Reliability of a clinical test for deep cervical flexor endurance. *J Manipulative Physiol Therapeutics.* 2006;29:134–138.

20. Rey-Einz G, Alburquerque-Sendin F, Barrera-Mellado I, Martin-Vallejo F, Fenandez-de-las-Penas C. Validity of the posterior-anterior middle cervical spine gliding test for the examination of intervertebral joint hypermobility in mechanical neck pain. *J Manipulative Physiol Ther.* 2010;33:279–285.

21. Sandmark H, Nisell R. Validity of five common manual neck pain provoking tests. *Scand J Rehabil Med.* 1995;27(3):131–136.

22. Shah KC, Rajshekhar V. Reliability of diagnosis of soft cervical disc prolapse using Spurling's test. *Br J Neurosurg.* 2004;18(5):480–483.

23. Sharp J, Purser DW, Lawrence JS. Rheumatoid arthritis of the cervical spine in the adult. *Ann Rheum Dis.* 1958;17(3):303–313.

24. Smedmark V, Wallin M, Arvidsson I. Inter-examiner reliability in assessing passive intervertebral motion of the cervical spine. *Man Ther.* 2000;5(2):97–101.

25. Spurling RG, Scoville WB. Lateral rupture of the cervical intervertebral disc. *Surg Gynecol Obstet.* 1944;78: 350–358.

26. Stiell IG, Clement CM, McKnight RD, Brison R, Schull MJ, Rowe BH, Worthington JR, Eisenhauer MA, Cass D, Greenberg G, MacPhail I, Dreyer J, Lee JS, Bandiera G, Reardon M, Holroyd B, Lesiuk H, Wells GA. The Canadian C-spine rule versus the NEXUS low-risk criteria in patients with trauma. *N Engl J Med.* 2003;349(26): 2510–2518.

27. Stiell IG, Wells GA, Vandemheen KL, Clement CM, Lesiuk H, De Maio VJ, Laupacis A, Schull M, McKnight RD, Verbeek R, Brison R, Cass D, Dreyer J, Eisenhauer MA, Greenberg GH, MacPhail I, Morrison L, Reardon M, Worthington J. The Canadian C-spine rule for radiography in alert and stable trauma patients. *JAMA.* 2001;286(15):1841–1848.

28. Tong HC, Haig AJ, Yamakawa K. The Spurling test and cervical radiculopathy. *Spine.* 2002;27(2):156–159.

29. Uchihara T, Furukawa T, Tsukagoshi H. Compression of brachial plexus as a diagnostic test of cervical cord lesion. *Spine.* 1994;19(19):2170–2173.

30. Uitvlugt G, Indenbaum S. Clinical assessment of atlantoaxial instability using the Sharp-Purser test. *Arthritis Rheum.* 1988;31(7): 918–922.

31. Van Suijlekom HA, De Vet HC, Van Den Berg SG, Weber WE. Interobserver reliability in physical examination of the cervical spine in patients with headache. *Headache.* 2000;40 (7):581–586.

32. Viikari-Juntura E, Porras M, Laasonen EM. Validity of clinical tests in the diagnosis of root compression in cervical disc disease. *Spine.* 1989;14(3):253–257.

33. Wainner RS, Fritz JM, Irrgang JJ, Boninger ML, Delitto A, Allison S. Reliability and diagnostic accuracy of the clinical examination and patient self-report measures for cervical radiculopathy. *Spine* 2003;28(1):52–62.

34. Zito G, Jull G, Story I. Clinical tests of musculoskeletal dysfunction in the diagnosis of cervicogenic headache. *Man Ther.* 2006;11:118–129.

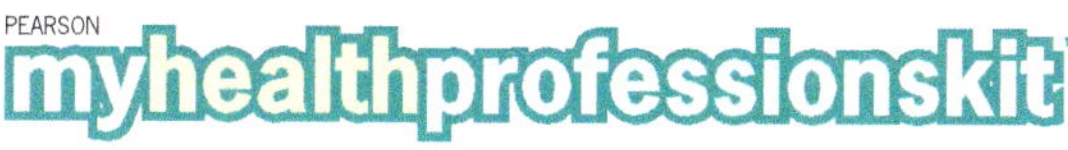

Use this address to access the Companion Website created for this textbook. Simply select "Physical Therapy" from the choice of disciplines. Find this book and log in using your username and password to access video clips of selected tests.

Physical Examination Tests for the Temporomandibular Joint

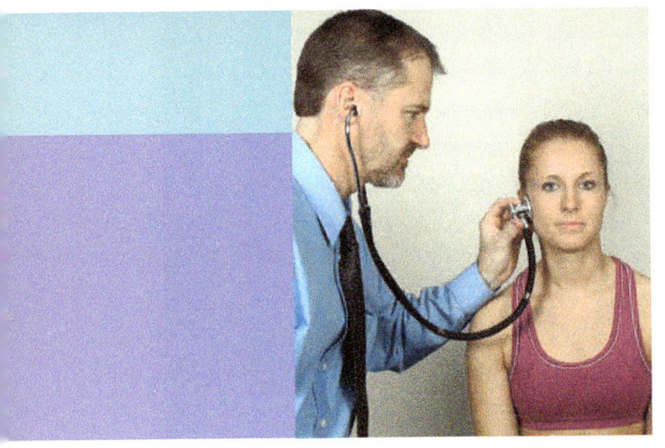

Physical Examination Tests for the Temporomandibular Joint

Jennifer Reneker and Chad E. Cook

Please refer to the chapter "Introduction to Diagnostic Accuracy" before reading this chapter.

Index of Tests

Tests for Temporomandibular Joint Dysfunction

TESTS FOR TEMPOROMANDIBULAR JOINT DYSFUNCTION

Pain During Active Movements

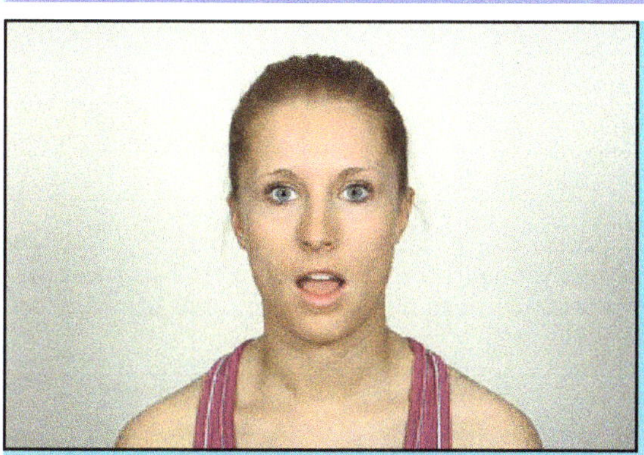

1) The patient is seated with the mouth partially closed, near its resting position.

2) The patient is instructed to open his or her mouth and report if the concordant pain is present during the opening process or near the end range.

3) A positive test finding is concordant (familiar) pain during any of the active movements.

UTILITY SCORE 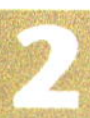

Study	Reliability	Sensitivity	Specificity	LR+	LR−	QUADAS Score (0–14)
Manfredini et al.[5] (effusion)	NT	81.9	60.6	2.08	0.30	10
Stegenga et al.[9] (DDR)	NT	44	31	0.64	1.81	8
Stegenga et al.[9] (DDNR)	NT	74	57	1.72	0.46	8
Yatani et al.[12] (DDR)	NT	17	69.9	0.56	1.19	8
Yatani et al.[12] (DDNR)	NT	59.1	87.9	4.90	0.47	8
Comments: DDR = disc displacement with reduction; DDNR = disc displacement without reduction. Note that in all instances the movements are used to differentiate one form of TMD classification from another.						

Pain During Active-Assistive Opening

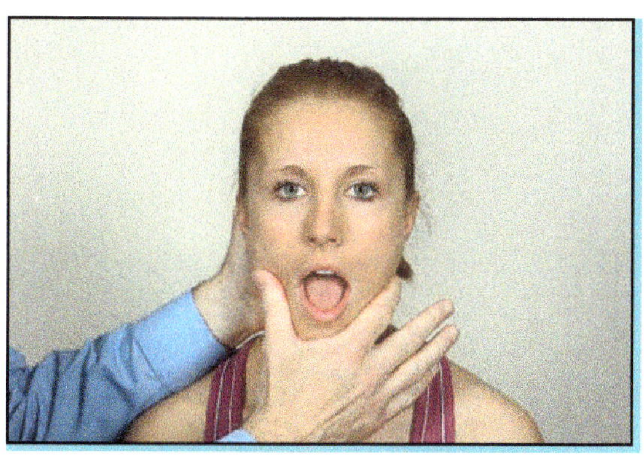

1) The patient is seated with the mouth partially closed, near its resting position.

2) The patient is instructed to open his or her mouth and report if the concordant pain is present during the opening process or near the end range.

3) The clinician furthers the opening movement with an active-assistive facilitation.

4) A positive test finding is concordant (familiar) pain during any of the active movements.

(continued)

TESTS FOR TEMPOROMANDIBULAR JOINT DYSFUNCTION

UTILITY SCORE 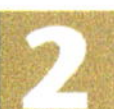

Study	Reliability	Sensitivity	Specificity	LR+	LR−	QUADAS Score (0–14)
Manfredini et al.[5] (effusion)	NT	93.4	1.6	0.95	4.13	10
Orsini et al.[7] (DDNR)	NT	55.4	90.8	6.02	0.49	10
Stegenga et al.[9] (DDR)	NT	47	29	0.66	1.83	8
Stegenga et al.[9] (DDNR)	NT	78	57	1.81	0.39	8
Comments: DDR = disc displacement with reduction; DDNR = disc displacement without reduction. Note that in all instances the movements are used to differentiate one form of TMD classification from another. Appears to only have value during identification of DDNR.						

Pain During Palpatory Testing

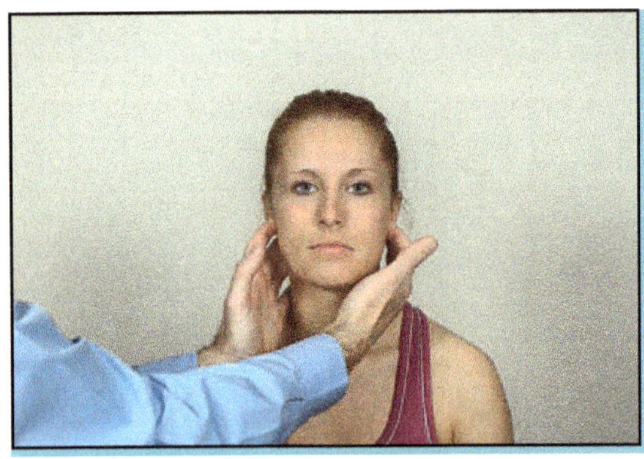

1) The patient is seated with the mouth partially closed, near its resting position.

2) The clinician instructs the patient to bite down and initiates the palpation sequence by palpating the temporalis and masseter muscles.

3) The clinician instructs the patient to fully open his or her mouth and initiates the palpation sequence by palpating the submandibular muscles.

4) The clinician then instructs the patient to relax.

5) The clinician palpates the joints of the TMJ externally, both laterally and posteriorly.

6) A positive test finding is concordant (familiar) pain during any of the palpatory tests.

TESTS FOR TEMPOROMANDIBULAR JOINT DYSFUNCTION

UTILITY SCORE 2

Study	Reliability	Sensitivity	Specificity	LR+	LR−	QUADAS Score (0–14)
Holmlund & Axelsson[2] (synovitis)	NT	88	36	1.38	0.33	7
Manfredini et al.[5] (effusion)	NT	(P)85.2 (L)83.6	62.2 68.8	2.25 2.68	0.24 0.24	10
Stegenga et al.[9] (DDR)	NT	38	41	0.64	1.51	8
Stegenga et al.[9] (DDNR)	NT	66	67	2.00	0.51	8
Usumez et al.[10] (DDR)	NT	100	11.9	1.14	0	7
Usumez et al.[10] (DDNR)	NT	100	7.9	1.09	0	7
Visscher et al.[11] (full region)	NT	75	67	2.3	0.4	6
Lobbezoo-Scholte et al.[4] (full region)	NT	86	64	2.4	0.2	8
Comments: P = posterior; L = lateral; DDR = disc displacement with reduction; DDNR = disc displacement without reduction. Note that in all instances the movements are used to differentiate one form of TMD classification from another. Appears to only have value during identification of DDNR. The finding may be very useful to rule out TMD when differentiating the disorder from a competing problem.						

Pain During Resistive Testing

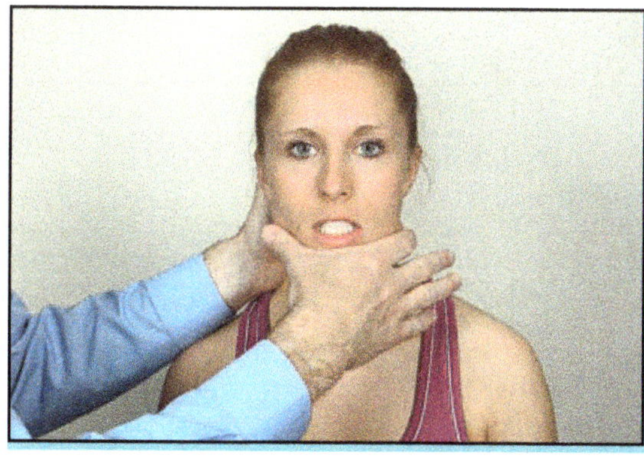

1) The patient is seated with the mouth partially closed, near its resting position.

2) The clinician instructs the patient to bite down, open, laterally deviate, protrude, and to perform retrusion, all with resistance.

3) A positive test finding is concordant (familiar) pain during any of the resistive testing.

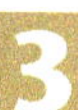

UTILITY SCORE 3

Study	Reliability	Sensitivity	Specificity	LR+	LR−	QUADAS Score (0–14)
Manfredini et al.[5] (effusion)	NT	73.7	44.2	1.32	0.60	10
Comments: Resistive testing was only used to differentiate effusion from other forms of TMD.						

TESTS FOR TEMPOROMANDIBULAR JOINT DYSFUNCTION

Limitations of Mouth Opening (Active)

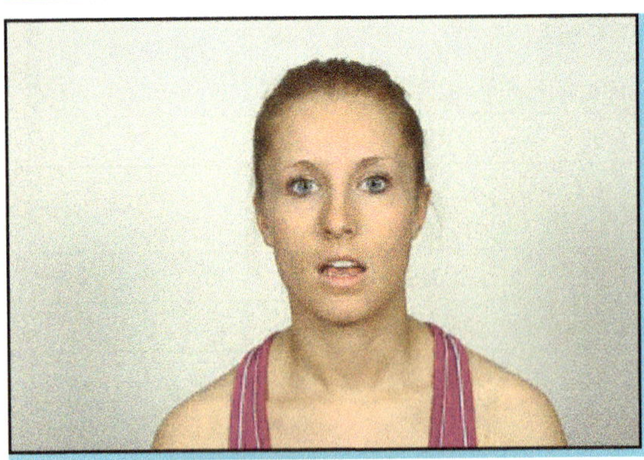

1) The patient is seated with the mouth partially closed, near its resting position.

2) The patient is instructed to open his or her mouth to its limit.

3) A positive test is a reduction in full mouth opening.

UTILITY SCORE 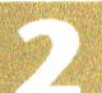

Study	Reliability	Sensitivity	Specificity	LR+	LR−	QUADAS Score (0–14)
Orsini et al.[7] (DDNR)	NT	32.4	83.2	1.93	0.81	10
Stegenga et al.[9] (DDR)	NT	38	21	0.48	2.95	8
Stegenga et al.[9] (DDNR)	NT	86	62	2.26	0.23	8
Usumez et al.[10] (DDR)	NT	10.5	59.5	0.26	1.50	7
Usumez et al.[10] (DDNR)	NT	76.5	87.3	6.02	0.27	7
Yatani et al.[12] (DDR)	NT	5.4	69.8	0.18	1.36	8
Yatani et al.[12] (DDNR)	NT	43.3	83.6	2.64	0.68	8

Comments: DDR = disc displacement with reduction; DDNR = disc displacement without reduction. It's very difficult to determine the value of restricted mouth opening. It does appear to slightly differentiate DDNR from DDR, in the one study of higher quality.

Limitations in Protrusion

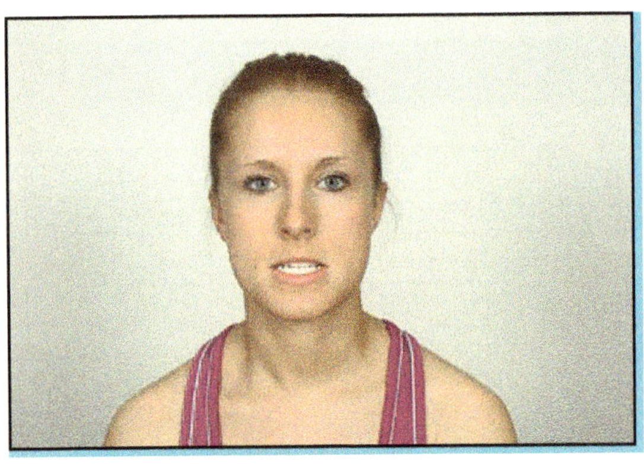

1) The patient is seated with the mouth partially closed, near its resting position.

2) The patient is instructed to protrude his or her mouth to its limit.

3) A positive test is a reduction in full protrusion.

TESTS FOR TEMPOROMANDIBULAR JOINT DYSFUNCTION

UTILITY SCORE 3

Study	Reliability	Sensitivity	Specificity	LR+	LR−	QUADAS Score (0–14)
Holmlund & Axelsson[2] (any disc dysfunction)	NT	90	40	1.5	0.25	6
Stegenga et al.[9] (DDR)	NT	29	38	0.47	1.87	8
Stegenga et al.[9] (DDNR)	NT	62	64	1.7	0.59	8

Comments: DDR = disc displacement with reduction; DDNR = disc displacement without reduction. Low quality studies reduce the likelihood of truly knowing the value of this clinical finding.

Limitations in Lateral Condylar Translation

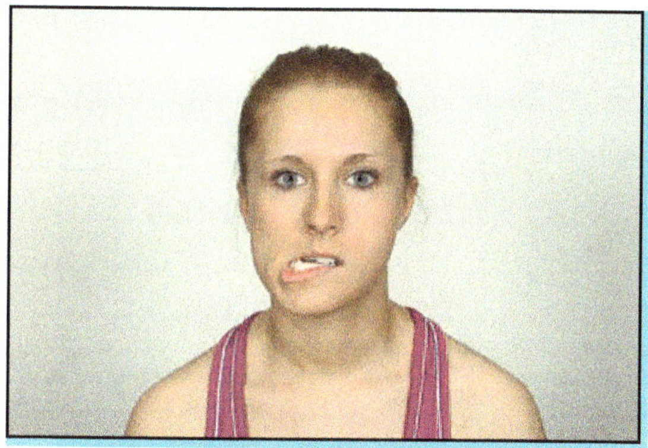

1) The patient is seated with the mouth partially closed, near its resting position.

2) The patient is instructed to laterally transfer his or her mandible to its limit.

3) A positive test is a reduction of lateral transfer.

UTILITY SCORE 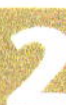

Study	Reliability	Sensitivity	Specificity	LR+	LR−	QUADAS Score (0–14)
Orsini et al.[7] (DDNR)	NT	68.9	80.7	3.57	0.39	10
Stegenga et al.[9] (DDR)	NT	15	38	2.4	2.24	8
Stegenga et al.[9] (DDNR)	NT	66	81	3.47	0.42	8
Yatani et al.[12] (DDR)	NT	10.7	56.1	0.24	1.59	8
Yatani et al.[12] (DDNR)	NT	77.8	82.5	4.44	0.27	8

Comments: DDR = disc displacement with reduction; DDNR = disc displacement without reduction. There appears to be value in detecting a DDNR and differentiating this from a DDR or other classification.

TESTS FOR TEMPOROMANDIBULAR JOINT DYSFUNCTION

Limitations in Contralateral Movement

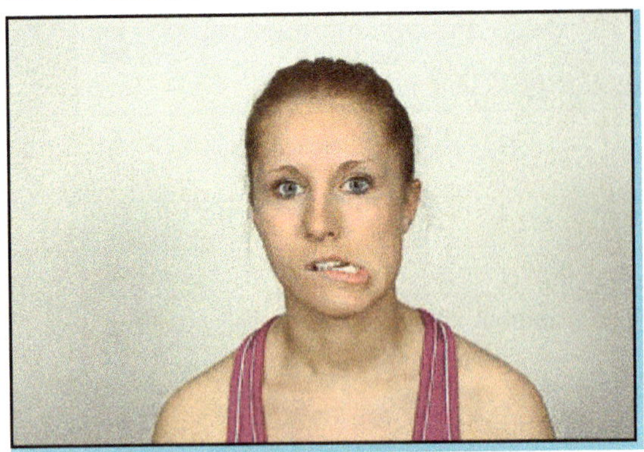

1) The patient is seated with the mouth partially closed, near its resting position.

2) The patient is instructed to laterally transfer the jaw, comparing one side to the other.

3) A positive test is a reduction of movement of one side of the jaw in comparison to the other.

UTILITY SCORE 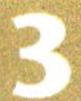

Study	Reliability	Sensitivity	Specificity	LR+	LR−	QUADAS Score (0–14)
Holmlund & Axelsson[2] (ID)	NT	60	54	1.3	0.74	6
Stegenga et al.[9] (DDR)	NT	15	34	0.22	2.5	8
Stegenga et al.[9] (DDNR)	NT	66	76	2.75	0.45	8

Comments: ID = internal dysfunction; DDR = disc displacement with reduction; DDNR = disc displacement without reduction. Poorly designed studies reduce the assumptions of this finding. There appears to be marginal value in differentiating classifications.

Limitations on Mouth Opening (Passive)

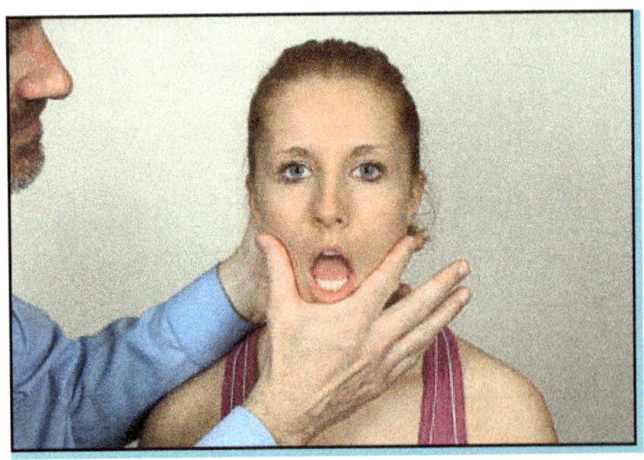

1) The patient is seated with the mouth partially closed, near its resting position.

2) The clinician passively opens the patient's mouth to its limit.

3) A positive finding is a reduction of mouth opening.

UTILITY SCORE 

Study	Reliability	Sensitivity	Specificity	LR+	LR−	QUADAS Score (0–14)
Stegenga et al.[9] DDR	NT	29	29	0.41	2.4	8
Stegenga et al.[9] DDNR	NT	76	69	2.45	0.35	8

Comments: DDR = disc displacement with reduction; DDNR = disc displacement without reduction. It is certainly not useful in discriminating DDR.

TESTS FOR TEMPOROMANDIBULAR JOINT DYSFUNCTION

Deviation from Symmetrical during Mouth Opening

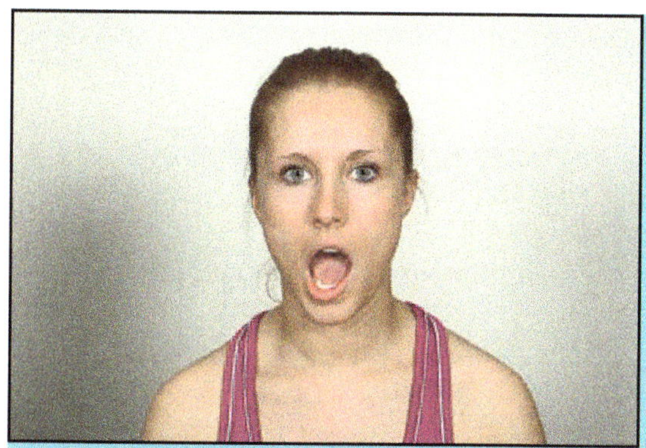

1) The patient is seated with the mouth partially closed, near its resting position.

2) The patient is instructed to open their mouth near end range.

3) The patient is instructed to deviate laterally their mouth (left and right) near end range.

4) The patient is instructed to close their mouth to end range.

5) A positive finding is any deviation from midline or a variation in lateral excursion from right to left.

UTILITY SCORE 2

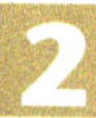

Study	Reliability	Sensitivity	Specificity	LR+	LR−	QUADAS Score (0–14)
Orsini et al.[7] (DDNR)	NT	32.4	87	2.49	0.78	10
Stegenga et al.[9] (DDR with correction)	NT	44	83	2.59	0.67	8
Stegenga et al.[9] (DDNR with correction)	NT	14	57	0.33	1.51	8
Stegenga et al.[9] (DDR without correction)	NT	18	41	0.30	2.0	8
Stegenga et al.[9] (DDNR without correction)	NT	66	83	3.88	0.41	8
Usumez et al.[10] (DDR)	NT	92.1	31	1.33	0.25	7
Usumez et al.[10] (DDNR)	NT	35.3	7.9	0.38	8.19	7
Lobbezoo-Scholte et al.[4] (any deviation)	NT	56	83	3.3	0.5	8
Lobbezoo-Scholte et al.[4] (any deviation)	NT	95	45	1.7	0.1	8

Comments: DDR = disc displacement with reduction; DDNR = disc displacement without reduction. Several studies have looked at this and there does appear to be value in looking at deviation during movement.

TESTS FOR TEMPOROMANDIBULAR JOINT DYSFUNCTION

Maximal Mouth Opening

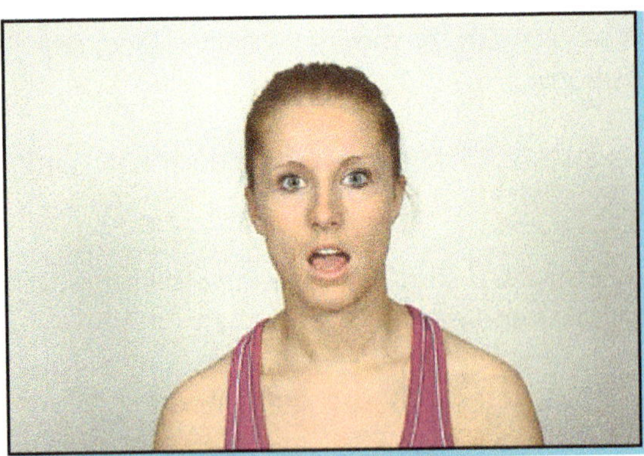

1) The patient is seated with the mouth partially closed, near its resting position.

2) The patient is instructed to open his or her mouth to the widest possible tolerated level.

3) The clinician measures the height of the opening by measuring the space between the bottom of the top teeth and the top of the bottom teeth.

4) A positive test finding is concordant (familiar) pain during maximal mouth opening or measured limitations in opening.

UTILITY SCORE 

Study	Reliability	Sensitivity	Specificity	LR+	LR−	QUADAS Score (0–14)
Visscher et al.[11] (overpressure during maximal mouth opening)	NT	80	64	2.2	0.3	6
Dworkin et al.[1] (maximal mouth opening of < 35mm for men and < 30mm for women)	NT	22	98	11	0.8	8
Comments: Low quality studies but there does appear to be some value in recognition of TMD when maximal mouth opening is limited.						

Audible Sounds During Temporomandibular Joint Movement (Crepitus)

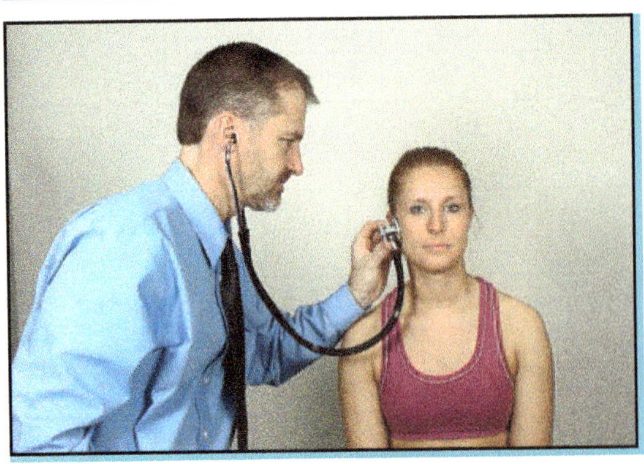

1) The patient is seated with the mouth partially closed, near its resting position.

2) The clinician places a stethoscope over the temporomandibular joint.

3) The patient is instructed to open his or her mouth, deviate the mouth laterally, and bite down.

4) A positive test finding is sounds during the movements.

TESTS FOR TEMPOROMANDIBULAR JOINT DYSFUNCTION

UTILITY SCORE 2

Study	Reliability	Sensitivity	Specificity	LR+	LR−	QUADAS Score (0–14)
Holmlund & Axelsson[2] (OA)	NT	45	86	3.21	0.64	7
Holmlund & Axelsson[2] (OA)	NT	67	84	4.19	0.39	7
Manfredini et al.[5] (Effusion)	NT	85.2	29.5	1.21	0.50	10
Usumez et al.[10] (DDR)	NT	10.5	64.3	0.29	1.39	7
Usumez et al.[10] (DDNR)	NT	70.6	88.9	6.36	0.33	7
Yatani et al.[9] (DDR)	NT	1.8	91.3	0.21	1.08	8
Yatani et al.[9] (DDNR)	NT	96.7	69.2	3.14	0.05	8
Israel et al.[3] (presence of crepitus during auscultation)	NT	70	43	1.2	0.7	6
Holmlund & Axelsson[2] (presence of crepitus during auscultation)	NT	67	86	4.8	0.4	6
Dworkin et al.[1] (digital palpation of crepitus)	NT	8	92	1	1	8
Comments: OA = osteoarthritis; DDR = disc displacement with reduction; DDNR = disc displacement without reduction. Design quality is low but the accuracy scores are very promising. The one study with a QUADAS of 10 demonstrated marginal value for detection of effusion, but didn't test other classifications.						

Audible Sounds During Temporomandibular Joint Movement (Presence of a Click)

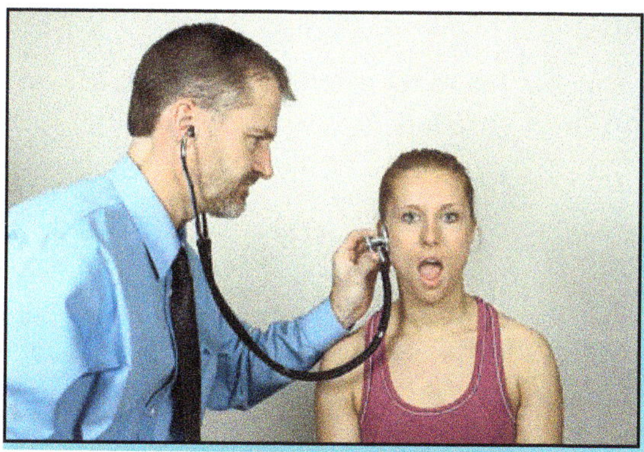

1) The patient is seated with the mouth partially closed, near its resting position.

2) The clinician places a stethoscope over the temporomandibular joint.

3) The patient is instructed to open his or her mouth, deviate the mouth laterally, and bite down.

4) A positive test finding is sounds during the movements.

(continued)

TESTS FOR TEMPOROMANDIBULAR JOINT DYSFUNCTION

UTILITY SCORE 2

Study	Reliability	Sensitivity	Specificity	LR+	LR−	QUADAS Score (0–14)
Manfredini et al.[5] (effusion)	N/T	68.8	50.8	1.40	0.61	10
Manfredini et al.[6] (DDR)	N/T	45.6	59.4	1.12	0.92	12
Manfredini et al.[6] (DDNR)	N/T	48.8	62	1.28	0.83	12
Orsini et.al.[7] (DDR)	N/T	50.8	83.1	3.01	0.59	10
Stegenga et al.[9] (DDR)	N/T	71	90	7.1	0.32	8
Stegenga et al.[9] (DDNR)	N/T	10	40	0.17	2.25	8
Usumez et al.[10] (DDR)	N/T	89.4	40.5	1.50	02.6	7
Usumez et al.[10] (DDNR)	N/T	29.4	14.3	0.34	4.93	7
Dworkin et al.[1] (digital palpation of a click)	N/T	43	75	1.7	0.8	8
Comments: DDR = disc displacement with reduction; DDNR = disc displacement without reduction. Studies with lower bias suggest only marginal benefit with presence of a click.						

Audible Sounds During Temporomandibular Joint Movement (Presence of a Grating)

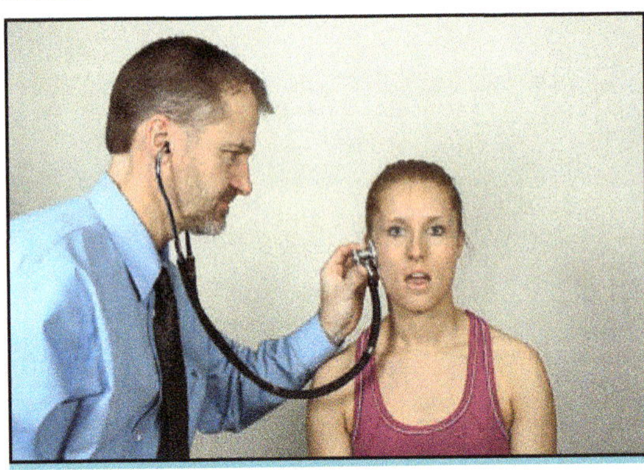

1) The patient is seated with the mouth partially closed, near its resting position.

2) The clinician places a stethoscope over the temporomandibular joint.

3) The patient is instructed to repeatedly open and close his or her mouth, with an effort toward going through full range.

4) A positive test finding is the sound of grating during the movements.

UTILITY SCORE 

Study	Reliability	Sensitivity	Specificity	LR+	LR−	QUADAS Score (0–14)
Dworkin et al.[1] (presence of grating)	NT	6	99	6	0.9	8
Comments: Grating is a very specific finding. How grating differs from crepitus is less known.						

TESTS FOR TEMPOROMANDIBULAR JOINT DYSFUNCTION

Pain During Joint Play

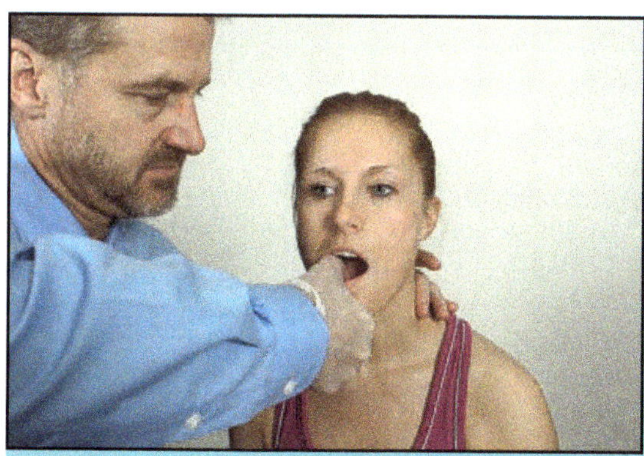

1) The patient is seated with the mouth partially closed, near its resting position.

2) The clinician places his or her thumb on top of the molars and grasps the jaw with the fingers.

3) The clinician applies a downward and slight anterior glide to the TMJ.

4) A positive test finding is a reduction of joint play during this passive assessment.

UTILITY SCORE 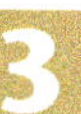

Study	Reliability	Sensitivity	Specificity	LR+	LR−	QUADAS Score (0–14)
Manfredini et al.[5] (effusion)	NT	80.3	39.3	1.3	0.50	10
Comments: No apparent benefit of joint play to detect effusion.						

Composite Examination Results for Classifications

1) A composite examination includes combined findings that represent pre-set criteria for diagnosis.

2) The composite examination includes palpation, pain during movement, maximal mouth opening deficits, and/or asymmetrical movements.

UTILITY SCORE 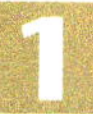

Study	Reliability	Sensitivity	Specificity	LR+	LR−	QUADAS Score (0–14)
Paesani et al.[8] (combined examination for arthrosis)	NT	42	90	4.2	0.6	8
Paesani et al.[8] (combined examination for internal derangement)	NT	78	52	1.6	0.4	8
Israel et al.[3] (combined examination for osteoarthritis)	NT	98	71	3.4	0.3	6
Israel et al.[3] (combined examination for synovitis)	NT	92	21	1.2	0.4	6
Lobbezoo-Scholte et al.[4] (full region for myositis)	NT	56	83	3.3	0.5	8
Comments: As with most composite findings, the full examination tends to provide somewhat better diagnostics than individual clinical tests and measures. Unfortunately, most articles were not descriptive in their explanation of total tests needed or distinct combinations.						

Key Points

1. The majority of tests differentiate subclassifications of TMD and not whether one has TMD.
2. The majority of tests for TMD provide little value in differentiation.

References

1. Dworkin S, LeResche L, DeRouen T. Assessing clinical signs of temporomandibular disorders: reliability of clinical examiners. *J Prosthet Dent.* 1990; 63:574–579.
2. Holmlund AB, Axelsson S. Temporomandibular arthropathy: correlation between clinical signs and symptoms and arthroscopic findings. *Int J Oral Maxillofac.* 1996; 25:178–181.
3. Israel HA, Diamond B, Saed-Nejad F, Ratcliffe A. Osteoarthritis and synovitis as major pathoses of the temporomandibular joint: comparison of clinical diagnosis with arthroscopic morphology. *J Oral Maxillo Surg.* 1998;56:1023–1028.
4. Lobbezoo-Scholte AM, Steenks MH, Faber JA, Bosman F. Diagnostic value of orthopedic tests in patients with temporomandibular disorders. *J Dent Res.* 1993;72:1443–1453.
5. Manfredini D, Tognini F, Zampa V, Bosco M. Predictive value of clinical findings for temporomandibular joint effusion. *Oral Surg Oral Med Oral Pathol Oral Radiol Endod.* 2003;96:521–526.
6. Manfredini D, Basso D, Salmaso L, Guarda-Nardini L. Temporomandibular joint click sound and magnetic resonance-depicted disk position: which relationship? *J Dentistry.* 2008;36:256–260.
7. Orsini MG, Kuboki T, Terada S, Matsuka Y, Yatani H, Yamachita A. Clinical predictability of temporomandibular joint disc displacement. *J Dent Res.* 1999;78:650–660.
8. Paesani D, Westesson PL, Hatala MP, Tallents RH, Brooks SL. Accuracy of clinical diagnosis for TMJ internal derangement and arthrosis. *Oral Surg Oral Med Oral Pathol.* 1992;73:360–363.
9. Stegenga B, de Bont LGM, van der Kuijl B, Boering G. Classification of temporomandibular joint osteoarthritis and internal derangement. Part I Diagnostic significance of clinical and radiographic symptoms and signs. *J Craniomandibular Pract.* 1992;10:96–117.
10. Usumez S, Oz F, Guray E. Comparison of clinical and magnetic resonance imaging diagnoses in patients with TMD history. *J Oral Rehab.* 2004; 31:52–56.
11. Visscher CM, Naeije M, De Laat A, et al. Diagnostic accuracy of temporomandibular disorder pain tests: a multicenter study. *J Orofacial Pain.* 2009;23:108–114.
12. Yatani H, Suzuki K, Kuboki T, Matsuka Y, Maekawa K, Yamashita A. The validity of clinical examination for diagnosing anterior disk displacement without reduction. *Oral Surg Oral Med Oral Pathol Oral Radiol Endod.* 1998;85:654–660.

PEARSON myhealthprofessionskit™

Use this address to access the Companion Website created for this textbook. Simply select "Physical Therapy" from the choice of disciplines. Find this book and log in using your username and password to access video clips of selected tests.

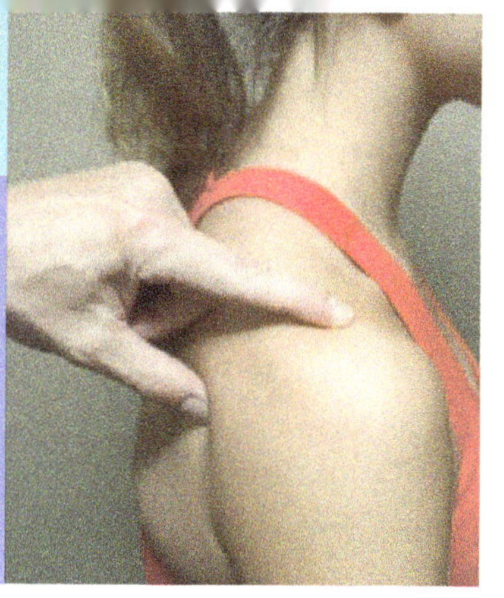

Physical Examination Tests for the Shoulder Complex

Eric J. Hegedus

Please refer to the chapter "Introduction to Diagnostic Accuracy" before reading this chapter.

Index of Tests

Torn Labrum/Instability Tests

Biceps Load Test II (SLAP Lesion)

Yergason's Test (Subacromial Impingement, Superior Labral Anterior to Posterior (SLAP) Lesion, Any Labral Lesion, Long Head of Biceps Pathology)

Crank Test (Labral Tear, SLAP Lesion)

Kim Test (Posteroinferior Labral Lesion)

Jerk Test (Posteroinferior Labral Lesion)

Anterior Release/Surprise Test (Anterior Instability)

Pain Provocation Test (SLAP Lesion)

Passive Compression Test (SLAP Lesion)

Apprehension Test (Anterior Instability, All Instabilities of the Glenohumeral Joint, Labral Tear, SLAP Lesion)

Modified Dynamic Labral Shear Test (Labral Tear)

Modified Relocation/Modified Jobe Relocation Test (Labral Pathology, Traumatic Anterior Instability)

Apprehension-Relocation/Jobe Relocation Test (Anterior Instability, Labral Tear, SLAP Lesion)

Supine Flexion Resistance Test (Type II SLAP Lesion)

Speed's Test [All Stages of Subacromial Impingement, Superior Labral Anterior to Posterior (SLAP) Lesion, Any Labral Lesion, Biceps Pathology]

Forced Shoulder Abduction and Elbow Flexion Test (Superior Labral Tear)

Sulcus Sign (Inferior Laxity, Superior Labral Tear)

Active Compression Test/O'Brien's Test [Labral Tear, SLAP Lesion, Labral Abnormality, Acromioclavicular (AC) Joint Pathology]

Resisted Supination External Rotation Test (RSERT) (SLAP Lesion)

Compression-Rotation Test (SLAP Lesion)

Anterior Slide Test (SLAP Lesion)

Biceps Load Test (SLAP Lesion with Anterior Shoulder Dislocation)

Clunk Test (Labral Tear, Superior Labral Tear)

Anterior Drawer Test (Anterior Laxity, Anterior Instability)

Biceps Tension Test (Unstable Superior Labrum—Lesions/SLAP Lesions)

Hyperabduction Test (Inferior Laxity)

Posterior Drawer Test (Posterior Laxity)

Load and Shift Test (Anterior, Posterior, Inferior Laxity)

Diagnostic Clusters—Instability

Diagnostic Clusters—Labral Tears

Acromioclavicular (AC) Dysfunction Tests

AC Resisted Extension Test (AC Joint Abnormality)

AC Joint Palpation (AC Joint Pain)

Paxinos Sign (AC Joint Pain)

Diagnostic Clusters—AC Joint Pathology

Nerve Palsies

Active Elevation Lag Sign (Spinal Accessory Nerve Palsy)

The Triangle Sign (Spinal Accessory Nerve Palsy)

Deltoid Extension Lag Sign (Axillary Nerve Palsy)

Stiffness-Related Disorders [Osteoarthritis (OA) & Adhesive Capsulitis]

Shrug Sign (OA & Adhesive Capsulitis)

Coracoid Pain Test (Adhesive Capsulitis)

Diagnostic Clusters—Adhesive Capsulitis

Test For Scapular Dysfunction

Lateral Scapular Slide Test (Shoulder Dysfunction)

Tests For Biceps Tendinopathy

Upper Cut Test (Biceps Tendinopathy)

Biceps Palpation (Biceps Tear, Type II SLAP)

Diagnostic Clusters—Biceps Tendinopathy

SCREENING FOR BONY ABNORMALITY

Olecranon-Manubrium Percussion Test (Fracture or Dislocation between the Elbow and Manubrium)

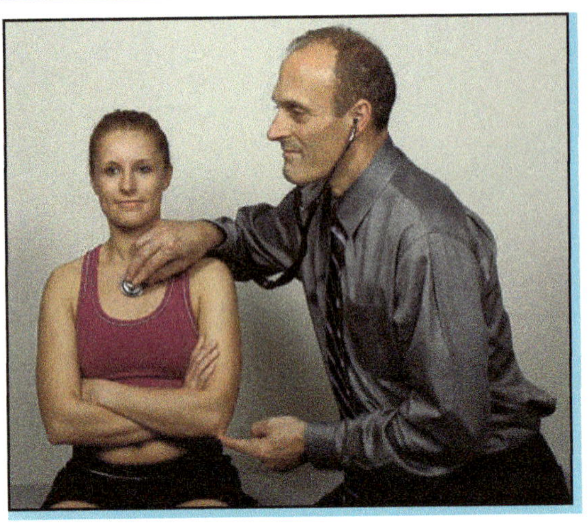

1. The patient is seated or standing with arms crossed.
2. The examiner taps on the involved side olecranon while using a stethoscope placed on the patient's manubrium.
3. Repeat step 2 but on the uninvolved side.
4. A positive test for fracture or dislocation is indicated by a difference in the quality of sound on the involved vs. the uninvolved side.

UTILITY SCORE 2

Study	Reliability	Sensitivity	Specificity	LR+	LR−	QUADAS Score (0–14)
Adams et al.[1]	NT	84	99	84.0	0.27	13
Comments: According to Adams et al., when the Olecranon-Manubrium Percussion Test[1] is positive, the clinician should order an x-ray. More research needs to be done to raise the Utility Score to a "1."						

SCREENING FOR BONY ABNORMALITY

The Bony Apprehension Test (A Bony Lesion Causing Anterior Instability of the Shoulder)

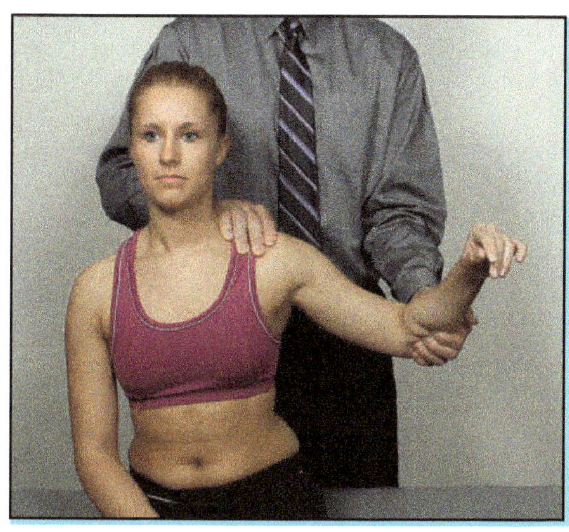

1) The patient is seated or standing.

2) The examiner stands behind the patient and grasps the suprascapular/supraclavicular region with one hand and the patient's proximal forearm with the other hand.

3) With the elbow flexed to 90 degrees, the examiner abducts the shoulder to 45 degrees or less and externally rotates the shoulder to 45 degrees or less.

4) A positive test for anterior instability due to a bony lesion is indicated by the patient registering apprehension with the test.

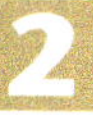

UTILITY SCORE 2

Study	Reliability	Sensitivity	Specificity	LR+	LR−	QUADAS Score (0–14)
Bushnell et al.[7]	NT	94	84	5.88	0.07	9
Comments: The Bony Apprehension Test[7] appears to be a screen for instability due to a Bankart or Hill-Sachs lesion but also has moderate diagnostic ability. More research needs to be done to raise the Utility Score to a "1."						

TORN ROTATOR CUFF/IMPINGEMENT

External Rotation Lag Sign (Supraspinatus/Infraspinatus Tear)

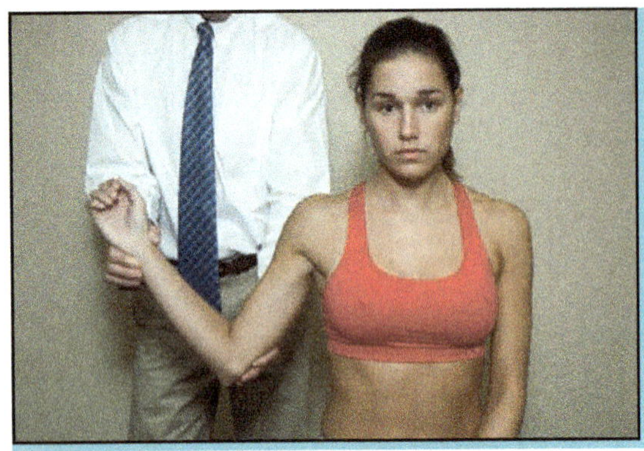

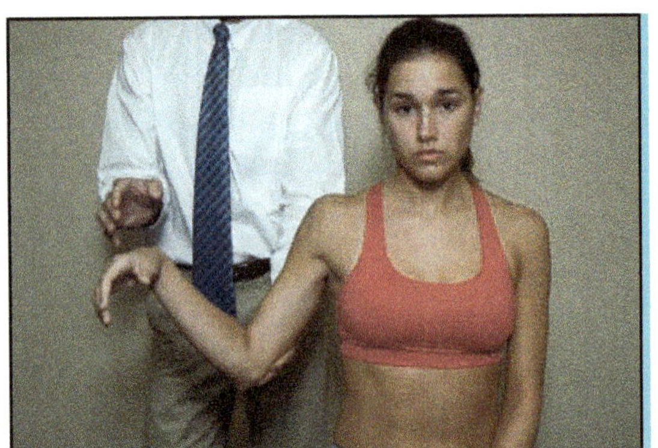

1. The patient is seated with the examiner standing to the rear.
2. The examiner grasps the patient's elbow with one hand and the wrist with the other.
3. The examiner places the elbow in 90 degrees of flexion and the shoulder in 20 degrees of elevation in the scapular plane.
4. The examiner passively externally rotates the shoulder to near end-range.
5. The examiner asks the patient to maintain this position as the patient's wrist is released.
6. A positive test for supraspinatus/infraspinatus tear is indicated by a lag that occurs with the inability of the patient to maintain his or her arm near full external rotation.

UTILITY SCORE 

Study	Reliability	Sensitivity	Specificity	LR+	LR−	QUADAS Score (0–14)
Hertel et al.[27] (Infraspinatus)	NT	70	100	NA	NA	8
Walch et al.[82] (Teres Minor)	NT	100	100	NA	NA	6
Jia et al.[34] (Massive RC Tear Biceps Tendinopathy)	NT NT	35 20	89 88	3.18 1.67	0.73 0.91	6
Miller et al.[60] (Full Thickness Tear)	NT	46	94	7.2	0.60	11
Bak et al.[4] (Full Thickness Supraspinatus Tear)	NT	45	91	5.00	0.61	13
Castoldi et al.[10] (Full Thickness-Supraspinatus Full Thickness Rotator Cuff Tears Teres Minor Tear)	NT	 56 97 100	 98 93 93	 28.0 13.86 14.29	 0.45 0.03 0.00	10

Comments: The External Rotation Lag Sign appears to be specific for more severe rotator cuff tears.

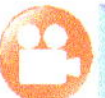

Rent Test [Rotator Cuff (RC) Tear]

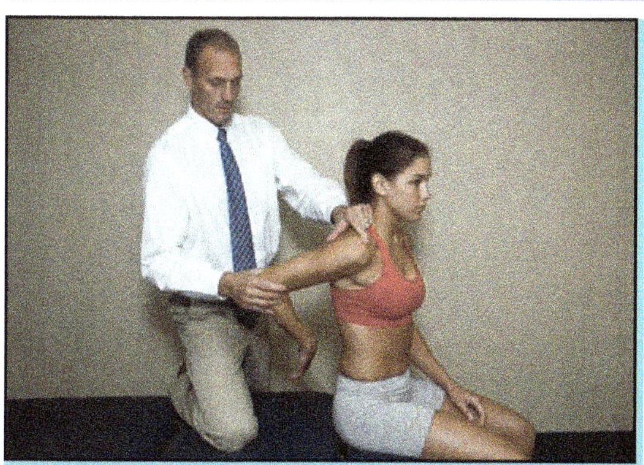

1) The patient is seated with arm relaxed and the examiner stands to the rear.

2) The examiner palpates anterior to the anterior edge of the acromion with one hand while grasping the patient's flexed elbow with the other.

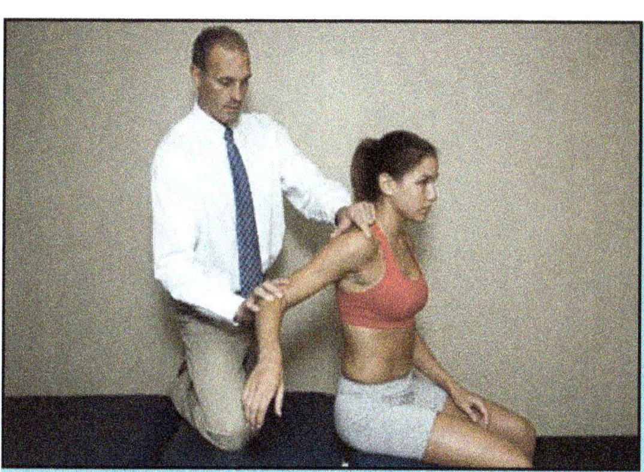

3) The examiner extends the patient's arm and then slowly internally and externally rotates the shoulder.

4) An eminence (prominent greater tuberosity) and a rent (depression of about 1 finger width) will be felt in the presence of a rotator cuff tear.

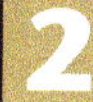

UTILITY SCORE 2

Study	Reliability	Sensitivity	Specificity	LR+	LR−	QUADAS Score (0–14)
Wolf & Agrawal[85]	NT	96	97	32	0.04	9
Lyons & Tomlinson[53]	NT	91	75	3.64	0.12	6
Comments: The Rent Test[12] should not be used to judge the size of a rotator cuff tear but rather the absence or presence of a rotator cuff tear. The quality of the studies keeps this Utility Score from being a 1.						

Supine Impingement Test[49] (RC Tear)

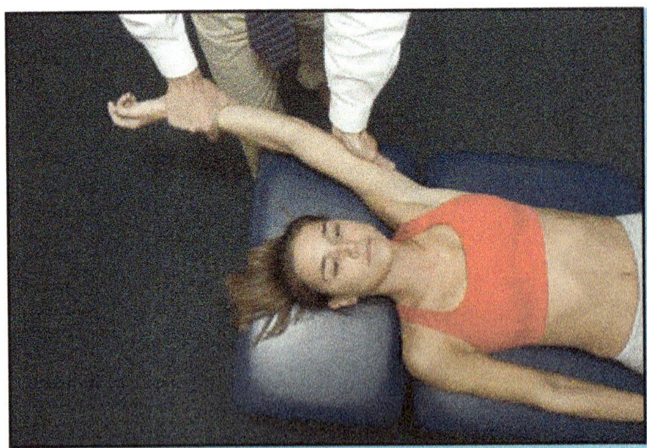

1) The patient assumes a supine position. The examiner stands to the side of the patient's involved shoulder.

2) The examiner grasps the patient's wrist and distal humerus and elevates the patients arm to end-range (170 degrees or greater).

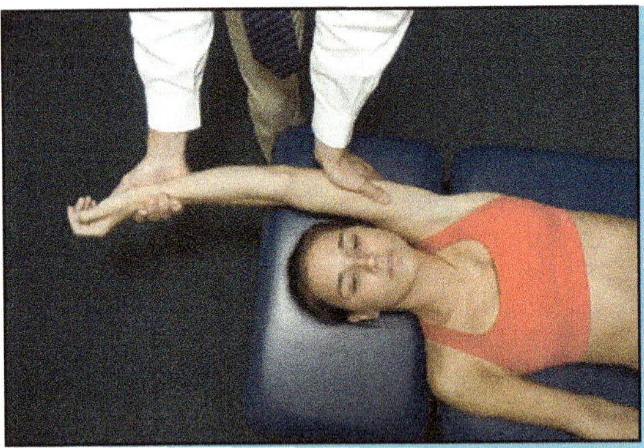

3) The examiner next moves the patient's arm into external rotation then adducts the arm to the patient's ear.

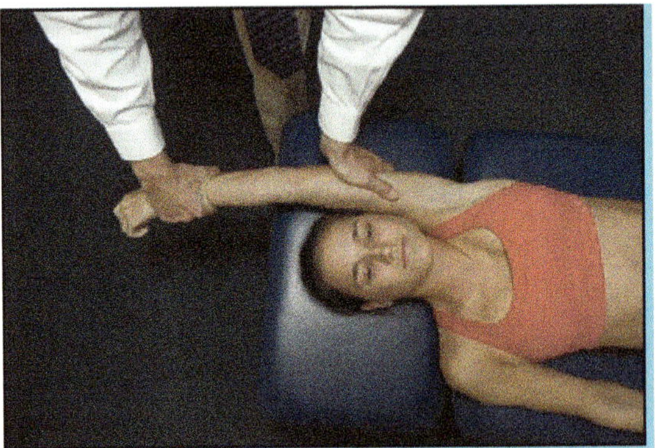

4) The examiner now internally rotates the patient's arm.

5) The supine impingement test is positive if the patient reports a significant increase in shoulder pain.

UTILITY SCORE 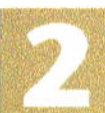

Study	Reliability	Sensitivity	Specificity	LR+	LR−	QUADAS Score (0–14)
Litaker et al.[49]	NT	97	9	1.07	0.33	11
Comments: This study was done well but retrospectively. The supine impingement test does not appear diagnostic but may have value as a screen because a negative finding may rule out a rotator cuff tear. Further research needs to be performed.						

TORN ROTATOR CUFF/IMPINGEMENT

Lift-Off Test[20] (Subscapularis Tear)

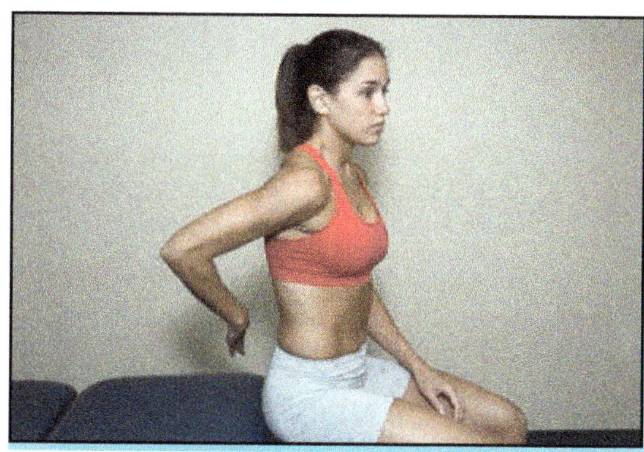

1) The patient is seated with affected arm behind his or her back.

2) The patient is asked to lift the arm off the back.

3) A positive test for subscapularis tear is indicated by inability of the patient to lift the arm off the back.

UTILITY SCORE 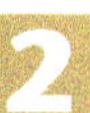

Study	Reliability	Sensitivity	Specificity	LR+	LR−	QUADAS Score (0–14)
Gerber & Krushell[20]	NT	89	98	44.5	0.11	8
Hertel et al.[27]	NT	62	100	NA	NA	8
Ostor et al.[69]	κ = .28–.32	NT	NT	NT	NT	NA
Jia et al.[34] (Massive RC Tear,Glenohumeral OA Biceps Tendinopathy)	NT NT NT	28 29 28	86 89 90	2.0 2.7 2.8	0.84 0.80 0.80	6
Barth et al.[5]	NT	18	100	NA	NA	11
Gill et al.[21] (Partial Biceps Tear)	NT	28	89	2.61	0.90	12
Itoi et al.[31] (Pain Weakness)	NT NT	46 79	69 59	1.48 1.93	0.78 0.36	8

Comments: The study by Gerber and Krushell[20] had only 16 patients, all of whom were male. Two studies show high specificity, meaning this test has value, when positive, of ruling in a subscapularis tear or biceps pathology but more research needs to be performed incorporating larger sample sizes. Of some concern is fair interobserver agreement.

Internal Rotation Lag Sign[27] (Subscapularis Tear)

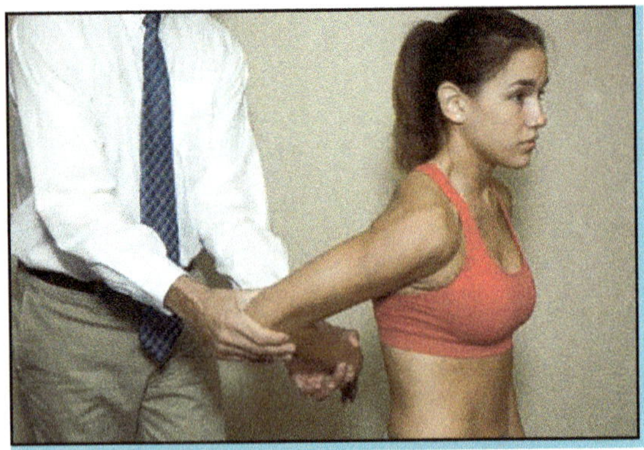

1) The patient is seated with affected arm behind his or her back.

2) The examiner grasps the patient's elbow with one hand and the wrist with the other.

3) The examiner lifts the patient's arm off the back.

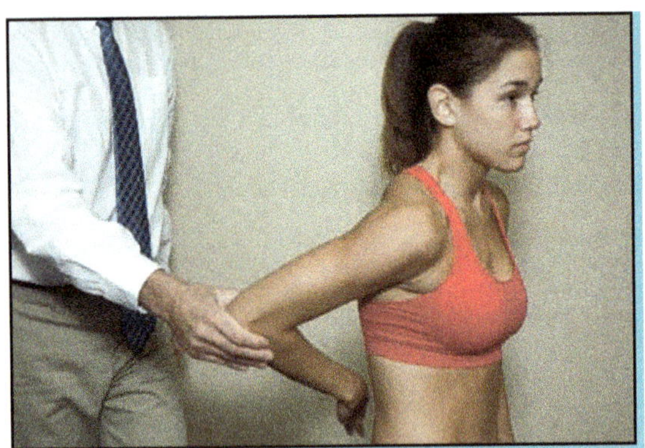

4) The examiner asks the patient to maintain this position as the patient's wrist is released.

5) A positive test for subscapularis tear is indicated by a lag that occurs with the inability of the patient to maintain the arm off the back.

UTILITY SCORE  **2**

Study	Reliability	Sensitivity	Specificity	LR+	LR−	QUADAS Score (0–14)
Hertel et al.[27]	NT	97	96	24.25	0.03	8
Scheibel et al.[75]	NT	75	NT	NT	NT	6
Miller et al.[60] (Full Thickness Tear)	NT	100	84	6.2	0.00	11
Bak et al.[4] (Full Thickness Supraspinatus Tear)	NT	31	87	2.38	0.79	13

Comments: Despite the solid statistical numbers, the Utility Score is only a 2 due to potential for bias in the conducting of the Hertel et al.[27] study or incomplete reporting of the study findings. More research still needs to be performed as the Miller et al.[60] study used diagnostic ultrasound as the criterion standard on a small sample size and Bak et al.[4] did not use the test to detect subscapularis tears.

Drop Sign[27] (Infraspinatus Tear, Irreparable Fatty Degeneration of Infraspinatus)

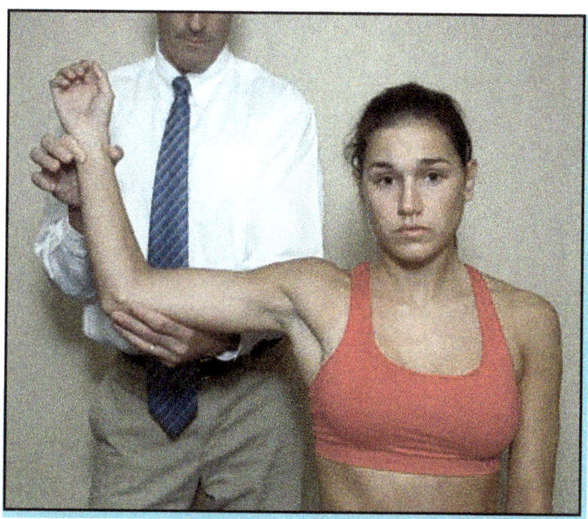

1) The patient is seated with the examiner standing to the rear.

2) The examiner grasps the patient's elbow with one hand and the wrist with the other.

3) The examiner places the elbow in 90 degrees of flexion and the shoulder in 90 degrees of elevation in the scapular plane.

4) The examiner passively externally rotates the shoulder to near end-range

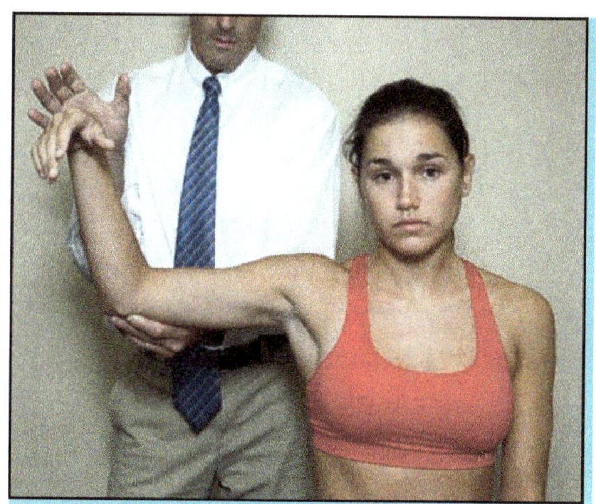

5) The examiner asks the patient to maintain this position as the patient's wrist is released.

6) A positive test for infraspinatus tear is indicated by a lag that occurs with the inability of the patient to maintain the arm near full external rotation.

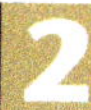

UTILITY SCORE 2

Study	Reliability	Sensitivity	Specificity	LR+	LR−	QUADAS Score (0–14)
Hertel et al.[27]	NT	20	100	NA	NA	8
Walch et al.[82]	NT	100	100	NA	NA	6
Miller et al.[60](Full Thickness Tear)	NT	73	77	3.2	0.30	11
Bak et al.[4] (Full Thickness Supraspinatus Tear)	NT	45	70	1.50	0.79	13

Comments: More research needs to be performed, especially in light of the quality of the first two studies and because the Miller et al.[60] study used diagnostic ultrasound as the criterion standard on a small sample size. Further, the two stronger studies did not report the test value in patients with infraspinatus tears as was the original design.

Empty Can Test/Supraspinatus Test[36] (Rotator Cuff Tear, All Stages of Impingement Syndrome from Bursitis through a Rotator Cuff Tear)

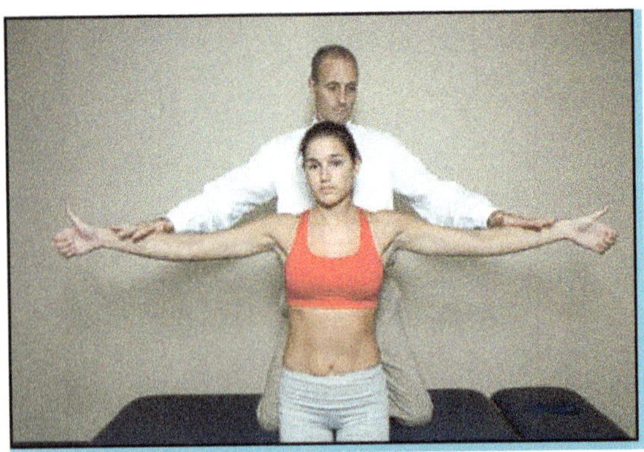

1) The patient elevates the arms to 90 degrees with thumbs up (full can position).

2) The examiner provides downward pressure on the arms and notes the patient's strength.

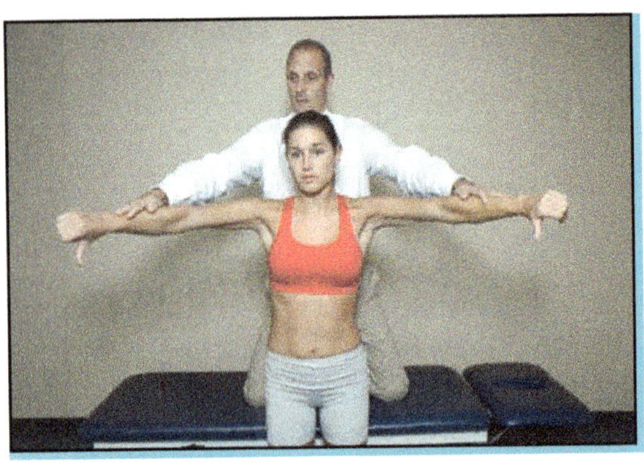

3) The patient elevates the arms to 90 degrees and horizontally adducts 30 degrees (scapular plane) with thumbs pointed down as if "emptying a can."

4) The examiner provides downward pressure on the arms and notes the patient's strength.

5) A positive test for rotator cuff tear is examiner assessment of more weakness in the empty can position vs. the full can position, patient complaint of pain, or both.

UTILITY SCORE 2

Study	Reliability	Sensitivity	Specificity	LR+	LR−	QUADAS Score (0–14)
Itoi et al.[30] (Supraspinatus Tear)	NT	89	50	1.78	0.22	9
Park et al.[72] (Impingement or Rotator Cuff Disease)	NT	44	90	4.2	0.63	10
Ostor et al.[69] (Supraspinatus Tear)	κ = .44–.49	NT	NT	NA	NA	NA
Michener et al.[59] (Impingement)	κ = .47	50	87	3.90	0.57	11
Kim et al.[42] Full Thickness Tear (Pain or Weak) Full Thickness Tear (Pain & Weak) Any Tear (Pain or Weak) Any Tear (Pain & Weak)	NT	 84 60 99 71	 59 91 43 74	 2.05 6.67 1.74 2.73	 0.27 0.44 0.02 0.39	9
Kelly et al.[38] (Impingement, Weakness, Pain)	NT	52 52	67 33	1.58 0.78	0.63 1.45	11
Itoi et al.[31] (Pain Weakness)	NT NT	78 87	40 43	1.30 1.53	0.55 0.30	8
Bak et al.[4] (Full Thickness Supraspinatus Tear)	NT	76	39	1.25	0.62	13

Comments: This test was originally described by Jobe & Moynes[36] as a supraspinatus strength test only, without a provocation component. Itoi et al.[30] used weakness, pain, or both as a positive sign and looked at the ability of the test to detect damage in any of the rotator cuff muscles. Kim et al.[42] gave different estimates of diagnostic accuracy depending on the definition of a tear and of a positive test. The Empty Can is sensitive for a rotator cuff tear when the definition of a positive test is broad and specific as the definition of a positive test narrows.

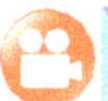

Belly Press/Napoleon Test[19] (Subscapularis Tear)

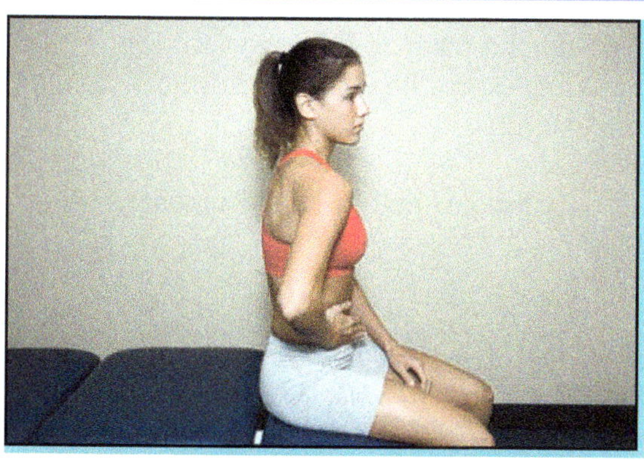

1) The patient can sit or stand with elbow flexed to 90 degrees.

2) The patient internally rotates the shoulder, causing the palm of the hand to be pressed into the stomach.

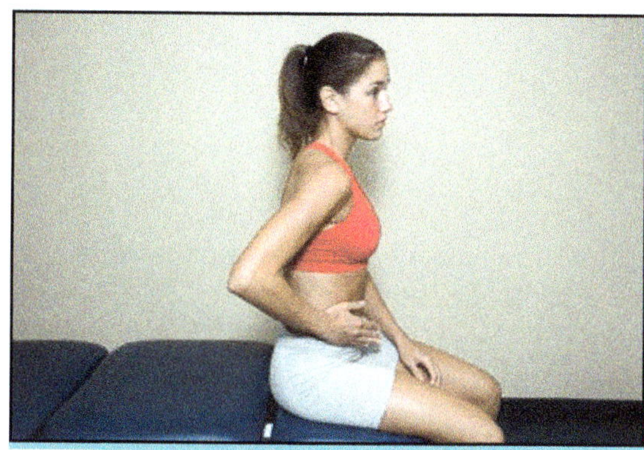

3) A positive test is indicated by the elbow dropping behind the body into extension.

UTILITY SCORE 2

Study	Reliability	Sensitivity	Specificity	LR+	LR−	QUADAS Score (0–14)
Gerber et al.[19]	NT	NT	NT	NA	NA	NA
Scheibel et al.[75]	NT	69	NR	NA	NA	6
Barth et al.[5] (Belly Press Subscapularis Tear)	NT	40	98	20.0	0.61	11
Barth et al.[5] (Napoleon Subscapularis Tear)	NT	25	98	12.50	0.77	11
Gill et al.[21] (Belly Press Partial Biceps Tear)	NT	17	92	2.01	0.90	12

Comments: The Belly Press Test[19] was originally described as an alternative to the Lift-off Test in those patients without adequate internal shoulder rotation but still with a suspected subscapularis tear. The Napoleon Test is performed in the same fashion as the Belly Press except the definition of a positive Napoleon Test is wrist flexion substituting for humeral internal rotation. In addition to a subscapularis tear, pain in the anterior shoulder with the Napoleon Test may be specific for a partial biceps tear.

TORN ROTATOR CUFF/IMPINGEMENT

Bear-Hug Test[62] (Subscapularis Tear)

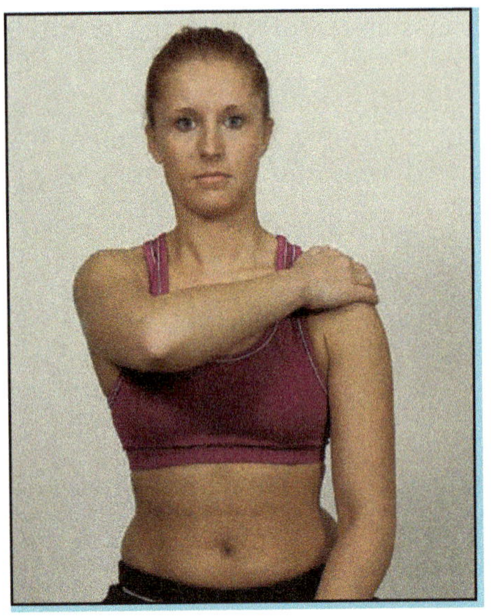

1) The patient places the palm of the involved side on the opposite shoulder, elbow flexed and pointing straight ahead, fingers extended.

2) The examiner attempts to pull the hand upward and off the opposite shoulder.

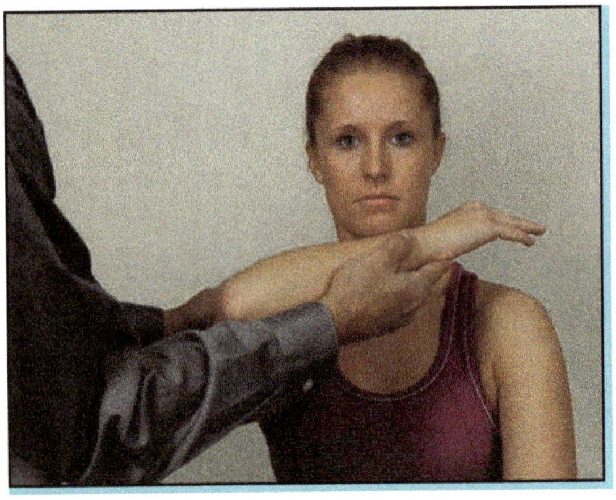

3) A positive test for subscapularis tear is if the patient cannot hold the hand against the shoulder.

UTILITY SCORE 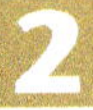

Study	Reliability	Sensitivity	Specificity	LR+	LR−	QUADAS Score (0–14)
Barth et al.[5] (Subscapularis Tear)	NT	60	92	7.23	0.44	11
Kibler et al.[41] (Biceps Pathology Labral Tear)	NT	79 37	60 32	1.94 0.54	0.74 1.98	9

Comment: The Bear Hug Test[5] appears to be specific for a torn subscapularis tear but one study does not a special test make. Further, the test is of no use in detecting biceps pathology or a labral tear but that is not the purpose of the test anyway.

TORN ROTATOR CUFF/IMPINGEMENT

Lateral Jobe Test (RC Tear)

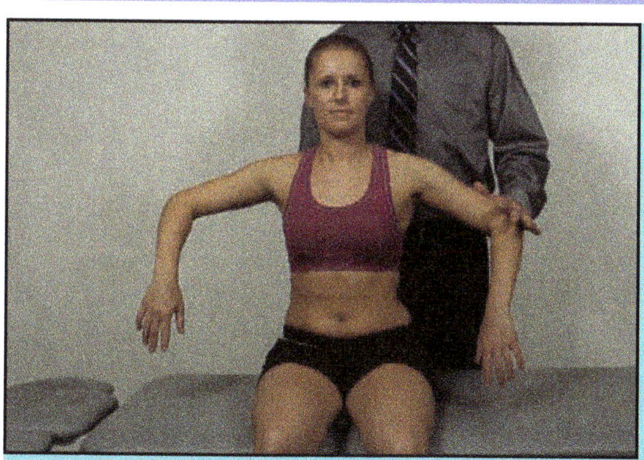

1) The patient is standing with arms abducted to 90 degrees.

2) The patient internally rotates to end-range humeral motion.

3) The examiner applies an inferior force to the patient's elbows as the patient resists.

4) A positive test is indicated by pain reproduction or weakness or inability to perform the test.

UTILITY SCORE 2

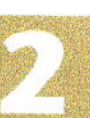

Study	Reliability	Sensitivity	Specificity	LR+	LR−	QUADAS Score (0–14)
Gillooly et al.[22]	NT	81	89	7.36	0.10	10
Comments: Based on this one well-performed study, the Lateral Jobe Test[22] modifies the posttest probability of diagnosing a rotator cuff tear a moderate to large amount and could be used as a diagnostic tool. More research needs to be performed to confirm these statistical numbers.						

TORN ROTATOR CUFF/IMPINGEMENT

Drop Arm Test (Supraspinatus Tear, Subacromial Impingement)

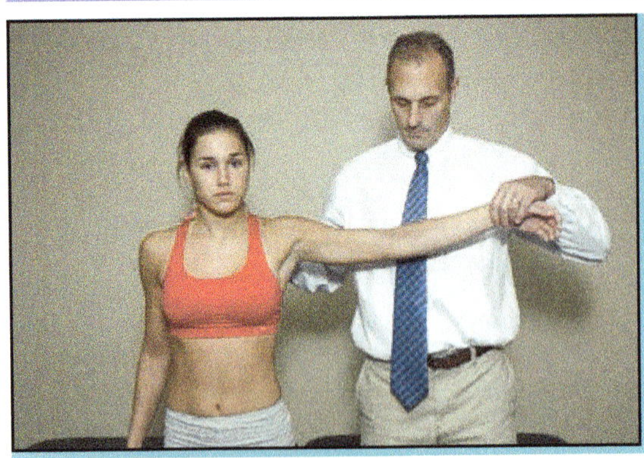

1) The patient is standing with the examiner, standing to the front.

2) The examiner grasps the patient's wrist and passively abducts the patient's shoulder to 90 degrees.

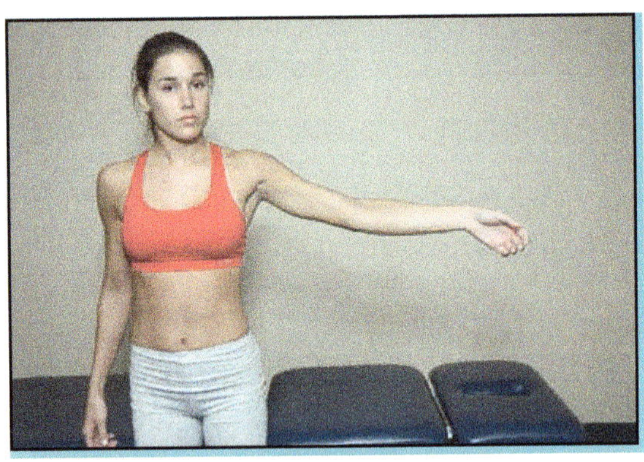

3) The examiner releases the patient's arm with instructions to slowly lower the arm.

4) A positive test for supraspinatus tear is the inability by the patient to lower the arm.

UTILITY SCORE 3

Study	Reliability	Sensitivity	Specificity	LR+	LR−	QUADAS Score (0–14)
Calis et al.[8] (Supraspinatus Tear Impingement)	NT NT	15 8	100 97	NA 2.66	NA .94	8 8
Murrell & Walton[63] (Rotator Cuff Tear)	NT	10	98	5.00	.92	5
Park et al.[72] (Impingement or Rotator Cuff Disease)	NT	27	88	2.25	.83	10
Ostor et al.[69] (Supraspinatus Tear)	κ = .28–.66	NT	NT	NA	NA	NA
Jia et al.[34] (RC Tendinopathy Full Thickness Tear Massive Tear)	NT	74 35 44	66 88 82	2.15 2.79 2.48	0.39 0.74 0.68	6
Bak et al.[4] Full Thickness Supraspinatus Tear	NT	41	83	2.41	0.71	13

Comments: Calis et al.[8] used subacromial injection as the criterion standard when surgery is the better choice. Park et al.[72] used this as an active test where the patient moved the arm through "elevation" and looked for a "drop" as the patient lowered the arm. If this test has value, it is in a positive finding to rule in either a rotator cuff tear or impingement. The likelihood ratios indicate this is only a modest diagnostic test at best despite fair to significant interobserver agreement.

TORN ROTATOR CUFF/IMPINGEMENT

Full Can/Supraspinatus Test (Supraspinatus Tear)

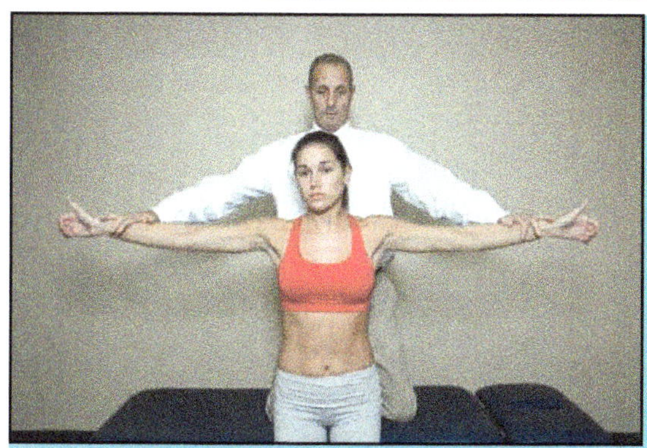

1) The patient elevates the arms to 90 degrees with thumbs up (full can position).

2) The examiner provides downward pressure on the arms and notes the patient's strength.

3) A positive test for rotator cuff tear is examiner assessment of more weakness in the involved shoulder, patient complaint of pain, or both.

UTILITY SCORE 3

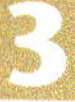

Study	Reliability	Sensitivity	Specificity	LR+	LR−	QUADAS Score (0–14)
Itoi et al.[30]	NT	86	57	2.00	0.25	9
Kim et al.[42]	NT					9
Full Thickness Tear (Pain or Weak)		74	68	2.31	0.38	
Full Thickness Tear (Pain & Weak)		42	91	4.67	0.64	
Any Tear (Pain or Weak)		90	54	1.96	0.19	
Any Tear (Pain & Weak)		59	82	3.28	0.50	
Kelly et al.[38] (Impingement	NT					11
Weakness		45	75	1.8	0.73	
Pain)		35	25	0.45	2.60	
Itoi et al.[31] Pain	NT	80	50	2.67	0.40	8
Weakness	NT	83	53	1.77	0.32	

Comments: Kelly et al.[37] first described this test as a less painful alternative test to the Empty Can Test. Like the Empty Can Test, this test was originally designed as a supraspinatus strength test only, but as the definition of a positive test broadens, the test becomes more sensitive and as the definition narrows, the test becomes more specific. The Full Can has limited ability to modify the probability of diagnosing or ruling out a rotator cuff tear.

TORN ROTATOR CUFF/IMPINGEMENT

Posterior Impingement Sign (Rotator Cuff Tear and/or Posterior Labral Tear)

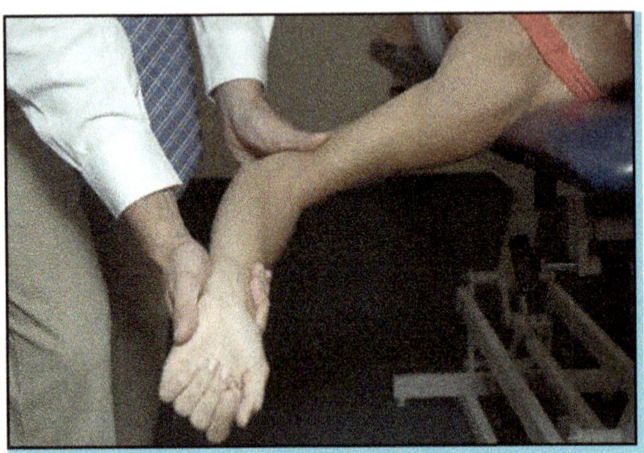

1) With the patient in supine, the shoulder is placed in 90–110 degrees of abduction, 10–15 degrees of extension, and maximum external rotation.

2) A positive test is indicated by complaints of pain in the deep posterior shoulder.

UTILITY SCORE 3

Study	Reliability	Sensitivity	Specificity	LR+	LR−	QUADAS Score (0–14)
Meister et al.[58]	NT	76	85	5.06	0.28	6
Comments: Despite good statistical numbers, the gender of the patients in this study was not specified and other design flaws leave a great potential for bias. More research needs to be performed, especially in light of the quality of this study.						

Hornblower's Sign (Irreparable Fatty Degeneration of Teres Minor)

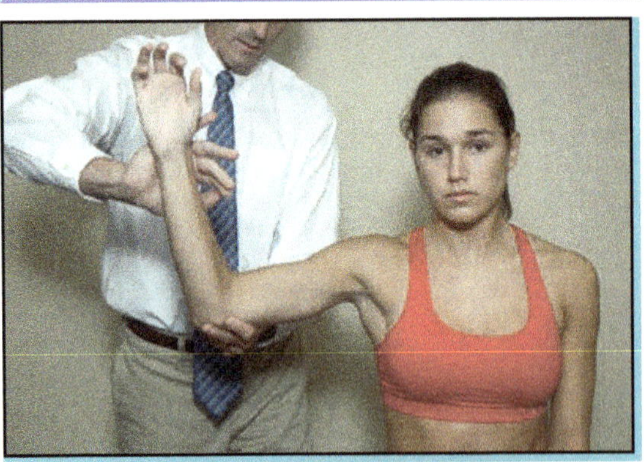

1) The patient is seated and the examiner supports the patients shoulder in 90 degrees of abduction in the scapular plane.

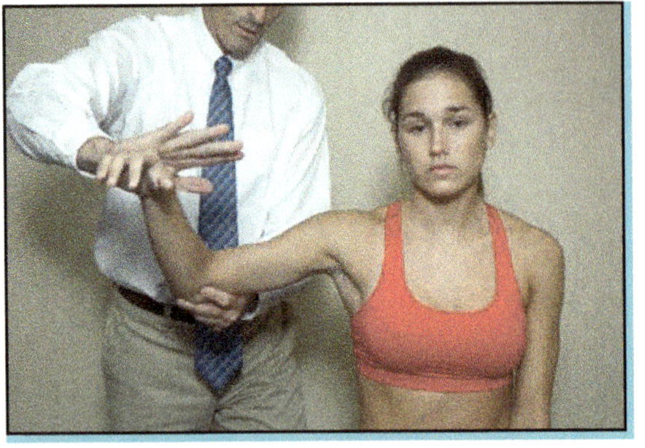

2) The elbow is flexed to 90 degrees and the patient is asked to forcefully externally rotate the shoulder against the examiner's resistance.

3) A positive test is indicated by the inability of the patient to externally rotate in this position.

UTILITY SCORE 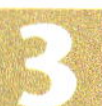

Study	Reliability	Sensitivity	Specificity	LR+	LR−	QUADAS Score (0–14)
Walch et al.[82]	NT	100	93	NA	NA	6
Comments: Despite the solid statistical numbers, the Utility Score is only a 3 due to potential for bias in the conduct of this study or incomplete reporting of the study findings. More research needs to be performed, especially in light of the quality of this study.						

Whipple Test[74] (Supraspinatus Tear)

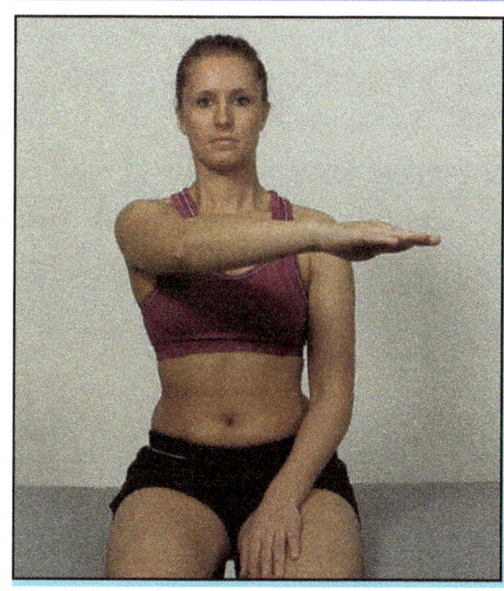

1) The patient is seated, arm flexed 90 degrees and adducted until hand is opposite the contralateral shoulder.

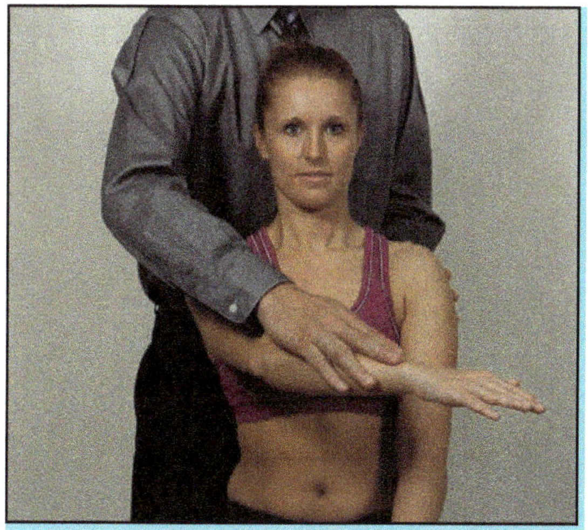

2) The examiner places downward pressure on the forearm of the involved side.

3) A positive test is indicated by reproduction of shoulder pain.

(continued)

TORN ROTATOR CUFF/IMPINGEMENT

UTILITY SCORE 3

Study	Reliability	Sensitivity	Specificity	LR+	LR−	QUADAS Score (0–14)
Jia et al.[34] (Massive Rotator Cuff Tear, Glenohumeral OA, AC Joint OA)	NT NT NT	100 88 88	26 25 25	NA 1.17 1.17	NA 0.48 0.48	6
Oh et al.[68] (Type II SLAP)	NT	65	42	1.12	0.83	11

Comments: The Whipple Test[74] was originally described as detecting a supraspinatus tear as part of a superior labral, anterior cuff (SLAC) lesion. The Whipple Test appears to be a good screen for a massiverotator cuff tear, but this conclusion should be viewed with caution due to the potential for bias in the one study to investigate this test.

Diagnostic Clusters—Rotator Cuff Tear

UTILITY SCORE 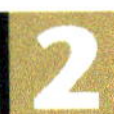

Study	Cluster	Reliability	Sensitivity	Specificity	LR+	LR−	QUADAS Score (0–14)
Malhi & Khan[55]	Supraspinatus weakness or impairment of abduction	NT	100	99	NA	NA	5
Litaker et al.[49]	Age ≥ 65 and weakness in external rotation (Infraspinatus test) and night pain	NT	49	95	9.84	0.54	10
MacDonald et al.[54] (Rotator Cuff Tendinopathy)	Hawkins or Neer Hawkins and Neer	NT	88 83	38 56	1.42 1.89	0.32 0.31	7
Ardic et al.[2]	Hawkins or Neer	NT	78	50	1.56	0.44	12
Park et al.[72]	Painful Arc, Drop Arm, and Infraspinatus test	NT	NT	NT	15.57	0.16	10
Park et al.[72]	Age ≥ 60, Painful Arc, Drop Arm, and Infraspinatus test	NT	NT	NT	28.00	0.09	10
Bak et al.[4] (Full Thickness, Supraspinatus Tear)	Active abduction < 90 degrees + Empty Can + ERLS test	NT	54	65	1.20	0.71	13
Bak et al.[4] (Full Thickness Supraspinatus Tear)	Active abduction < 90 degrees + Empty Can + Hawkins	NT	72	39	1.18	0.72	13
Murrell & Walton[63]	Empty Can and Infraspinatus Test and Hawkins or Neer	NT	NT	NT	48.0	0.76	4

Comments: Based on the higher quality studies, key ingredients to diagnostic clusters to detect a rotator cuff tear seem to be age and external rotation weakness plus either the Drop Arm or Empty Can. The Murrell & Walton[63] study scored poorly because it was published as a brief report without much detail. These authors reported that patients who present with shoulder pain, and who test positive for supraspinatus weakness, weakness in external rotation, and impingement, have a 98 percent chance of rotator cuff tear.

IMPINGEMENT TESTS

Internal Rotation Resisted Strength Test[87] (Internal/Intraarticular vs. External/Subacromial Impingement)

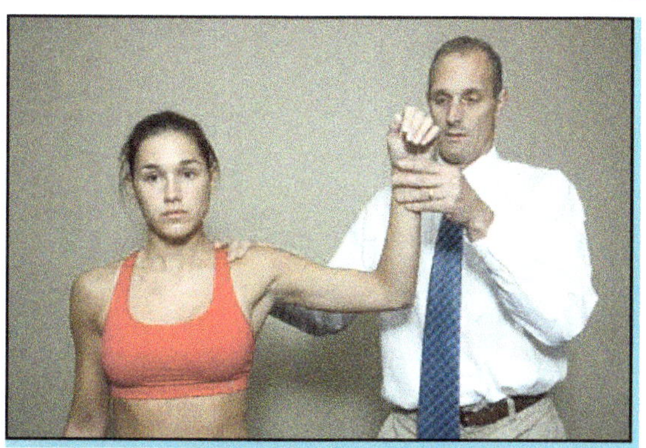

1) The patient is instructed to stand. The examiner stands behind the patient.

2) The examiner places the patient's shoulder in 90 degrees of abduction and 80 degrees of external rotation with the elbow at 90 degrees flexion.

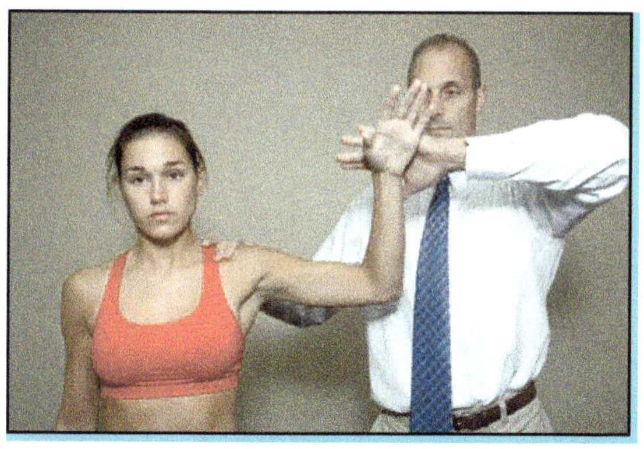

3) The examiner applies manual resistance to the wrist; first to test isometric external rotation.

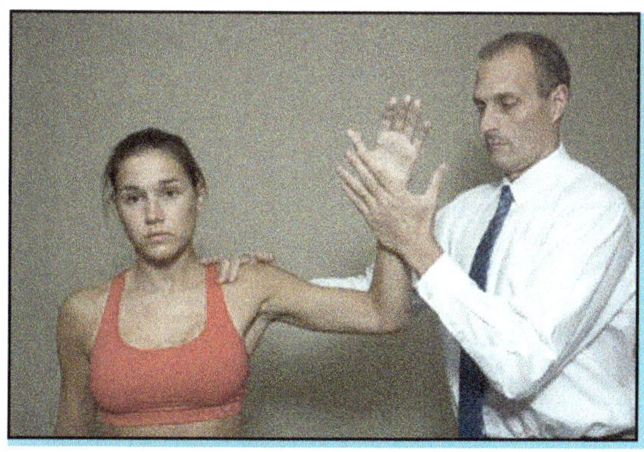

4) The examiner applies manual resistance to the wrist next to test isometric internal rotation.

5) The examiner compares the results of this isometric test. If internal rotation strength is weaker than external rotation, the IRRST test is considered positive and the patient purportedly has internal impingement.

UTILITY SCORE 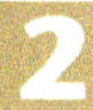

Study	Reliability	Sensitivity	Specificity	LR+	LR−	QUADAS Score (0–14)
Zaslav[87]	NT	88	96	22	0.12	8

Comments: Despite the great statistical numbers, the Utility Score is only a two because of potential for bias in the conduct of this study and/or incomplete reporting of the study findings. More research needs to be performed, especially in light of the quality of this study.

IMPINGEMENT TESTS

Infraspinatus/External Rotation Resistance Test[72] (All Stages of Subacromial Impingement)

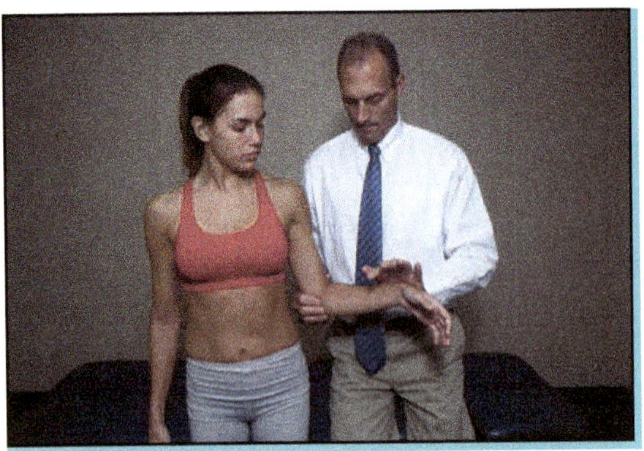

1. The patient is standing with elbow in 90 degrees flexion, neutral forearm rotation, and elbow adducted against the body.
2. The examiner stands to the side of the patient and provides an internal rotation force while the patient resists.

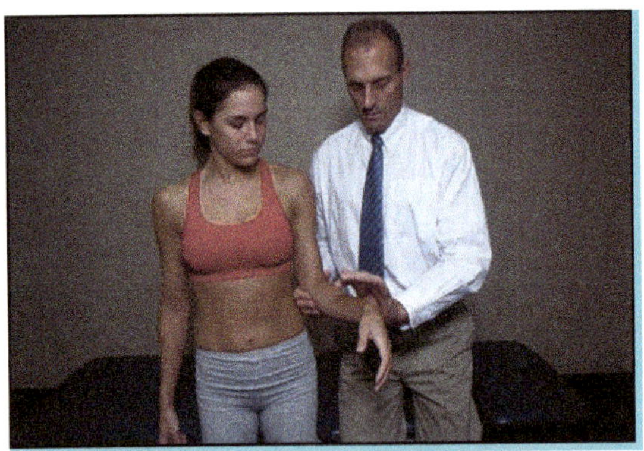

3. A positive test is indicated by patient giving way due to either pain or weakness.

UTILITY SCORE 

Study	Reliability	Sensitivity	Specificity	LR+	LR−	QUADAS Score (0–14)
Park et al.[72]	NT	42	90	4.20	0.65	10
Ostor et al.[69]	κ = 0.18–0.45	NT	NT	NA	NA	NA
Michener et al.[59]	κ = 0.67	56	87	4.39	0.50	11
Kelly et al.[38] (Weakness Pain)	NT	55 35	25 100	0.73 NA	1.80 NA	11
Itoi et al.[31] (Infraspinatus Tear Pain, Weakness)	NT NT	54 84	54 53	1.17 1.79	0.85 0.30	8

Comments: Park et al.[72] incorporated the External Rotation Lag Sign as part of the assessment of the infraspinatus, in effect combining two tests. Unfortunately, the test has only a small effect on posttest probability when trying to find any stage of impingement (bursitis through full-thickness rotator cuff tear). Pain may be a more specific sign than weakness.

IMPINGEMENT TESTS

Neer Test (Subacromial Impingement, Subacromial Bursitis (SAB), Rotator Cuff Tear, Superior Labral Tear)

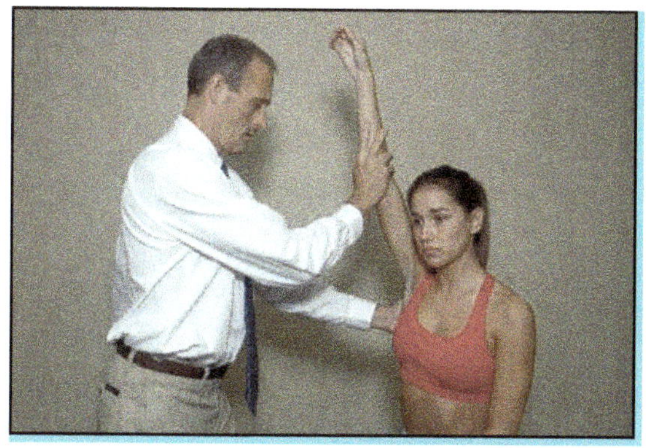

1. The patient is seated while the examiner stands to the side of the involved shoulder.
2. The examiner raises the patient's arm into flexion with one hand while the other hand stabilizes the scapula.
3. The examiner applies forced flexion toward end-range in an attempt to reproduce the shoulder pain.
4. If concordant shoulder pain is present, the test is positive.

UTILITY SCORE 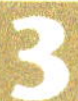 3

Study	Reliability	Sensitivity	Specificity	LR+	LR−	QUADAS Score (0–14)
MacDonald et al.[54] (SAB, Rotator Cuff Tear)	NT NT	75 83	48 51	1.40 1.69	0.52 0.33	7 7
Park et al.[72]	NT	68	69	2.20	0.46	10
Calis et al.[8]	NT	89	31	1.28	0.35	8
Parentis et al.[71] (Superior Labral Tear)	NT	48	51	0.98	1.02	5
Bak & Fauno[3] (Impingement)	NT	0	100	NA	NA	6
Nakagawa et al.[65] (Superior Labral Tear)	NT	33	60	0.83	1.11	10
Jia et al.[34] (Stage I Impingement All Stages of RC Tendinopathy)	NT NT	86 64	49 43	1.69 1.12	0.29 0.84	6
Michener et al.[59](Impingement)	κ = .40	81	54	1.76	0.35	11
Kelly et al.[38] (Impingement)	NT	62	0	NA	NA	11
Gill et al.[21] (Biceps Partial Tear)	NT	64	41	1.08	0.88	12
Bak et al.[4] (Full Thickness Supraspinatus Tear)	NT	60	35	0.92	1.14	13
Silva et al.[78] (Impingement)	NT	68	30	0.98	1.07	11

Comments: The test was originally described by Neer in 1983 and a positive test was confirmed by injecting 10 ml of xylocaine into the subacromial space and repeating steps 1–4 above in a pain free fashion. Newer and better designed studies show this test is of little to no use in diagnosing impingement syndrome. The ability of this test to detect a superior labral tear is worse than chance.

IMPINGEMENT TESTS

Hawkins-Kennedy Test[26] (Subacromial Impingement, Subacromial Bursitis, Rotator Cuff Tear, Superior Labral Tear)

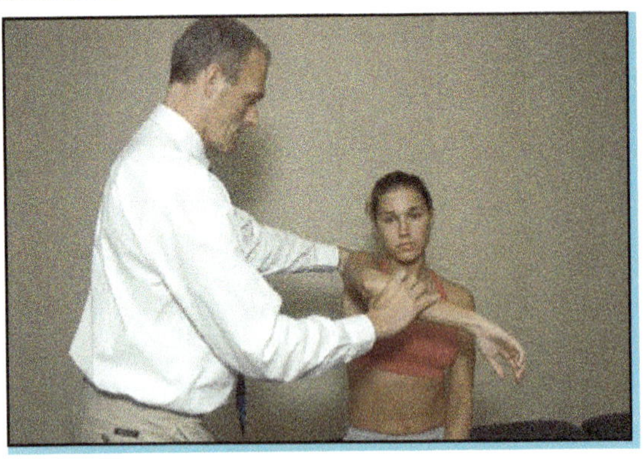

1) The patient is seated while the examiner stands anteriorly to the involved shoulder.

2) The examiner first raises the patient's arm into approximately 90 degrees of shoulder flexion or abduction with one hand while the other hand stabilizes the scapula (typically superiorly).

3) The examiner applies forced humeral internal rotation in an attempt to reproduce the concordant shoulder pain. If concordant shoulder pain is present, the test is positive.

UTILITY SCORE 3 

Study	Reliability	Sensitivity	Specificity	LR+	LR−	QUADAS Score (0–14)
MacDonald et al.[54] (Bursitis Rotator Cuff Tear)	NT NT	92 88	44 43	1.64 1.54	0.18 0.27	7 7
Park et al.[72] (Impingement)	NT	72	66	2.11	0.42	10
Calis et al.[8] (Impingement Rotator Cuff Tear)	NT NT	92 100	25 36	1.22 NA	0.32 NA	8 8
Parentis et al.[71] (Superior Labral Tear)	NT	65	30	0.94	1.15	5
Bak & Fauno[3] (Impingement)	NT	80	76	3.33	0.26	6
Ostor et al.[69] (Impingement)	κ = .18–.43	NT	NT	NA	NA	NA
Nakagawa et al.[65] (Superior Labral Tear)	NT	50	67	1.52	0.75	10
Jia et al.[33] (Stage I Impingement All Stages of RC Tendinopathy)	NT NT	76 71	45 42	1.38 1.22	0.53 0.69	6
Michener et al.[59]	κ = .39	63	62	1.63	0.61	11
Kelly et al.[38] (Impingement)	NT	74	50	1.48	0.52	11
Gill et al.[21] (Biceps Partial Tear)	NT	55	38	0.89	1.18	12
Bak et al.[4] (Full Thickness Supraspinatus Tear)	NT	77	26	1.04	0.88	13

Comments: The Hawkins-Kennedy Test[26] is probably a more sensitive test suitable for screening for either impingement or rotator cuff tear than it is a specific test suitable for diagnosis. Further, in the four best performed/reported studies, the test has mediocre value and may not be a good screening or diagnostic test for impingement.

IMPINGEMENT TESTS

Painful ARC Test[39] (All Stages of Subacromial Impingement)

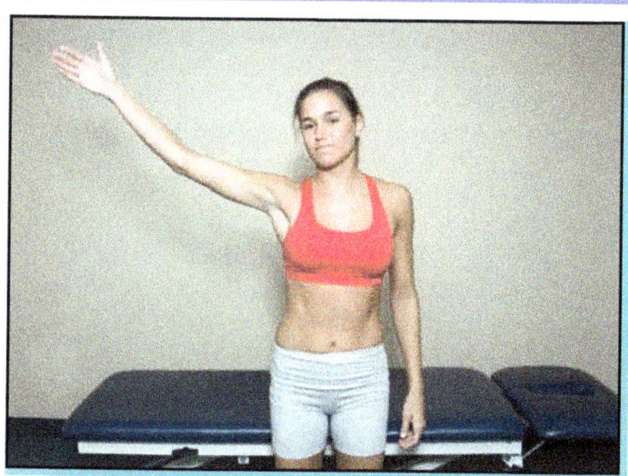

1) The patient is standing. The examiner faces the patient to observe shoulder motion.

2) The patient is instructed to actively abduct the involved shoulder.

3) A positive test is indicated by patient report of concordant pain in the 60–120 degree range. Pain outside of this range is considered a negative test. Pain that increases in severity as the arm reaches 180 degrees is indicative of "a disorder of the acromioclavicular joint."

UTILITY SCORE 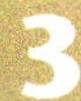

Study	Reliability	Sensitivity	Specificity	LR+	LR–	QUADAS Score (0–14)
Park et al.[72] Impingement	NT	74	81	3.89	0.32	10
Calis et al.[8] (Impingement Rotator Cuff Tear)	NT NT	33 45	81 79	1.73 2.14	0.82 0.70	8 8
Litaker et al.[49] (Rotator Cuff Tear)	NT	98	10	1.09	0.20	11
Jia et al.[34] (Rotator Cuff Tendinopathy)	NT	67	50	1.34	0.66	6
Michener et al[59]	κ = .45	75	67	2.25	0.38	11
Kelly et al.[38] (Impingement)	NT	30	50	0.60	1.40	11
Bak et al.[4] (Full Thickness Supraspinatus Tear)	NT	96	4	1.00	1.00	13
Silva et al.[78] (Impingement)	NT	74	40	1.23	0.65	11

Comments: This test modifies posttest probability very little. Further, the broad cluster of diagnoses captured under "impingement" may not aid the examiner with prognosis or intervention.

IMPINGEMENT TESTS

Cross-Body Adduction Test[57] [Subacromial Impingement, Acromioclavicular (AC) Joint Damage]

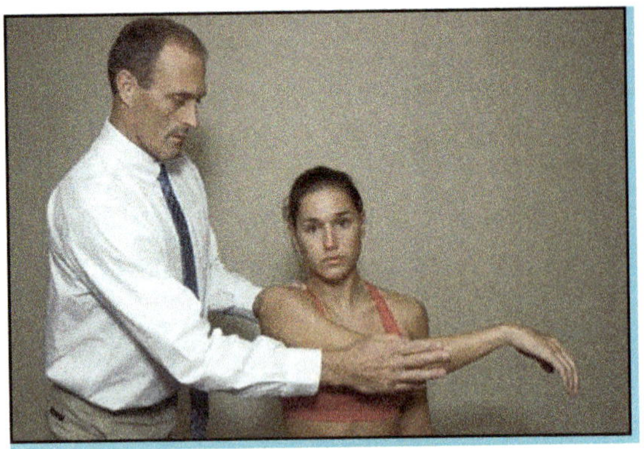

1. The patient assumes a sitting position. The patient is instructed to elevate the arm to 90 degrees of shoulder flexion.
2. The examiner stands in front of the patient and horizontally adducts the patient's arm to end range, maintaining the flexion at the shoulder.
3. If shoulder pain is present, the test is positive.

UTILITY SCORE 3

Study	Reliability	Sensitivity	Specificity	LR+	LR−	QUADAS Score (0–14)
Park et al.[72] (Impingement)	NT	23	82	1.27	0.93	10
Calis et al.[8] (Impingement, Rotator Cuff Tear)	NT NT	82 90	28 29	1.13 1.27	0.64 0.35	8 8
Chronopoulos et al.[11] (AC Joint Pathology)	NT	77	79	3.66	0.29	10
Ostor et al.[69] (AC Joint Pathology)	κ = .08–.29	NT	NT	NT	NT	NA
Jia et al.[34] (AC Joint OA)	NT	77	79	3.67	0.29	6
Comments: The Cross-Body Test[57] appears to be a stronger indicator of AC joint pathology than impingement but the inter–observer agreement for this test may negatively affect clinical application.						

Diagnostic Clusters—Impingement

UTILITY SCORE 2

Study	Cluster	Reliability	Sensitivity	Specificity	LR+	LR−	QUADAS Score (0–14)
Malhi & Khan[55]	Hawkins or Neer or Painful Arc or Subacromial Crepitus	NT	84	76	3.5	0.21	5
Calis et al.[8]	At least 3 of 6: Hawkins, Neer, Horizontal Adduction, Speed, Yergason, Painful Arc, Drop Arm	NT	84	44	1.5	0.36	8
Park et al.[72]	Hawkins, Painful Arc, and Infraspinatus test	NT	NT	NT	10.56	0.17	10
Michener et al.[59]	3 or more positive of: Hawkins, Neer, Painful Arc, Empty Can, External Rotation Weakness	NT	75	74	2.93	0.34	11
Comments: Despite the strong numbers in the Park et al.[46] study, the impingement tests themselves are not strong diagnostic tools and the diagnosis of impingement is not helpful in prognosis nor treatment.							

TORN LABRUM/INSTABILITY TESTS

Biceps Load Test II[44] (SLAP Lesion)

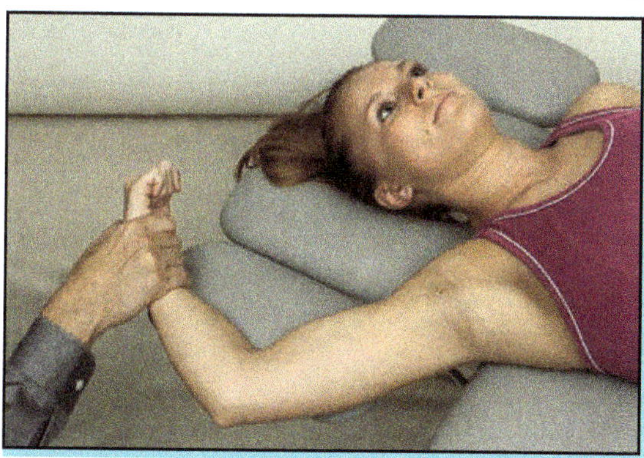

1) The patient assumes a supine position. The examiner sits on the side of the patient's involved extremity.

2) The examiner places the patient's shoulder in 120 degrees of abduction, the elbow in 90 degrees of flexion, and the forearm in supination.

3) The examiner moves the patient's shoulder to end-range external rotation (apprehension position).

4) At end-range external rotation, the examiner asks the patient to flex his or her elbow while the examiner resists this movement.

5) A positive test is indicated as a reproduction of concordant pain during resisted elbow flexion.

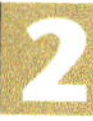

UTILITY SCORE 2

Study	Reliability	Sensitivity	Specificity	LR+	LR−	QUADAS Score (0–14)
Kim et al.[44] (SLAP)	κ = .82	90	97	26.38	0.11	10
Oh et al.[68] (Type II SLAP)	NT	30	78	1.36	0.90	11

Comments: This sequel to the Biceps Load Test[45] was performed in a broader spectrum of patients with blinding of the testers. Newest research casts at least some doubt on the original numbers.

TORN LABRUM/INSTABILITY TESTS

Yergason's Test[86] (Subacromial Impingement, Superior Labral Anterior to Posterior (SLAP) Lesion, Any Labral Lesion, Long Head of Biceps Pathology)

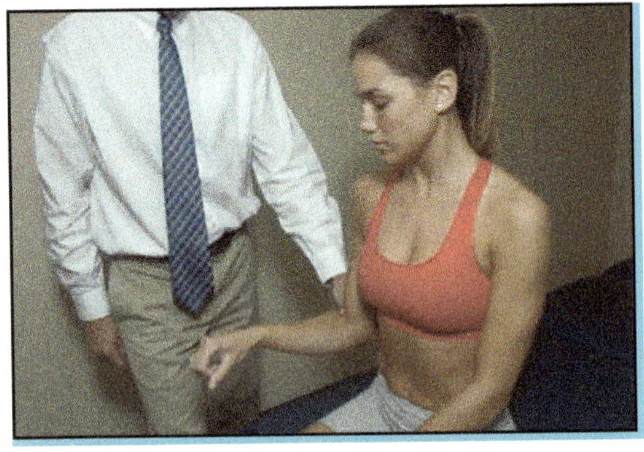

1) The patient may sit or stand. The examiner stands in front of the patient.

2) The patient's elbow is flexed to 90 degrees and the forearm is in a pronated position while maintaining the upper arm at the side.

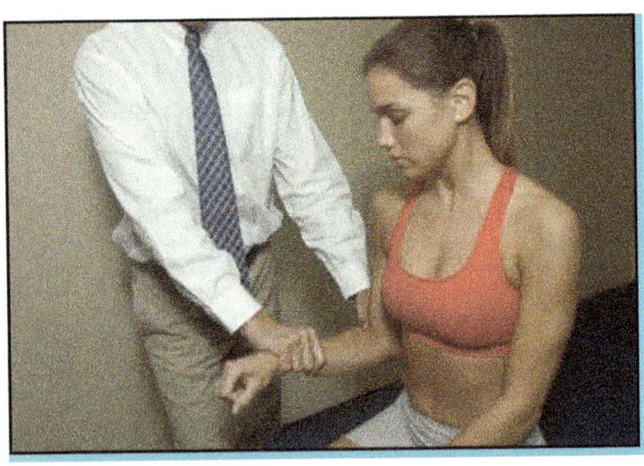

3) The patient is instructed to supinate his or her forearm, while the examiner concurrently resists forearm supination at the wrist.

4) If the patient localizes concordant pain to the bicipital groove, the test is positive.

UTILITY SCORE 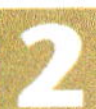

Study	Reliability	Sensitivity	Specificity	LR+	LR−	QUADAS Score (0–14)
Calis et al.[8] (Impingement Rotator Cuff Tear)	NT NT	37 50	86 86	2.64 3.57	0.73 0.58	8 8
Holtby & Razmjou[29] (SLAP)	NT	43	79	2.05	0.72	12
Guanche & Jones[24] (SLAP Any Labral Lesion)	NT NT	12 9	96 93	3.00 1.29	0.92 0.98	12 12
Parentis et al.[71] (SLAP)	NT	13	93	1.78	0.94	5
Parentis et al.[70] (SLAP)	NT	13	94	1.9	0.9	9
Kibler et al.[41] (Biceps Tendinopathy, Labral Tear)	NT	41 26	79 70	1.94 0.88	0.74 1.05	9
Oh et al.[68] (Type II SLAP)	NT	12	87	0.92	1.01	11
Ostor et al.[69] (Long Head of Biceps Pathology)	κ = .28	NT	NT	NA	NA	NA

Comments: The better studies show Yergason's Test[86] to have high specificity and therefore, a positive test may help rule in a labral tear but the likelihood ratios indicate that overall, the test is minimally helpful in diagnosis of a SLAP lesion. The interobserver agreement of this test is fair when detecting pathology of the long head of the biceps.

TORN LABRUM/INSTABILITY TESTS

Crank Test[51] (Labral Tear, SLAP Lesion)

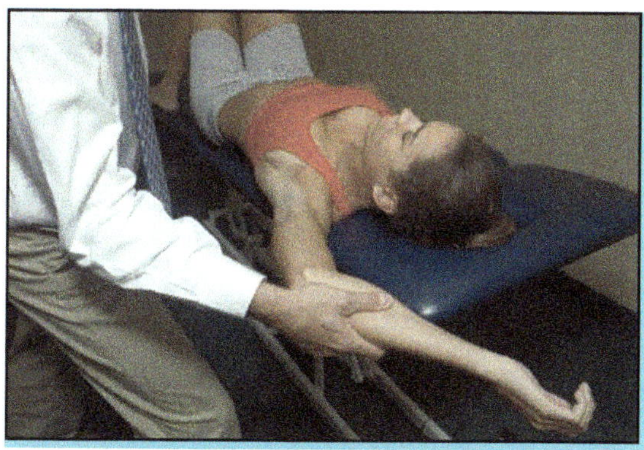

1) The patient assumes either a sitting or supine position. The examiner typically stands at the side of the involved extremity.

2) The examiner places the patient's shoulder in 160 degrees of abduction and elbow in 90 degrees of flexion.

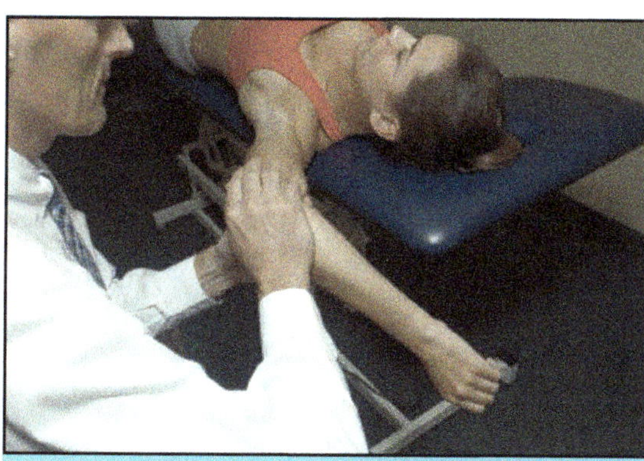

3) The examiner first applies a compression force to the humerus and then rotates the humerus repeatedly into internal rotation and external rotation in an attempt to pinch the torn labrum.

4) A positive test is indicated by the production of pain either with or without a click in the shoulder or by reproduction of the patient's concordant complaint (usually pain or catching).

UTILITY SCORE 

Study	Reliability	Sensitivity	Specificity	LR+	LR−	QUADAS Score (0–14)
Parentis et al.[71] SLAP	NT	9	83	0.50	1.10	5
Stetson & Templin[81] (Labral Tear)	NT	46	56	1.04	0.96	10
Myers et al.[64] (SLAP)	NT	35	70	0.87	2	8
Liu et al.[51] (Labral Tear)	NT	91	93	7.0	0.10	9
Nakagawa et al.[65] (Superior Labral Tear)	NT	58	72	2.1	0.58	10
Gill et al.[21] (Biceps Partial Tear)	NT	34	77	1.49	0.86	12
Walsworth et al.[83] (Any Labral Tear)	$\kappa = 0.20$	61	55	1.35	0.71	11

Comments: There is uncertainty in use for the Crank Test[51] in diagnosing SLAP lesions according to available research and its use to detect any labral tear is mixed according to two stronger studies. More well-designed research is needed.

Kim Test[46] (Posteroinferior Labral Lesion)

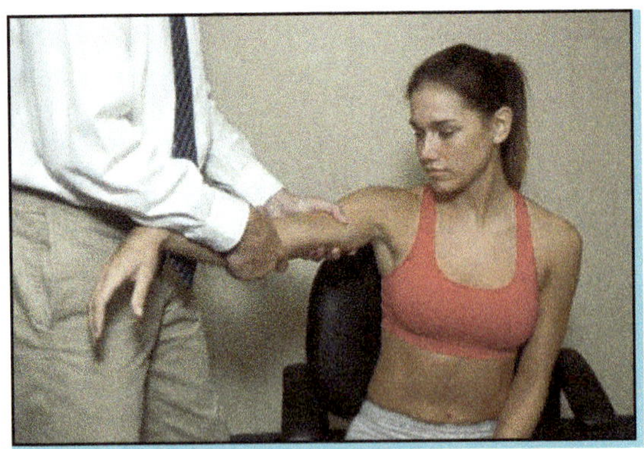

1) The patient is seated in a chair with his or her back supported.

2) The examiner stands to the side of the involved shoulder and faces the patient. The examiner grasps the elbow with one hand and the mid-humeral region with the other and elevates the patient's arm to 90 degrees abduction.

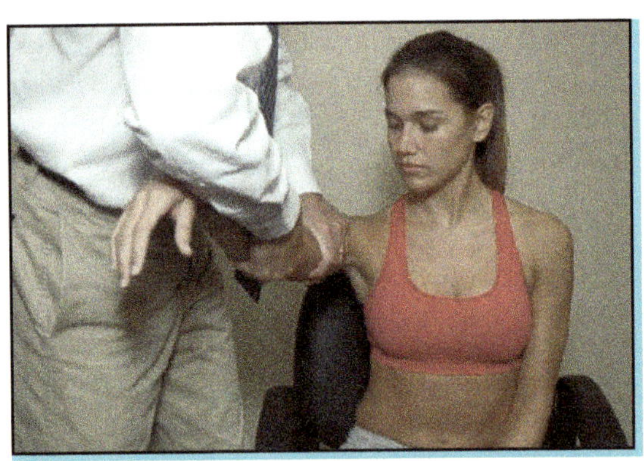

3) Simultaneously the examiner provides an axial load to the humerus and a 45-degree diagonal elevation to the distal humerus concurrent with a posteroinferior glide to the proximal humerus.

4) A positive test is indicated by a sudden onset of posterior shoulder pain.

UTILITY SCORE 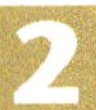

Study	Reliability	Sensitivity	Specificity	LR+	−LR	QUADAS Score (0–14)
Kim et al[46]	NT	80	94	13.33	0.21	9
Comments: More research with more strict methodology needs to be done to corroborate these statistics, but as of now, the Kim Test is a significant indicator of a posteroinferior labral lesion. However, the Jerk Test[46] is easier to perform and performs better statistically.						

TORN LABRUM/INSTABILITY TESTS

Jerk Test[46] (Posteroinferior Labral Lesion)

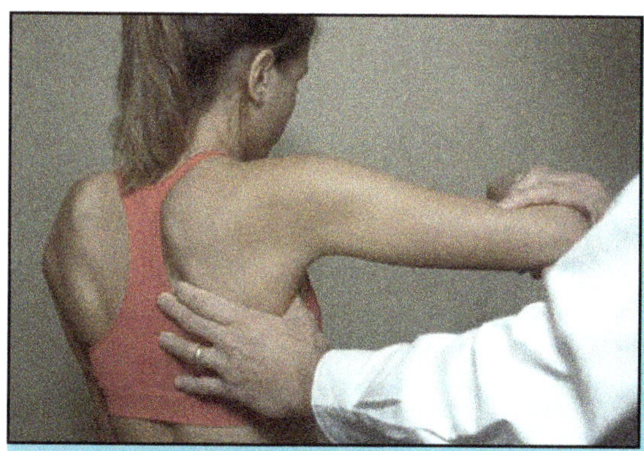

1) The patient assumes a sitting position. The examiner stands behind the patient.

2) The examiner grasps the elbow with one hand and the scapula with the other and elevates the patient's arm to 90 degrees abduction and internal rotation.

3) The examiner provides an axial compression-based load to the humerus through the elbow maintaining the horizontally abducted arm.

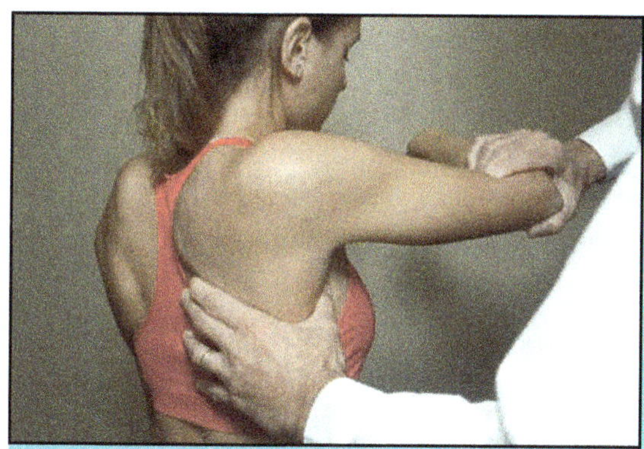

4) The axial compression is maintained as the patient's arm is moved into horizontal adduction.

5) A positive test is indicated by a sharp shoulder pain with or without a clunk or click.

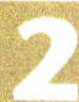

UTILITY SCORE 2

Study	Reliability	Sensitivity	Specificity	LR+	LR−	QUADAS Score (0–14)
Kim et al.[43]	NT	73	98	36.5	0.27	9
Nakagawa et al.[65] (Superior Labral Tear)	NT	25	80	1.25	0.94	10
Comments: More research with more strict methodology needs to be done to corroborate these statistics, but as of now, the Jerk Test[43] is a significant indicator of a posteroinferior labral lesion and a nondescript test for superior labral tear (not the original purpose of the test).						

TORN LABRUM/INSTABILITY TESTS

Anterior Release/Surprise Test[23] (Anterior Instability)

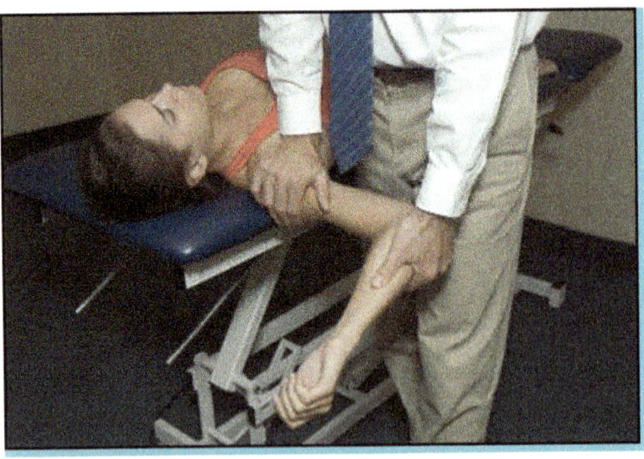

1) The patient assumes a supine position. The examiner stands beside the patient.

2) The examiner grasps the forearm with one hand and provides a posterior force on the humerus with the other.

3) The posterior force on the proximal humerus is maintained while the examiner moves the patient's shoulder into the apprehension position of 90 degrees abduction and end-range external rotation.

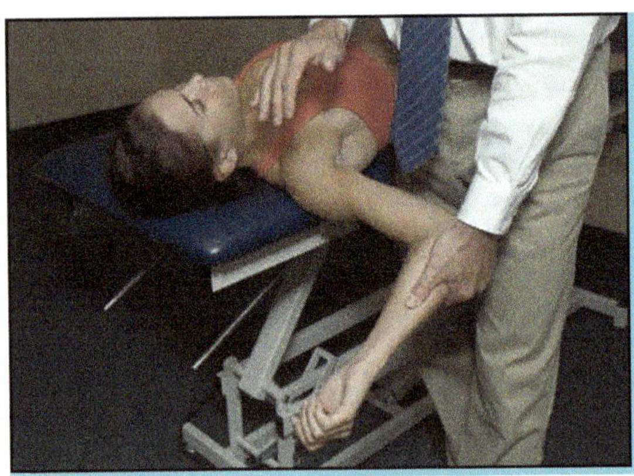

4) The posterior force on the humerus is then released.

5) A positive test is indicated if the patient reports sudden pain, an increase in pain, or by reproduction of the patient's concordant symptoms.

UTILITY SCORE 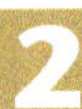

Study	Reliability	Sensitivity	Specificity	LR+	LR−	QUADAS Score (0–14)
Gross & Distefano[23]	NT	92	89	8.36	0.08	9
Lo et al.[52]	NT	64	99	64	0.36	7
Comments: Despite the apparently good statistics, the quality of these two studies is poor so the examiner should be guarded about the results.						

TORN LABRUM/INSTABILITY TESTS

Pain Provocation Test[61] (SLAP Lesion)

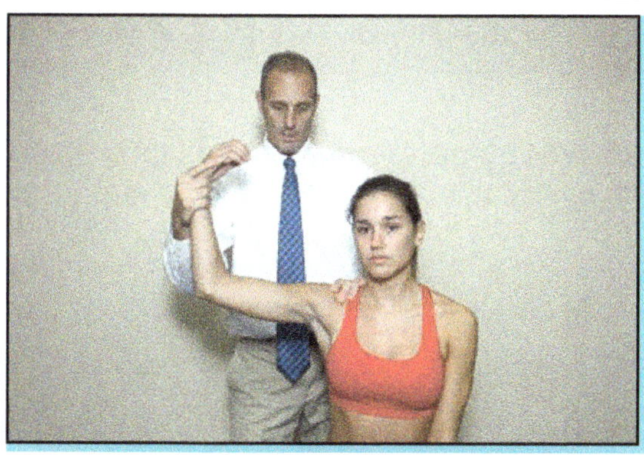

1) The patient assumes a sitting position. The examiner stands behind the patient.

2) The examiner places the patient's shoulder in 90 degrees of abduction and toward end-range external rotation. The elbow is placed at 90 degrees of flexion and the forearm in maximum pronation.

3) The examiner asks the patient to rate his or her pain in this position.

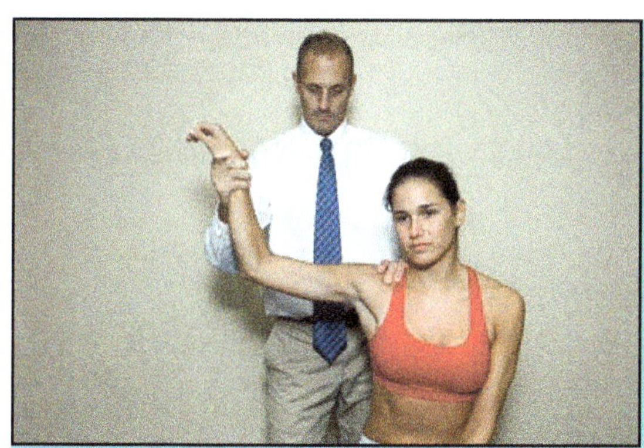

4) The examiner then fully pronates the patient's forearm and asks the patient to, again, rate his or her pain.

5) A positive test is indicated by production of the patient's concordant pain in the forearm-pronated position or when the patient's pain is worse in pronation than in supination.

UTILITY SCORE 2

Study	Reliability	Sensitivity	Specificity	LR+	LR−	QUADAS Score (0–14)
Mimori et al.[61] SLAP	NT	100	90	NA	NA	7
Parentis et al.[71] SLAP	NT	17	90	1.72	0.92	5
Parentis et al.[70] SLAP	NT	15	90	1.5	0.9	9

Comments: Despite the great numbers reported by Mimori et al.[61], their study had many design faults including a criterion standard (arthroscopy) which was given to only 11 of 32 patients. The newer work by Parentis et al.[70] in 2006 shows that the Pain Provocation test may be a specific test for a SLAP lesion with application to a wider population.

Passive Compression Test[58] (SLAP Lesion)

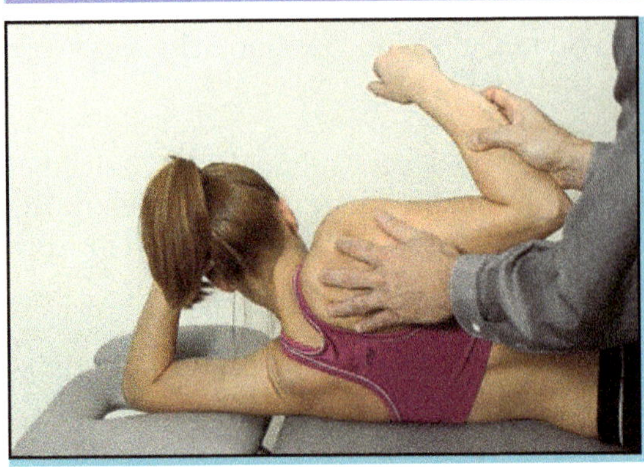

1) The patient lies on the uninvolved side. The examiner stands behind the patient.

2) The examiner stabilizes the superior aspect of the scapula with one hand while using the other hand to grasp the elbow.

3) The examiner externally rotates the arm and abducts the arm 30 degrees.

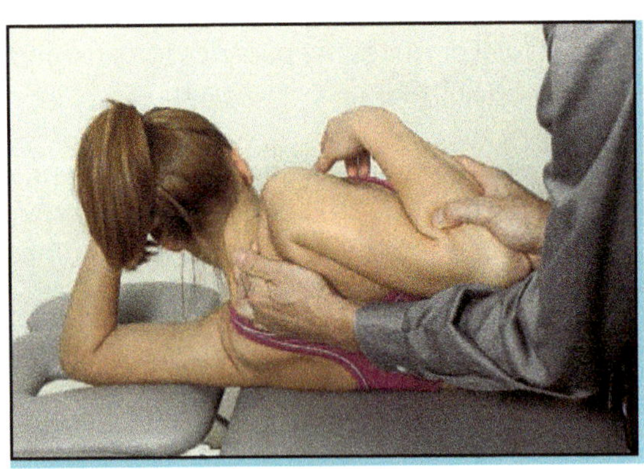

4) The examiner applies a superior compressive force while extending the arm.

5) A positive test is indicated by pain reproduction or a painful click.

UTILITY SCORE 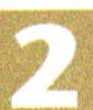

Study	Reliability	Sensitivity	Specificity	LR+	LR−	QUADAS Score (0–14)
Kim et al.[47]	κ = .77	82	86	5.72	0.21	8
Comments: Based on this one study of moderate quality, the Passive Compression Test[47] appears to be both an accurate and reliable clinical diagnostic tool. However, a sample size of 61 subjects means that more research needs to be done.						

Apprehension Test[73] (Anterior Instability, All Instabilities of the Glenohumeral Joint, Labral Tear, SLAP Lesion)

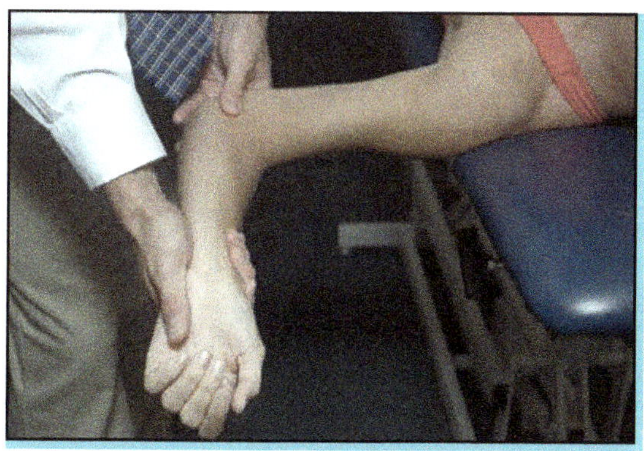

1) The patient is either standing or supine. The examiner stands either behind or at the involved side of the patient.

2) The examiner grasps the wrist with one hand and maximally externally rotates the humerus with the shoulder in 90 degrees of abduction.

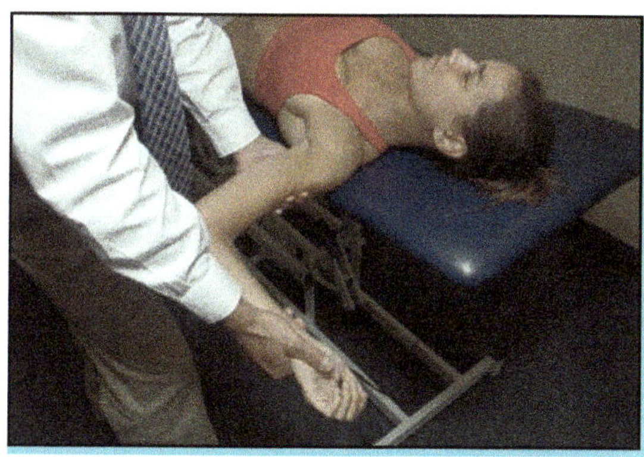

3) Forward pressure is then applied to the posterior aspect of the humeral head by either the examiner (if patient is standing) or the examination table (if the patient is in supine).

4) A positive test for anterior instability is indicated by a show of apprehension by the patient or a report of pain.

UTILITY SCORE 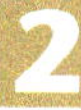

Study	Reliability	Sensitivity	Specificity	LR+	LR−	QUADAS Score (0–14)
Guanche & Jones[24] (SLAP	NT	30	63	0.81	1.11	12
Any Labral Lesion)	NT	40	87	3.08	0.69	12
Lo et al.[52]	NT	53	99	53	0.47	7
Jia et al.[34] (Any Instability	NT	58	96	14.5	0.65	6
Anterior Instability	NT	72	96	18.0	0.29	
Posterior Instability	NT	20	85	1.33	0.94	
Multidirectional Instability)	NT	43	85	2.87	0.67	
Farber et al.[15] (Pain	NT	50	56	1.14	0.89	11
Apprehension)	NT	72	96	18.0	0.29	
Oh et al.[68] (Type II SLAP)	NT	62	42	1.07	0.90	11

Comments: The Apprehension Test was originally described in 1981 by Rowe and Zarins[73] to detect anterior instability. The test appears to be specific for that pathology when apprehension (not pain) is used as the definition of a positive test.

TORN LABRUM/INSTABILITY TESTS

Modified Dynamic Labral Shear Test[80] (Labral Tear)

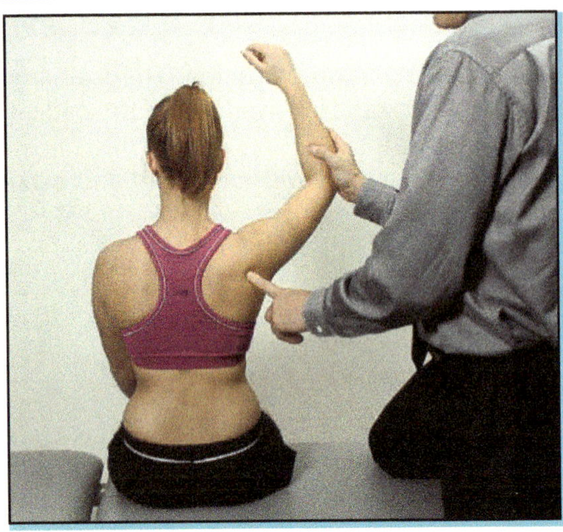

1) The patient is standing with the involved elbow flexed 90 degrees and the shoulder abducted in the scapular plane to above 120 degrees and externally rotated to end-range.

2) The examiner moves the involved shoulder into maximum horizontal abduction.

3) The examiner applies a posterior-to-anterior force to the posterior humeral head while lowering the arm from 120 degrees to 60 degrees abduction.

4) A positive test is indicated by reproduction of the pain and/or a painful click or catch in the posterior joint line between 120 degrees and 90 degrees abduction.

UTILITY SCORE 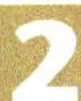

Study	Reliability	Sensitivity	Specificity	LR+	LR−	QUADAS Score (0–14)
Kibler et al.[41]	NT	72	98	31.57	0.29	9
Comments: This test appears to be specific for a labral tear but more research needs to be done by other than the inventor of the test.						

TORN LABRUM/INSTABILITY TESTS

Modified Relocation/Modified Jobe Relocation Test[25] (Labral Pathology, Traumatic Anterior Instability)

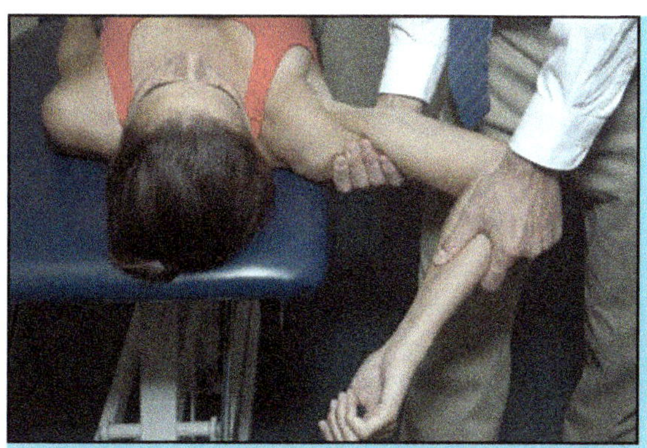

1) The patient assumes a supine position. The examiner stands beside the patient.

2) The examiner pre-positions the shoulder at 120 degrees of abduction then grasps the patient's forearm and maximally externally rotates the humerus.

3) A posterior to anterior force is then applied to the posterior aspect of the humeral head by the examiner.

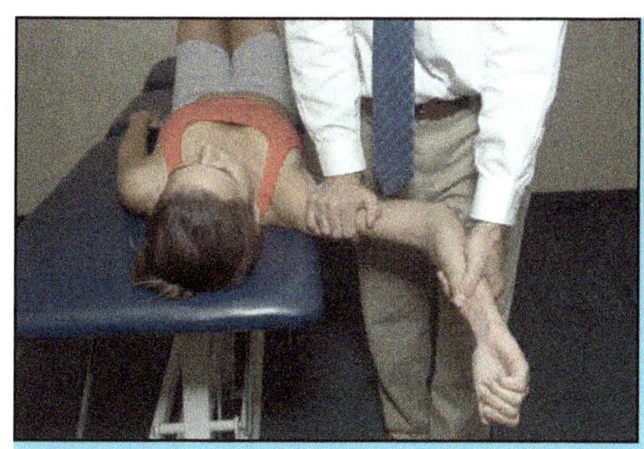

4) If the patient reports pain, a posterior force is then applied to the proximal humerus.

5) A positive test for labral pathology is indicated by a report of pain with the anterior-directed force and relief of pain with the posterior-directed force.

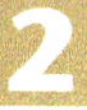

UTILITY SCORE 2

Study	Reliability	Sensitivity	Specificity	LR+	LR−	QUADAS Score (0–14)
Hamner et al.[25]	NT	92	100	92	0.08	7
Farber et al.[15] (Pain Apprehension)	NT	30 81	90 92	3.0 10.13	0.78 0.10	11

Comments: There were only 14 subjects in the Hamner et al.[25] study—all overhead throwing athletes between the ages of 21 and 31, and there were many other design faults that lead to potential bias. The Farber et al.[15] study is a nice addition with a sample size of 363 but the group in their study with traumatic anterior instability was younger and more athletic which may have a great deal to do with the numbers. Nevertheless, when apprehension is used as a positive sign, the Relocation Test[25] may be a strong diagnostic tool.

TORN LABRUM/INSTABILITY TESTS

Apprehension-Relocation/Jobe Relocation Test[35] (Anterior Instability, Labral Tear, SLAP Lesion)

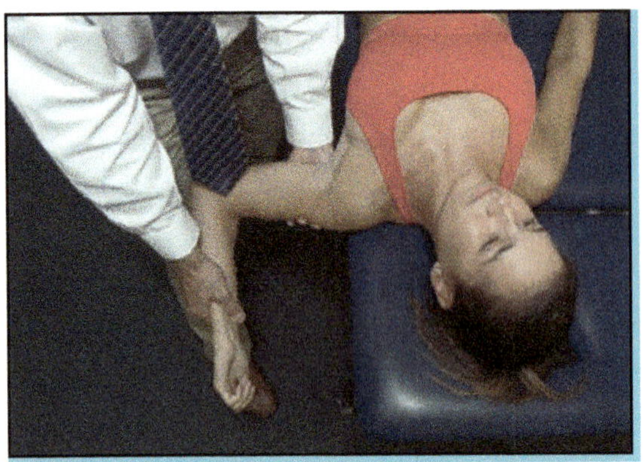

1) The patient assumes a supine position. The examiner stands beside the patient.

2) The examiner pre-positions the shoulder at 90 degrees of abduction then grasps the patient's forearm and maximally externally rotates the humerus.

3) A posterior to anterior force is then applied to the posterior aspect of the humeral head by the examiner

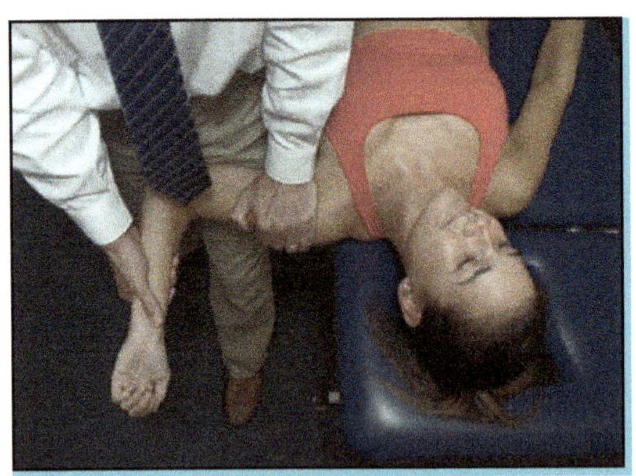

4) If the patient displays apprehension or reports pain, a posterior force is then applied to the proximal humerus.

5) A positive test for anterior instability is indicated by a decrease in the pain or apprehension whereas no change in pain symptoms indicates impingement.

UTILITY SCORE 3

Study	Reliability	Sensitivity	Specificity	LR+	−LR	QUADAS Score (0–14)
Guanche & Jones[24] (SLAP Any Labral Lesion)	NT NT	36 44	63 87	.97 3.38	1.02 .64	12 12
Morgan et al.[62] Anterior Labral Tear Posterior Labral Tear Combined (SLAP)	NT NT NT	4 85 59	27 68 54	.05 2.67 1.28	3.52 .21 .76	11 11 11
Parentis et al.[71] (SLAP)	NT	44	51	.90	1.10	5
Nakagawa et al.[65] (Superior Labral Tear)	NT	75	40	1.25	.63	10
Lo et al.[52]	NT	46	54	1.0	1.0	7
Speer et al.[80] (Pain Apprehension)	NT NT	54 68	44 100	.96 NA	1.05 NA	9 9
Parentis et al.[70]	NT	50	53	1.1	0.9	9

Comments: Originally described by Jobe et al. in 1989[21], the Relocation Test was supposed to differentiate between impingement and anterior instability. The Speer et al.[50] study would seem to indicate that the Relocation Test has value as a positive test in ruling in anterior instability when the patient emotes "apprehension." However, the Speer et al.[50] study had significant limitations with regard to blinding and description of the spectrum of patients so the numbers are to be taken with caution. Research does not support the use of this test to differentiate impingement from instability or to diagnose any type of labral tear.

Supine Flexion Resistance Test (Type II SLAP Lesion)

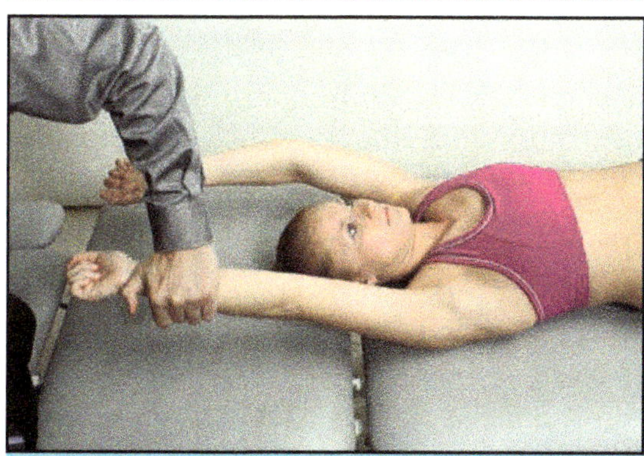

1) The patient is supine with arms above head in full elevation and palms facing up.

2) The examiner, standing on the involved side, grasps the patient's arm just distal to the elbow.

3) The examiner provides resistance as the patient tries to flex the arm/raise the arm off the table.

4) A positive test for a Type II SLAP lesion is indicated by reproduction of pain deep inside the shoulder or the dorsal aspect of the glenohumeral joint line.

UTILITY SCORE 3

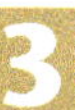

Study	Reliability	Sensitivity	Specificity	LR+	LR−	QUADAS Score (0–14)
Ebinger et al.[14]	NT	80	69	2.58	0.29	12
Comments: An important note is that the Supine Flexion Resistance Test[14] was tested for Type II SLAP lesions only as Type I lesions were eliminated from final analysis; perhaps an unrealistic situation for most clinicians.						

Speed's Test[13] [All Stages of Subacromial Impingement, Superior Labral Anterior to Posterior (SLAP) Lesion, Any Labral Lesion, Biceps Pathology]

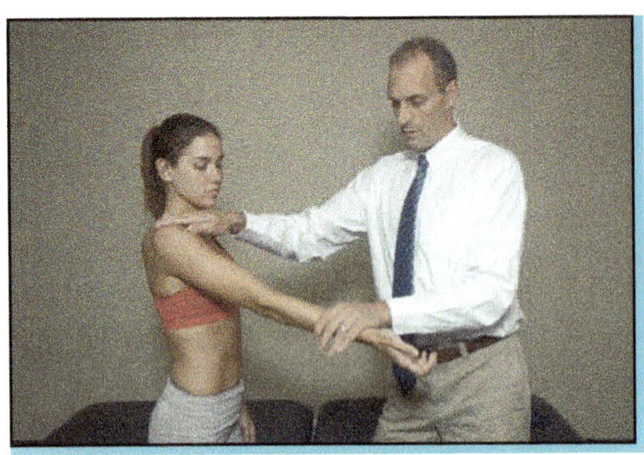

1. The patient assumes a standing position. The patient is instructed to extend his/her elbow and fully supinate the forearm.
2. The examiner, standing in front of the patient, resists shoulder flexion from zero to 60 degrees.
3. If the patient localizes concordant pain to the bicipital groove, the test is positive.

UTILITY SCORE 3

Study	Reliability	Sensitivity	Specificity	LR+	LR−	QUADAS Score (0–14)
Park et al.[72] (Impingement)	NT	38	83	2.23	0.74	10
Calis et al.[8] (Impingement Rotator Cuff Tear)	NT NT	69 85	56 57	1.56 1.98	0.55 0.26	8 8
Holtby & Razmjou[29] (SLAP)	NT	32	75	1.28	0.91	12
Bennett[6] (SLAP and Biceps Pathology)	NT	90	14	1.04	0.72	9
Guanche & Jones[24] (SLAP Any Labral Lesion)	NT NT	9 18	74 87	0.35 1.38	1.23 0.94	12 12
Morgan et al.[62] (Anterior Labrum Posterior Labrum SLAP)	NT NT NT	100 29 78	70 11 37	NA 0.32 1.23	NA 6.32 0.60	11 11 11
Parentis et al.[71] (SLAP)	NT	48	68	1.49	0.77	5
Ostor et al.[69] (Long Head of Biceps Pathology)	κ = .17–.32	NT	NT	NT	NT	NA
Nakagawa et al.[65] (Superior Labral Tear)	NT	4	100	NA	NA	10
Parentis et al.[70] (SLAP)	NT	48	67	1.5	0.8	9
Jia et al.[34] (Biceps Tendinopathy)	NT	50	67	1.51	0.75	6
Ebinger et al.[14] (SLAP)	NT	60	38	0.97	1.05	12
Gill et al.[21] (Biceps Partial Tear)	NT	50	67	1.51	0.75	12
Ardic et al.[2] (Biceps Tendinopathy)	NT	69	60	1.73	0.52	12
Kibler et al.[41] (Biceps Tendinopathy Labral Tear)	NT	54 29	81 69	2.77 0.93	0.58 1.03	9
Oh et al.[68] (Type II SLAP)	NT	32	66	0.94	1.03	11

Comments: Speed's Test was originally used to test for long head bicipital tenosynovitis but the use of the test expanded to many pathologies. Unfortunately, in the well-performed studies this test seems a poor test for any of those pathologies with the exception of an anterior labral tear, where one study showed it may be used as a screening tool due to high sensitivity.

TORN LABRUM/INSTABILITY TESTS

Forced Shoulder Abduction and Elbow Flexion Test[65] (Superior Labral Tear)

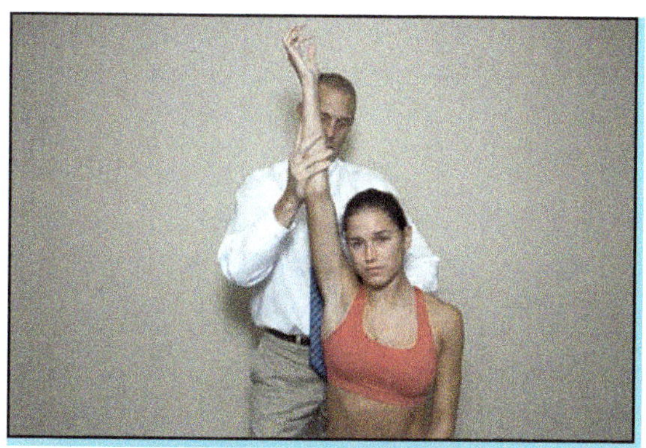

1) The patient assumes a sitting position. The examiner typically stands at the side of the involved extremity.

2) The examiner places the patient's shoulder in maximum abduction with full elbow extension and notes pain in the posterior-superior aspect of the shoulder.

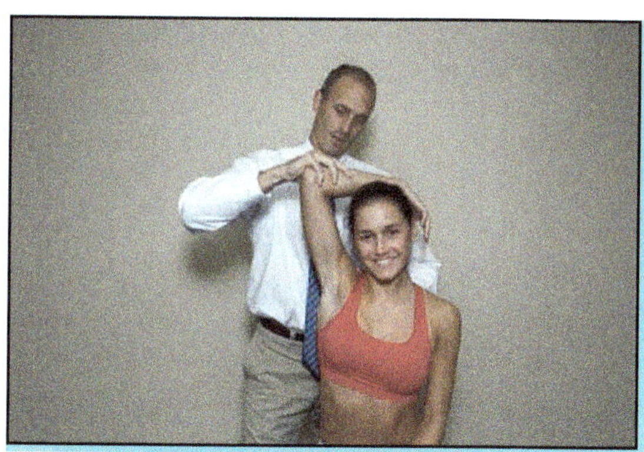

3) The examiner then flexes the patient's elbow.

4) A positive test is indicated by the production of pain in the posterior-superior aspect of the shoulder during shoulder abduction with elbow extension that is diminished or relieved by elbow flexion.

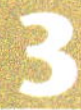

UTILITY SCORE 3

Study	Reliability	Sensitivity	Specificity	LR+	LR−	QUADAS Score (0–14)
Nakagawa et al.[65]	NT	67	67	2.0	0.49	10

Comments: The one study to examine the Forced Shoulder Abduction and Elbow Flexion Test[65] had some design /reporting flaws. Most notably, all subjects were young throwing athletes and only 2 of 54 subjects were female leading to spectrum bias. More well-designed research is needed.

Sulcus Sign[77] (Inferior Laxity, Superior Labral Tear)

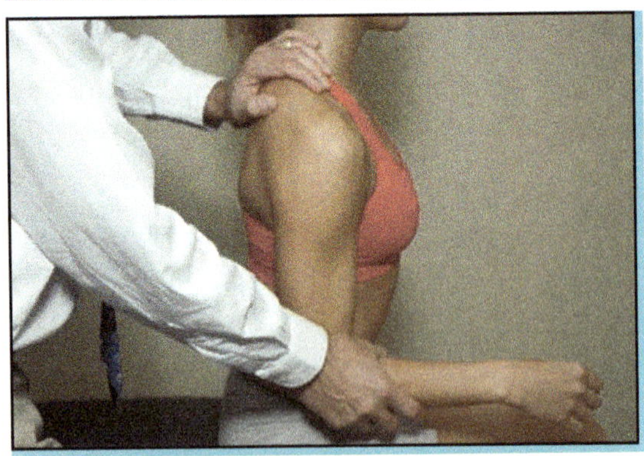

1) The patient assumes a sitting position. The examiner stands behind the patient.

2) The examiner grasps the elbow and pulls down causing an inferior traction force.

3) The examiner notes, in centimeters, the distance between the inferior surface of the acromion and the superior portion of the humeral head.

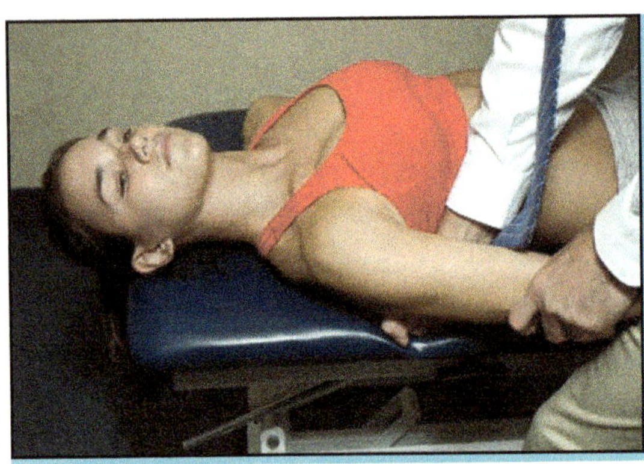

4) The examiner repeats the test in supine with the shoulder in 20 degrees of abduction and in forward flexion while maintaining a neutral rotation.

UTILITY SCORE 

Study	Reliability	Sensitivity	Specificity	LR+	LR−	QUADAS Score (0–14)
Silliman & Hawkins[77]	ND	ND	ND	ND	ND	NA
Nakagawa et al.[65] (Superior Labral Tear)	NT	17	93	2.43	0.89	10
Comments: The Sulcus Sign is often used clinically but amazingly, has been researched in only one study.[65] The use of this sign to detect inferior instability is not supported but the Sulcus Sign may be a specific test that rules in a superior labral tear when positive.						

TORN LABRUM/INSTABILITY TESTS

Active Compression Test/O'Brien's Test[66] [Labral Tear, SLAP Lesion, Labral Abnormality, Acromioclavicular (AC) Joint Pathology]

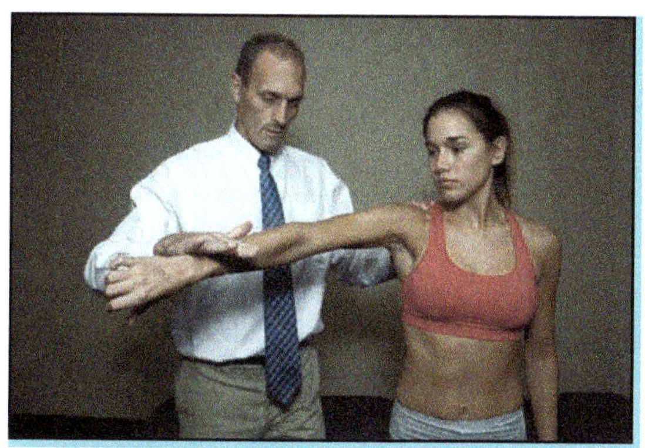

1) The patient is instructed to stand with his or her involved shoulder at 90 degrees of flexion, 10 degrees of horizontal adduction, and maximum internal rotation with the elbow in full extension. The examiner stands directly behind the patient's involved shoulder.

2) The examiner applies a downward force at the wrist of the involved extremity. The patient is instructed to resist the force.

3) The patient resists the downward force and reports any pain as either "on top of the shoulder" (acromioclavicular joint) or "inside the shoulder" (SLAP lesion).

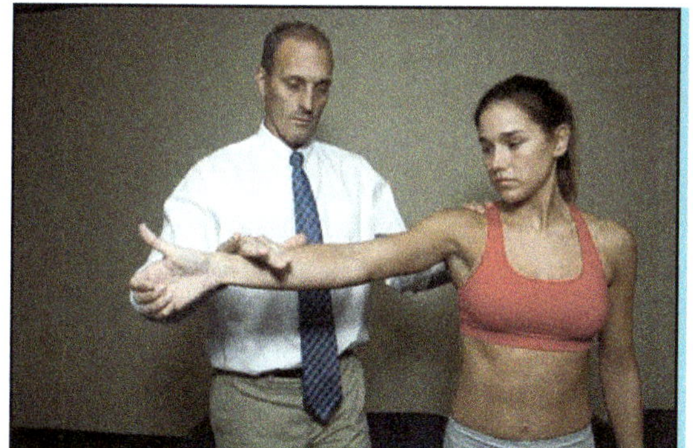

4) The patient's shoulder is then moved to a position of maximum external rotation, and the downward force is repeated.

5) A positive test is indicated by pain or painful clicking in shoulder internal rotation and less or no pain in external rotation.

UTILITY SCORE 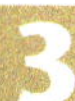

Study	Reliability	Sensitivity	Specificity	LR+	LR−	QUADAS Score (0–14)
O'Brien et al.[66] (Labral Abnormality AC Joint Pathology)	NT NT	100 100	99 97	NA NA	NA NA	3 3
Guanche & Jones[24] (SLAP Any Labral Lesion)	NT NT	54 63	47 73	1.01 2.33	0.98 0.51	12 12
Morgan et al.[62] [Anterior Labral Posterior Labral Tear Combined (SLAP)]	NT	88 32 85	42 13 41	1.52 0.37 1.44	0.28 5.14 0.36	11 11 11
Parentis et al.[71] (SLAP)	NT	65	49	1.27	0.72	5
McFarland et al.[56] (SLAP)	NT	47	55	1.04	0.96	11
Stetson & Templin[81] (Labral Tear)	NT	54	31	0.78	1.48	10
Myers et al.[64] (SLAP)	NT	78	11	0.88	2	8
Walton et al.[84] (AC Joint)	NT	16	90	1.6	0.93	13

(continued)

TORN LABRUM/INSTABILITY TESTS

Study	Reliability	Sensitivity	Specificity	LR+	LR−	QUADAS Score (0–14)
Nakagawa et al.[65] (Superior Labral Tear)	NT	54	60	1.35	0.77	10
Parentis et al.[70] (SLAP)	NT	63	50	1.3	0.7	9
Jia et al.[34] (SLAP AC Joint)	NT NT	47 41	55 95	1.04 8.2	0.96 0.62	6
Ebinger et al.[14] (Type II SLAP)	NT	94	28	1.30	0.21	13
Kibler et al.[41] (Labral Tear)	NT	61	84	3.83	0.84	9
Oh et al.[68] (Type II SLAP)	NT	63	53	1.34	0.70	11
Walsworth et al.[83] (Any Labral Tear)	$\kappa = 0.24$	55	18	0.67	2.5	11

Comments: The original optimistic statistical numbers presented by O'Brien et al.[66] were most likely the result of poor study design. Better conducted studies may be showing that the Active Compression Test is sensitive for SLAP tears and specific for an AC joint problem or that the test may be of no clinical utility.

Resisted Supination External Rotation Test (RSERT)[64] (SLAP Lesion)

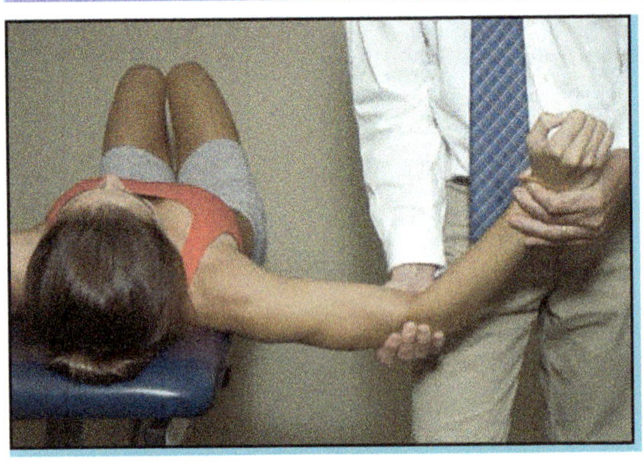

1. The patient assumes a supine position. The examiner stands beside the patient's involved extremity.
2. The examiner grasps the patient's hand and supports the elbow. The examiner then places the patient's shoulder in 90 degrees of abduction and neutral rotation, the elbow in 65–70 degrees of flexion, and the forearm in neutral pronation/supination.
3. The examiner instructs the patient to attempt to supinate his or her arm.

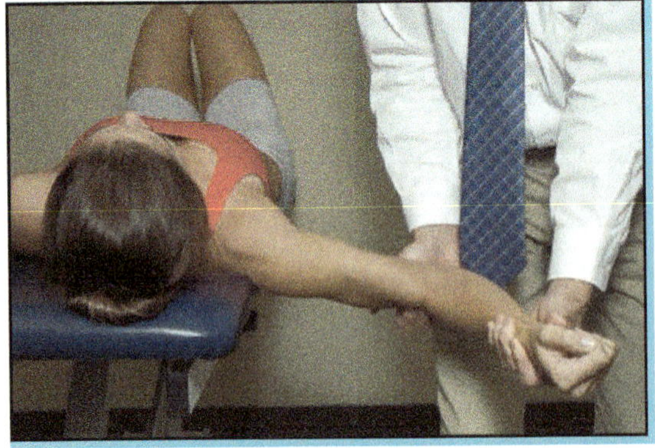

4. The examiner resists supination while gradually moving the patient's shoulder to end-range of external rotation.
5. A positive test is indicated by the production of pain in the anterior or deep shoulder, clicking or catching in the shoulder, or by reproduction of the patient's concordant symptoms.

TORN LABRUM/INSTABILITY TESTS

UTILITY SCORE 3

Study	Reliability	Sensitivity	Specificity	LR+	LR−	QUADAS Score (0–14)
Myers et al.[64] SLAP	NT	83	82	4.61	.20	8

Comments: The RSERT has only a small to moderate effect on the posttest probability of having a SLAP lesion. Additionally, there is only one study, with numerous design/reporting limitations, which looked at this test. More research needs to be performed, especially in light of the quality of this study.

Compression-Rotation Test[79] (SLAP Lesion)

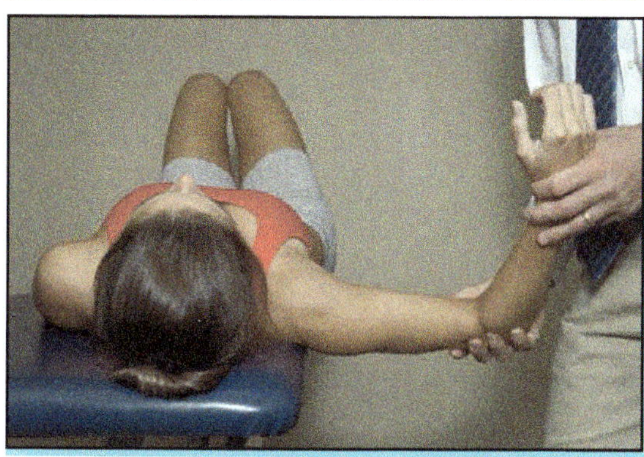

1) The patient assumes a supine position. The examiner stands to the side of the involved extremity.

2) The examiner passively places the patient's shoulder in 90 degrees of abduction and the elbow in 90 degrees of flexion.

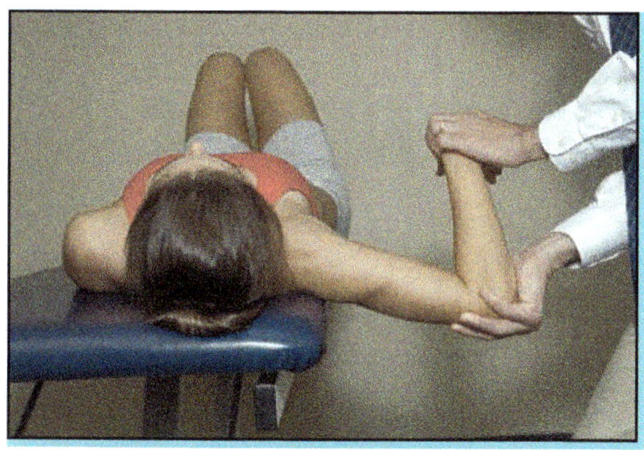

3) The examiner first applies a compression force to the humerus and rotates the humerus back and forth from internal rotation to external rotation in an attempt to pinch the torn labrum.

4) A positive test is indicated by the production of a catching or snapping in the shoulder.

UTILITY SCORE 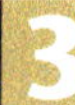

Study	Reliability	Sensitivity	Specificity	LR+	LR−	QUADAS Score (0–14)
McFarland et al.[56] (SLAP)	NT	24	76	1.0	1.0	11
Oh et al.[68] (Type II SLAP)	NT	61	54	1.33	0.72	11

Comments: The Compression-Rotation Test was originally reported by Snyder et al.[79] Both studies to examine the Compression-Rotation Test were performed well. There appears to be little use for this test in the clinic to detect SLAP lesions.

TORN LABRUM/INSTABILITY TESTS

Anterior Slide Test[40] (SLAP Lesion)

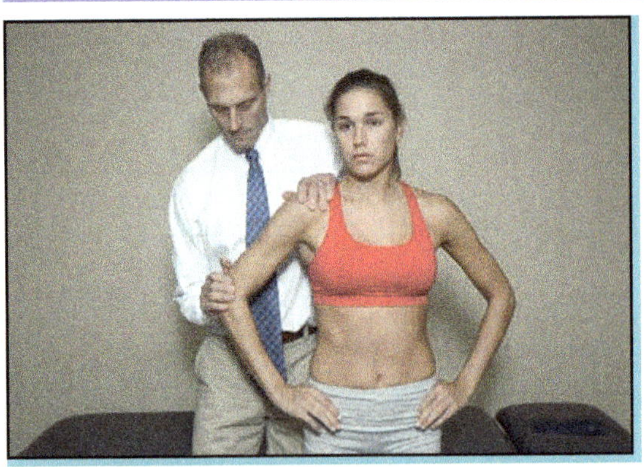

1) The patient is in either standing or sitting with his or her hands on his or her hips so that the thumb is positioned posteriorly. The examiner stands behind the patient.

2) The examiner places one hand superior on the shoulder to stabilize the scapula and clavicle.

3) The examiner places his or her opposite hand on the patient's elbow with the palm of the hand cupping the olecranon.

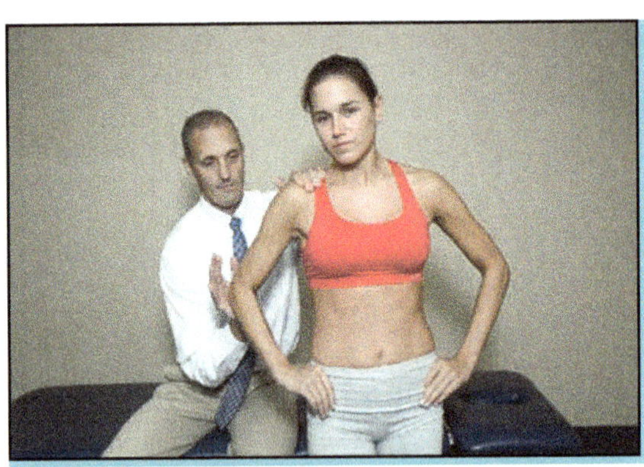

4) The examiner provides an anterior-superior force through the elbow to the glenohumeral joint while the patient resists this movement.

5) A positive test is indicated by the production of pain in the anterior shoulder, by the production of a pop or click in the shoulder, or by reproduction of the patient's concordant symptoms.

UTILITY SCORE 

Study	Reliability	Sensitivity	Specificity	LR+	LR−	QUADAS Score (0–14)
McFarland et al.[56] (SLAP)	NT	8	84	0.50	1.10	11
Kibler[40] (SLAP)	NT	78	92	9.75	0.24	6
Parentis et al.[71] (SLAP)	NT	13	84	0.79	1.04	5
Nakagawa et al.[65] (Superior Labral Tear)	NT	5	93	0.71	1.0	10
Parentis et al.[70] (SLAP)	NT	10	82	0.56	1.1	9
Jia et al.[34] (SLAP Biceps Tendinopathy)	NT NT	19 50	81 81	1.03 2.68	1.0 0.62	6
Gill et al.[21] (Belly Press, Partial Biceps Tear)	NT	23	84	1.40	0.92	12
Kibler et al.[41] (Labral Tear)	NT	48	82	2.63	0.64	9
Oh et al.[68] (Type II SLAP)	NT	21	70	0.70	1.13	11
Walsworth et al.[83] (Any Labral Tear)	κ = 0.21	43	82	2.38	0.69	11

Comments: The original author's solid statistical numbers may be the result of poor study design/reporting. The well-performed studies seem to indicate that there is little use for this test in the clinic to detect SLAP lesions, partial biceps tears, or labral tears in general.

TORN LABRUM/INSTABILITY TESTS

Biceps Load Test[45] (SLAP Lesion with Anterior Shoulder Dislocation)

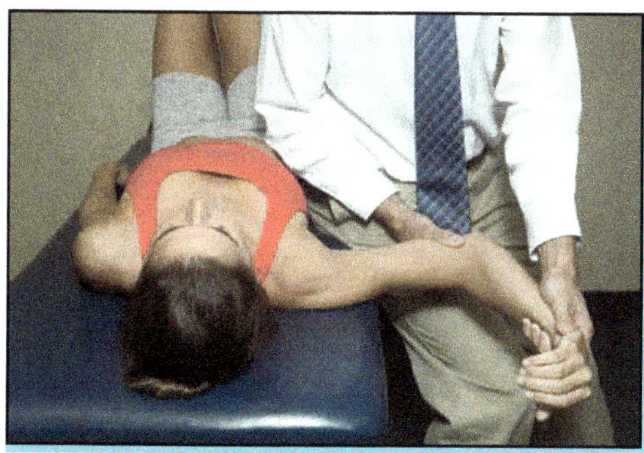

1) The patient assumes a supine position. The examiner sits on the side of the patient's involved extremity.

2) The examiner places the patient's shoulder in 90 degrees of abduction, the elbow in 90 degrees of flexion, and the forearm in supination.

3) The examiner moves the patient's shoulder to end-range external rotation (apprehension position).

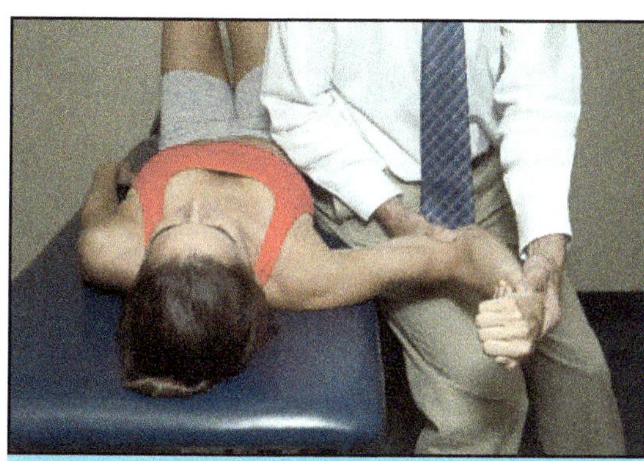

4) At end-range external rotation, the examiner asks the patient to flex his or her elbow while the examiner resists this movement.

5) The examiner queries the patient if and how his or her apprehension has changed after flexion of the elbow.

6) A positive test is indicated by either no change in apprehension or pain that is worsened with resisted elbow flexion.

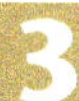

UTILITY SCORE 3

Study	Reliability	Sensitivity	Specificity	LR+	LR−	QUADAS Score (0–14)
Kim et al.[45] (SLAP)	κ = .85	91	97	29.32	.09	9

Comments: The great numbers reported by Kim et al[45] would seem to warrant a better "Utility Score," but their study had many design faults including the fact that only patients with repeated anterior dislocations were studied. The fact that all patients had repetitive dislocations may have been a more important predictor of a SLAP lesion than the Biceps Load Test.[45] The authors may have recognized these shortcomings because they developed the Biceps Load Test II.[44]

Clunk Test (Labral Tear, Superior Labral Tear)

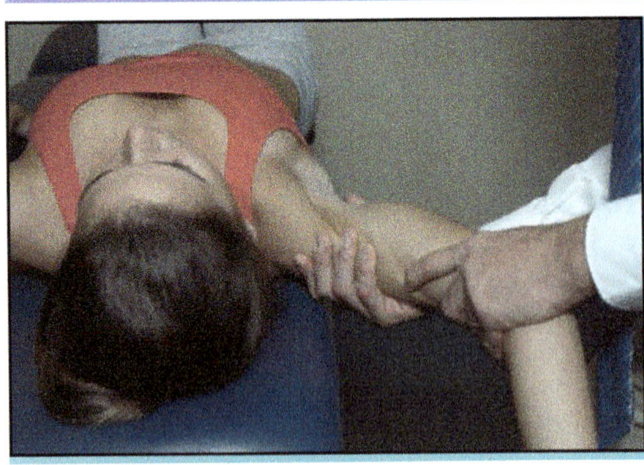

1) The patient is supine. The examiner stands to the involved side of the patient with one hand on the posterior humeral head and the other on the medial distal humerus.

2) The examiner abducts the patient's shoulder to end-range.

3) A posterior to anterior force is then applied to the posterior aspect of the humeral head by the examiner's one hand while the hand at the elbow provides a lateral rotation of the humerus.

4) A positive test is indicated by a "clunk" or a grinding.

UTILITY SCORE 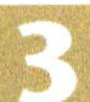 3

Study	Reliability	Sensitivity	Specificity	LR+	LR−	QUADAS Score (0–14)
Nakagawa et al.[65] (Superior Labral Tear)	NT	44	68	1.38	.82	10
Comments: Based on this one study with a limited patient population (52 male, 2 female throwing athletes), this often-used clinical test for labral tear has little merit.						

TORN LABRUM/INSTABILITY TESTS

Anterior Drawer Test[18] (Anterior Laxity, Anterior Instability)

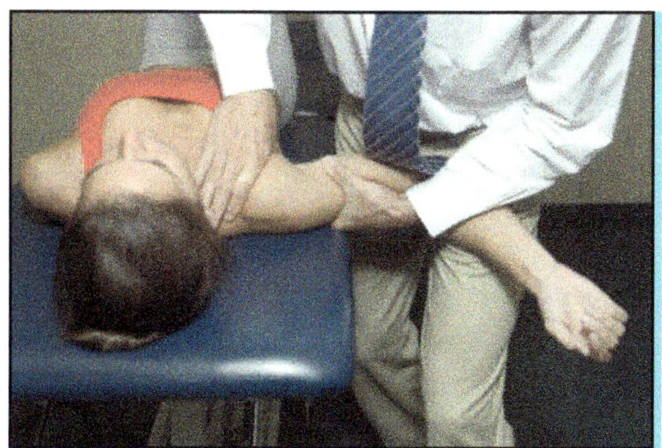

1) The patient assumes a supine position. The examiner stands behind the patient.

2) The examiner secures the distal arm of the patient in his/her axillary region.

3) The examiner's hands are placed so that one hand stabilizes the scapula and the other grasps the proximal humerus.

4) The examiner abducts the patient's arm to between 80 and 100 degrees, and then applies a posterior-to-anterior force to the humerus. The examiner carefully notes the amount of translation of the glenohumeral joint compared to the uninvolved shoulder.

UTILITY SCORE 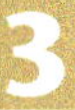

Study	Reliability	Sensitivity	Specificity	LR+	LR−	QUADAS Score (0–14)
Gerber & Ganz[18]	NT	NT	NT	NA	NA	NA
Farber et al.[15] (Pain Reproduction of Instability Symptoms)	NT NT	28 53	71 85	0.97 3.53	1.01 0.55	11
Comments: The Anterior Drawer[18] is often used clinically but one study of high quality shows this test to be of limited clinical value.						

Biceps Tension Test[16] (Unstable Superior Labrum—Lesions/SLAP Lesions)

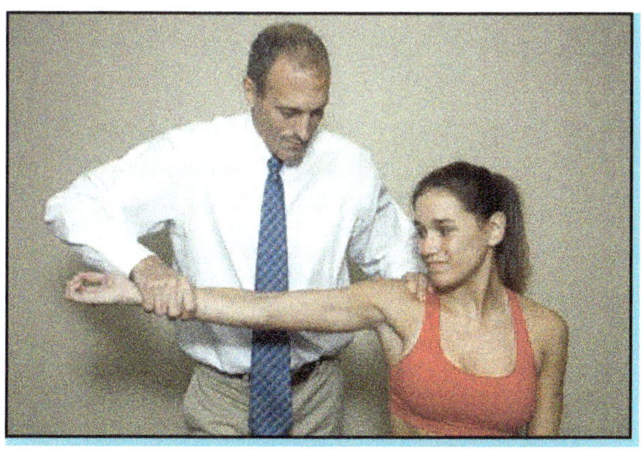

1) The patient assumes a sitting or standing position. The examiner stands in front of the patient.

2) The patient places their arm in 90 degrees of shoulder abduction, with a fully extended elbow and forearm supinated.

3) The examiner applies a downward-directed force to the distal forearm.

4) A positive test is indicated by patient report of pain.

UTILITY SCORE 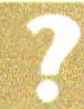

Study	Reliability	Sensitivity	Specificity	LR+	LR−	DOR	QUADAS Score (0–14)
Field & Savoie[16]	NT	NT	NT	NA	NA	NA	NA
Comments: Research needs to be performed to validate this test. The original description of the test is very limited.							

TORN LABRUM/INSTABILITY TESTS

Hyperabduction Test[17] (Inferior Laxity)

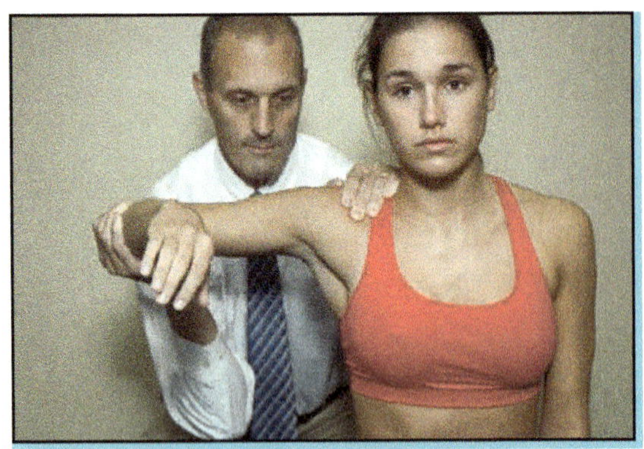

1) The patient assumes a sitting position. The examiner stands behind the patient.

2) The examiner stabilizes the scapula with a downward force on the supraclavicular region and passively places the patient's elbow in 90 degrees of flexion and the patient's forearm in pronation.

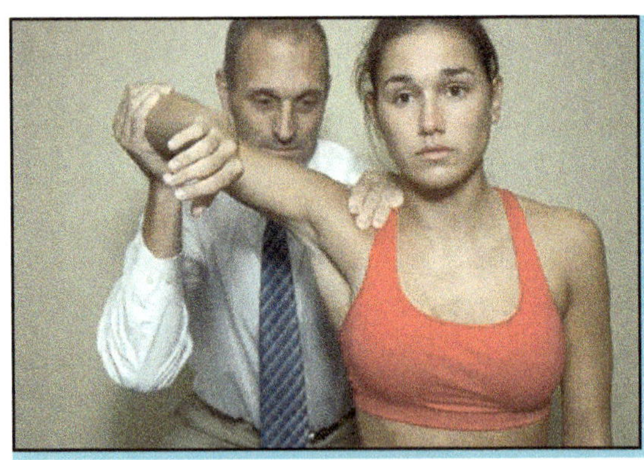

3) The examiner moves the patient's arm to maximum abduction stabilizing the scapula to reduce rotation.

4) A positive test is indicated by passive abduction greater than 105 degrees.

UTILITY SCORE

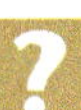

Study	Reliability	Sensitivity	Specificity	LR+	LR−	QUADAS Score (0–14)
Gagey & Gagey[17]	NT	NT	NT	NA	NA	NA
Comments: This is a very interesting test studied in cadavers, normal volunteers, and patients undergoing surgery for instability but neither diagnostic accuracy nor reliability was established.						

TORN LABRUM/INSTABILITY TESTS

Posterior Drawer Test[18] (Posterior Laxity)

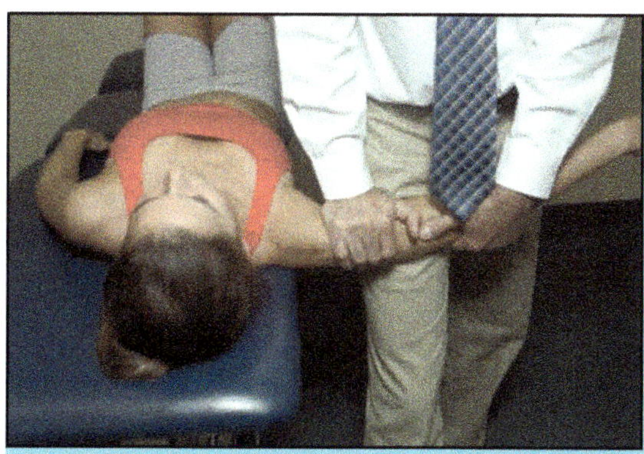

1) The patient assumes a supine position. The examiner stands beside the patient to the side of the involved shoulder.

2) The examiner secures the distal arm of the patient in his/her axillary region.

3) The examiner's hands are placed so that the upper arm is stabilized.

4) The examiner abducts the patient's arm to between 80 and 100 degrees, and then applies an anterior-to-posterior force to the humerus. The examiner carefully notes the amount of translation of the glenohumeral joint compared to the uninvolved shoulder.

UTILITY SCORE 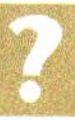

Study	Reliability	Sensitivity	Specificity	LR+	LR−	QUADAS Score (0–14)
Gerber & Ganz[18]	NT	NT	NT	NA	NA	NA
Comments: The Posterior Drawer is often used clinically but, amazingly, has never been researched, perhaps because of the difficulty of establishing a criterion standard for "instability."						

TORN LABRUM/INSTABILITY TESTS

Load and Shift Test[77] (Anterior, Posterior, Inferior Laxity)

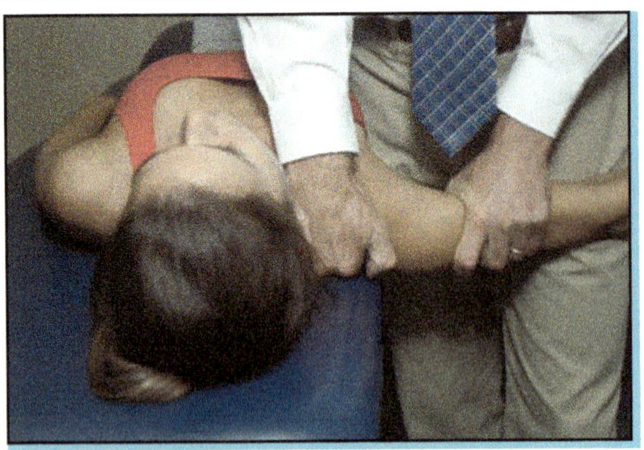

1) The patient assumes a supine position. The examiner stands to the side of the patient's involved shoulder.

2) The examiner grasps the proximal humerus with one hand providing a compression force and "loading" the humerus into the glenoid fossa. The examiner's other hand stabilizes the scapula.

3) The examiner applies an anterior-to-posterior force noting the amount of translation as either (1) to the posterior rim of the glenoid, or (2) beyond the rim of the glenoid.

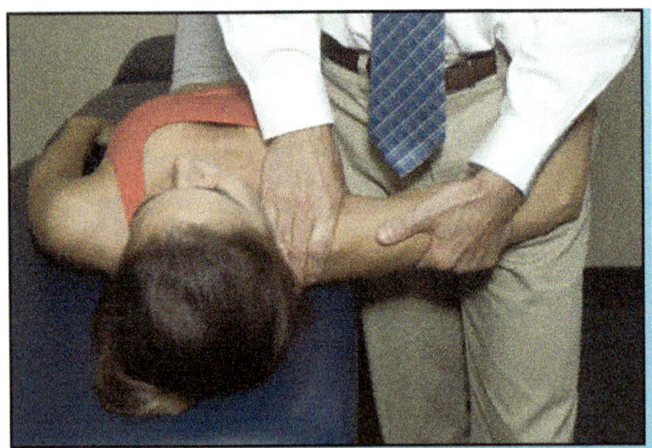

4) The examiner applies a posterior-to-anterior force noting the amount of translation as either (1) to the anterior rim of the glenoid, or (2) beyond the rim of the glenoid.

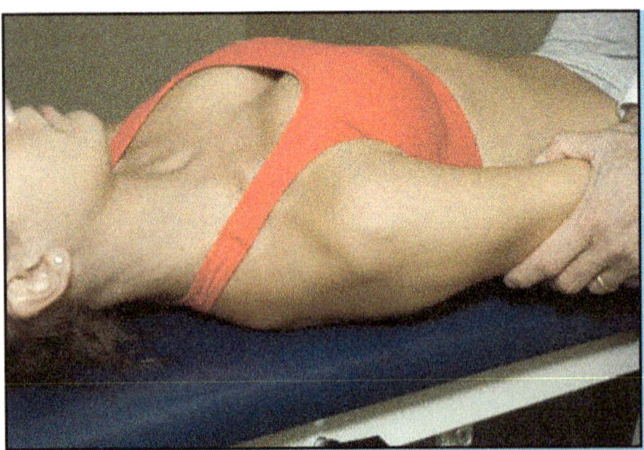

5) A Sulcus Sign (see Figure 6.64 is then performed to assess the full excursion of the humeral head in the glenoid fossa.

UTILITY SCORE 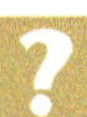

Study	Reliability	Sensitivity	Specificity	LR+	LR−	QUADAS Score (0–14)
Silliman & Hawkins[77]	NT	NT	NT	NA	NA	NA
Comments: Uh . . . Happy twentieth birthday to the Load and Shift?[77]						

TORN LABRUM/INSTABILITY TESTS

Diagnostic Clusters—Instability

UTILITY SCORE 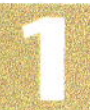

Study	Cluster	Reliability	Sensitivity	Specificity	LR+	LR−	QUADAS Score (0–14)
Malhi & Khan[55]	Apprehension or Relocation	NT	81	100	NA	19.0	5
Lo et al.[52]	Apprehension and Relocation and Surprise	NT	40	100	NA	NA	7
Farber et al.[15]	Apprehension and Relocation	NT	81	98	36.98	0.19	11
Comments: Clearly the combination of Apprehension followed by Relocation is a winning combination but may not be as good as the Surprise test by itself, based on the statistics.							

Diagnostic Clusters—Labral Tears

UTILITY SCORE 

Study	Cluster	Reliability	Sensitivity	Specificity	LR+	LR−	QUADAS Score (0–14)
Malhi & Khan[55]	Apprehension or Relocation	NT	81	1.0	NA	19.0	5
Liu et al.[50]	Apprehension or Relocation or Clicking with Load and Shift or Sulcus	NT	90	85	6.00	0.12	9
Liu et al.[50]	Age < 35 and failed conservative care	NT	66	85	4.40	0.40	9
Guanche and Jones[24]	Relocation and Active Compression	NT	41	91	4.56	0.65	12
Guanche and Jones[24]	Relocation and Apprehension	NT	38	93	5.43	0.67	12
Guanche and Jones[24]	Relocation or Active Compression	NT	72	73	2.67	0.38	12
Guanche and Jones[24]	Relocation or Apprehension	NT	72	73	2.67	0.38	12
Oh et al.[68]	Compression Rotation and Active Compression and Biceps Load II	NT	22	95	4.40	0.82	11
Oh et al.[68]	Compression Rotation or Anterior Apprehension or Speed's	NT	80	28	1.11	0.71	11
Walsworth et al.[83] (Any Labral Tear)	History of pop, click, or catch and Anterior Slide and Crank	NT	21	100	NA	0.91	11

Comments: A large majority (64%) of the patients in the Liu et al[50] study were throwing athletes and all had failed conservative therapy. Active Compression, Relocation, and Apprehension seem to be the most popular tests as part of clusters but demographic data like age, onset, and overhead work or sport may be more important in diagnosing a SLAP lesion.

ACROMIOCLAVICULAR (AC) DYSFUNCTION TESTS

AC Resisted Extension Test[32] (AC Joint Abnormality)

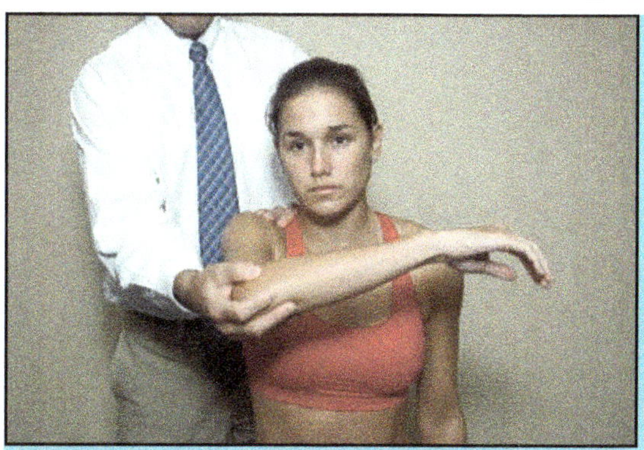

1) The patient is seated with his or her shoulder in 90 degrees of flexion and internal rotation, and his or her elbow in 90 degrees of flexion.

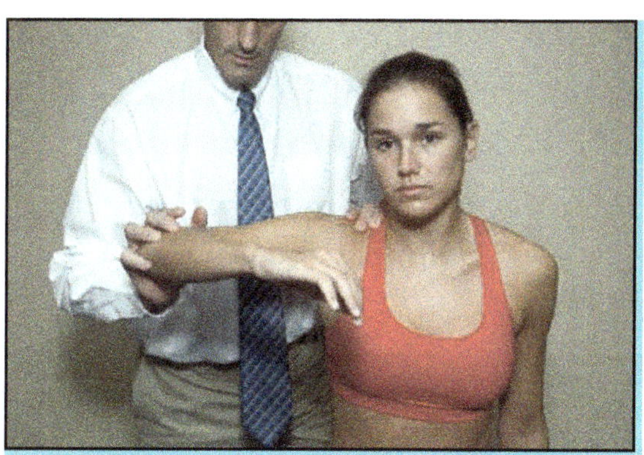

2) The examiner, standing beside the patient, asks the patient to horizontally abduct his or her arm while the examiner provides an isometric resistance to this movement.

3) A positive test is indicated by pain at the AC joint.

UTILITY SCORE 2

Study	Reliability	Sensitivity	Specificity	LR+	LR−	QUADAS Score (0–14)
Chronopoulos et al.[11]	NT	72	85	4.80	0.32	10
Jia et al.[34] (AC Joint OA)	NT	72	85	4.80	0.32	6

Comments: The AC Resisted Extension Test has a moderate effect on the posttest probability of the patient having an AC joint pathology.

ACROMIOCLAVICULAR (AC) DYSFUNCTION TESTS

AC Joint Palpation[84] (AC Joint Pain)

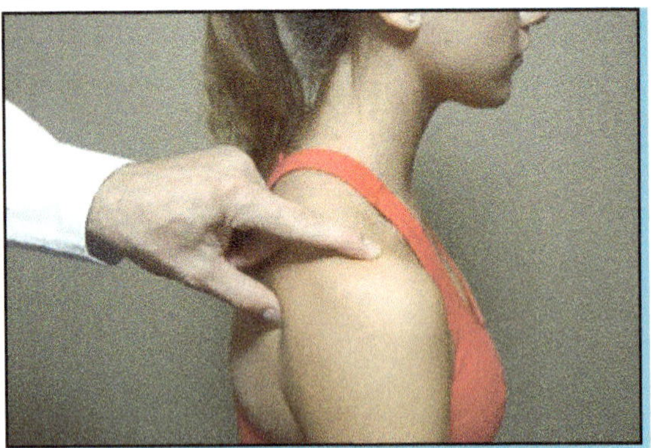

1) The patient is seated with the involved arm at his or her side. The examiner stands behind the patient and palpates the AC joint.

UTILITY SCORE 2

Study	Reliability	Sensitivity	Specificity	LR+	LR−	QUADAS Score (0–14)
Walton et al.[84]	NT	96	10	1.07	.40	13

Comments: Based on this one well-performed study, AC joint palpation should not be used as a diagnostic tool but may be a valuable screen as negative test to rule out the AC joint. More research needs to be performed.

Paxinos Sign[84] (AC Joint Pain)

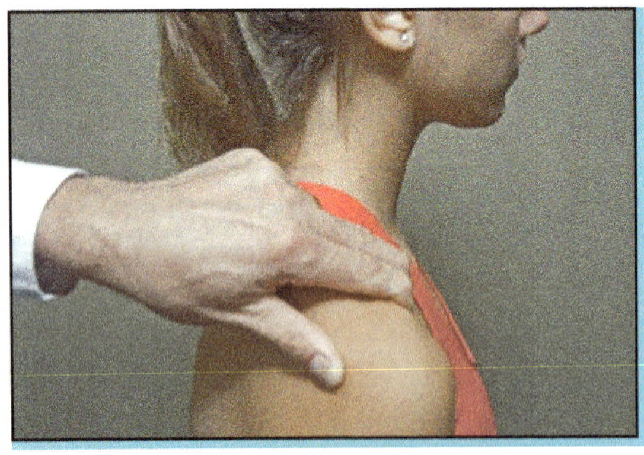

1) The patient is seated with the involved arm at his or her side. The examiner stands behind the patient.

2) The examiner places his or her thumb under the posterolateral aspect of the acromion and the index and middle fingers of the same hand on the distal clavicle.

3) The examiner applies an anterosuperior force with the thumb while concurrently applying an inferior force with the index and middle fingers.

4) A positive test is indicated by pain reproduction or an increase in pain at the AC joint.

UTILITY SCORE 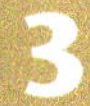

Study	Reliability	Sensitivity	Specificity	LR+	LR−	QUADAS Score (0–14)
Walton et al.[84]	NT	79	50	1.58	0.42	13

Comments: Based on this one well-performed study, the Paxinos Test/Sign[84] modifies the posttest probability of detecting AC joint pain minimally and should not be used as a diagnostic tool.

Diagnostic Clusters—AC Joint Pathology

UTILITY SCORE 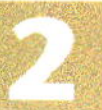

Study	Cluster	Reliability	Sensitivity	Specificity	LR+	LR−	QUADAS
Chronopoulos et al.[11]	2 or more of: Cross-body Adduction, AC Resisted Extension, and Active Compression	NT	81	89	7.36	0.21	10
Comments: There is only a small improvement in diagnostic ability of a cluster of AC joint tests when compared to the AC Resisted Extension test alone							

NERVE PALSIES

Active Elevation Lag Sign (Spinal Accessory Nerve Palsy)

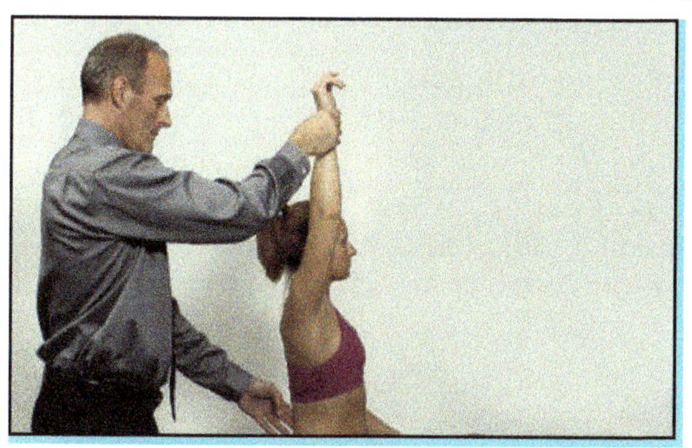

1) The patient is standing. The examiner takes each of the patient's arms into full flexion passively to make sure stiffness is not an issue. If stiffness is the reason for limited flexion, the Active Elevation Lag Sign cannot be performed.

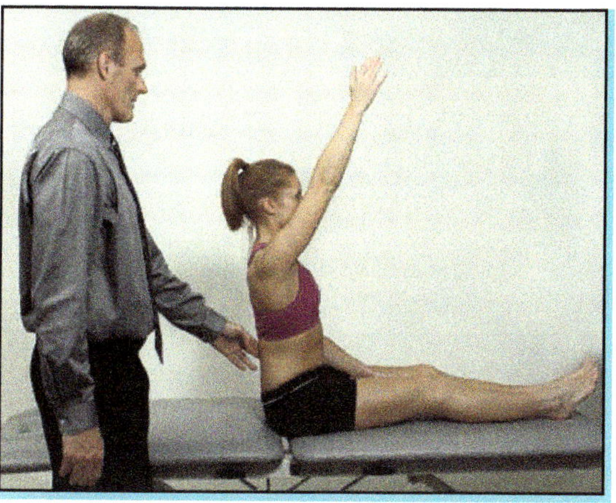

2) The examiner stands beside the patient on the unaffected side palpating the lumbar spine for hyperextension

3) The examiner asks the patient to flex their arm to end-range which is defined as the maximum elevation of the shoulder until the lumbar spine hyperextends

4) Steps two and three are repeated on the affected side

5) A positive test is indicated by decreased flexion on the involved vs. the uninvolved side.

NERVE PALSIES

UTILITY SCORE 3

Study	Reliability	Sensitivity	Specificity	LR+	LR−	QUADAS Score (0–14)
Levy et al.[48]	NT	100	95	NA	NA	7
Comments: This study was performed on only 10 patients (demographics unknown) but the authors derived their numbers by having 8 assessors look at video of the test. The quality and methodology of this study are questionable.						

The Triangle Sign (Spinal Accessory Nerve Palsy)

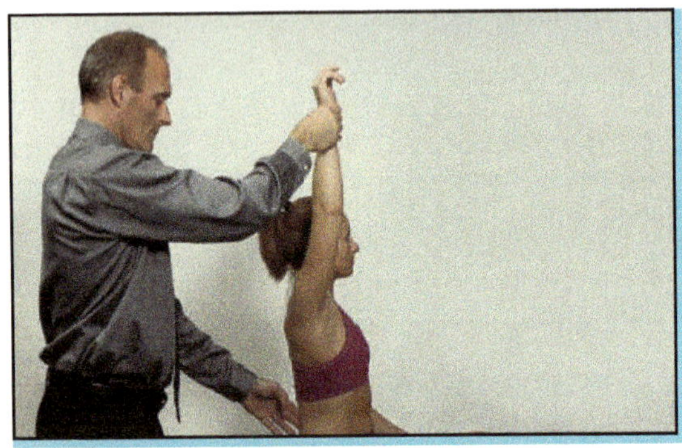

1) The patient is standing. The examiner takes each of the patient's arms into full flexion passively to make sure stiffness is not an issue. If stiffness is the reason for limited flexion, the Triangle Sign cannot be performed.

2) The examiner stands beside the patient who is lying prone with arms overhead.

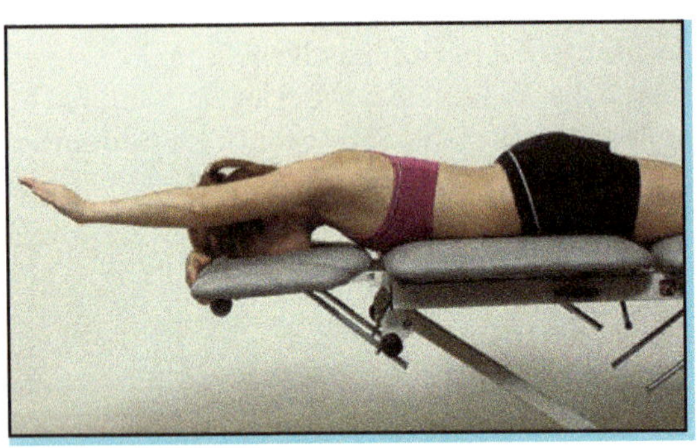

3) The examiner asks the patient to flex their arm to end-range which is defined as the maximum elevation of the shoulder until the lumbar spine hyperextends.

4) A positive sign is indicated by the compensatory strategy of lumbar extension to lift the affected arm from the table.

UTILITY SCORE 3

Study	Reliability	Sensitivity	Specificity	LR+	LR−	QUADAS Score (0–14)
Levy et al.[48]	NT	100	95	NA	NA	7
Comments: This study was performed on only 10 patients (demographics unknown) but the authors derived their numbers by having 8 assessors look at video of the test. The quality and methodology of this study are questionable.						

NERVE PALSIES

Deltoid Extension Lag Sign[28] (Axillary Nerve Palsy)

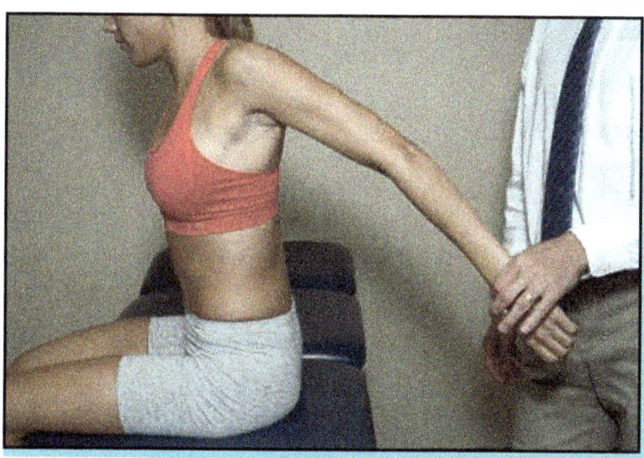

1) The patient assumes a supine position. The examiner stands behind the patient.

2) The examiner grasps the patient's wrist and pulls the arm into near full extension.

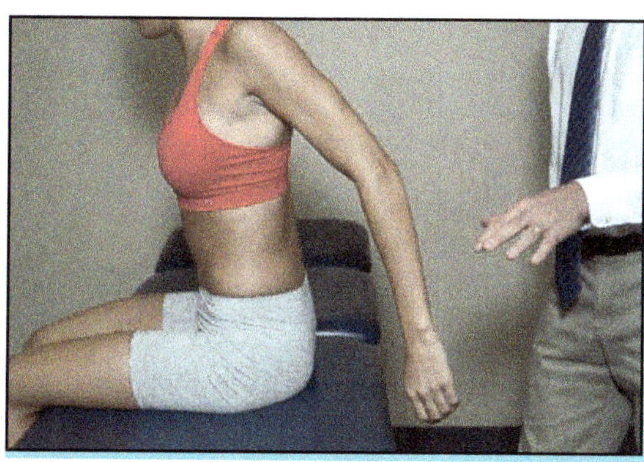

3) The examiner then releases the wrists.

4) A positive test is indicated by an angular drop or lag. The inability to maintain the shoulder extension is considered a positive test.

5) The examiner records any lag to the nearest five degrees.

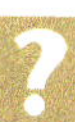

UTILITY SCORE ?

Study	Reliability	Sensitivity	Specificity	LR+	LR−	QUADAS Score (0–14)
Hertel et al.[28]	NT	NT	NT	NA	NA	NA
Comments: This study was performed with only five male patients after acute traumatic anterior dislocation of the shoulder to track recovery of the axillary nerve.						

STIFFNESS-RELATED DISORDERS [OSTEOARTHRITIS (OA) & ADHESIVE CAPSULITIS]

Shrug Sign (OA & Adhesive Capsulitis)

1. The patient is asked to elevate the involved arm overhead or as high as possible
2. A positive test is indicated when the patient elevates the entire shoulder girdle as if "shrugging" the shoulder.

UTILITY SCORE 2

Study	Reliability	Sensitivity	Specificity	LR+	LR−	QUADAS Score (0–14)
Jia et al.[33] (Glenohumeral OA Adhesive Capsulitis Rotator Cuff Tendinopathy)	NT NT NT	91 95 96	57 50 53	2.12 1.90 2.04	0.16 0.10 0.08	10
Comments: Based on this one study of high quality and a sample size of 982 patients, the Shrug Sign[84] is a screen for pathologies that create stiffness and weakness. More research is needed.						

Coracoid Pain Test (Adhesive Capsulitis)

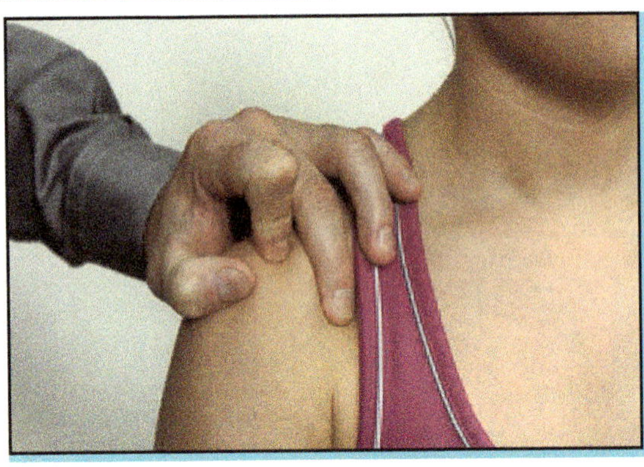

1. The examiner palpates the coracoid, the AC joint, and the anterolateral subacromial region all on the involved side.
2. The patient is asked to rate their pain on a 0 (no pain) to 10 (most severe pain) scale.
3. A positive test is indicated when the coracoids pain is three points or greater above the other two palpated areas.

UTILITY SCORE 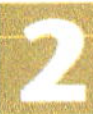

Study	Reliability	Sensitivity	Specificity	LR+	LR−	QUADAS Score (0–14)
Carbone et al.[9] (Adhesive Capsulitis)	NT	96	89	8.73	0.04	6
Comments: Statistical gymnastics in this article required recalculation of sensitivity and specificity. Based on this one study of moderate quality but with a sample size of 680 patients, the Coracoid Pain Test[9] is diagnostic for adhesive capsulitis. More research is needed.						

Diagnostic Clusters—Adhesive Capsulitis

UTILITY SCORE 3

Study	Cluster	Reliability	Sensitivity	Specificity	LR+	LR−	QUADAS
Malhi & Khan[55]	Global reduction of motion	NT	100	95	NA	NA	5
Comments: Clinically, this cluster would seem most appropriate, especially in Stage 2 and 3 but the quality of the research to back this clinical assumption is poor.							

TEST FOR SCAPULAR DYSFUNCTION

Lateral Scapular Slide Test (Shoulder Dysfunction)

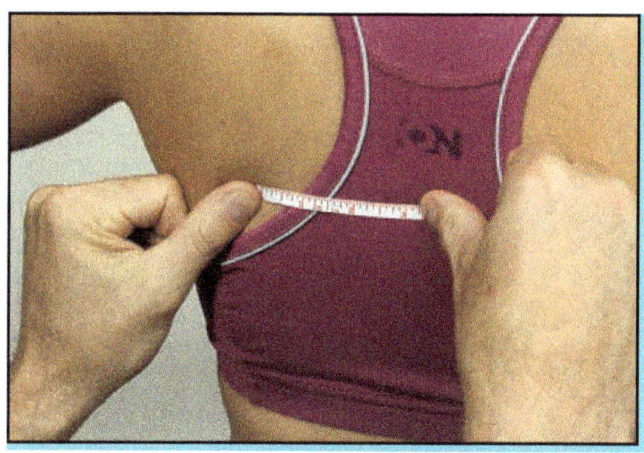

1) The patient is asked to abduct the involved arm to 0, 45 (with medial rotation), then 90 (with maximal medial rotation) degrees.

2) The examiner measures the distance from the inferior angle of the scapula to the thoracic spinous process at the same level.

3) The examiner repeats steps one and two on the uninvolved side.

4) A positive test is indicated when a side-to-side difference of 1–1.5 cm is detected.

(*continued*)

TEST FOR SCAPULAR DYSFUNCTION

UTILITY SCORE 3

Study	Reliability	Sensitivity	Specificity	LR+	LR−	QUADAS Score (0–14)
Odom et al.[67] 1 cm Threshold	Inter-rater					11
0° Abduction	ICC = .79	35	48	0.67	1.35	
45° Abduction	ICC = .45	41	54	0.89	1.09	
90° Abduction	ICC = .57	43	56	0.98	1.02	
1.5 cm Threshold	Intra-rater					
0° Abduction	ICC = .52	28	53	0.60	1.36	
45° Abduction	ICC = .66	50	58	1.19	0.86	
90° Abduction	ICC = .62	34	52	0.71	1.27	
Shadmehr et al.[76] 1 cm Threshold	Inter-rater					6
0° Abduction	ICC = .79	93–100	8–23	1.01–1.21	0–0.88	
45° Abduction	ICC = .70	90–93	4–23	0.97–1.17	0.43–1.75	
90° Abduction	ICC = .63	86–96	4–15	0.98–1.13	0.27–1.17	
1.5 cm Threshold	Intra-rater					
0° Abduction	ICC = .88	90–96	12–26	1.02–1.22	0.21–0.83	
45° Abduction	ICC = .96	83–90	15–26	1.02–1.22	0.38–0.89	
90° Abduction	ICC = .90	80–90	4–19	0.94–0.99	1.05–2.5	

Comments: The Odom et al.[67] study used a case-control design which artificially elevates sensitivity and specificity—a sobering thought considering how poor those statistics show the Lateral Scapular Slide Test to be. The Shadmehr et al.[76] study was not well done.

TESTS FOR BICEPS TENDINOPATHY

Upper Cut Test (Biceps Tendinopathy)

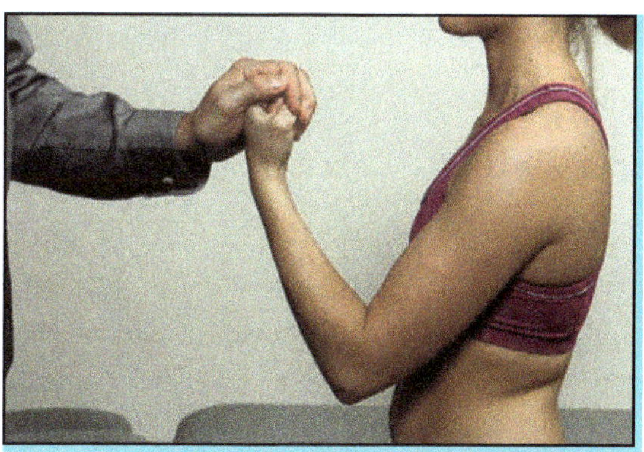

1) The patient is standing with the involved shoulder in a neutral position, the elbow flexed to 90 degrees, the forearm supinated, and the patient making a fist.

2) The examiner stands on the involved side with one hand on the patient's elbow and one hand covering the patient's fist.

3) The examiner asks the patient to rapidly bring the hand up and toward the chin—a boxing "upper cut" punch—while resisting this motion

4) A positive test is indicated by pain or a painful pop over the anterior shoulder.

UTILITY SCORE 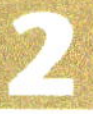

Study	Reliability	Sensitivity	Specificity	LR+	LR−	QUADAS Score (0–14)
Kibler et al.[41]	NT	73	78	3.38	0.34	9

Biceps Palpation (Biceps Tear, Type II SLAP)

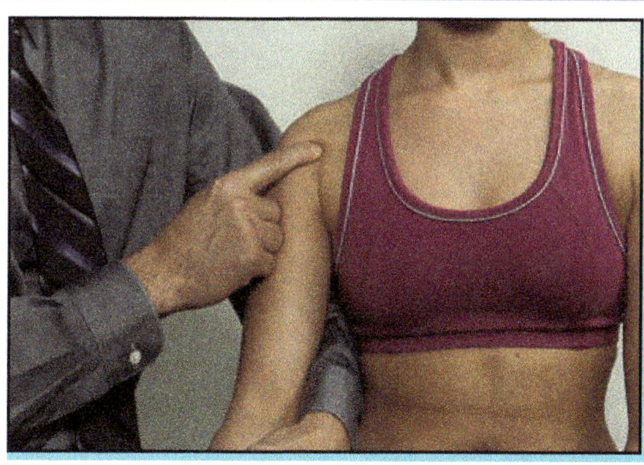

1) The examiner palpates the proximal long head of the biceps over the anterior shoulder region.

2) A positive test is indicated by pain.

UTILITY SCORE 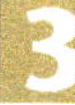

Study	Reliability	Sensitivity	Specificity	LR+	LR−	QUADAS Score (0–14)
Oh et al.[68] (Type II SLAP)	NT	27	66	0.79	1.11	11
Gill et al.[21] (Biceps Tear)	NT	53	54	1.13	0.87	12
Comments: Biceps palpation does not appear to be a useful clinical tool.						

Diagnostic Clusters—Biceps Tendinopathy

UTILITY SCORE  3

Study	Cluster	Reliability	Sensitivity	Specificity	LR+	LR−	QUADAS Score (0–14)
Kibler et al.[41]	Upper Cut and Speed's	NT	NT	NT	NT	NT	9
Gill et al.[21] (Biceps Tear)	Speed's and Biceps Palpation	NT	68	49	1.31	0.65	12

Comments: Kibler et al.[41] performed a binary logistic regression to discover that the Upper Cut and Speed's explained 40% of the variance (R^2) in detecting biceps tendinopathy.

Key Points

1. Screening and diagnosis for bony abnormality and bony instability can be accomplished with the Olecranon-Manubrium Percussion test and the Bony Apprehension test, respectively.
2. For rotator cuff tears:
   - The Rent Test and the Lateral Jobe test appear to be the best tests for a rotator cuff tear generally.
   - The Supine Impingement Test has promise as a screening examination technique where a negative test would rule out a rotator cuff tear.
   - The External Rotation Lag sign may have value as a positive test to rule in a full thickness rotator cuff tear.
   - The Lift-Off, Internal Rotation Lag, Belly Press, and Bear Hug tests may all be appropriate when trying to detect a subscapularis tear.
3. Impingement is a broad diagnosis that captures a range of pathologies from subacromial bursitis, to partial rotator cuff tear, to a full thickness rotator cuff tear making its value as a diagnostic label questionable.
4. There are no clinical examination tests of diagnostic value in cases of impingement.
5. For detecting laxity/instability, the Anterior Release/Surprise Test shows some promise. Also, the Apprehension, Relocation, and Modified Dynamic Labral Shear tests are specific for instability, especially when apprehension is used as a positive sign over pain.
6. For SLAP lesions, the Biceps Load Test II and the Passive Compression may be appropriate diagnostic tools and the Pain Provocation test appears to have value in ruling in the SLAP when positive.
7. For posteroinferior labral tears, both the Kim Test and Jerk Test show promise, but more/better research is needed.
8. Pain with palpation is a good screen as a negative test to rule out AC joint pathology.
9. The Resisted Extension Test may be of some use in diagnosing AC joint pathology, but more/better research needs to be performed.

References

1. Adams SL, Yarnold PR, Mathews JJ. Clinical use of the olecranon-manubrium percussion sign in shoulder trauma. *Ann Emerg Med.* May 1988;17(5):484–487.
2. Ardic F, Kahraman Y, Kacar M, Kahraman MC, Findikoglu G, Yorgancioglu ZR. Shoulder impingement syndrome: relationships between clinical, functional, and radiologic findings. *Am J Phys Med Rehabil.* Jan 2006;85(1):53–60.
3. Bak K, Fauno P. Clinical findings in competitive swimmers with shoulder pain. *Am J Sports Med.* Mar–Apr 1997;25(2):254–260.
4. Bak K, Sorensen AK, Jorgensen U, et al. The value of clinical tests in acute full-thickness tears of the supraspinatus tendon: does a subacromial lidocaine injection help in the clinical diagnosis? A prospective study. *Arthroscopy.* Jun 2010;26(6):734–742.
5. Barth JR, Burkhart SS, De Beer JF. The bear-hug test: a new and sensitive test for diagnosing a subscapularis tear. *Arthroscopy.* Oct 2006;22(10):1076–1084.
6. Bennett WF. Specificity of the Speed's test: arthroscopic technique for evaluating the biceps tendon at the level of the bicipital groove. *Arthroscopy.* Nov–Dec 1998;14(8):789–796.
7. Bushnell BD, Creighton RA, Herring MM. The bony apprehension test for instability of the shoulder: a prospective pilot analysis. *Arthroscopy.* Sep 2008;24(9):974–982.
8. Calis M, Akgun K, Birtane M, Karacan I, Calis H, Tuzun F. Diagnostic values of clinical diagnostic tests in subacromial impingement syndrome. *Ann Rheum Dis.* Jan 2000;59(1):44–47.
9. Carbone S, Gumina S, Vestri AR, Postacchini R. Coracoid pain test: a new clinical sign of shoulder adhesive capsulitis. *Int Orthop.* Mar 2010;34(3):385–388.
10. Castoldi F, Blonna D, Hertel R. External rotation lag sign revisited: accuracy for diagnosis of full thickness supraspinatus tear. *J Shoulder Elbow Surg.* Jul–Aug 2009;18(4):529–534.
11. Chronopoulos E, Kim TK, Park HB, Ashenbrenner D, McFarland EG. Diagnostic value of physical tests for isolated chronic acromioclavicular lesions. *Am J Sports Med.* Apr–May 2004;32(3):655–661.
12. Codman EA. Rupture of the supraspinatus tendon. 1911. *Clin Orthop Relat Res.* May 1990(254):3–26.
13. Crenshaw AH, Kilgore WE. Surgical treatment of bicipital tenosynovitis. *J Bone Joint Surg Am.* Dec 1966;48(8):1496–1502.
14. Ebinger N, Magosch P, Lichtenberg S, Habermeyer P. A new SLAP test: the supine flexion resistance test. *Arthroscopy.* May 2008;24(5):500–505.
15. Farber AJ, Castillo R, Clough M, Bahk M, McFarland EG. Clinical assessment of three common tests for traumatic anterior shoulder instability. *J Bone Joint Surg Am.* Jul 2006;88(7):1467–1474.
16. Field LD, Savoie FH, 3rd. Arthroscopic suture repair of superior labral detachment lesions of the shoulder. *Am J Sports Med.* Nov–Dec 1993;21(6):783–790; discussion 790.
17. Gagey OJ, Gagey N. The hyperabduction test. *J Bone Joint Surg Br.* Jan 2001;83(1):69–74.
18. Gerber C, Ganz R. Clinical assessment of instability of the shoulder. With special reference to anterior and posterior drawer tests. *J Bone Joint Surg Br.* Aug 1984;66(4):551–556.
19. Gerber C, Hersche O, Farron A. Isolated rupture of the subscapularis tendon. *J Bone Joint Surg Am.* Jul 1996;78(7):1015–1023.
20. Gerber C, Krushell RJ. Isolated rupture of the tendon of the subscapularis muscle. Clinical features in 16 cases. *J Bone Joint Surg Br.* May 1991;73(3):389–394.
21. Gill HS, El Rassi G, Bahk MS, Castillo RC, McFarland EG. Physical examination for partial tears of the biceps tendon. *Am J Sports Med.* Aug 2007;35(8):1334–1340.
22. Gillooly JJ, Chidambaram R, Mok D. The lateral Jobe test: a more reliable method of diagnosing rotator cuff tears. *Int J Shoulder Surg.* Apr 2010;4(2):41–43.
23. Gross ML, Distefano MC. Anterior release test. A new test for occult shoulder instability. *Clin Orthop Relat Res.* Jun 1997(339):105–108.
24. Guanche CA, Jones DC. Clinical testing for tears of the glenoid labrum. *Arthroscopy.* May–Jun 2003;19(5):517–523.
25. Hamner DL, Pink MM, Jobe FW. A modification of the relocation test: arthroscopic findings associated with a positive test. *J Shoulder Elbow Surg.* Jul–Aug 2000;9(4):263–267.
26. Hawkins RJ, Kennedy JC. Impingement syndrome in athletes. *Am J Sports Med.* May–Jun 1980;8(3):151–158.
27. Hertel R, Ballmer FT, Lombert SM, Gerber C. Lag signs in the diagnosis of rotator cuff rupture. *J Shoulder Elbow Surg.* Jul Aug 1996;5(4):307–313.
28. Hertel R, Lambert SM, Ballmer FT. The deltoid extension lag sign for diagnosis and grading of axillary nerve palsy. *J Shoulder Elbow Surg.* Mar–Apr 1998;7(2):97–99.
29. Holtby R, Razmjou H. Accuracy of the Speed's and Yergason's tests in detecting biceps pathology and SLAP lesions: comparison with arthroscopic findings. *Arthroscopy.* Mar 2004;20(3):231–236.
30. Itoi E, Kido T, Sano A, Urayama M, Sato K. Which is more useful, the "full can test" or the "empty can test," in detecting the torn supraspinatus tendon? *Am J Sports Med.* Jan–Feb 1999;27(1):65–68.
31. Itoi E, Minagawa H, Yamamoto N, Seki N, Abe H. Are pain location and physical examinations useful in locating a tear site of the rotator cuff? *Am J Sports Med.* Feb 2006;34(2):256–264.

32. Jacob AK, Sallay PI. Therapeutic efficacy of corticosteroid injections in the acromioclavicular joint. *Biomed Sci Instrum.* 1997;34:380–385.

33. Jia X, Ji JH, Petersen SA, Keefer J, McFarland EG. Clinical evaluation of the shoulder shrug sign. *Clin Orthop Relat Res.* Nov 2008;466(11):2813–2819.

34. Jia X, Petersen SA, Khosravi AH, Almareddi V, Pannirselvam V, McFarland EG. Examination of the shoulder: the past, the present, and the future. *J Bone Joint Surg Am.* Nov 2009;91 Suppl 6:10–18.

35. Jobe FW, Kvitne RS, Giangarra CE. Shoulder pain in the overhand or throwing athlete. The relationship of anterior instability and rotator cuff impingement. *Orthop Rev.* Sep 1989;18(9):963–975.

36. Jobe FW, Moynes DR. Delineation of diagnostic criteria and a rehabilitation program for rotator cuff injuries. *Am J Sports Med.* Nov–Dec 1982;10(6):336–339.

37. Kelly BT, Kadrmas WR, Speer KP. The manual muscle examination for rotator cuff strength. An electromyographic investigation. *Am J Sports Med.* Sep–Oct 1996;24(5):581–588.

38. Kelly SM, Brittle N, Allen GM. The value of physical tests for subacromial impingement syndrome: a study of diagnostic accuracy. *Clin Rehabil.* Feb 2010;24(2):149–158.

39. Kessel L, Watson M. The painful arc syndrome. Clinical classification as a guide to management. *J Bone Joint Surg Br.* May 1977;59(2):166–172.

40. Kibler WB. Specificity and sensitivity of the anterior slide test in throwing athletes with superior glenoid labral tears. *Arthroscopy.* Jun 1995;11(3):296–300.

41. Kibler WB, Sciascia AD, Hester P, Dome D, Jacobs C. Clinical utility of traditional and new tests in the diagnosis of biceps tendon injuries and superior labrum anterior and posterior lesions in the shoulder. *Am J Sports Med.* Sep 2009;37(9):1840–1847.

42. Kim E, Jeong HJ, Lee KW, Song JS. Interpreting positive signs of the supraspinatus test in screening for torn rotator cuff. *Acta Med Okayama.* Aug 2006;60(4):223–228.

43. Kim KH, Cho JG, Lee KO, et al. Usefulness of physical maneuvers for prevention of vasovagal syncope. *Circ J.* Sep 2005;69(9):1084–1088.

44. Kim SH, Ha KI, Ahn JH, Kim SH, Choi HJ. Biceps load test II: A clinical test for SLAP lesions of the shoulder. *Arthroscopy.* Feb 2001;17(2):160–164.

45. Kim SH, Ha KI, Han KY. Biceps load test: a clinical test for superior labrum anterior and posterior lesions in shoulders with recurrent anterior dislocations. *Am J Sports Med.* May–Jun 1999;27(3):300–303.

46. Kim SH, Park JS, Jeong WK, Shin SK. The Kim test: a novel test for posteroinferior labral lesion of the shoulder—a comparison to the jerk test. *Am J Sports Med.* Aug 2005;33(8):1188–1192.

47. Kim YS, Kim JM, Ha KY, Choy S, Joo MW, Chung YG. The passive compression test: a new clinical test for superior labral tears of the shoulder. *Am J Sports Med.* Sep 2007;35(9):1489–1494.

48. Levy O, Relwani JG, Mullett H, Haddo O, Even T. The active elevation lag sign and the triangle sign: new clinical signs of trapezius palsy. *J Shoulder Elbow Surg.* Jul–Aug 2009;18(4):573–576.

49. Litaker D, Pioro M, El Bilbeisi H, Brems J. Returning to the bedside: using the history and physical examination to identify rotator cuff tears. *J Am Geriatr Soc.* Dec 2000;48(12):1633–1637.

50. Liu SH, Henry MH, Nuccion S, Shapiro MS, Dorey F. Diagnosis of glenoid labral tears. A comparison between magnetic resonance imaging and clinical examinations. *Am J Sports Med.* Mar–Apr 1996;24(2):149–154.

51. Liu SH, Henry MH, Nuccion SL. A prospective evaluation of a new physical examination in predicting glenoid labral tears. *Am J Sports Med.* Nov–Dec 1996;24(6):721–725.

52. Lo IK, Nonweiler B, Woolfrey M, Litchfield R, Kirkley A. An evaluation of the apprehension, relocation, and surprise tests for anterior shoulder instability. *Am J Sports Med.* Mar 2004;32(2):301–307.

53. Lyons AR, Tomlinson JE. Clinical diagnosis of tears of the rotator cuff. *J Bone Joint Surg Br.* May 1992;74(3):414–415.

54. MacDonald PB, Clark P, Sutherland K. An analysis of the diagnostic accuracy of the Hawkins and Neer subacromial impingement signs. *J Shoulder Elbow Surg.* Jul–Aug 2000;9(4):299–301.

55. Malhi AM, Khan R. Correlation between clinical diagnosis and arthroscopic findings of the shoulder. *Postgrad Med J.* Oct 2005;81(960):657–659.

56. McFarland EG, Kim TK, Savino RM. Clinical assessment of three common tests for superior labral anterior-posterior lesions. *Am J Sports Med.* Nov–Dec 2002;30(6):810–815.

57. McLaughlin H. On the frozen shoulder. *Bull Hosp Joint Dis.* Oct 1951;12(2):383–393.

58. Meister K, Buckley B, Batts J. The posterior impingement sign: diagnosis of rotator cuff and posterior labral tears secondary to internal impingement in overhand athletes. *Am J Orthop.* Aug 2004;33(8):412–415.

59. Michener LA, Walsworth MK, Doukas WC, Murphy KP. Reliability and diagnostic accuracy of 5 physical examination tests and combination of tests for subacromial impingement. *Arch Phys Med Rehabil.* Nov 2009;90(11):1898–1903.

60. Miller CA, Forrester GA, Lewis JS. The validity of the lag signs in diagnosing full-thickness tears of the rotator cuff: a preliminary investigation. *Arch Phys Med Rehabil.* Jun 2008;89(6):1162–1168.

61. Mimori K, Muneta T, Nakagawa T, Shinomiya K. A new pain provocation test for superior labral tears of the shoulder. *Am J Sports Med.* Mar–Apr 1999;27(2):137–142.

62. Morgan CD, Burkhart SS, Palmeri M, Gillespie M. Type II SLAP lesions: three subtypes and their relationships to superior instability and rotator cuff tears. *Arthroscopy.* Sep 1998;14(6):553–565.

63. Murrell GA, Walton JR. Diagnosis of rotator cuff tears. *Lancet.* Mar 10 2001;357(9258):769–770.

64. Myers TH, Zemanovic JR, Andrews JR. The resisted supination external rotation test: a new test for the diagnosis of superior labral anterior posterior lesions. *Am J Sports Med.* Sep 2005;33(9):1315–1320.

65. Nakagawa S, Yoneda M, Hayashida K, Obata M, Fukushima S, Miyazaki Y. Forced shoulder abduction and elbow flexion test: a new simple clinical test to detect superior labral injury in the throwing shoulder. *Arthroscopy.* Nov 2005;21(11):1290–1295.

66. O'Brien SJ, Pagnani MJ, Fealy S, McGlynn SR, Wilson JB. The active compression test: a new and effective test for diagnosing labral tears and acromioclavicular joint abnormality. *Am J Sports Med.* Sep–Oct 1998;26(5):610–613.

67. Odom CJ, Taylor AB, Hurd CE, Denegar CR. Measurement of scapular asymetry and assessment of shoulder dysfunction using the Lateral Scapular Slide Test: a reliability and validity study. *Phys Ther.* Feb 2001;81(2):799–809.

68. Oh JH, Kim JY, Kim WS, Gong HS, Lee JH. The evaluation of various physical examinations for the diagnosis of type II superior labrum anterior and posterior lesion. *Am J Sports Med.* Feb 2008;36(2):353–359.

69. Ostor AJ, Richards CA, Prevost AT, Hazleman BL, Speed CA. Interrater reproducibility of clinical tests for rotator cuff lesions. *Ann Rheum Dis.* Oct 2004;63(10):1288–1292.

70. Parentis MA, Glousman RE, Mohr KS, Yocum LA. An evaluation of the provocative tests for superior labral anterior posterior lesions. *Am J Sports Med.* Feb 2006;34(2):265–268.

71. Parentis MA, Mohr KJ, ElAttrache NS. Disorders of the superior labrum: review and treatment guidelines. *Clin Orthop Relat Res.* Jul 2002(400):77–87.

72. Park HB, Yokota A, Gill HS, El Rassi G, McFarland EG. Diagnostic accuracy of clinical tests for the different degrees of subacromial impingement syndrome. *J Bone Joint Surg Am.* Jul 2005;87(7):1446–1455.

73. Rowe CR, Zarins B. Recurrent transient subluxation of the shoulder. *J Bone Joint Surg Am.* Jul 1981;63(6):863–872.

74. Savoie FH, 3rd, Field LD, Atchinson S. Anterior superior instability with rotator cuff tearing: SLAC lesion. *Orthop Clin North Am.* Jul 2001;32(3):457–461, ix.

75. Scheibel M, Magosch P, Pritsch M, Lichtenberg S, Habermeyer P. The belly-off sign: a new clinical diagnostic sign for subscapularis lesions. *Arthroscopy.* Oct 2005;21(10):1229–1235.

76. Shadmehr A, Bagheri H, Ansari NN, Sarafraz H. The reliability measurements of lateral scapular slide test at three different degrees of shoulder joint abduction. *Br J Sports Med.* Mar 2010;44(4):289–293.

77. Silliman JF, Hawkins RJ. Current concepts and recent advances in the athlete's shoulder. *Clin Sports Med.* Oct 1991;10(4):693–705.

78. Silva L, Andreu JL, Munoz P, et al. Accuracy of physical examination in subacromial impingement syndrome. *Rheumatology (Oxford).* May 2008;47(5):679–683.

79. Snyder SJ, Karzel RP, Del Pizzo W, Ferkel RD, Friedman MJ. SLAP lesions of the shoulder. *Arthroscopy.* 1990;6(4):274–279.

80. Speer KP, Hannafin JA, Altchek DW, Warren RF. An evaluation of the shoulder relocation test. *Am J Sports Med.* Mar–Apr 1994;22(2):177–183.

81. Stetson WB, Templin K. The crank test, the O'Brien test, and routine magnetic resonance imaging scans in the diagnosis of labral tears. *Am J Sports Med.* Nov–Dec 2002;30(6):806–809.

82. Walch G, Boulahia A, Calderone S, Robinson AH. The 'dropping' and 'Hornblower's' signs in evaluation of rotator-cuff tears. *J Bone Joint Surg Br.* Jul 1998;80(4):624–628.

83. Walsworth MK, Doukas WC, Murphy KP, Mielcarek BJ, Michener LA. Reliability and diagnostic accuracy of history and physical examination for diagnosing glenoid labral tears. *Am J Sports Med.* Jan 2008;36(1):162–168.

84. Walton J, Mahajan S, Paxinos A, et al. Diagnostic values of tests for acromioclavicular joint pain. *J Bone Joint Surg Am.* Apr 2004;86-A(4):807–812.

85. Wolf EM, Agrawal V. Transdeltoid palpation (the rent test) in the diagnosis of rotator cuff tears. *J Shoulder Elbow Surg.* Sep–Oct 2001;10(5):470–473.

86. Yergason R. Supination sign. *J Bone Joint Surg.* 1931;13:160–165.

87. Zaslav KR. Internal rotation resistance strength test: a new diagnostic test to differentiate intra-articular pathology from outlet (Neer) impingement syndrome in the shoulder. *J Shoulder Elbow Surg.* Jan–Feb 2001;10(1):23–27.

PEARSON **myhealthprofessionskit**™

Use this address to access the Companion Website created for this textbook. Simply select "Physical Therapy" from the choice of disciplines. Find this book and log in using your username and password to access video clips of selected tests.

Physical Examination Tests for the Elbow and Forearm

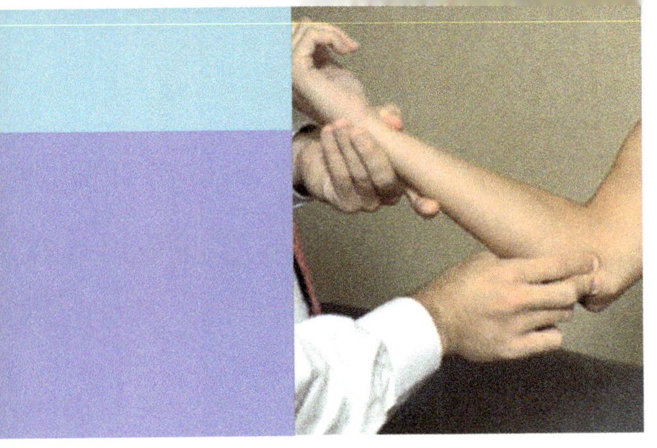

Physical Examination Tests for the Elbow and Forearm

Adam Goode and Chad E.Cook

Please refer to the chapter "Introduction to Diagnostic Accuracy" before reading this chapter.

Index of Tests

Tests for Ulnar Nerve Entrapment

Elbow Flexion Test (Cubital Tunnel Syndrome)

Pressure Provocation Test (Cubital Tunnel Syndrome)

Elbow Flexion Test (Ulnar Nerve Neuropathy)

Tinel's Sign (Cubital Tunnel Syndrome)

Elbow Scratch Collapse Test

Tests for Elbow Fracture

Elbow Extension Test

Elbow Flexion Test

Elbow Pronation Test

Elbow Supination Test

Tests for Elbow Instability

Moving Valgus Stress Test (Chronic Medial Collateral Ligament Tear of the Elbow)

Posterior Lateral Rotary Instability (Posterior Lateral Instability of the Radius)

Varus Stress Test (Integrity of the Lateral Collateral Complex)

Valgus Stress Test

Tests for Biceps Tear

Biceps Squeeze Test (Distal Bicep Tendon Rupture)

Biceps Crease Index (Distal Bicep Tendon Rupture)

Hook Test (Distal Bicep Tendon Rupture)

Tests for Lateral Epicondylitis

Cozen's Test

Resisted Tennis Elbow Test

Passive Tennis Elbow Test

Lateral Epicondylitis/Maudsley's Test

TESTS FOR ULNAR NERVE ENTRAPMENT

Elbow Flexion Test (Cubital Tunnel Syndrome)

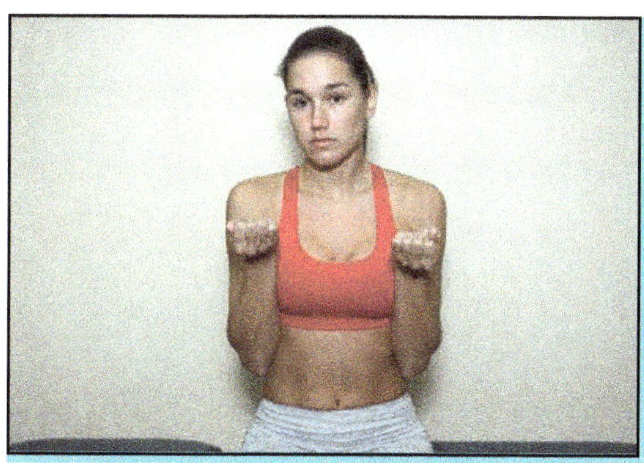

1) Patient is sitting with both arms and shoulders in the anatomic position. Both elbows are fully but not forcibly flexed with full wrist extension.

2) Patients are asked to describe any symptoms following holding this position for 3 minutes.

3) A positive test is the reproduction of pain, tingling, or numbness along the ulnar nerve distribution.

UTILITY SCORE 2

Study	Reliability	Sensitivity	Specificity	LR+	LR−	QUADAS Score (0–14)
Buehler & Thayer[2]	NT	93	NT	NA	NA	NT
Novak et al.[8]	NT	75	99	75	0.25	7

Comments: Buehler & Thayer[2] studied 15 subjects with suspected cubital tunnel syndrome confirmed by NCS without a control group. Novak et al.[8] performed the elbow flexion test without wrist extension and with wrist supination held for 60 seconds.

Pressure Provocation Test (Cubital Tunnel Syndrome)

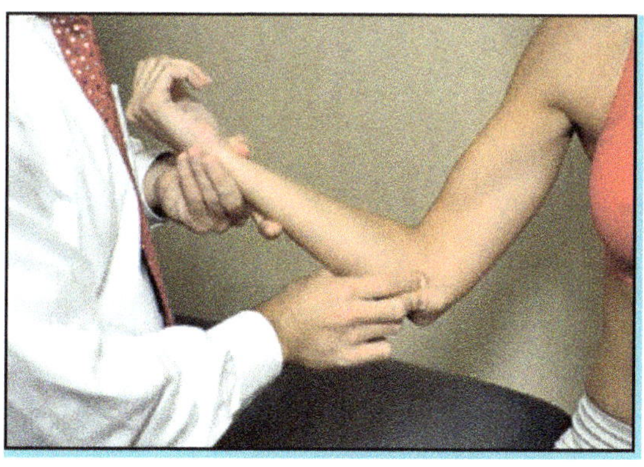

1) The examiner places his or her first and second fingers over the patient's ulnar nerve proximal to the cubital tunnel with the elbow in 20 degrees flexion and forearm supination.

2) The test is held for 60 seconds.

3) A positive test is the reproduction of symptoms along the ulnar nerve.

UTILITY SCORE 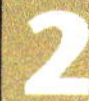

Study	Reliability	Sensitivity	Specificity	LR+	LR−	QUADAS Score (0–14)
Novak et al.[8]	NT	89	98	45	0.11	7
Cheng et al.[4]	NT	46	99	46	0.54	6

Comments: This test should be used with caution secondary to potential bias of the two studies.

TESTS FOR ULNAR NERVE ENTRAPMENT

Elbow Flexion Test (Ulnar Nerve Neuropathy)

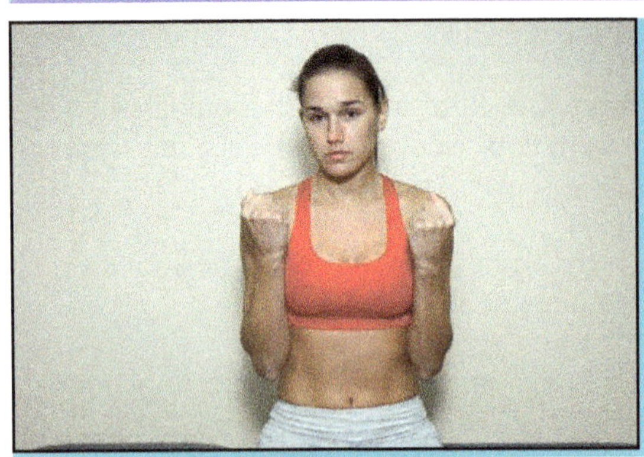

1) Patient is instructed to fully flex the elbows with the wrists and shoulders in neutral. This position is held for 60 seconds.

2) Full elbow flexion is maintained for 60 seconds with the shoulders in neutral and wrists in full extension.

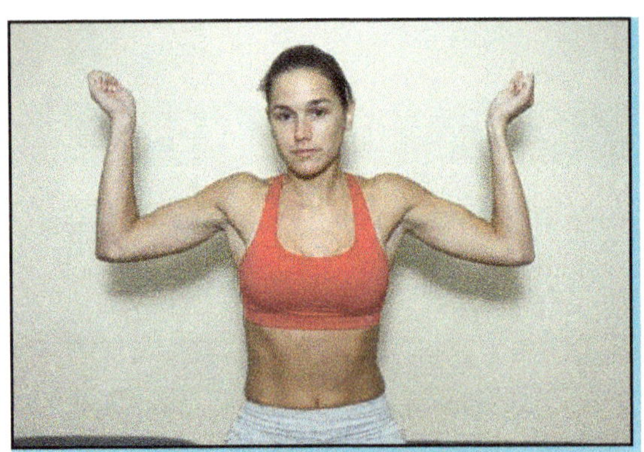

3) The patient is asked to abduct the shoulders to 90 degrees with the elbows in full flexion and wrist in full extension for 90 seconds.

4) A positive test is reproduction of ulnar nerve symptoms (paresthesia) along the ulnar nerve distribution.

UTILITY SCORE 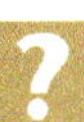

Study	Reliability	Sensitivity	Specificity	LR+	LR−	QUADAS Score (0–14)
Rayan et al.[12]	NT	NT	13	NA	NA	NT

Comments: Rayan et al.[12] studied this test in a population of 204 elbows of patients without an upper extremity-related diagnosis. The study used a combination of four movements: (1) full elbow flexion passively with wrist in neutral was positive in 10%; (2) same test with the wrist in full extension was positive in 7%; (3) same test with the shoulder in 90 degrees of abduction was positive in 11%; (4) same test with the shoulder in 90 degrees of abduction and wrist in full extension was positive in 13%.

TESTS FOR ULNAR NERVE ENTRAPMENT

Tinel's Sign (Cubital Tunnel Syndrome)

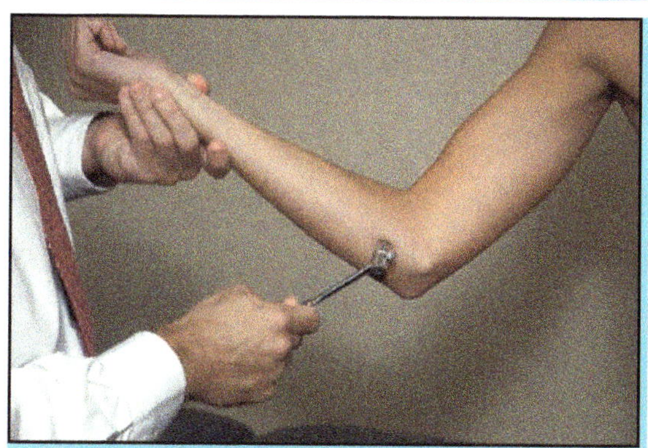

1) The examiner applies four to six taps to the patient's ulnar nerve just proximal to the cubital tunnel.

2) A positive test is the reproduction of symptoms along the ulnar nerve.

UTILITY SCORE 

Study	Reliability	Sensitivity	Specificity	LR+	LR−	QUADAS Score (0–14)
Novak et al.[8]	NT	70	98	35	0.31	7
Rayan et al.[12]	NT	NT	24	NA	NA	NT
Cheng et al.[4]	NT	54	99	54	0.46	6
Comments: Rayan et al.[12] observed the presence of a positive elbow percussion test in 48 of 204 asymptomatic elbows. The Cheng et al.[4] study was poorly performed.						

Elbow Scratch Collapse Test

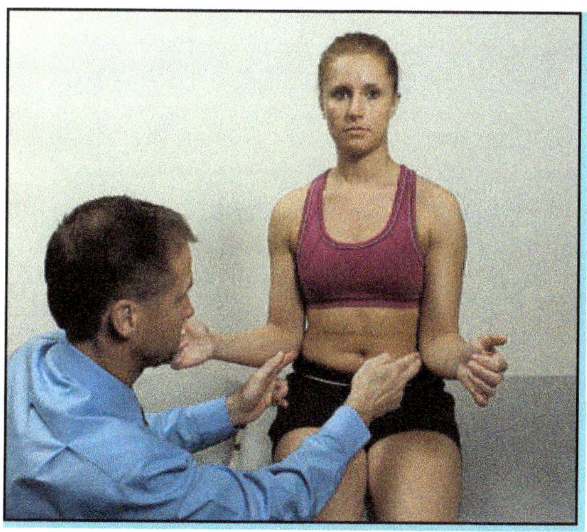

1) The examiner sits directly in front of the patient.

2) The patient resists bilateral shoulder external rotation movement (internal rotation force provided by the clinician).

3) The examiner scratches or swipes the fingertips over the area of the compressed ulnar nerve.

4) The patient again resists bilateral shoulder external (same as step 2).

5) A positive finding is weakness (unilaterally) in the affected area.

UTILITY SCORE 

Study	Reliability	Sensitivity	Specificity	LR+	LR−	QUADAS Score (0–14)
Cheng et al.[4]	NT	69	99	69	0.31	6
Comments: The finding is doubtful and the bias is very high.						

TESTS FOR ELBOW FRACTURE

Elbow Extension Test

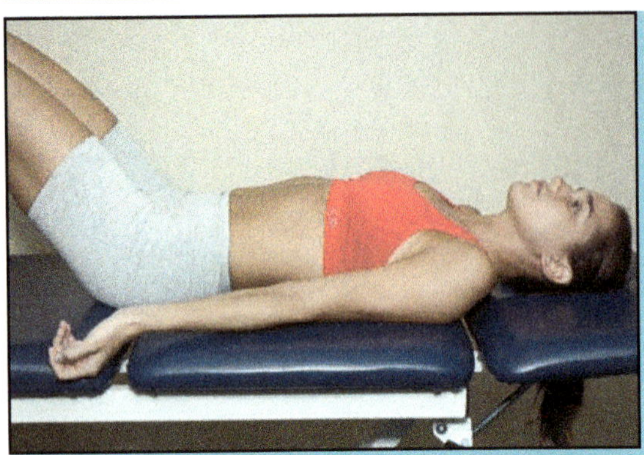

1) Patient lies supine and is asked to fully extend the elbow.

2) A positive test is indicated by the patient's inability to fully extend the elbow.

UTILITY SCORE 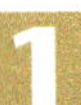

Study	Reliability	Sensitivity	Specificity	LR+	LR−	QUADAS Score (0–14)
Docherty et al.[6]	NT	97	69	3.1	0.04	10
Appelboam et al.[1]	NT	96.8	48.5	1.88	0.06	8
Darracq et al.[5]	NT	100	100	NA	NA	11
Comments: This test was designed as a clinical screening test for radiographic evaluation of elbow fractures. A single false positive was present in the Docherty et al.[6] study with the patient being able to fully extend the elbow with radiographic evidence of a non-displaced radial head fracture.						

Elbow Flexion Test

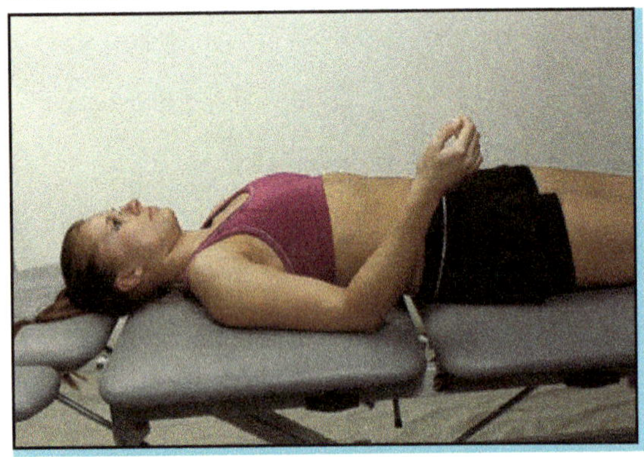

1) Patient lies supine and is asked to fully flex the elbow.

2) A positive test is indicated by the patient's inability to fully flex the elbow in comparison to the opposite side.

UTILITY SCORE 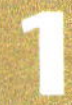

Study	Reliability	Sensitivity	Specificity	LR+	LR−	QUADAS Score (0–14)
Darracq et al.[5]	NT	64	100	Inf	0.36	11
Comments: This was a well designed study. Comparative assessment using the opposite, unaffected limb was used. A wide variety of ages were included in the very large sample size.						

TESTS FOR ELBOW FRACTURE

Elbow Pronation Test

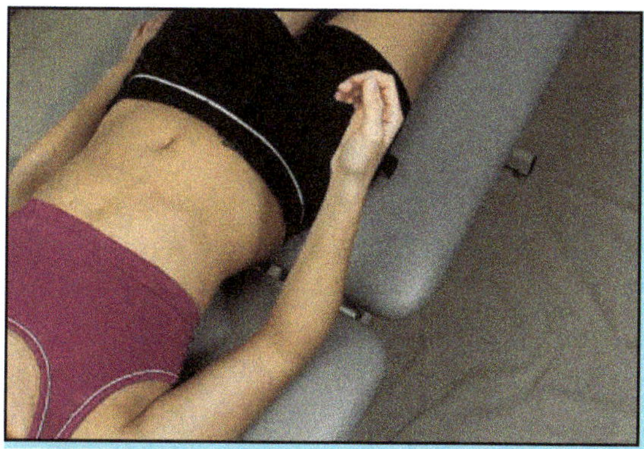

1) Patient lies supine and is asked to fully pronate the elbow.

2) A positive test is indicated by the patient's inability to fully pronate the elbow in comparison to the opposite side.

UTILITY SCORE 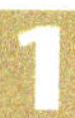

Study	Reliability	Sensitivity	Specificity	LR+	LR−	QUADAS Score (0–14)
Darracq et al.[5]	NT	34	100	Inf	0.66	11
Comments: This was a well designed study. Comparative assessment using the opposite, unaffected limb was used. A wide variety of ages were included in the very large sample size.						

Elbow Supination Test

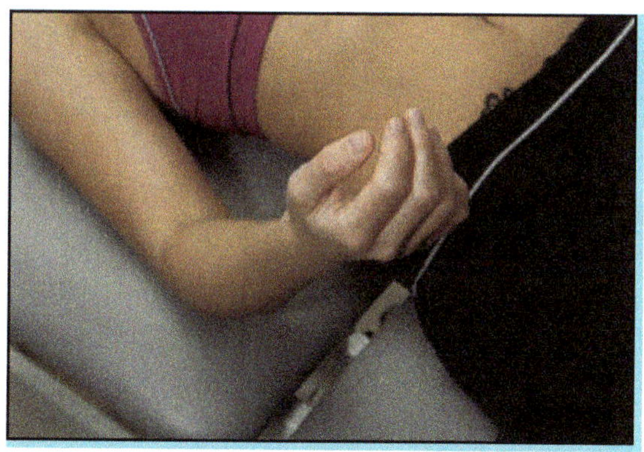

1) Patient lies supine and is asked to fully supinate the elbow.

2) A positive test is indicated by the patient's inability to fully supinate the elbow in comparison to the opposite side.

UTILITY SCORE 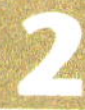

Study	Reliability	Sensitivity	Specificity	LR+	LR−	QUADAS Score (0–14)
Darracq et al.[5]	NT	43	97	14.3	0.58	11
Comments: This was a well designed study. Comparative assessment using the opposite, unaffected limb was used. A wide variety of ages were included in the very large sample size.						

TESTS FOR ELBOW INSTABILITY

Moving Valgus Stress Test (Chronic Medial Collateral Ligament Tear of the Elbow)

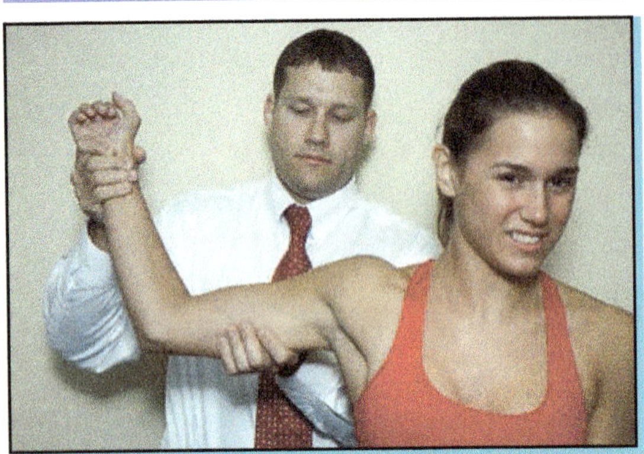

1) The patient is in an upright position and the shoulder is abducted to 90 degrees. With the elbow in full flexion of 120 degrees, modest valgus torque is applied to the elbow until the shoulder reaches full external rotation.

2) With a constant valgus torque the elbow is quickly extended to 30 degrees.

3) A positive test is reproduction of medial elbow pain when forcibly extending the elbow from a flexed position between 120 to 70 degrees.

UTILITY SCORE 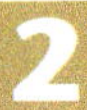

Study	Reliability	Sensitivity	Specificity	LR+	LR−	QUADAS Score (0–14)
O'Driscoll et al.[10]	NT	100	75	4	0	10
Comments: Spectrum bias exists within this study: low study population with 19 of 21 patients being male.						

Posterior Lateral Rotary Instability (Posterior Lateral Instability of the Radius)

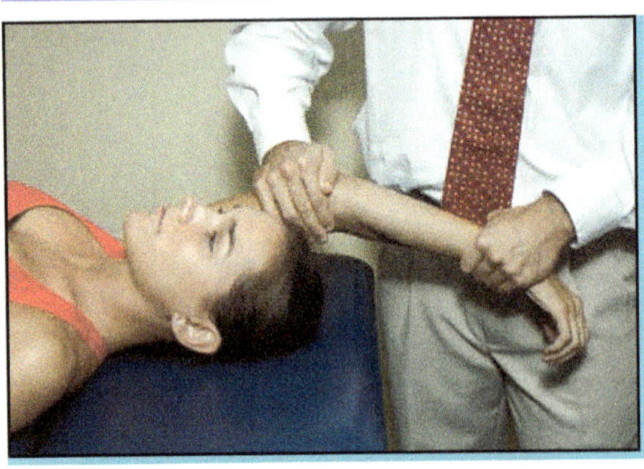

1) The patient lies supine.

2) The examiner flexes the shoulder until the arm is above the patient's head with the elbow in full extension. One hand of the examiner prevents external rotation of the humerus.

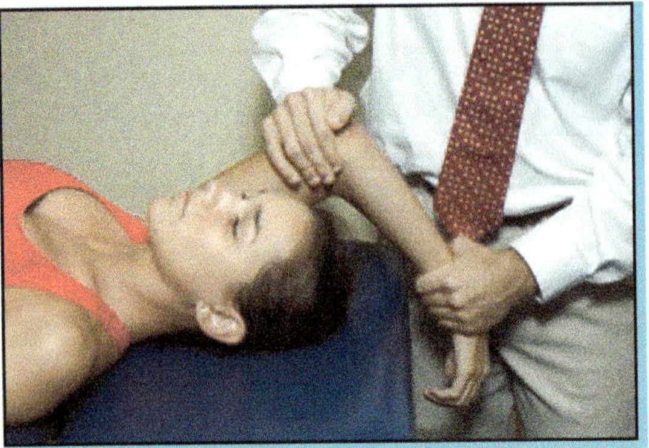

3) The examiner's other hand grasps the patient's forearm into full supination.

4) The examiner brings the patient's elbow into flexion while applying a supinatory force at the forearm and a valgus stress and axial compression at the elbow.

5) A positive test is posterior lateral displacement or apprehension of the radius followed by reduction of the radius as the elbow approaches 90 degrees.

TESTS FOR ELBOW INSTABILITY

UTILITY SCORE 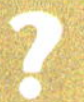

Study	Reliability	Sensitivity	Specificity	LR+	LR−	QUADAS Score (0–14)
O'Driscoll et al.[9]	NT	NT	NT	NA	NA	NT
Comments: O'Driscoll et al.[9] performed this test on a case series of five patients who demonstrated apprehension with testing and posterolateral dislocation of the radial head under anesthesia. All five patients underwent operative restoration to improve functional integrity of the ulnar part of the lateral collateral ligament. Four of the five patients returned to normal function.						

Varus Stress Test (Integrity of the Lateral Collateral Complex)

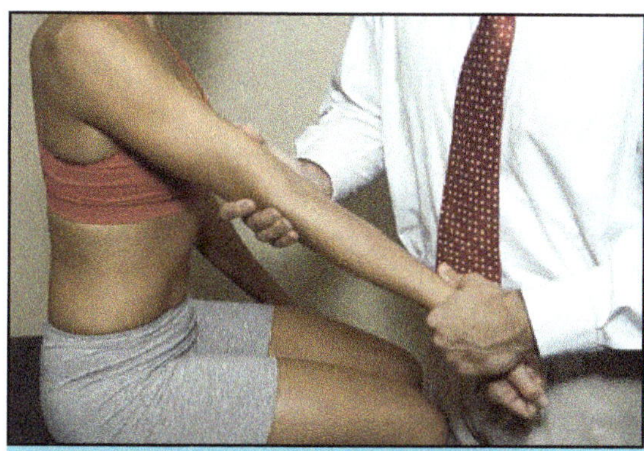

1) With the patient seated or standing, the examiner places one hand at the elbow and the other hand is placed over the patient's wrist. With the patient's elbow in a fully extended position, an adduction or varus force is applied while palpating the lateral collateral ligament of the elbow.

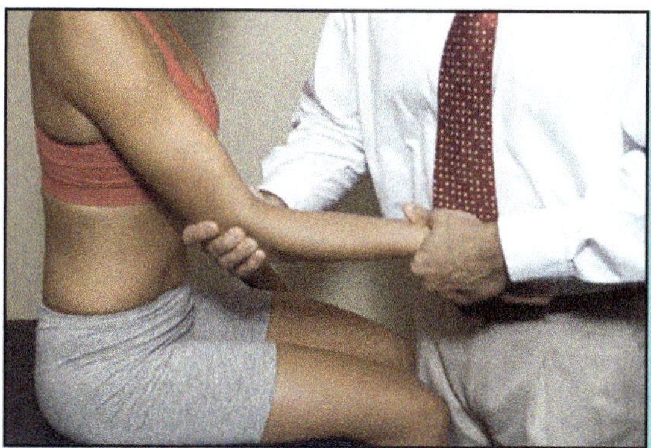

2) The examiner places one hand at the elbow and the other hand is placed over the patient's wrist. With the patient's elbow in 20–30 degrees of flexion, an adduction or varus force is applied while palpating the lateral collateral ligament of the elbow.

3) A positive test is reproduction of distraction pain laterally and compression pain medially at the joint line and laxity with stress.

UTILITY SCORE 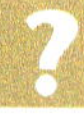

Study	Reliability	Sensitivity	Specificity	LR+	LR−	QUADAS Score (0–14)
NA	NT	NT	NT	NA	NA	NT
Comments: No diagnostic accuracy studies have been performed to determine the sensitivity or specificity of the Varus Stress Test of the elbow. Authors have suggested that placing the elbow in a slight degree of flexion will assist in differentiating ligamentous versus bony joint involvement.						

TESTS FOR ELBOW INSTABILITY

Valgus Stress Test

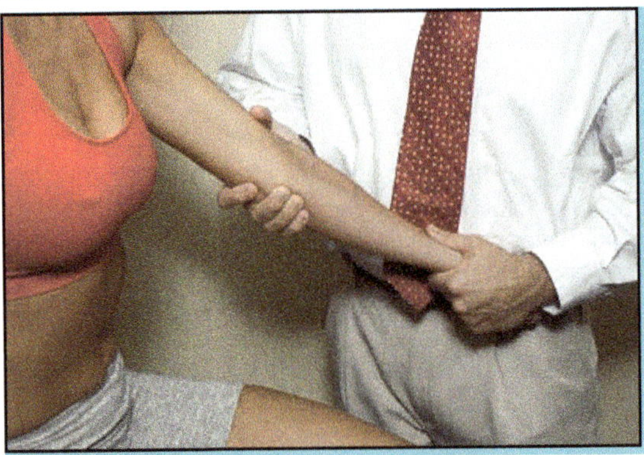

1) With the patient seated or standing, the examiner places one hand at the elbow and the other hand is placed over the patient's wrist. With the patient's elbow in a fully extended position, an abduction or valgus force is applied while palpating the medial collateral ligament of the elbow.

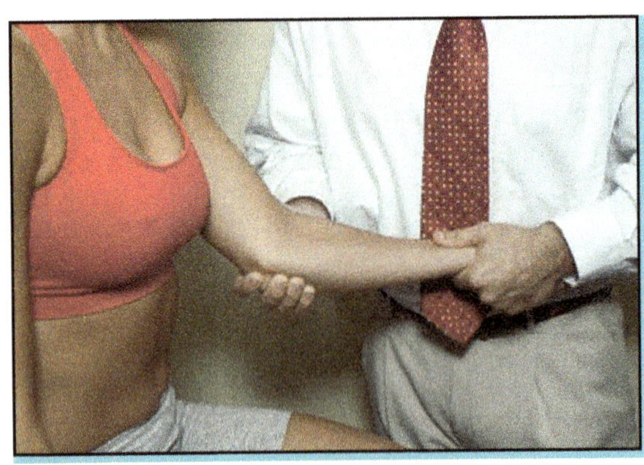

2) The examiner places one hand at the elbow and the other hand is placed over the patient's wrist. With the patient's elbow in 20–30 degrees of flexion, an abduction or valgus force is applied while palpating the medial collateral ligament of the elbow.

3) A positive test is reproduction of distraction pain medially and compression pain laterally at the elbow joint line with stress.

UTILITY SCORE 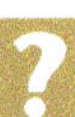

Study	Reliability	Sensitivity	Specificity	LR+	LR−	QUADAS Score (0–14)
None	NT	NT	NT	NA	NA	NT
Comments: No diagnostic accuracy studies have been performed to determine the sensitivity or specificity of the Valgus Stress Test of the elbow. It is suggested that placing the elbow in a slight degree of flexion will assist in differentiating ligamentous versus bony joint involvement.						

TESTS FOR BICEPS TEAR

Biceps Squeeze Test (Distal Bicep Tendon Rupture)

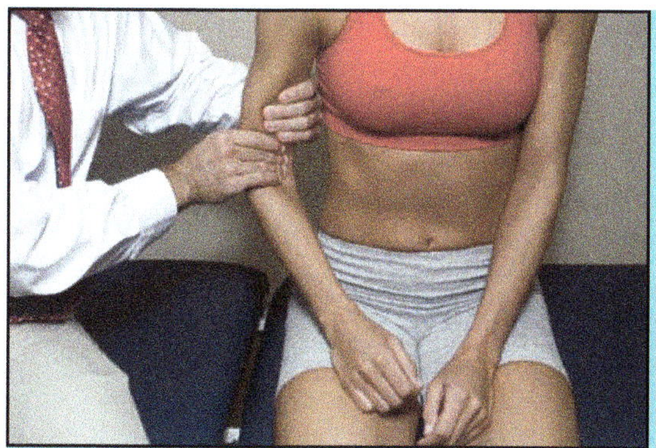

1) Patient is seated with the forearm resting comfortably in the patient's lap with the elbow flexed to approximately 60–80 degrees and forearm in slight pronation.

2) The examiner stands on the affected side and squeezes the biceps firmly with both hands with one hand at the distal myotendinous junction and the other around the belly of the biceps brachii.

3) A positive test is lack of forearm supination as the biceps brachii is squeezed, indicating a biceps brachii tendon or muscle belly rupture.

UTILITY SCORE 

Study	Reliability	Sensitivity	Specificity	LR+	LR−	QUADAS Score (0–14)
Ruland et al.[13]	NT	96	100	NA	0.04	9
Comment: This study included only 25 male patients referred for suspected biceps tendon rupture. The interpretation of the index and reference test is unclear without knowledge of results.						

Biceps Crease Index (Distal Bicep Tendon Rupture)

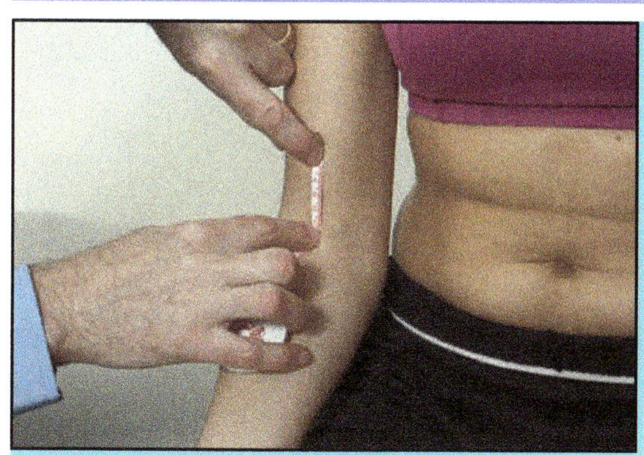

1) The biceps crease index is the measurement of the distance, in centimeters, between the biceps cusp and the antecubital crease.

2) A positive test is a distance of 6 cm or more.

UTILITY SCORE 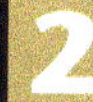

Study	Reliability	Sensitivity	Specificity	LR+	LR−	QUADAS Score (0–14)
El Maraghy et al.[7]	NT	92	100	Inf	0.08	5
Comment: Poor quality study, use caution is assuming the test has value.						

TESTS FOR BICEPS TEAR

Hook Test (Distal Bicep Tendon Rupture)

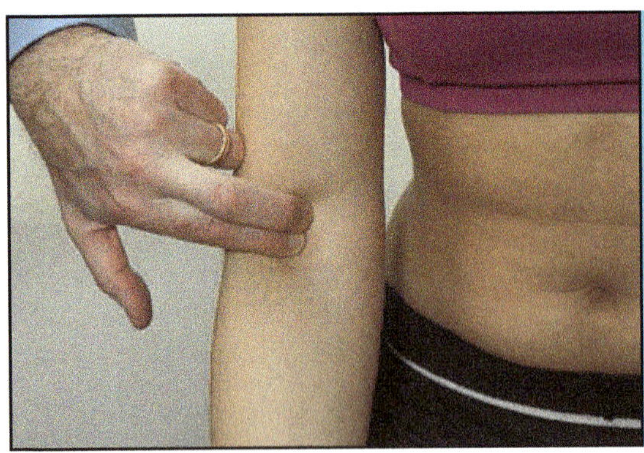

1. The patient is asked to actively flex the elbow to 90 degress while sitting or standing and to fully supinate the forearm to its end point of supination.
2. The examiner attempts to hook the biceps tendon laterally.
3. A positive test is the inability to hook the tendon (by at least 1 cm) under the tendon attachment.

UTILITY SCORE 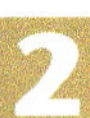

Study	Reliability	Sensitivity	Specificity	LR+	LR−	QUADAS Score (0–14)
O'Driscoll et al.[11]	NT	100	100	Inf	Inf	6
Comment: It was a small sample size and a relatively low quality study.						

TESTS FOR LATERAL EPICONDYLITIS

Cozen's Test

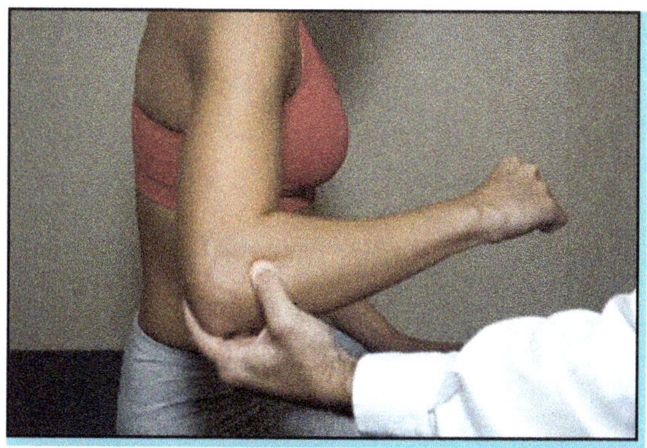

1) With the patient sitting or standing, the examiner palpates the lateral epicondyle with his or her thumb. The patient makes a fist with the forearm in pronation and radial deviation of the wrist.

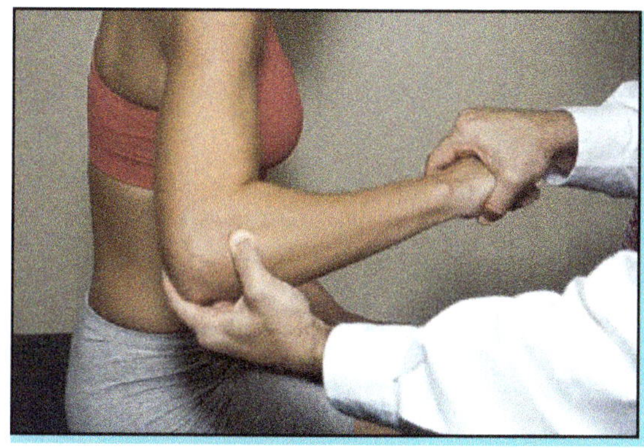

2) The patient extends the wrist against a force applied by the examiner.

3) A positive test is reproduction of pain along the lateral epicondyle.

UTILITY SCORE 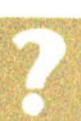

Study	Reliability	Sensitivity	Specificity	LR+	LR−	QUADAS Score (0–14)
Cozen[3]	NT	NT	NT	NA	NA	NT
Comments: No diagnostic accuracy studies have been performed to determine the sensitivity and specificity of this test.						

Resisted Tennis Elbow Test

1) The patient is placed in a seated position.

2) The patient extends his/her third digit against resistance applied by the clinician.

3) A positive test is reproduction of pain along the lateral epicondyle.

(continued)

TESTS FOR LATERAL EPICONDYLITIS

UTILITY SCORE 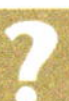

Study	Reliability	Sensitivity	Specificity	LR+	LR−	QUADAS Score (0–14)
None	NT	NT	NT	NA	NA	NT
Comments: No diagnostic accuracy studies have been performed to determine the sensitivity and specificity of this test.						

Passive Tennis Elbow Test

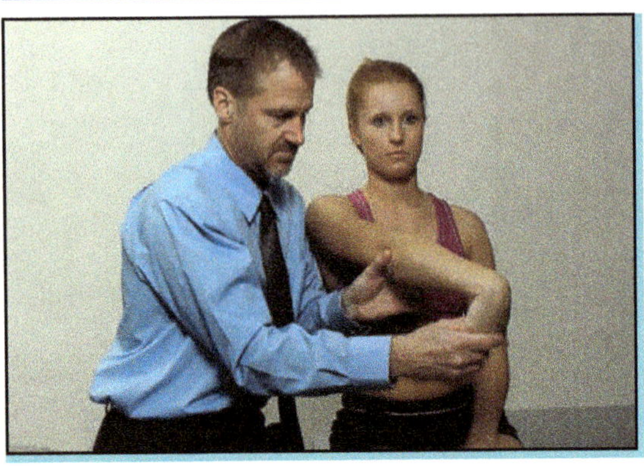

1) The patient is seated and the elbow is placed in full extension.
2) The examiner passively pronates the forearm and flexes the wrist to end-range.
3) A positive test is reproduction of pain along the lateral epicondyle.

UTILITY SCORE 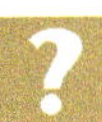

Study	Reliability	Sensitivity	Specificity	LR+	LR−	QUADAS Score (0–14)
None	NT	NT	NT	NA	NA	NT
Comments: No diagnostic accuracy studies have been performed to determine the sensitivity and specificity of this test.						

Lateral Epicondylitis/Maudsley's Test

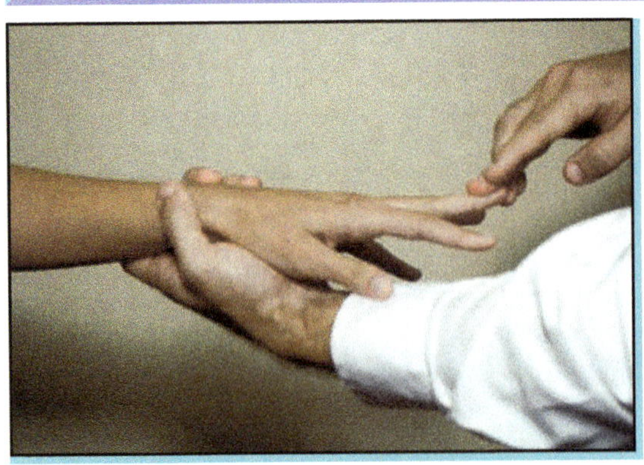

1) The examiner resists third digit extension, stressing the extensor digitorum muscle.
2) A positive test is reproduction of pain along the lateral epicondyle.

TESTS FOR LATERAL EPICONDYLITIS

UTILITY SCORE ?

Study	Reliability	Sensitivity	Specificity	LR+	LR−	QUADAS Score (0–14)
None	NT	NT	NT	NA	NA	NT
Comments: No diagnostic accuracy testing has been performed to determine the sensitivity or specificity of this test.						

Key Points

1. There are few well-designed diagnostic accuracy studies assessing the elbow for pathology.
2. The common diagnostic clinical tests used in clinical practice for the elbow, such as the varus and valgus stress and medial and lateral epicondylitis, have not been studied for diagnostic accuracy.
3. Those tests that have been studied for diagnostic accuracy, such as cubital tunnel syndrome and moving valgus stress testing, demonstrate several procedural biases.

References

1. Appelboam A, Reuben AD, Benger JR, et al. Elbow extension test to rule out elbow fracture: multicentre, prospective validation and observational study of diagnostic accuracy in adults and children. *BMJ* 2008;337:a2428.
2. Buehler MJ, Thayer DT. The elbow flexion test. A clinical test for the cubital tunnel syndrome. *Clin Orthop Relat Res.* 1988:213–216.
3. Cozen L. The painful elbow. *Ind Med Surg.* 1962; 31:369–371.
4. Cheng C, Mackinnon-Patterson B, Beck J, Mackinnon S. Scratch collapse test for evaluation of carpal and cubital tunnel syndrome. *J Hand Surg.* 2008;33A:1518–1524.
5. Darracq M, Vinson D, Panacek E. Preservation of active range of motion after acute elbow trauma predicts absence of elbow fracture. *Am J Emerg Med.* 2008;26:779–782.
6. Docherty MA, Schwab RA, Ma OJ. Can elbow extension be used as a test of clinically significant injury? *South Med J.* 2002;95:539–541.
7. El Maraghy A, Devereaux M. The biceps crease interval for diagnosing complete distal biceps tendon ruptures. *Clin Orthop Relat Res.* 2008;466:2255–2262.
8. Novak CB, Lee GW, Mackinnon SE, Lay L. Provocative testing for cubital tunnel syndrome. *J Hand Surg [Am].* 1994;19:817–820.
9. O'Driscoll SW, Bell DF, Morrey BF. Posterolateral rotatory instability of the elbow. *J Bone Joint Surg Am.* 1991;73:440–446.
10. O'Driscoll SW, Lawton RL, Smith AM. The "moving valgus stress test" for medial collateral ligament tears of the elbow. *Am J Sports Med.* 2005;33:231–239.
11. O'Driscoll SW, Goncalves LB, Dietz P. The hook test for distal biceps tendon avulsion. *Am J Sports Med.* 2007;35:1865–1869.
12. Rayan GM, Jensen C, Duke J. Elbow flexion test in the normal population. *J Hand Surg [Am].* 1992;17:86–89.
13. Ruland RT, Dunbar RP, Bowen JD. The biceps squeeze test for diagnosis of distal biceps tendon ruptures. *Clin Orthop Relat Res.* 2005;437:128–131.

PEARSON myhealthprofessionskit™

Use this address to access the Companion Website created for this textbook. Simply select "Physical Therapy" from the choice of disciplines. Find this book and log in using your username and password to access video clips of selected tests.

Physical Examination Tests for the Wrist and Hand

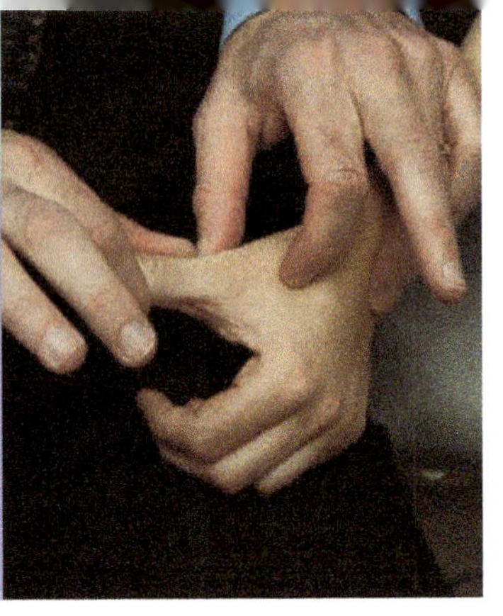

Physical Examination Tests for the Wrist and Hand

Adam Goode, Alyson Cadman, and Chad E. Cook

Please refer to the chapter "Introduction to Diagnostic Accuracy" before reading this chapter.

Index of Tests

Special Tests for the Wrist and Hand

Test for Thumb Instability

Gamekeeper's or Skier's Thumb/ Ulnar Collateral Ligament (UCL) Test

Test for Thumb Tenosynivitis

Finkelstein's Test

Test for Extensor Carpi Ulnaris Tendinosis

ECU Synergy Test

Tests for a Scaphoid Fracture

Scaphoid Compression Test
Anatomical Snuffbox Tenderness
Scaphoid Tubercle Tenderness
Pronation with Ulnar Deviation of the Wrist
Abduction of the Thumb
Radial Deviation of the Wrist
Axial Loading of the Thumb
Flexion of the Wrist
Extension of the Wrist
Power Grip of the Hand
Ulnar Deviation of the Wrist
Pronation of the Forearm
Supination of the Forearm
Thumb-Index Finger Pinch

Test for Wrist Laxity

Garcia-Elias Test
Beighton Method
AROM Method

Test for Central Slip Rupture

Integrity of the Central Slip Test

Tests for Wrist Instability

- Watson Scaphoid Test (Scaphoid Instability)
- Ulnomeniscotriquetral Dorsal Glide (TFCC Tear or Triquetral Instability)
- Ballottement (Reagan's) Test (Lunotriquetral Ligament Integrity)
- Wrist-Flexion and Finger-Extension Test (Scapholunate Pathology)
- Dorsal Capitate Displacement Apprehension Test (To Determine Stability of the Capitate Bone)
- Clinical Stress Test (Distal Radius Fracture)
- Ulno-carpal Stress Test
- Grind Test
- Press Test
- Supination Lift Test

Tests for Carpal Tunnel Syndrome

- Composite Physical Exam and History
- Katz Hand Diagram
- Wrist Ratio Index
- Thenar Atrophy
- Wrist Flexion (Phalen's)
- Modified Phalen's Test
- Flick Maneuver
- Percussion (Tinel's)
- Scratch Collapse Test
- Wrist Flexion and Median Nerve Compression
- Median Nerve Compression Test/ Pressure Provocation Test
- Two-Point Discrimination
- Semmes-Weinstein Monofilament Test
- Hypoesthesia
- Therapeutic Ultrasound
- Hand Elevation Test
- Carpal Compression Test
- Modified Carpal Compression Test
- Closed Fist/Lumbrical Provocation Test (Carpal Tunnel Syndrome from Lumbrical Excursion)
- Wrist Extension (Reverse Phalen's)
- Tethered Stress Test
- Gilliat Tourniquet Test
- Abnormal Vibration
- Abductor Pollicis Brevis Weakness
- Nocturnal Paresthesia
- Wainner's Clinical Prediction Rule for Carpal Tunnel Syndrome
- Hems' Questionnaire for Carpal Tunnel Syndrome
- Purdue Pegboard Test
- Subjective Swelling

SPECIAL TESTS FOR THE WRIST AND HAND

TEST FOR THUMB INSTABILITY

Gamekeeper's or Skier's Thumb/Ulnar Collateral Ligament (UCL) Test

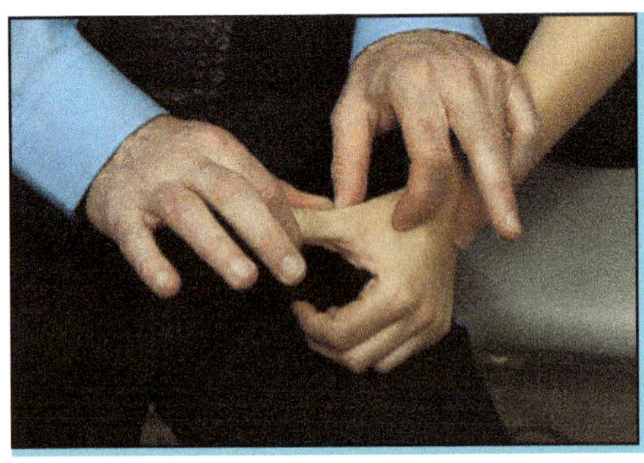

1) The patient sits and the examiner stabilizes the patient's hand with one hand and takes the patient's thumb into extension with the other hand.

2) While holding the thumb into extension, the examiner applies a valgus stress to the metacarpalphalangeal joint of thumb to stress the ulnar collateral ligament.

3) A positive test is present if the valgus movement is greater than 30 to 35 degrees, indicating a complete tear of the ulnar collateral ligament and accessory collateral ligaments.

UTILITY SCORE 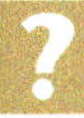

Study	Reliability	Sensitivity	Specificity	LR+	LR−	QUADAS Score (0–14)
Heyman et al.[44]	NT	94	NT	NA	NA	NT
Comments: Heyman et al.[44] reported a 100% sensitivity and 46% specificity for detection of a palpable mass proximal to the metacarpophalangeal (MCP) joint to indicate a complete tear of the UCL of the thumb.						

TEST FOR THUMB TENOSYNIVITIS

Finkelstein's Test

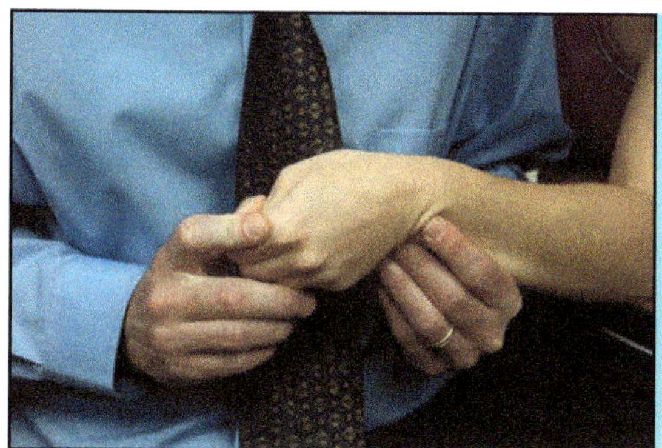

1. The patient makes a fist with the thumb inside the fingers.
2. The examiner stabilizes the forearm and deviates the wrist toward the ulnar side.
3. A positive test is indicated by pain over the abductor pollicis longus and extensor pollicis brevis tendons at the wrist, and is indicative of paratendonitis.

UTILITY SCORE 3

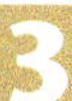

Study	Reliability	Sensitivity	Specificity	LR+	LR−	QUADAS Score (0–14)
Finkelstein[30]	NT	NT	NT	NA	NA	NT
Alexander et al.[2]	NT	81	50	1.62	0.38	9
Dawson & Mudgal [21]	NT	NT	NT	NA	NA	NT
Forman et al. [32]	NT	NT	NT	NA	NA	NT

Comments: No diagnostic accuracy studies have been performed in order to determine the sensitivity and specificity of the original Finkelstein Test for de Quervain's syndrome. Alexander et al.[2] performed an extensor pollicis brevis test to determine a septum between the EPB and APL, which led to the diagnosis and surgical intervention for de Quervain's disease. Testing consisted of two parts: the examiner resisted thumb metacarpalphalangeal joint extension, then the examiner resisted thumb palmar abduction. A positive test was indicated if pain was reproduced during resistance of thumb extension greater than abduction. A positive test may indicate a separate compartment for the EPB.

TEST FOR EXTENSOR CARPI ULNARIS TENDINOSIS

ECU Synergy Test

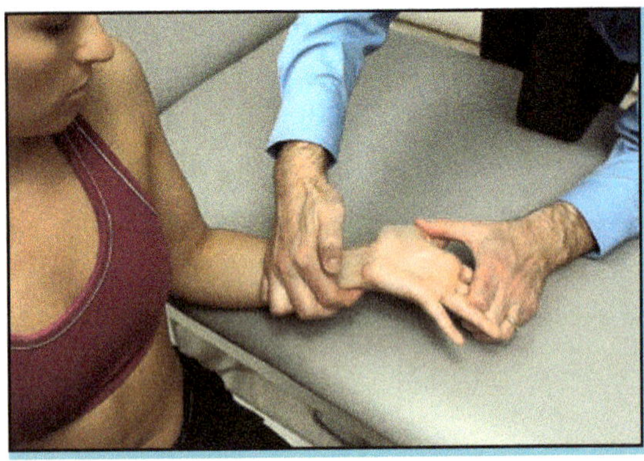

1) The patient is asked to rest his or her arm on a table with the elbow flexed at 90 degrees and forearm in full supination.

2) The patient holds the wrist in neutral position with the fingers fully extended.

3) The examiner grasps the patient's thumb and middle finger with one hand and palpates the ECU tendon with the other hand.

4) The patient then radially abducts the thumb against resistance.

5) Recreation of pain along the dorsal ulnar aspect of the wrist is considered to be a positive test for ECU tendonitis.

UTILITY SCORE 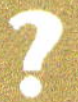

Study	Reliability	Sensitivity	Specificity	LR+	LR−	QUADAS Score (0–14)
Ruland & Hogan [77]	NT	NT	NT	NA	NA	NA
Comments: No diagnostic accuracy studies have been performed to determine sensitivity and specificity of this clinical test.						

TESTS FOR A SCAPHOID FRACTURE

Scaphoid Compression Test

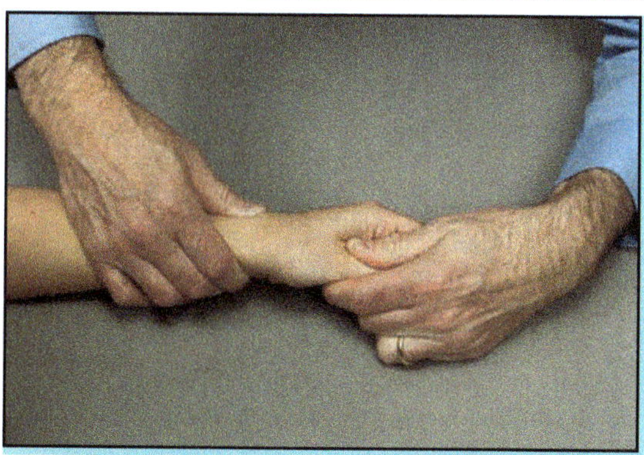

1) The examiner exerts longitudinal pressure down the thumb of the patient, in order to compress the scaphoid.

2) A positive test is reproduction of pain in the patient's wrist.

UTILITY SCORE 3

Study	Reliability	Sensitivity	Specificity	LR+	LR−	QUADAS Score (0–14)
Esberger[28]	NT	70.0	21.8	0.90	1.38	9
Comments: Of the 25 patients with a negative compression test, 13 were shown to have a scaphoid fracture through x-ray and/or bone scan.						

Anatomical Snuffbox Tenderness

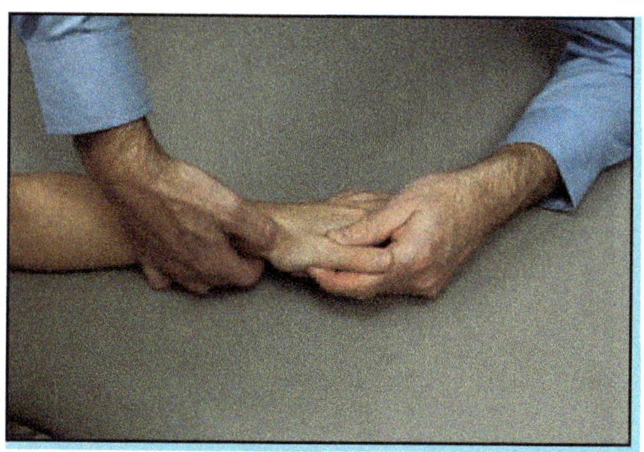

1) The examiner exerts pressure on the anatomical snuffbox.

2) A positive test is pain/tenderness when the pressure is exerted.

UTILITY SCORE 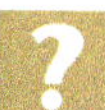

Study	Reliability	Sensitivity	Specificity	LR+	LR−	QUADAS Score (0–14)
Phillips et al.[72]	NT	NT	NT	NA	NA	NT
Comments: Phillips et al.[72] referred to Freeland[31] for sensitivity and specificity on this test. They were 90 and 40, respectively.						

TESTS FOR A SCAPHOID FRACTURE

Scaphoid Tubercle Tenderness

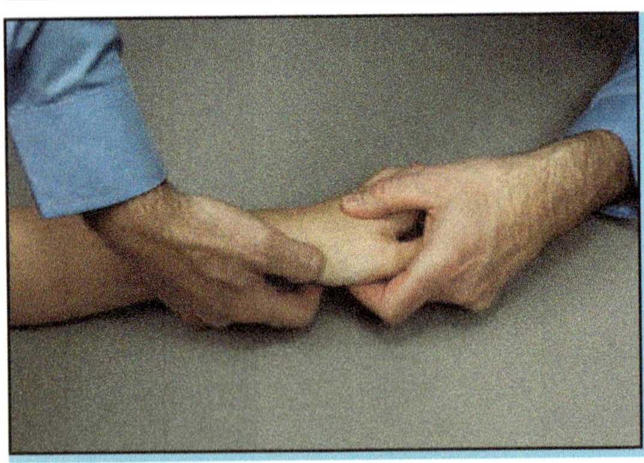

1) The examiner extends the patient's wrist with one hand and applies pressure to the tuberosity at the proximal wrist crease with the opposite hand.

2) A positive test is pain/tenderness when the pressure is exerted.

UTILITY SCORE 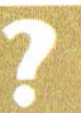

Study	Reliability	Sensitivity	Specificity	LR+	LR−	QUADAS Score (0–14)
Phillips et al.[72]	NT	NT	NT	NA	NA	NT
Comments: Phillips et al.[72] referred to Freeland[31] for sensitivity and specificity on this test. They were 87 and 57, respectively.						

Pronation with Ulnar Deviation of the Wrist

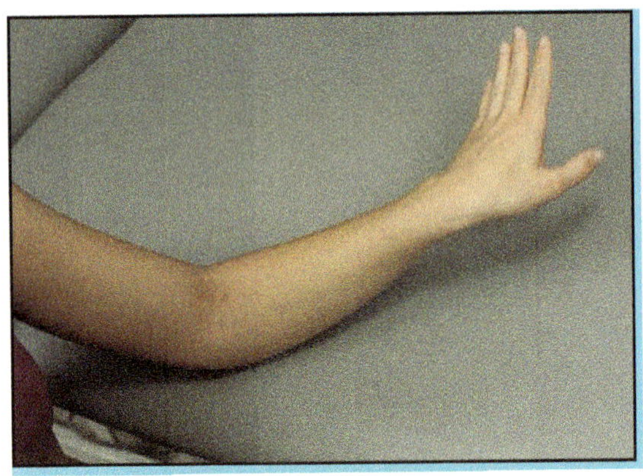

1) The patient pronates the wrist, followed by ulnar deviation.

2) A positive test is pain in the anatomical snuffbox.

UTILITY SCORE 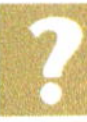

Study	Reliability	Sensitivity	Specificity	LR+	LR−	QUADAS Score (0–14)
Phillips et al.[72]	NT	NT	NT	NA	NA	NT
Comments: No diagnostic accuracy studies have been performed to determine sensitivity and specificity of this clinical test.						

TESTS FOR A SCAPHOID FRACTURE

Abduction of the Thumb

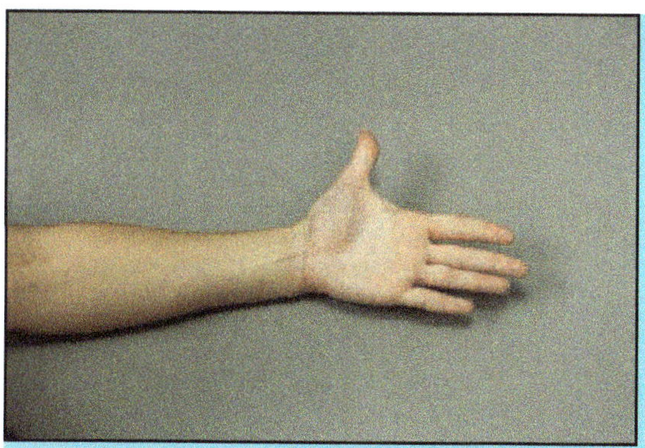

1) The patient actively abducts the thumb.

2) A positive test is reproduction of pain during abduction.

UTILITY SCORE 

Study	Reliability	Sensitivity	Specificity	LR+	LR−	QUADAS Score (0–14)
Unay et al.[88]	NT	73	50	1.45	0.55	11
Comments: The MRI results were reviewed by three orthopedic surgeons with at least 10 years of clinical experience in treating trauma. They were provided with the results of the clinical test prior to interpreting the MRI results. This test was performed first out of 10 during the physical examination. This may have an effect on pain tolerance.						

Radial Deviation of the Wrist

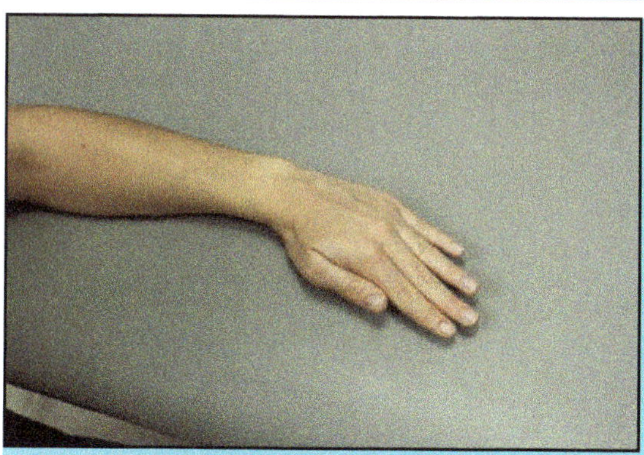

1) The patient actively performs radial deviation of the wrist.

2) A positive test is reproduction of pain during radial deviation.

UTILITY SCORE 

Study	Reliability	Sensitivity	Specificity	LR+	LR−	QUADAS Score (0–14)
Unay et al.[88]	NT	68	33	1.03	0.95	11
Comments: The MRI results were reviewed by three orthopedic surgeons with at least 10 years of clinical experience in treating trauma. They were provided with the results of the clinical test prior to interpreting the MRI results. This test was performed second out of 10 during the physical examination. This may have an effect on pain tolerance.						

TESTS FOR A SCAPHOID FRACTURE

Axial Loading of the Thumb

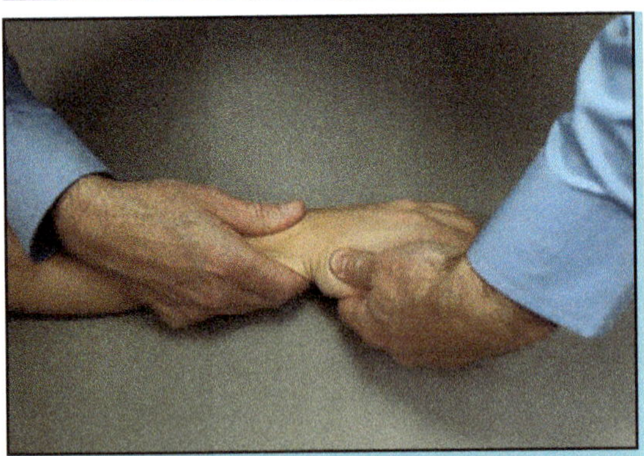

1) The clinician applies an active compression load to the thumb.

2) A positive test is reproduction of pain during loading.

UTILITY SCORE 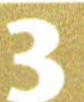

Study	Reliability	Sensitivity	Specificity	LR+	LR−	QUADAS Score (0–14)
Unay et al.[88]	NT	71	35	1.10	0.82	11
Comments: The MRI results were reviewed by three orthopedic surgeons with at least 10 years of clinical experience in treating trauma. They were provided with the results of the clinical test prior to interpreting the MRI results. This test was performed third out of 10 during the physical examination. This may have an effect on pain tolerance.						

Flexion of the Wrist

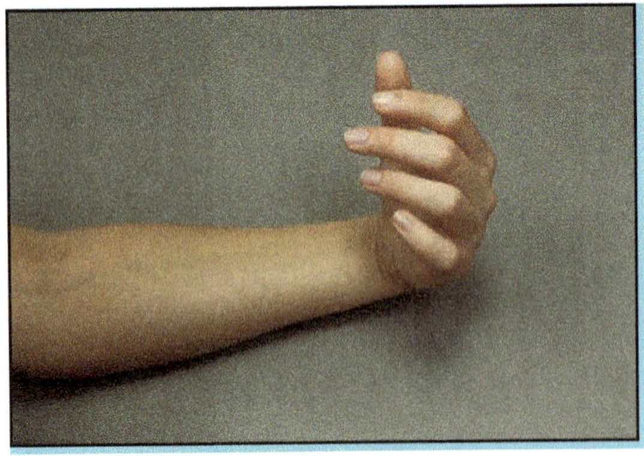

1) The patient actively flexes the wrist.

2) A positive test is reproduction of pain during wrist flexion.

UTILITY SCORE 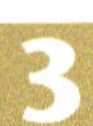

Study	Reliability	Sensitivity	Specificity	LR+	LR−	QUADAS Score (0–14)
Unay et al.[88]	NT	71	50	1.43	0.57	11
Comments: The MRI results were reviewed by three orthopedic surgeons with at least 10 years of clinical experience in treating trauma. They were provided with the results of the clinical test prior to interpreting the MRI results. This test was performed fourth out of 10 during the physical examination. This may have an effect on pain tolerance.						

TESTS FOR A SCAPHOID FRACTURE

Extension of the Wrist

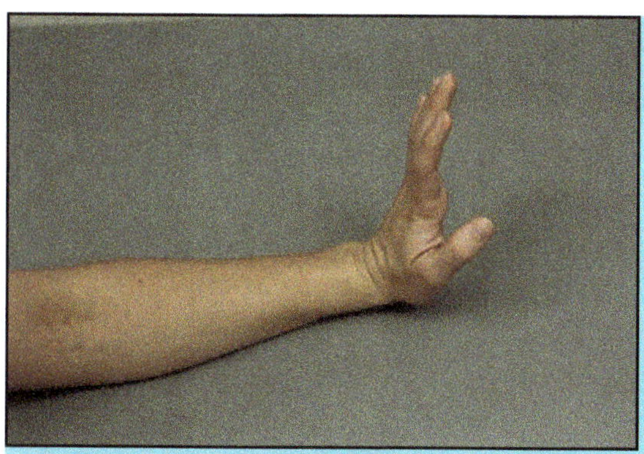

1) The patient actively extends the wrist.

2) A positive test is reproduction of pain during wrist extension.

UTILITY SCORE 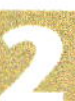

Study	Reliability	Sensitivity	Specificity	LR+	LR−	QUADAS Score (0–14)
Unay et al.[88]	NT	72	60	1.81	0.46	11

Comments: The MRI results were reviewed by three orthopedic surgeons with at least 10 years of clinical experience in treating trauma. They were provided with the results of the clinical test prior to interpreting the MRI results. This test was performed fifth out of 10 during the physical examination. This may have an effect on pain tolerance.

Power Grip of the Hand

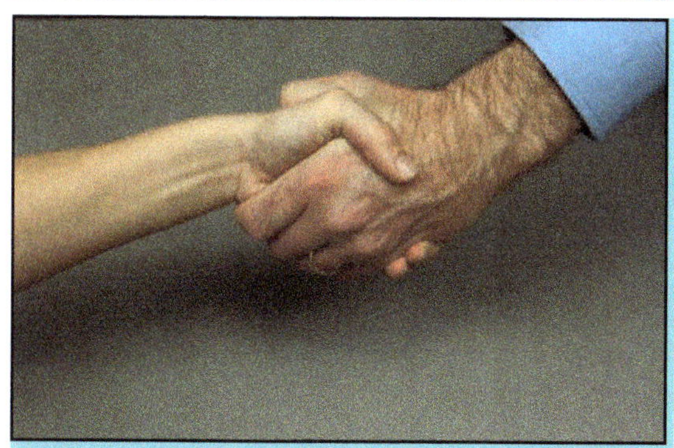

1) The clinician assumes a handshake position with the patient.

2) The patient is instructed to squeeze the hand of the clinician.

3) A positive test is pain during squeezing.

UTILITY SCORE 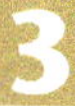

Study	Reliability	Sensitivity	Specificity	LR+	LR−	QUADAS Score (0–14)
Unay et al.[88]	NT	67	20	0.83	1.67	11

Comments: The MRI results were reviewed by three orthopedic surgeons with at least 10 years of clinical experience in treating trauma. They were provided with the results of the clinical test prior to interpreting the MRI results. This test was performed sixth out of 10 during the physical examination. This may have an effect on pain tolerance.

TESTS FOR A SCAPHOID FRACTURE

Ulnar Deviation of the Wrist

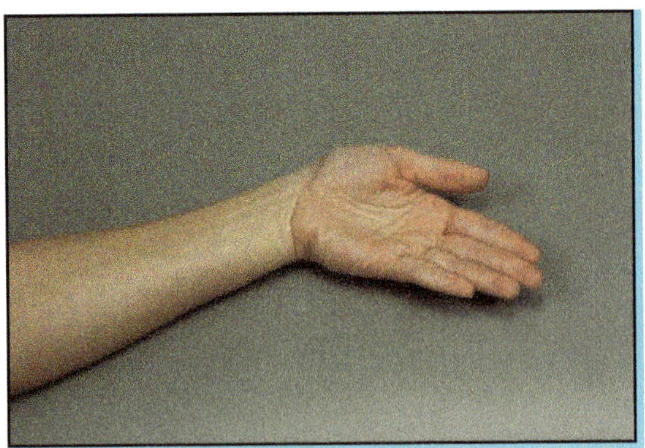

1) The patient actively performs ulnar deviation of the wrist.

2) A positive test is reproduction of pain during ulnar deviation.

UTILITY SCORE 3

Study	Reliability	Sensitivity	Specificity	LR+	LR−	QUADAS Score (0–14)
Unay et al.[88]	NT	70	36	1.10	0.83	11
Comments: The MRI results were reviewed by three orthopedic surgeons with at least 10 years of clinical experience in treating trauma. They were provided with the results of the clinical test prior to interpreting the MRI results. This test was performed seventh out of 10 during the physical examination. This may have an effect on pain tolerance.						

Pronation of the Forearm

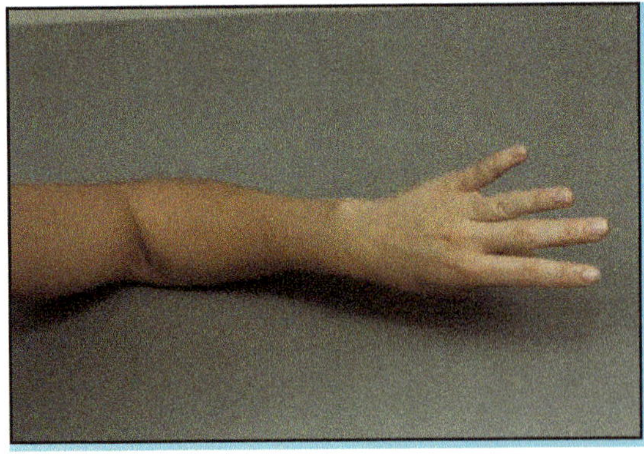

1) The patient actively performs pronation of the forearm.

2) A positive test is reproduction of pain during wrist pronation.

UTILITY SCORE 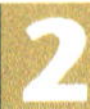

Study	Reliability	Sensitivity	Specificity	LR+	LR−	QUADAS Score (0–14)
Unay et al.[88]	NT	79	58	1.90	0.35	11
Comments: The MRI results were reviewed by three orthopedic surgeons with at least 10 years of clinical experience in treating trauma. They were provided with the results of the clinical test prior to interpreting the MRI results. This test was performed eighth out of 10 during the physical examination. This may have an effect on pain tolerance.						

TESTS FOR A SCAPHOID FRACTURE

Supination of the Forearm

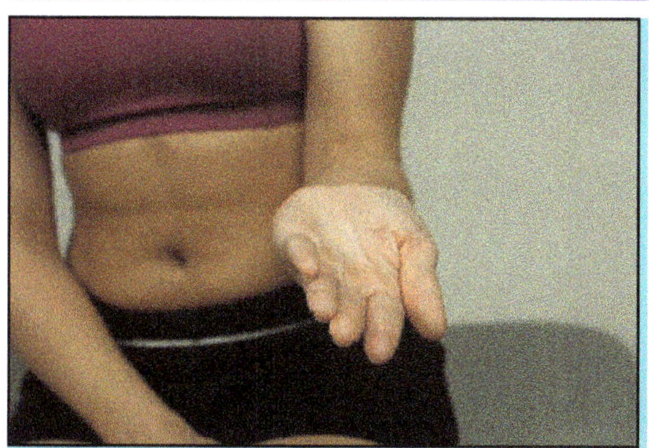

1) The patient actively performs supination of the forearm.

2) A positive test is reproduction of pain during forearm supination.

UTILITY SCORE 

Study	Reliability	Sensitivity	Specificity	LR+	LR−	QUADAS Score (0–14)
Unay et al.[88]	NT	76	50	1.52	0.48	11
Comments: The MRI results were reviewed by three orthopedic surgeons with at least 10 years of clinical experience in treating trauma. They were provided with the results of the clinical test prior to interpreting the MRI results. This test was performed ninth out of 10 during the physical examination. This may have an effect on pain tolerance.						

Thumb-Index Finger Pinch

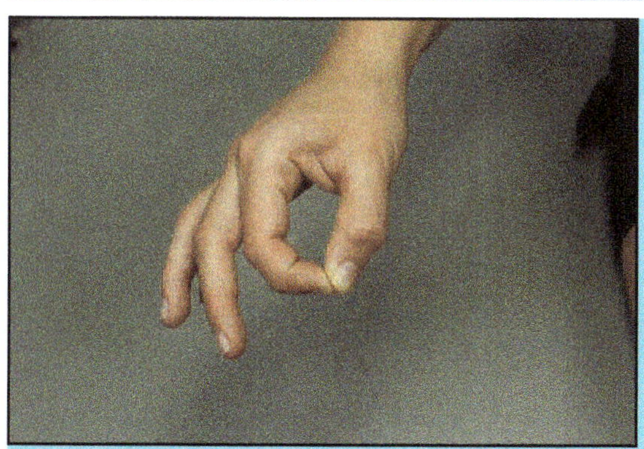

1) The patient actively pinches the thumb and index finger pads together.

2) A positive test is reproduction of pain.

UTILITY SCORE 

Study	Reliability	Sensitivity	Specificity	LR+	LR−	QUADAS Score (0–14)
Unay et al.[88]	NT	73	75	2.92	0.36	11
Comments: The MRI results were reviewed by three orthopedic surgeons with at least 10 years of clinical experience in treating trauma. They were provided with the results of the clinical test prior to interpreting the MRI results. This test was performed tenth out of 10 during the physical examination. This may have an effect on pain tolerance.						

TEST FOR WRIST LAXITY

Garcia-Elias Test

1) Patients perform four tests and are given a score of 1–50 points for each test.
2) A score of 50 indicates the highest joint laxity for that test.
3) All four test scores are added together for a point total of 4–200.
4) Patients are then ranked based on their laxity score.
5) A positive test is a rank in the top 25% of total patients.

UTILITY SCORE 3

Study	Reliability	Sensitivity	Specificity	LR+	LR–	QUADAS Score (0–14)
van Andel et al.[89]	NT	20	55	0.44	1.46	8

Comments: The tests include: (1) A measurement in millimeters of the shortest perpendicular distance between the center of the thumbnail and the forearm when the patient extends the wrist and maximally moves the thumb toward the forearm. (2) A measurement of the angle of the wrist when the subject was asked to extend the wrist maximally. (3) A measurement in millimeters of the shortest perpendicular distance between the center of the thumbnail and the forearm when the patient maximally flexes the wrist. (4) A measurement of the angle of the wrist when the subject was asked to flex the wrist maximally. This test was designed to test multiple patients. Only premenopausal women were chosen for this study.

Beighton Method

1) The patient performs five tests and receives a laxity score of 0–9.
2) A positive test is a score of 4 or more.

UTILITY SCORE 2

Study	Reliability	Sensitivity	Specificity	LR+	LR–	QUADAS Score (0–14)
van Andel et al.[89]	NT	67	77	2.88	0.43	8
Beighton et al.[8]	NT	NT	NT	NA	NA	NT

Comments: The five tests include: (1) The patient can put their hands on the ground with straight knees (1 point). (2) The elbow hyperextends greater than or equal to 10 degrees (1 point per elbow). (3) The knee hyperextends greater than or equal to 10 degrees (1 point per knee). (4) The thumb can be bent back to touch the front of the forearm (1 point per thumb). (5) The little finger hyperextends past 90 degrees (1 point per little finger). van Andel et al.[89] only examined premenopausal women. Beighton et al.[8] stated that a score of 4 or more is positive.

TEST FOR WRIST LAXITY

AROM Method

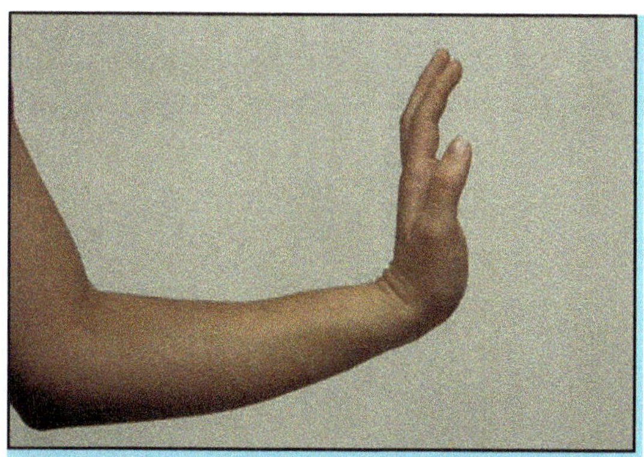

1) The patient's forearm and hand are in a fixed position.

2) The patient is asked to reach their maximal dorsal and palmar flexion angles.

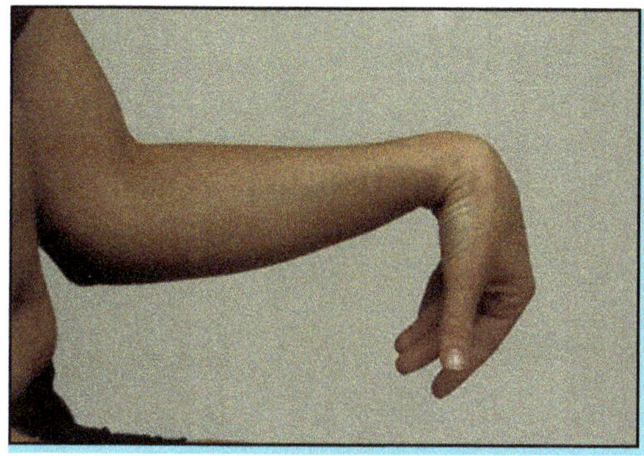

3) A positive test is a total active motion of 180 degrees or more.

UTILITY SCORE 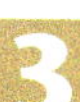

Study	Reliability	Sensitivity	Specificity	LR+	LR−	QUADAS Score (0–14)
van Andel et al.[89]	NT	54	67	1.61	0.69	8
Comments: A measurement device was created to record Active Range of Motion (AROM) while fixing the hand and forearm in place. Only premenopausal women were selected to participate in this study.						

TEST FOR CENTRAL SLIP RUPTURE

Integrity of the Central Slip Test

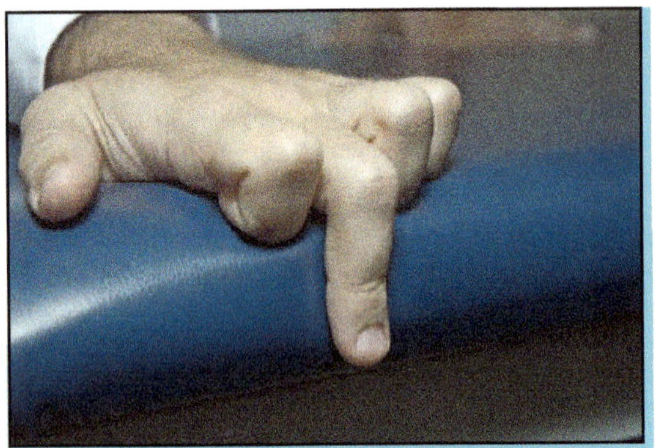

1) The patient flexes the finger to 90 degrees at the proximal interphalangeal joint over the edge of the table.

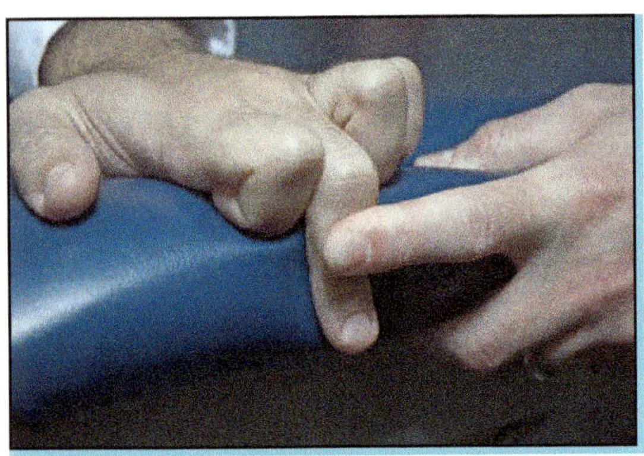

2) The patient is then asked to extend the proximal interphalangeal joint while the examiner palpates the middle phalanx.

3) A positive test is the examiner's feeling of little pressure from the middle phalanx while the distal interphalangeal joint is extending.

UTILITY SCORE 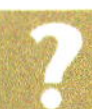

Study	Reliability	Sensitivity	Specificity	LR+	LR−	QUADAS Score (0–14)
Elson[27]	NT	NT	NT	NA	NA	NT
Comments: No diagnostic accuracy studies have been performed to determine sensitivity and specificity of this clinical test.						

TESTS FOR WRIST INSTABILITY

Watson Scaphoid Test (Scaphoid Instability)

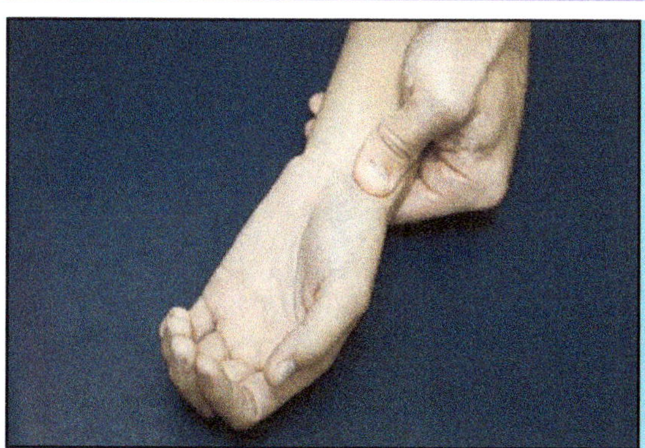

1) The patient's arm is slightly pronated. The examiner grasps the wrist from the radial side with thumb over the scaphoid tubercle.

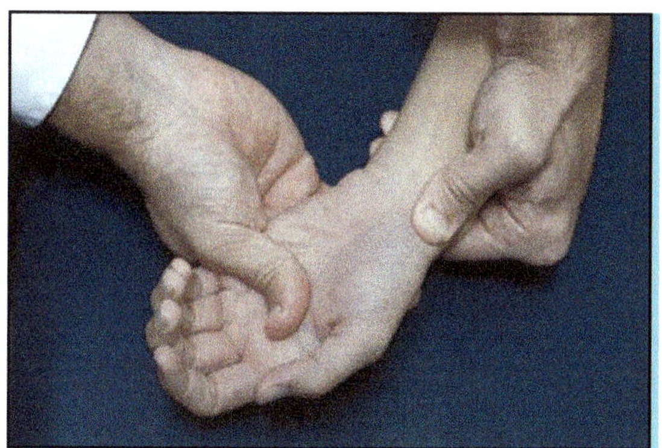

2) The examiner's other hand grasps the metacarpals. Starting in ulnar deviation and slight extension, the wrist is moved into radial deviation and slight flexion.

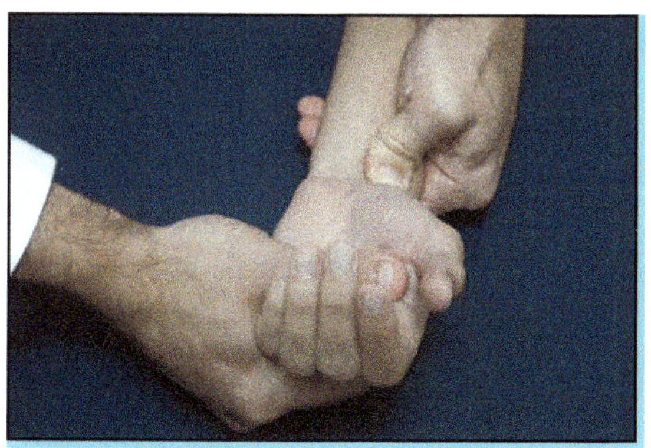

3) The examiner's thumb presses the scaphoid out of normal alignment when laxity exists and when the thumb is released there is a "thunk" as the scaphoid moves back in place.

4) A positive test is identified by subluxation or clunk over the examiner's thumb and patient reports pain.

(*continued*)

TESTS FOR WRIST INSTABILITY

UTILITY SCORE 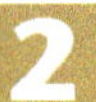

Study	Reliability	Sensitivity	Specificity	LR+	LR−	QUADAS Score (0–14)
LaStayo & Howell[57]	NT	69	66	2.0	0.47	12
Forman et al.[32]	NT	NT	NT	NA	NA	NT

Comments: Easterling & Wolfe[25] demonstrated a 34% prevalence of the painless but positive for laxity Watson tests in a population of 100 uninjured wrists. Lane[56] described a modification of the Watson Test and named this test the Scaphoid Shift Test. The positioning is the same as the Watson Test; however, with the wrist in neutral to a slight (0–10) degree of radial deviation and neutral wrist flexion/extension, the examiner quickly pushes the tubercle of the scaphoid in a dorsal direction, noting a clunk, crepitus, or pain in comparison to the opposite wrist.

Ulnomeniscotriquetral Dorsal Glide (TFCC Tear or Triquetral Instability)

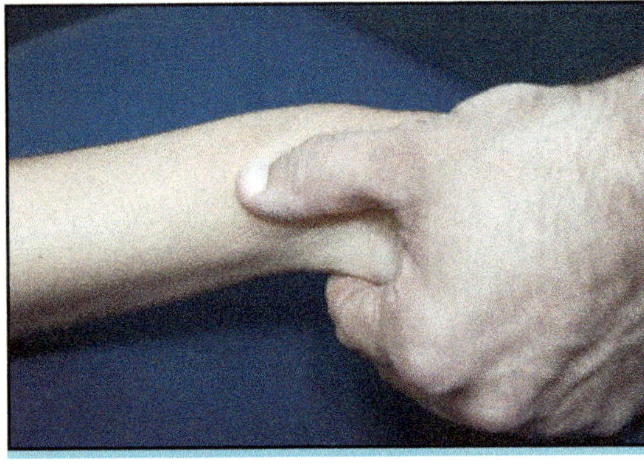

1) The examiner places his or her thumb dorsally over the ulna while placing the Proximal Interphalangeal Joints (PIP) of the index finger over the pisotriquetral complex.

2) The examiner then produces a dorsal glide of the pisotriquetral complex.

3) A positive test is reproduction of pain or laxity in the ulnomeniscotriquetral region.

UTILITY SCORE 

Study	Reliability	Sensitivity	Specificity	LR+	LR−	QUADAS Score (0–14)
LaStayo & Howell[57]	NT	66	64	1.8	0.5	12
Moriya et al.[65]	NT	NT	NT	NA	NA	NT
Forman et al.[32]	NT	NT	NT	NA	NA	NT

Comments: This test is commonly referred to as the Piano Key Test. Moriya et al.[65] used 11 cadaver specimens to examine this test. The triangular ligament was released to simulate instability of the distal radial ulnar joint (DRUJ).

TESTS FOR WRIST INSTABILITY

Ballottement (Reagan's) Test (Lunotriquetral Ligament Integrity)

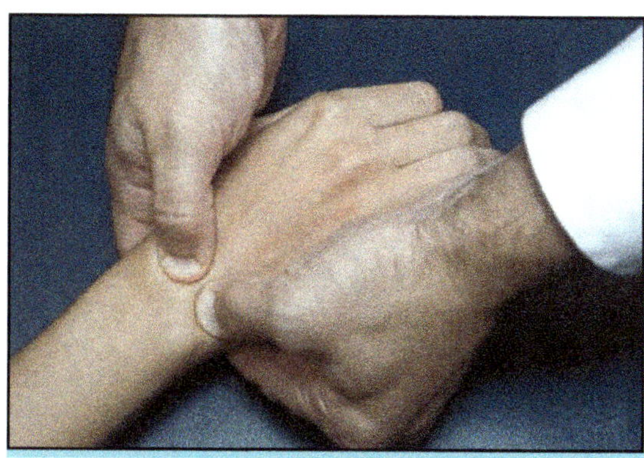

1) The examiner grasps the triquetrum between the thumb and second finger of one hand and the lunate with the thumb and second finger of the other hand.

2) The examiner moves the lunate palmar and dorsal with respect to the triquetrum.

3) A positive test is laxity, crepitus, or reproduction of the patient's pain during anteriorposterior movement.

UTILITY SCORE 3

Study	Reliability	Sensitivity	Specificity	LR+	LR−	QUADAS Score (0–14)
Reagan et al.[76]	NT	NT	NT	NA	NA	NT
LaStayo & Howell[57]	NT	64	44	1.14	0.82	12
Moriya et al.[65]	NT	NT	NT	NA	NA	NT
Forman et al.[32]	NT	NT	NT	NA	NA	NT

Comments: It is unclear if the index test and reference test was interpreted without knowledge of either result. Moriya et al.[65] used 11 cadaver specimens to examine this test. The triangular ligament was released to simulate instability of the DRUJ. This test demonstrated a statistically significant degree of accuracy when assessing DRUJ instability.

Wrist-Flexion and Finger-Extension Test (Scapholunate Pathology)

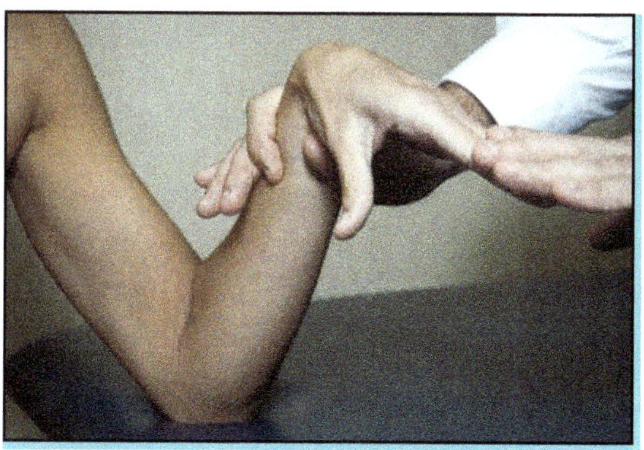

1) The patient is placed in the sitting position with the elbow placed on the table.

2) The examiner holds the patient's wrist in flexion and asks the patient to extend the fingers against resistance.

3) A positive test is identified by pain over the scaphoid.

UTILITY SCORE 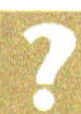

Study	Reliability	Sensitivity	Specificity	LR+	LR−	QUADAS Score (0–14)
Truong et al.[87]	NT	NT	NT	NA	NA	NT

Comments: No diagnostic accuracy studies have been performed to determine the sensitivity and specificity of this particular clinical test. Truong et al.[87] described this test for use in determining scapholunate pathology using a composite of five clinical exam techniques and tests.

TESTS FOR WRIST INSTABILITY

Dorsal Capitate Displacement Apprehension Test (To Determine Stability of the Capitate Bone)

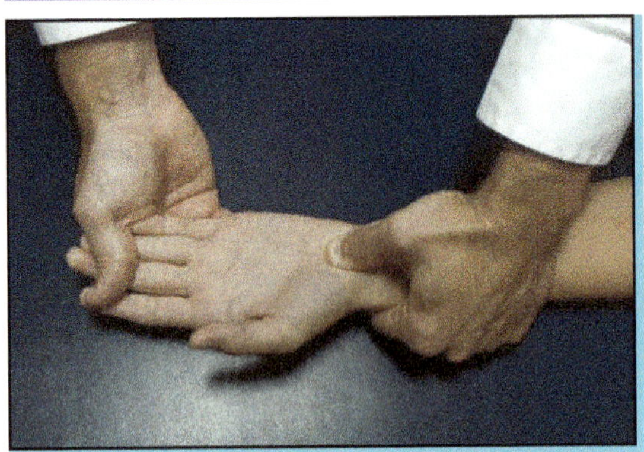

1) The patient sits facing the examiner.

2) The examiner holds the patient's hand with one hand. The thumb of the examiner is placed over the patient's palmar aspect of the capitate while the other hand holds the patient's hand in neutral and applies a counterpressure when the examiner pushes the capitate posterior with the thumb.

3) A positive test is identified by reproduction of the patient's concordant pain or apprehension. A positive test may also be if half of the proximal pole of the capitate is displaced outside of the lunate fossa.

UTILITY SCORE 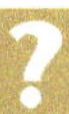

Study	Reliability	Sensitivity	Specificity	LR+	LR−	QUADAS Score (0–14)
Johnson & Carrera[45]	NT	NT	NT	NA	NA	NT

Comments: No diagnostic accuracy studies have been performed to determine sensitivity and specificity of this particular test in isolation. Truong et al.[87] performed a similar test named the Capitolunate Instability Pattern Wrist Maneuver in order to determine scapholunate instability in a series of tests. However, sensitivity and specificity cannot be calculated from this study. Johnson & Carrera[45] examined 12 patients under fluoroscopic control, demonstrating dorsal subluxation of the capitate out of the cup of the lunate. Eleven patients underwent surgical intervention in order to shorten the radiocapitate ligament.

Clinical Stress Test (Distal Radius Fracture)

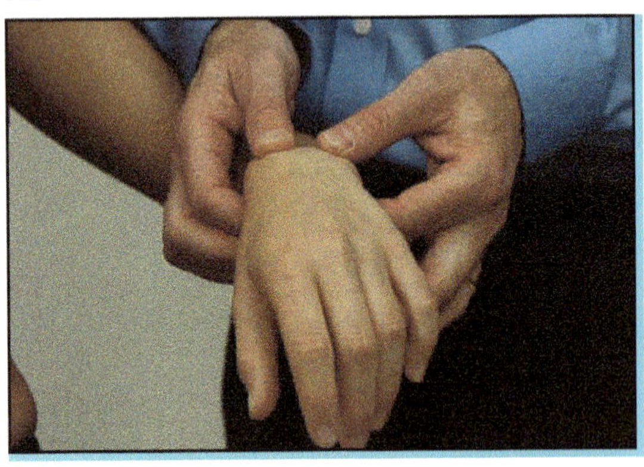

1) The patient's radius is grasped by the examiner with the forearm in neutral position.

2) The distal ulna is fixed between the examiner's thumb and index finger and is moved in dorsal and palmar directions with respect to the radius.

3) A positive test is when the ulna is conspicuously displaced relative to the contralateral side with presence of pain or apprehension.

UTILITY SCORE 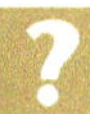

Study	Reliability	Sensitivity	Specificity	LR+	LR−	QUADAS Score (0–14)
Kim & Park[51]	0.33 (MRUL) 0.56 (Epicenter) 0.41 (RUR)	NT	NT	NA	NA	10

Comments: No diagnostic accuracy studies have been performed to determine sensitivity and specificity of this particular test. Reliability of this test was determined by comparing it to modified radioulnar line (MRUL), epicenter, and radioulnar ratio (RUR) computerized tomography (CT) diagnosis, respectively.

TESTS FOR WRIST INSTABILITY

Ulno-carpal Stress Test

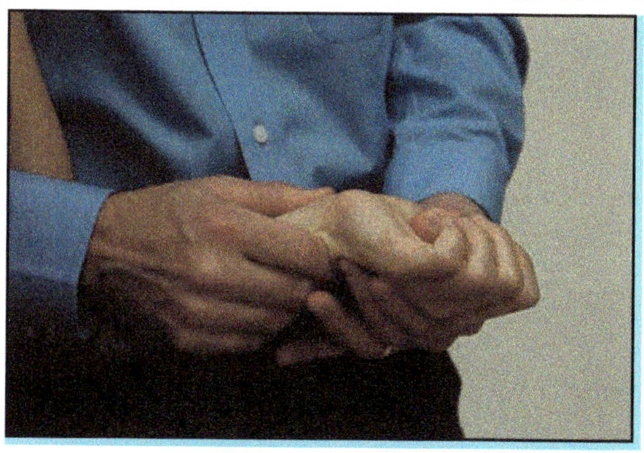

1) The patient is seated with their elbow fully flexed, with the wrist in full active ulnar deviation and the forearm in supination.

2) The examiner supports the patient's elbow and grasps the palm of the patient's hand.

3) The examiner then maintains ulnar deviation and produces supination and pronation of the wrist.

4) A positive test is a 'click' during the tests, along with pain on the medial aspect of the wrist within the ulno-carpal region.

UTILITY SCORE 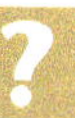

Study	Reliability	Sensitivity	Specificity	LR+	LR−	QUADAS Score (0–14)
Moriya et al.[65]	NT	NT	NT	NA	NA	NT
Comments: No diagnostic accuracy studies have been performed to determine sensitivity and specificity of this particular test. Moriya et al.[65] used 11 cadaver specimens to examine this test. The triangular ligament was released to simulate instability of the DRUJ.						

Grind Test

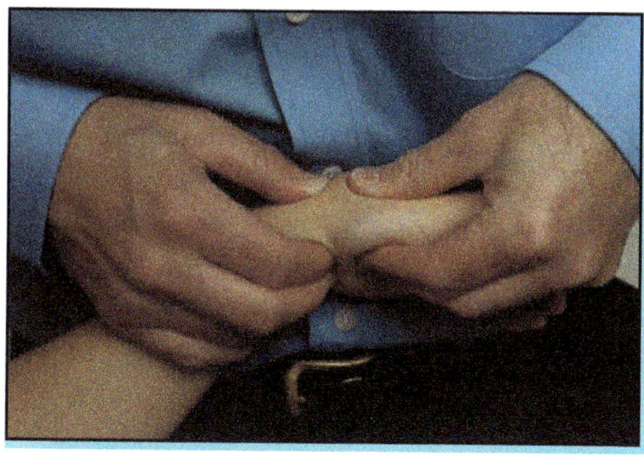

1) The examiner compresses and rotates the patient's first metacapal bone, along with the trapezium.

2) A positive test is pain and crepitus due to this movement.

UTILITY SCORE 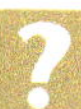

Study	Reliability	Sensitivity	Specificity	LR+	LR−	QUADAS Score (0–14)
Forman et al.[32]	NT	NT	NT	NA	NA	NT
Comments: No diagnostic accuracy studies have been performed to determine the sensitivity and specificity of this clinical test.						

TESTS FOR WRIST INSTABILITY

Press Test

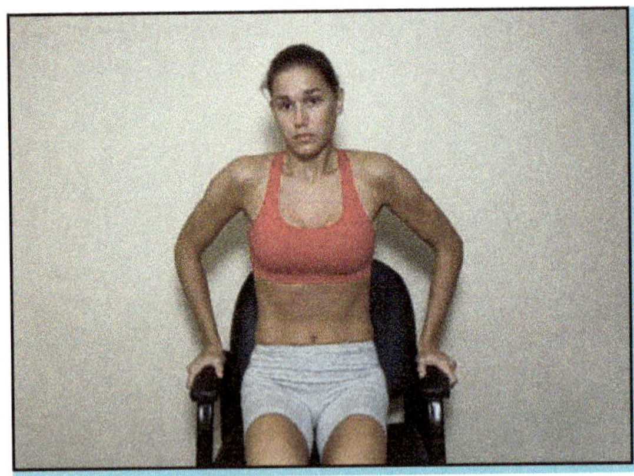

1) The patient places both hands on the arms of a stable chair and pushes off to suspend the body using only the hands.

2) A positive test is the reproduction of wrist pain while pressing up the patient's body weight.

UTILITY SCORE ?

Study	Reliability	Sensitivity	Specificity	LR+	LR−	QUADAS Score (0–14)
Lester et al.[58]	NT	100	NT	NA	NA	7
Comments: Lester et al.[58] reported 100% sensitivity compared with arthroscopic surgery and 79% sensitivity compared to MRI arthrogram. Specificity could not be determined based on the methodology of this test design.						

Supination Lift Test

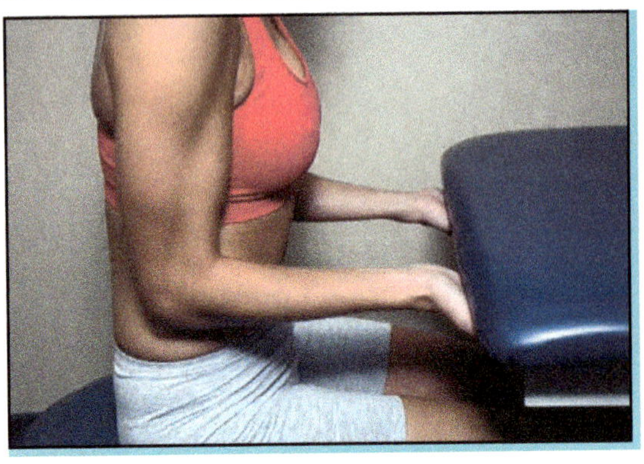

1) The patient is seated with elbows flexed to 90 degrees and forearms supinated. The patient is asked to place the palms flat on the underside of a heavy table or against the examiner's hands.

2) The patient is asked to lift the table or push up against the resisting examiner's hands.

3) A positive test is pain localized to the ulnar side of the wrist or difficulty applying force.

UTILITY SCORE 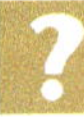

Study	Reliability	Sensitivity	Specificity	LR+	LR−	QUADAS Score (0–14)
Buterbaugh et al.[17]	NT	NT	NT	NA	NA	NT
Forman et al.[32]	NT	NT	NT	NA	NA	NT
Comments: No diagnostic accuracy studies have been performed to determine the sensitivity and specificity of this clinical test.						

TESTS FOR CARPAL TUNNEL SYNDROME

Composite Physical Exam and History

1) Examination by neurologist or standardized questionnaire to gather history of presenting symptoms prior to NCS.

2) A positive test is the ability of a physical exam, history, or questionnaire to predict the diagnosis of CTS in relation to the reference standard of NCS.

UTILITY SCORE 2

Study	Reliability	Sensitivity	Specificity	LR+	LR−	QUADAS Score (0–14)
*Katz & Stirrat[48]	NT	84	72	3.0	0.2	13
*Gunnarsson et al.[39]	NT	94	80	4.7	0.1	13
*Bland[9]	NT	79	56	1.8	0.4	11
*Wainner et al.[90]	NT	18	99	18	0.8	12
*Amirfeyz et al.[4]	NT	70	73	2.58	0.41	7
Hems et al.[42]	NT	71	61	1.82	0.48	7
Priganc & Henry[73]	0.91 0.95	NA	NA	NA	NA	11

Comments: No specific detail was given by Katz et al.[48] or Gunnarsson et al.[39] to the content of the physical exam other than an exam by a board-certified neurologist. The Bland[9] study provided a questionnaire, including the Levine Questionnaire and Symptoms Severity Scale, to describe a collection of CTS history symptoms and collect information from patients. Wainner et al.[90] developed a clinical prediction rule including a positive Flick sign, Symptom Severity Scale of greater than 1.9, decreased sensibility testing, age greater than 45, and wrist ratio index greater than 0.67 for the above diagnostic accuracy. Hems et al.[43] developed a questionnaire including age below 60, night pain, paresthesia median nerve distribution, relief of pain by shaking, relief of pain by splint, clumsiness, a positive Tinel's sign, Phalen's test, altered median nerve sensation, and wasting thenar eminence. Amirfeyz et al.[4] examined the Kamath-Stothard questionnaire. Priganc & Henry[73] examined reliability of the Spearman symptom severity scale and functional status, respectively.
*Indicates those studies using EMG/NCS as inclusion criteria.

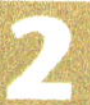

TESTS FOR CARPAL TUNNEL SYNDROME

Katz Hand Diagram

1) The patient is asked to fill out a diagram using a key of numbness, pain, tingling, and decreased sensation.

2) The Katz Hand Diagram is subdivided into those patients that have "classic," "probable," "possible," and "unlikely" carpal tunnel syndrome based on completion of the diagram.

UTILITY SCORE 2

Study	Reliability	Sensitivity	Specificity	LR+	LR−	QUADAS Score (0–14)
*Szabo et al.[84]	NT	76	98	38	0.2	9
*Katz et al.[47]	NT	61	71	2.1	0.5	13
*Katz & Stirrat[48]	NT	80	90	3.6	0.1	11
Atroshi et al.[7]	NT	80	90	8.0	0.2	8
*Gunnarsson et al.[39]	NT	66	69	2.1	0.5	13
O'Gradaigh & Merry[67]	NT	72	53	1.5	0.5	8
Priganc & Henry[73]	0.95	NA	NA	NA	NA	11

Comments: With the exception of reporting intermediate results, the Katz Hand Diagram is an excellent method of collecting patient information with consistent diagnostic accuracy to support its use. Priganc & Henry[73] examined the relationship between Katz Hand Diagram and severity of CTS.
*Indicates those studies using EMG/NCS as inclusion criteria.

Wrist Ratio Index

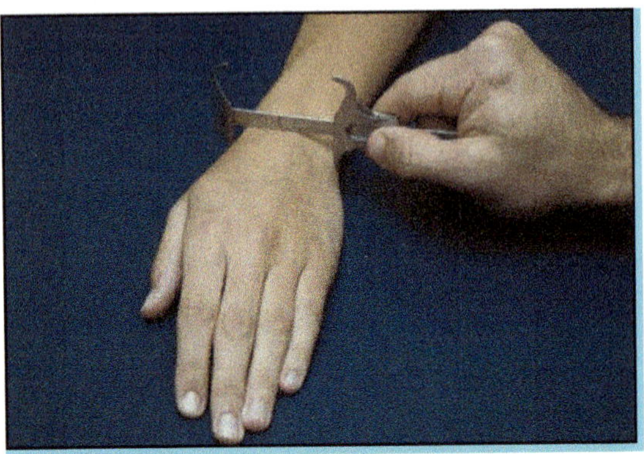

1) Sliding calipers are used to measure the mediolateral (ML) wrist width in centimeters.

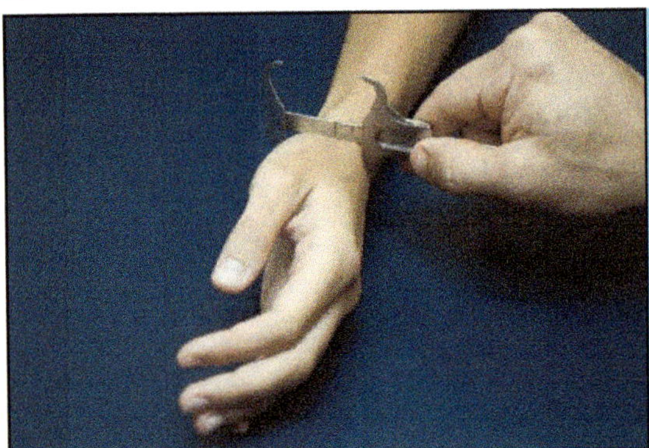

2) Next, sliding calipers are used to measure the anteroposterior height (AP) in centimeters. Caliper jaws are aligned with the distal wrist crease for both measurements.

3) Wrist ratio index is computed by dividing the AP wrist width by the ML wrist width.

4) A positive test is a wrist ratio of greater than 0.67.

TESTS FOR CARPAL TUNNEL SYNDROME

UTILITY SCORE 2

Study	Reliability	Sensitivity	Specificity	LR+	LR−	QUADAS Score (0–14)
*Kuhlman & Hennessey[53]	NT	69	73	2.6	0.4	10
Radecki[75]	NT	47	83	2.8	0.6	10
*Wainner et al.[90]	ICC 77 (AP) 86 (ML)	93	26	1.3	0.3	12
*Lim et al.[59]	NT	NT	NT	NA	NA	NT

Comments: Wainner et al.[90] used the wrist ratio index as part of the clinical prediction rule to diagnose CTS. As a test in isolation the wrist ratio index does not appear to have strong diagnostic accuracy. Lim et al.[59] also measured wrist palm ratio by dividing the AP wrist width by the palm length.
*Indicates those studies using EMG/NCS as inclusion criteria.

Thenar Atrophy

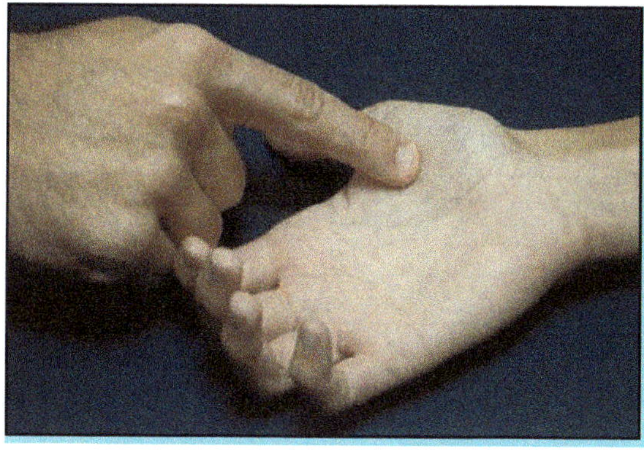

1) The examiner observes the patient's thenar eminence in comparison to the contralateral thenar eminence for signs of atrophy.

2) A positive test is the presence of observable atrophy in the thenar eminence.

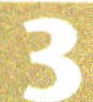

UTILITY SCORE 3

Study	Reliability	Sensitivity	Specificity	LR+	LR−	QUADAS Score (0–14)
*de Krom et al.[22]	NT	70	45	1.3	0.7	10
*Gerr & Letz[35]	NT	28	82	1.6	0.9	12
*Golding et al.[37]	NT	04	99	4.0	1.0	7
*Katz et al.[47]	NT	14	90	1.4	1.0	13

Comments: There is little evidence to support the use of thenar atrophy in the diagnosis of CTS. Thenar atrophy is a sign of CTS; however, these patients are generally in the later stages of CTS and have not been part of diagnostic accuracy studies.
*Indicates those studies using EMG/NCS as inclusion criteria.

TESTS FOR CARPAL TUNNEL SYNDROME

Wrist Flexion (Phalen's)

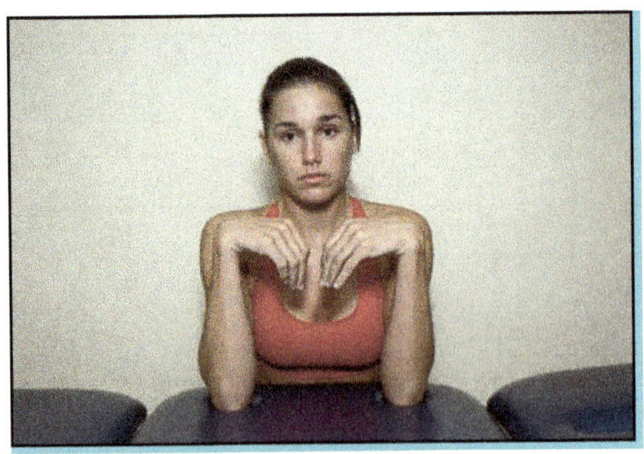

1) The patient is asked to hold the forearms vertically and allow both hands to drop into complete flexion at the wrist for approximately 60 seconds.

2) A positive test is the reproduction of symptoms along the distribution of the median nerve.

UTILITY SCORE 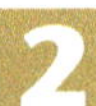

Study	Reliability	Sensitivity	Specificity	LR+	LR−	QUADAS Score (0–14)
Phalen[71]	NT	74	NT	NA	NA	NT
Mossman & Blau[66]	NT	33	NT	NA	NA	6
Seror[79]	NT	62	90?	6.2	0.42	6
Miedany et al.[62]	NT	47.00	17.00	0.57	3.12	9
*Buch-Jaeger & Foucher[14]	NT	58	54	1.3	0.8	9
*Gerr & Letz[35]	NT	75	33	1.1	0.7	12
*Heller et al.[42]	NT	67	59	1.6	0.6	5
*Katz et al.[47]	NT	75	47	1.4	0.5	13
*Kuhlman & Hennessey[53]	NT	51	76	2.1	0.6	10
*Golding et al.[37]	NT	10	86	0.7	1.0	7
Burke et al.[16]	NT	49	54	1.1	0.9	6
Ahn[1]	NT	68	91	7.4	0.4	8
*Amirfeyz et al.[3]	NT	83	98	41.5	0.17	7
*Hansen et al.[41]	NT	34	74	1.3	0.9	11
*Tetro et al.[86]	NT	61	83	3.6	0.5	9
*Gonzalez del Pino et al.[38]	NT	87	90	8.7	0.1	10
*de Krom et al.[22]	NT	49	48	0.9	1.1	10
*Mondelli et al.[64]	NT	59	93	8.4	0.4	8
LaJoie et al.[55]	NT	92	88	7.7	0.1	5
*Szabo et al.[84]	NT	75	95	15	0.3	9
*Gellman et al.[33]	NT	71	80	3.6	0.4	9
*Fertl et al.[29]	NT	79	92	9.9	0.2	13
*Durkan[24]	NT	70	84	4.4	0.4	7
Borg & Lindblom[12]	NT	83	67	2.5	0.3	7
Gunnarsson et al.[39]	NT	86	48	1.7	0.3	13

TESTS FOR CARPAL TUNNEL SYNDROME

Study	Reliability	Sensitivity	Specificity	LR+	LR−	QUADAS Score (0–14)
Williams et al.[95]	NT	88	100	NA	0.12	11
O'Gradaigh & Merry[67]	NT	72	53	1.5	0.5	8
*Yii & Elliot[96]	NT	87	93	12	0.1	8
*Wainner et al.[90]	0.79	77	40	1.29	0.58	12
*Boland & Kiernan[10]	NT	64	75	2.54	0.49	9
Cannon[18]	NT	NT	NA	NA	NA	NT
*Amirfeyz et al.[4]	NT	87	84	5.55	0.15	7
*Ansari et al.[6]	NT	NA	NA	NA	NA	9
Priganc & Henry[73]	0.58	NA	NA	NA	NA	11
*Bruske et al.[13]	NT	85	89	7.73	0.17	9
*Sawaya & Sakr[78]	NT	NA	NA	NA	NA	8

Comments: Phalen originally described this test for carpal tunnel syndrome in 1966. Some studies have varied this test to be performed by the patient with wrist in complete flexion and elbow extended, bilateral wrist flexion with the dorsal aspect of the hand pressing against one another, or passive wrist flexion by the examiner. However, there have been no studies to verify these alterations in wrist or elbow movement or studies that compare these alterations for the diagnostic accuracy of CTS. Priganc & Henry[73] examined the relationship between Phalen's test and severity of CTS. Sawaya & Sakr[78] found that Phalen's test was positive in 75% to 100% of moderate to severe cases of CTS. However, negative tests were found present in most mild cases of CTS.
*Indicates those studies using EMG/NCS as inclusion criteria.

Modified Phalen's Test

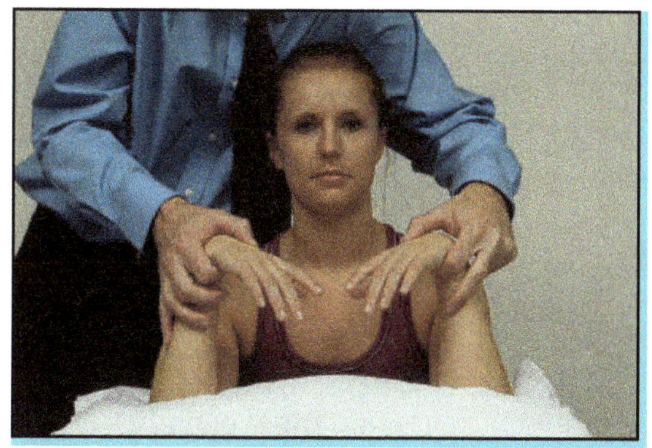

1) The patient rests both arms on a pillow or arm holder, with their hand floating at the end.

2) The examiner passively flexes the wrists up to 90 degrees.

3) A positive test is the reproduction of symptoms along the distribution of the median nerve.

UTILITY SCORE 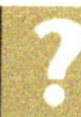

Study	Reliability	Sensitivity	Specificity	LR+	LR−	QUADAS Score (0–14)
Meek and Dellon[61]	NT	NT	NT	NA	NA	NA

Comments: No diagnostic accuracy studies have been performed to determine the sensitivity and specificity of this particular clinical test. This test differs from Phalen's original test by having the forearms vertical, rather than horizontal and the examiner performs the passive wrist flexion.

TESTS FOR CARPAL TUNNEL SYNDROME

Flick Maneuver

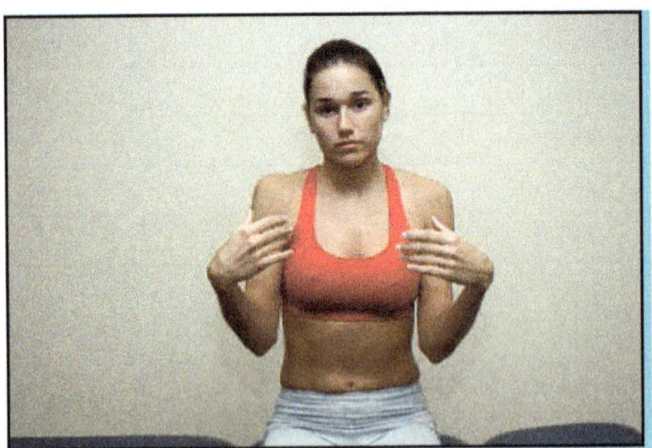

1) The patient vigorously shakes his or her hand(s).

2) A positive test is the resolution of paresthesia symptoms associated with carpal tunnel syndrome during or following administration of "flicking the wrist."

UTILITY SCORE 3

Study	Reliability	Sensitivity	Specificity	LR+	LR−	QUADAS Score (0–14)
*Hansen et al.[41]	NT	37	74	1.4	0.9	11
*Pryse-Phillips[74]	NT	93	96	23	0.1	6
*de Krom et al.[22]	NT	50	61	1.3	0.8	10
Gunnarsson et al.[39]	NT	90	30	1.3	0.3	13

Comments: These studies vary greatly in what constitutes a positive Flick Maneuver in the manner in which the data is collected. Some studies define a flick as a rapid, alternating movement up and down of the wrist, whereas others describe a positive flick with as little movement as elbow extension.
*Indicates those studies using EMG/NCS as inclusion criteria.

Percussion (Tinel's)

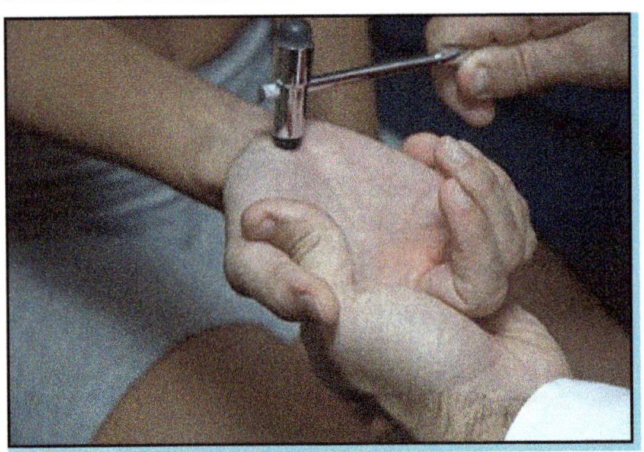

1) The patient's wrist is placed in a neutral position. The examiner uses his or her finger or a reflex hammer (pictured) to tap on the median nerve where it enters the carpal tunnel.

2) A positive test reproduces symptoms of paresthesia along the median nerve distribution.

TESTS FOR CARPAL TUNNEL SYNDROME

UTILITY SCORE 2

Study	Reliability	Sensitivity	Specificity	LR+	LR−	QUADAS Score (0–14)
*Gerr & Letz[35]	NT	25	67	0.7	1.1	12
Golding et al.[37]	NT	26	80	1.3	0.9	7
*Heller et al.[42]	NT	60	77	2.7	0.5	5
*Katz et al.[47]	NT	60	67	1.8	0.6	13
*Kuhlman & Hennessey[53]	NT	23	87	1.8	0.9	10
*Buch-Jaeger & Foucher[14]	NT	42	64	1.1	0.9	9
*Ahn[1]	NT	68	90	6.8	0.4	8
Amirfeyz et al.[3]	NT	48	94	8.0	0.6	7
*Hansen et al.[41]	NT	27	91	3.0	0.8	11
*Tetro et al.[86]	NT	74	91	8.2	0.3	9
**Gonzalez del Pino et al.[38]	NT	33	97	11	0.7	10
*de Krom et al.[22]	NT	35	53	0.7	1.2	10
*Mondelli et al.[64]	NT	41	90	4.1	0.7	8
LaJoie et al.[55]	NT	97	91	11	0.03	5
**Szabo et al.[84]	NT	64	99	64	0.4	9
*Gellman et al.[33]	NT	44	94	7.3	0.6	9
*MacDermid et al.[60]	0.81	59;41	92;94	7.4/ 6.8	0.5/ 0.6	9
*Seror[80]	NT	63	45	1.1	0.8	4
*Gunnarsson et al.[39]	NT	62	57	1.4	0.7	13
*Walters & Rice[92]	NT	64;57	40;31	1.1/ 0.8	0.9/ 1.4	9
*Durkan[24]	NT	56	80	2.8	0.6	7
*O'Gradaigh & Merry[67]	NT	55	72	2.0	0.6	8
Borg & Lindblom[12]	NT	64	62	1.7	0.6	7
*Gelmers[34]	NT	43	74	1.7	0.8	10
*Stewart & Eisen[82]	NT	40	71	1.4	0.8	8
*Mossman & Blau[66]	NT	79	NT	NA	NA	6
Williams et al.[95]	NT	67	100	NA	0.3	11
*Yii & Elliot[96]	NT	42	100	NA	0.6	8
*Wainner et al.[90]	0.47	41	58	0.98	1.01	12
*Cheng et al.[19]	NT	32	99	32	0.69	6
*Miedany et al.[62]	NT	30	65	0.86	1.08	9
*Amirfeyz et al.[4]	NT	53	93	7.45	0.51	7

(continued)

TESTS FOR CARPAL TUNNEL SYNDROME

Study	Reliability	Sensitivity	Specificity	LR+	LR−	QUADAS Score (0–14)
*Ansari et al.[6]	NT	NA	NA	NA	NA	9
Priganc & Henry[73]	0.51	NA	NA	NA	NA	11
*Bruske et al.[13]	NT	67	68	2.09	0.49	9

Comments: Variations exist between studies on the location and number of taps necessary to elicit a positive response. Some studies were performed by tapping the median nerve in 20 degrees of extension, others tapped along the path of the median nerve up to where the median nerve enters the carpal tunnel. In a few studies the examiners used a reflex hammer to tap rather than the examiner's finger. Gonzalez del Pino et al.[38] and Szabo et al.[84] used surgical outcomes as the reference standard. MacDermid et al.[60] calculated the sensitivity and specificity separately for two testers used in the reliability study. Walters & Rice[92] divided the sensitivity and specificity into groups of those patients with positive NCS for distal sensory latency and distal motor latency, respectively. This test is also referred to as the Nerve Percussion test. Priganc & Henry[73] examined the relationship between Tinel's test and severity of CTS.
*Indicates those studies using EMG/NCS as inclusion criteria.

Scratch Collapse Test

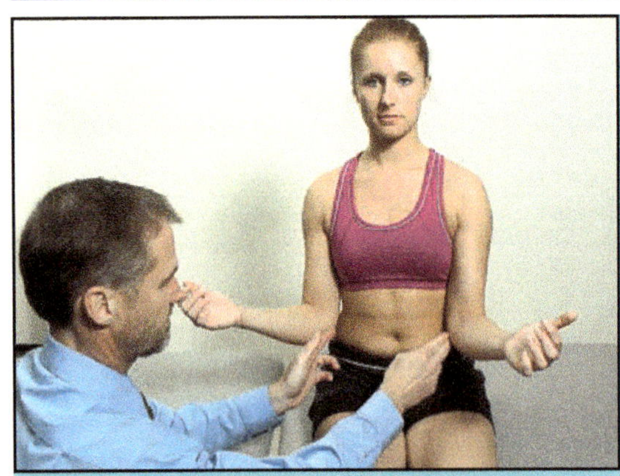

1) The patient faces the examiner with arms adducted, elbows flexed, and hands outstretched with wrists neutral.

2) The patient is asked to resist bilateral shoulder adduction/internal rotation to the forearms applied by the examiner.

3) The examiner "scratches" their fingertips over the ulnar nerve.

4) Step two is immediately repeated.

5) A positive test is brief temporary loss of the patient's external resistance tone.

UTILITY SCORE 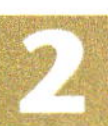

Study	Reliability	Sensitivity	Specificity	LR+	LR−	QUADAS Score (0–14)
Cheng et al.[19]	.98 (IRR) .18 (WF/NC)	64	99	64	0.32	6

Comments: Inter-rater reliability and correlation kappa values were reported, but only select values were reported. Cheng et al.[19] reported a kappa value of .98 when examining inter-rated reliability and .18 when examining the correlation between the scratch collapse and the wrist flexion/nerve compression tests.

TESTS FOR CARPAL TUNNEL SYNDROME

Wrist Flexion and Median Nerve Compression

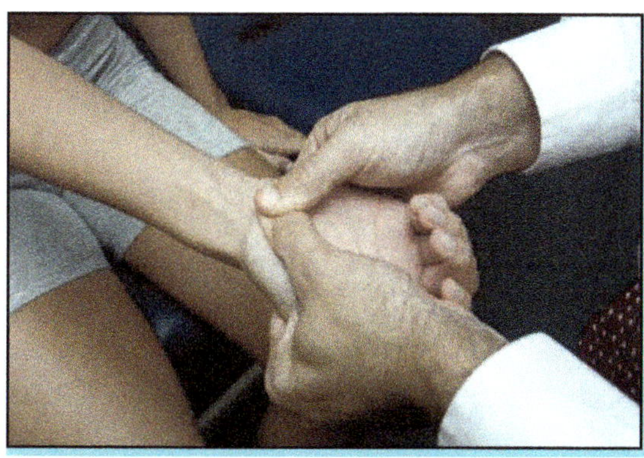

1) The patient sits with elbow fully extended, forearm in supination, and wrist flexed to 60 degrees. Even, constant pressure is applied by the examiner over the median nerve at the carpal tunnel.

2) A positive test is the reproduction of symptoms along the median nerve distribution within 30 seconds.

UTILITY SCORE 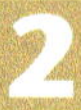

Study	Reliability	Sensitivity	Specificity	LR+	LR−	QUADAS Score (0–14)
*Tetro et al.[86]	NT	86	95	17	0.1	9
Edwards[26]	NT	62	92	7.8	0.4	4

Comments: Tetro et al.[86] originally performed this study to validate a new provocation test which involved wrist flexion and nerve compression. Edwards[26] studied a population of diabetic patients only without blinding. In addition, he used a reference standard of a questionnaire as inclusion criteria that would not accurately classify the target disorder.
*Indicates those studies using EMG/NCS as inclusion criteria.

Median Nerve Compression Test/Pressure Provocation Test

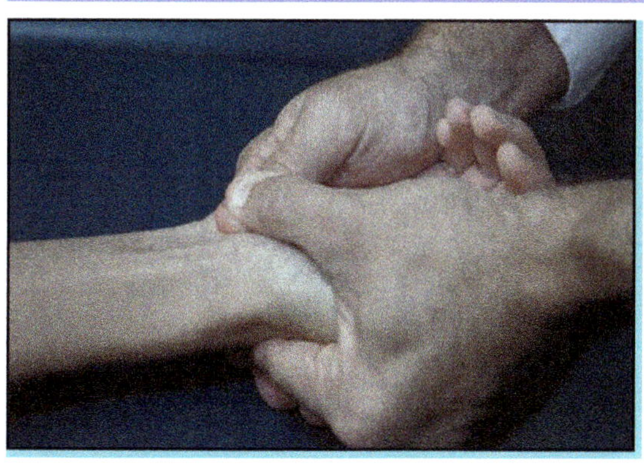

1) The examiner sits opposite the patient and holds the patient's hand with the examiner's thumbs directly over the course of the median nerve as it passes under the flexor retinaculum between the flexor carpi radialis and palmaris longus. The examiner places gentle sustained pressure with the thumbs for 15 seconds to 2 minutes.

2) The pressure of the examiner's thumbs is removed and the examiner questions the patient on the relief of symptoms, which may take a few minutes.

3) A positive test is the reproduction of pain, paresthesia, or numbness distal to the site of compression in the distribution of the median nerve.

(continued)

TESTS FOR CARPAL TUNNEL SYNDROME

UTILITY SCORE 1

Study	Reliability	Sensitivity	Specificity	LR+	LR−	QUADAS Score (0–14)
Paley & McMurtry[69]	NT	NT	NT	NA	NA	NT
*Williams et al.[95]	.92	100	97	33	0	11
*Mondelli et al.[64]	NT	42	99	42	0.6	8
*Kaul et al.[50]	NT	55	68	1.7	0.7	10
*Yii & Elliot[96]	NT	81	100	NA	0.2	8

Comments: This test differs from the carpal compression test in the location of pressure and in questioning the symptoms following the release of pressure.
*Indicates those studies using EMG/NCS as inclusion criteria.

Two-Point Discrimination

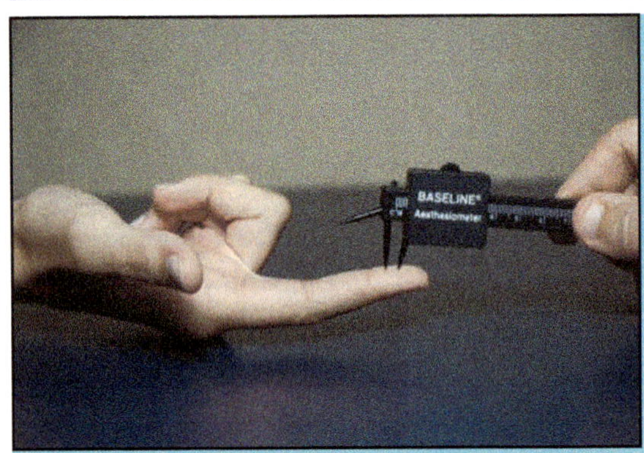

1. The examiner uses a two-point aesthesiometer on the index finger of the patient.
2. The smallest distance perceived as two separate points is recorded in millimeters.
3. A positive test is the inability of the patient to detect a distance of 6 mm or more.

UTILITY SCORE 

Study	Reliability	Sensitivity	Specificity	LR+	LR−	QUADAS Score (0–14)
*Buch-Jaeger & Foucher[14]	NT	06	99	6	0.9	9(Static)
*Katz et al.[47] (Moving)	NT	32	80	1.6	0.9	13
*Gerr & Letz[35] (Static)	NT	28	64	0.8	1.1	12
*Gellman et al.[33] (Static)	NT	33	100	NA	0.7	9
Patel & Bassini[70]	NT	30	92	3.8	0.8	3
*Szabo et al.[85] (Static)	NT	22	NT	NA	NA	NT
*Amirfeyz et al.[4]	NT	51	90	5.14	0.54	7

Comments: Moving two-point discrimination was performed by Katz et al.[47] with electrocardiograph calipers set at 4 mm apart. The index and fifth finger were stroked five times. A positive test was the inability to identify the number of points on two of the five strokes. Two-point discrimination appears to be a much more specific test that may be useful for ruling in CTS.
*Indicates those studies using EMG/NCS as inclusion criteria.

TESTS FOR CARPAL TUNNEL SYNDROME

Semmes-Weinstein Monofilament Test

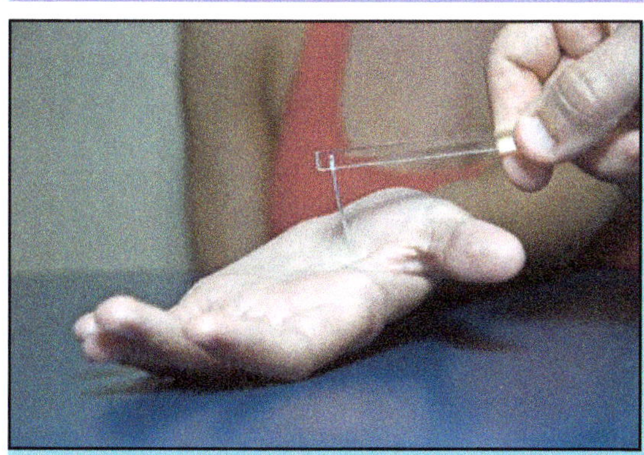

1) The examiner applies the monofilament perpendicular to the palmar digital surface and pressure is increased until the monofilament begins to bend.

2) A positive test is when the patient, with eyes closed, can verbally report which digit was receiving pressure at 2.83 milligrams.

UTILITY SCORE 

Study	Reliability	Sensitivity	Specificity	LR+	LR−	QUADAS Score (0–14)
*Buch-Jaeger & Foucher[14]	NT	59	59	1.4	0.7	9
*Szabo et al.[83]	NT	65	88	5.4	0.4	9
Pagel et al.[68]	NT	98	15	1.2	0.1	10
*Gellman et al.[33]	NT	91	80	4.6	0.1	9
*MacDermid et al.[60]	0.22	86/85	60/32	2.2/1.3	0.2/0.5	9
Patel & Bassini[70]	NT	71	40	1.2	0.7	3
*Koris et al.[52]	NT	82	86	5.9	0.2	11
*Szabo et al.[84]	NT	83	NT	NA	NA	NT
Borg & Lindblom[11]	NT	17	67	0.5	1.2	7
*Amirfeyz et al.[4]	NT	16	49	0.31	1.73	7

Comments: Koris et al.[52] assessed sensibility using Semmes-Weinstein Monofilament testing in combination with the wrist flexion test. Szabo et al.[83] also examined the combination of the wrist flexion test and Semmes-Weinstein Monofilament with similar results of sensitivity 83% and specificity 86%. MacDermid et al.[60] reported the diagnostic accuracy of both examiners used for the reliability studies.

*Indicates those studies using EMG/NCS as inclusion criteria.

Hypoesthesia

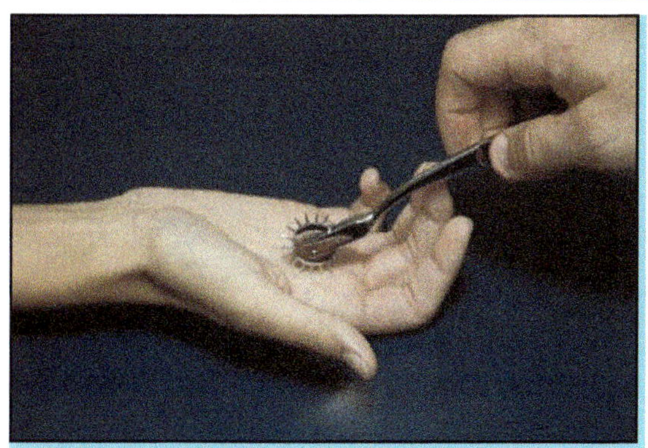

1) A pinwheel is rolled across the patient's hand in the distribution of the median nerve.

2) A positive test is the patient's ability to report a decrease in the ability to detect pain along the distribution of the median nerve.

(continued)

TESTS FOR CARPAL TUNNEL SYNDROME

UTILITY SCORE 2

Study	Reliability	Sensitivity	Specificity	LR+	LR−	QUADAS Score (0–14)
*de Krom et al.[22]	NT	46	48	0.9	1.1	10
*Kuhlman & Hennessey[53]	NT	51	85	3.4	0.6	10
*Golding et al.[37]	NT	15	93	2.1	0.9	7
Comments: * Indicates those studies using EMG/NCS as inclusion criteria.						

Therapeutic Ultrasound

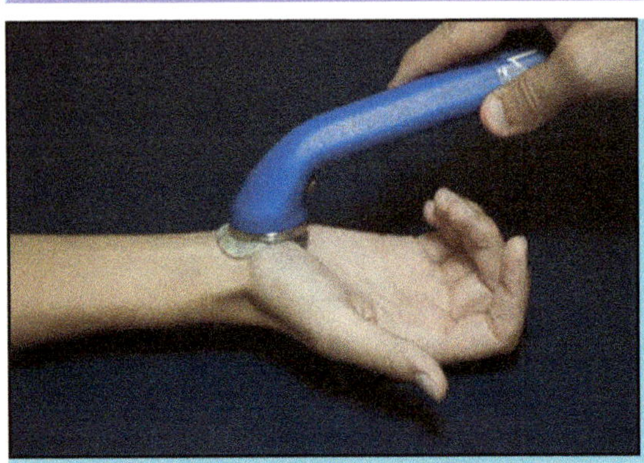

1. The examiner uses a 0.75 cm^2 sound head to apply 1 MHZ therapeutic ultrasound at intensity of 1.0 w/cm^2, 1.5 w/cm^2, and 2.0 w/cm^2 for a duration of 5 minutes.
2. The transducer is passed from the proximal wrist crease a distance of 5 cm distally in line with the ring finger in a slow movement.
3. A positive test is the experience of paresthesia, discomfort, or pain over the carpal tunnel or median nerve distribution.

UTILITY SCORE 

Study	Reliability	Sensitivity	Specificity	LR+	LR−	QUADAS Score (0–14)
Molitor[63]	NT	89	94	14	0.11	9
Comments: Several biases exist in this study including recruitment bias, as it is unclear how many male and female patients comprised the study group. In addition, the same examiner interpreted the reference and index test. This study has not been replicated for diagnostic accuracy.						

Hand Elevation Test

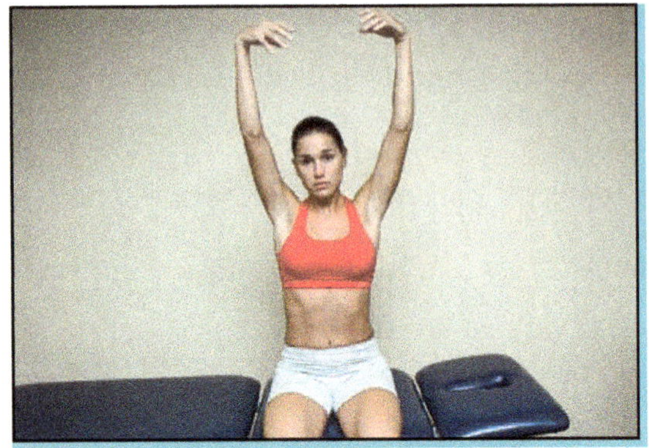

1. The patient raises both hands and maintains the position until the patient feels paresthesia or numbness in the distribution of the median nerve.
2. A positive test is the reproduction of symptoms such as tingling and numbness along the median nerve distribution after raising the arms for no greater than 2 minutes.

TESTS FOR CARPAL TUNNEL SYNDROME

UTILITY SCORE 2

Study	Reliability	Sensitivity	Specificity	LR+	LR−	QUADAS Score (0–14)
*Ahn[1]	NT	76	99	76	.24	8
Amirfeyz et al.[3]	NT	88	98	44	.12	7
*Amirfeyz et al.[4]	NT	99	91	11.47	0.02	7
Comments: Although this clinical test has high diagnostic values there are numerous procedural biases in both study designs. The test may be positive in patients with thoracic outlet syndrome. *Indicates those studies using EMG/NCS as inclusion criteria.						

Carpal Compression Test

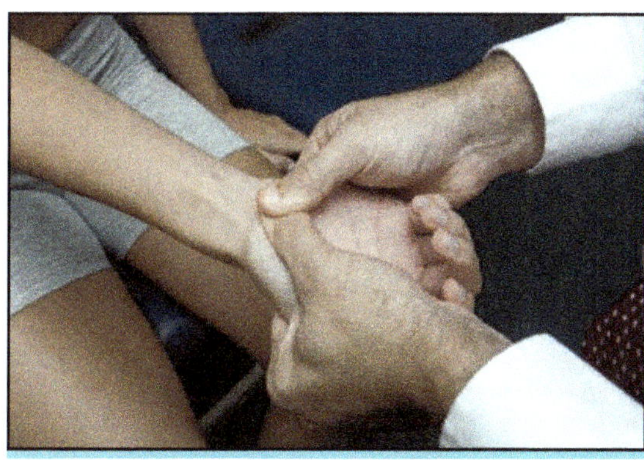

1) The examiner places even pressure with both thumbs directly over the patient's median nerve of the carpal tunnel for 30 seconds.

2) A positive test is the reproduction of pain, paresthesia, or numbness in the distribution of the median nerve distal to the carpal tunnel.

UTILITY SCORE 2

Study	Reliability	Sensitivity	Specificity	LR+	LR−	QUADAS Score (0–14)
*Kaul et al.[49]	NT	53	62	1.4	0.8	10
*Buch-Jaeger & Foucher[14]	NT	49	54	1.1	0.9	9
*Durkan[23]	NT	87	90	8.7	0.1	7
*Gonzalez del Pino et al.[38]	NT	87	95	17	0.1	10
**Szabo et al.[84]	NT	89	91	9.9	0.1	9
*Tetro et al.[86]	NT	82	99	11	0.3	9
*Fertl et al.[29]	NT	83	92	10	0.2	13
*Kuhlman & Hennessey[53]	NT	28	74	1.1	1.0	10
*Burke et al.[16]	NT	48	38	0.8	1.4	6
de Krom et al.[22]	NT	5	94	0.8	1.0	10
*Durkan[24]	NT	89	96	22	0.1	8
*Wainner et al.[90]	NT	36	57	0.8	1.1	11
*Wainner et al.[91]	0.77	64	30	0.9	1.2	12

(continued)

TESTS FOR CARPAL TUNNEL SYNDROME

Study	Reliability	Sensitivity	Specificity	LR+	LR−	QUADAS Score (0–14)
*Miedany et al.[62]	NT	46	25	0.61	2.16	9
*Amirfeyz et al.[4]	NT	84	79	3.94	0.20	7
*Tekeoglu et al.[85]	NT	82	98	41	0.18	8

Comments: There are some differences between studies in regard to time held for a positive test. Kuhlman & Hennessey[53] held this pressure for a total of 5 seconds. Tetro et al.[86] found the optimal cutoff to be 20 seconds of sustained pressure. Durkan[24] originally used a gauge to produce pressure over the median nerve at pressures of 11.94 pounds per square inch (psi) and 15.25 psi, as it was suggested that this would reproduce symptoms in patients with CTS.
*Indicates those studies using EMG/NCS as inclusion criteria.

Modified Carpal Compression Test

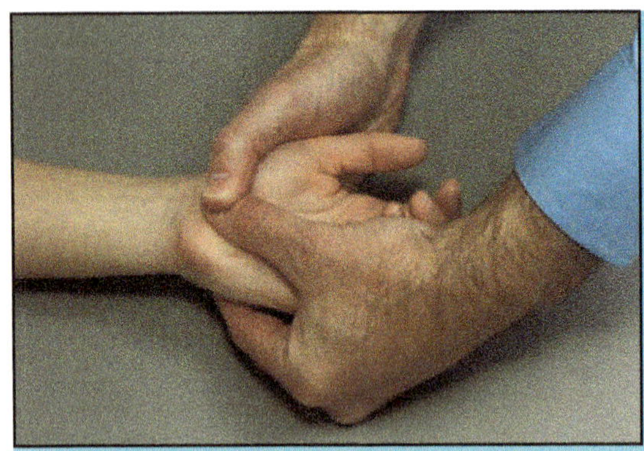

1) The patient is asked to rest both forearms, in supination, on a table with wrists in neutral alignment.

2) The examiner applies oscillary pressure over the palmar aspect of the carpal tunnel with adjacent thumbs.

3) A positive test is the reproduction of symptoms in the median distribution of the palmar hand within 5 seconds.

UTILITY SCORE 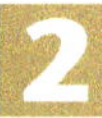

Study	Reliability	Sensitivity	Specificity	LR+	LR−	QUADAS Score (0–14)
*Boland & Kiernan[10]	NT	14	96	3.64	0.89	9
*Tekeoglu et al.[85]	NT	94	92	11.75	0.89	8
Priganc & Henry[73]	0.63	NA	NA	NA	NA	11

Comments: Priganc & Henry[73] examined the relationship between the modified carpal compression test and severity of CTS.
*Indicates those studies using EMG/NCS as inclusion criteria.

TESTS FOR CARPAL TUNNEL SYNDROME

Closed Fist/Lumbrical Provocation Test (Carpal Tunnel Syndrome from Lumbrical Excursion)

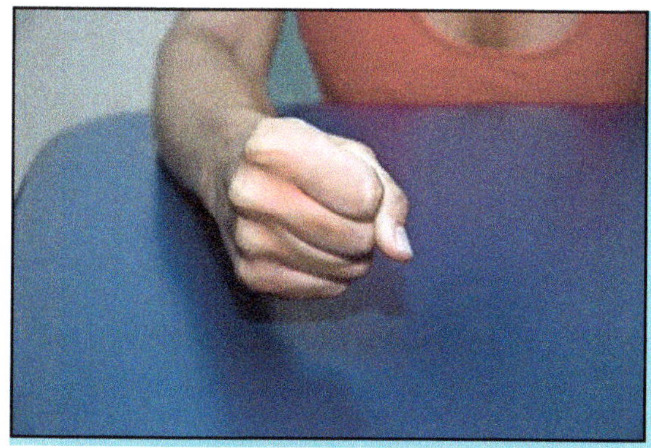

1) The patient is asked to make a fist for 1 minute.

2) A positive test is the reproduction of symptoms along the distribution of the median nerve.

UTILITY SCORE 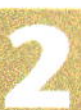

Study	Reliability	Sensitivity	Specificity	LR+	LR−	QUADAS Score (0–14)
*Karl et al.[46]	NT	37	71	1.3	0.9	8
*Yii & Elliot[96]	NT	97	93	14	0.03	7
Comments: Studies do not indicate the amount of force needed to reproduce the symptoms of CTS during administration of the test. This test is based on the possibility of excursion of the lumbricals into the carpal tunnel, which may increase tunnel pressures. *Indicates those studies using EMG/NCS as inclusion criteria.						

Wrist Extension (Reverse Phalen's)

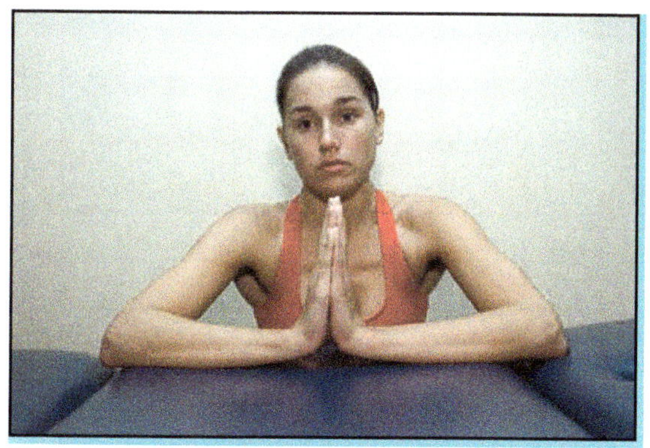

1) The patient is asked to keep both hands with the wrist in complete dorsal extension for 60 seconds.

2) A positive test is the reproduction of numbness or tingling in the distribution of the median nerve within 60 seconds.

(continued)

TESTS FOR CARPAL TUNNEL SYNDROME

UTILITY SCORE 3

Study	Reliability	Sensitivity	Specificity	LR+	LR−	QUADAS Score (0–14)
*Mondelli et al.[64]	NT	55	96	14	0.5	8
*MacDermid et al.[60]	0.72	65/75	96/85	16/5	0.4/0.3	9
*de Krom et al.[22]	NT	41	55	0.9	1.1	10
*Miedany et al.[62]	NT	42	35	0.65	1.66	9

Comments: One of several variations of the original wrist flexion test described by Phalen. MacDermid et al.[60] described the diagnostic accuracy of both examiners used in the reliability study.
*Indicates those studies using EMG/NCS as inclusion criteria.

Tethered Stress Test

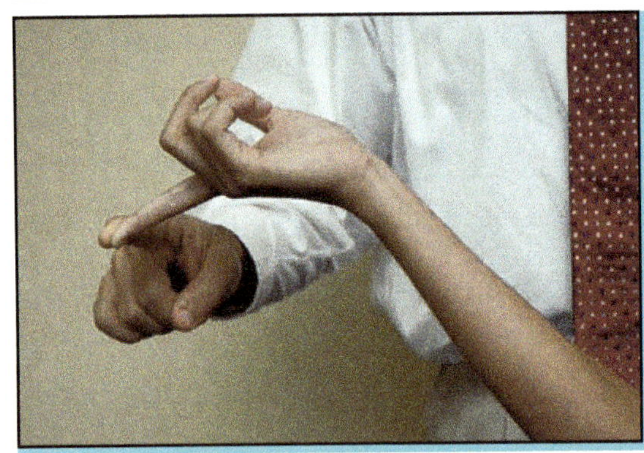

1) The examiner hyperextends the patient's supinated wrist by hyperextending the patient's index finger.

2) A positive test is the reproduction of dysesthesias in the hand with proximal radiation of pain to the volar forearm.

UTILITY SCORE 3

Study	Reliability	Sensitivity	Specificity	LR+	LR−	QUADAS Score (0–14)
*LaBan et al.[54]	NT	90	NT	NA	NA	NT
*Kaul et al.[49]	NT	50	51	1.0	1.0	11
*MacDermid et al.[60]	0.49	52/36	92/95	6.5/7.2	0.5/0.7	9

Comments: LaBan et al.[54] reported that extension of the index finger with a supinated wrist may produce greater excursion of the median nerve and be responsible for the symptoms. MacDermid et al.[60] provided the sensitivity and specificity for both examiners used in the reliability study.
*Indicates those studies using EMG/NCS as inclusion criteria.

TESTS FOR CARPAL TUNNEL SYNDROME

Gilliat Tourniquet Test

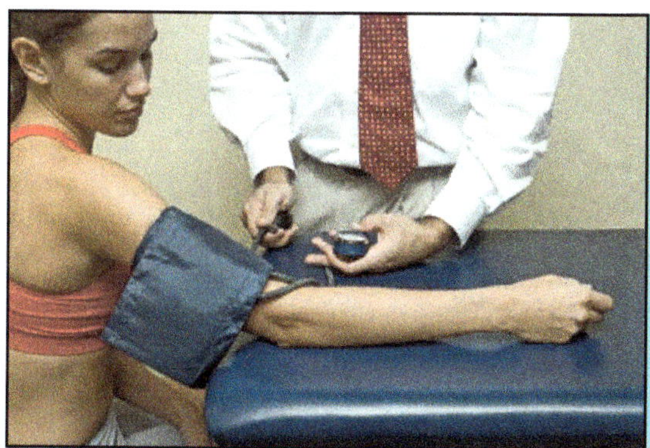

1) The examiner inflates a blood pressure cuff that has been placed over the patient's arm proximal to the elbow to a pressure above the patient's systolic pressure for 60 seconds.

2) A positive test is reproduction of paresthesia or numbness in the thumb or the index finger.

UTILITY SCORE 

Study	Reliability	Sensitivity	Specificity	LR+	LR−	QUADAS Score (0–14)
*Buch-Jaeger & Foucher[14]	NT	52	36	0.8	1.3	9
*Golding et al.[37]	NT	21	87	1.6	0.9	7
*de Krom et al.[22]	NT	44	62	1.2	0.9	10
*Gellman et al.[33]	NT	65	60	1.6	0.6	9
*Amirfeyz et al.[4]	NT	93	64	2.60	0.11	7

Comments: There is little diagnostic accuracy to support the use of this particular test.
*Indicates those studies using EMG/NCS as inclusion criteria.

Abnormal Vibration

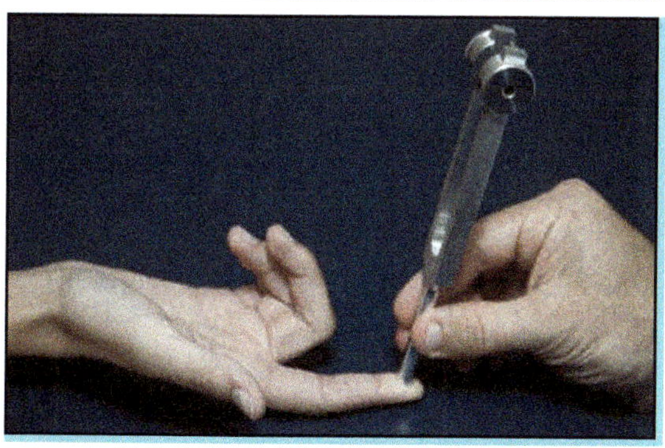

1) The test is performed utilizing a 256-cycle per second tuning fork struck against a firm object and then placed against the patient's fingertip.

2) Each digit is tested and compared to the contralateral limb.

3) A positive test is when perception to the stimulus was considered altered when the patient stated that the two stimuli felt different and could qualify the difference as being lesser or greater or some similar response.

(continued)

TESTS FOR CARPAL TUNNEL SYNDROME

UTILITY SCORE 3

Study	Reliability	Sensitivity	Specificity	LR+	LR−	QUADAS Score (0–14)
*Buch-Jaeger & Foucher[14]	NT	20	81	1.1	1.0	9
*MacDermid et al.[60]	0.71	77	80/72	3.9/2.8	0.3/0.3	9
*Szabo et al.[84]	NT	87	NT	NA	NA	NT
*Spindler & Dellon[81]	NT	78	NT	NA	NA	NT
*Cherniack et al.[20]	NT	21	85	1.4	0.9	10
*Borg & Lindblom[12]	NT	52	NT	NA	NA	NT
*Werner et al.[93]	NT	4	25	1	3.8	13
*Werner et al.[94]	NT	61	56	1.4	0.7	13
Gerr et al.[36]	NT	61	80	3.1	0.5	12
*Gerr & Letz[35]	NT	35	83	2.1	0.8	12

Comments: MacDermid et al.[60] calculated the sensitivity and specificity of both examiners used in determining the reliability. Werner et al.[93,94] used an electronic vibrometer in both studies in order to determine tolerance to vibration.
*Indicates those studies using EMG/NCS as inclusion criteria.

Abductor Pollicis Brevis Weakness

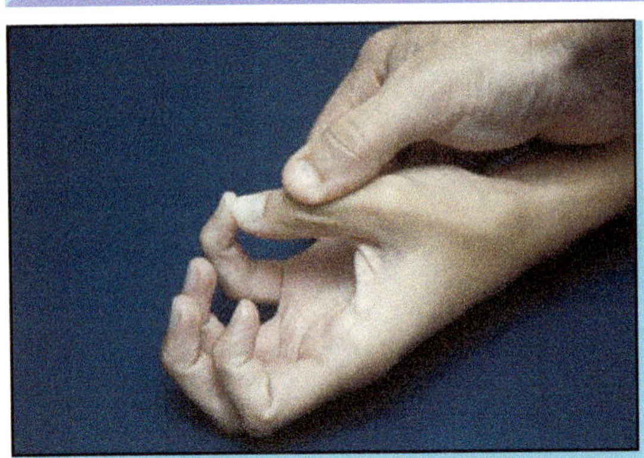

1) The examiner instructs the patient to touch the pads of the thumb and small finger together.

2) The examiner applies a strong force in order to resist thumb abduction and instructs the patient to keep the pads of the thumb and small finger together.

3) A positive test is weakness in thumb abduction with resisted testing.

UTILITY SCORE 3

Study	Reliability	Sensitivity	Specificity	LR+	LR−	QUADAS Score (0–14)
*de Krom et al.[22]	NT	63	41	1.1	0.9	10
*Gerr & Letz[35]	NT	63	62	1.7	0.6	12
*Kuhlman & Hennessey[53]	NT	66	66	2.0	0.5	10

Comments: Studies performed to determine weakness in the abductor pollicis brevis are relatively consistent, demonstrating moderate diagnostic accuracy.
*Indicates those studies using EMG/NCS as inclusion criteria.

TESTS FOR CARPAL TUNNEL SYNDROME

Nocturnal Paresthesia

1) The patient is asked if he or she experiences paresthesia which awakens him or her at night.

2) A positive test is the report of paresthesia along the median nerve distribution that awakens the patient at night.

UTILITY SCORE 3

Study	Reliability	Sensitivity	Specificity	LR+	LR−	QUADAS Score (0–14)
*Szabo et al.[84]	NT	96	100	NA	0.04	9
*Buch-Jaeger & Fouche[14]	NT	51	68	1.6	0.7	9
*Katz et al.[47]	NT	77	27	1.1	0.9	13
Gupta & Benstead[40]	NT	84	33	1.3	0.5	11

Comments: Gupta & Benstead[40] reported nocturnal pain rather than paresthesia, which was a sensitive test. Interestingly, the study design of those patients with "exclusive" carpal tunnel only reported nocturnal pain and no patients reported daytime pain. Although this is considered a classic symptom of CTS in isolation, it does appear to have significant diagnostic accuracy.
*Indicates those studies using EMG/NCS as inclusion criteria.

Wainner's Clinical Prediction Rule for Carpal Tunnel Syndrome

1) Five test variables are used to predict the presence of carpal tunnel syndrome.

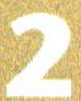

2) Two or more positive results are indicative of carpal tunnel syndrome.

UTILITY SCORE 2

Study	Reliability	Sensitivity	Specificity	LR+	LR−	QUADAS Score (0–14)
Wainner et al. 2 or greater[91]	NT	98	14	1.1	0.14	10
Wainner et al. 3 or greater[91]	NT	98	54	2.1	0.04	10
Wainner et al. 4 or greater[91]	NT	77	83	4.6	0.28	10
Wainner et al. all 5 positive[91]	NT	18	95	18.3	0.83	10

Comments: The five tests included: (1) Hand shaking does improve symptoms; (2) Wrist-ratio index > .67; (3) SSS score > 1.9; (4) Diminished sensation in median sensory field 1 (thumb); Age > 45 years.

TESTS FOR CARPAL TUNNEL SYNDROME

Hems' Questionnaire for Carpal Tunnel Syndrome

1) Examination by neurologist or standardized questionnaire to gather history of presenting symptoms prior to NCS.

2) A positive test is a score of 6 points or higher.

UTILITY SCORE 2

Study	Reliability	Sensitivity	Specificity	LR+	LR−	QUADAS Score (0–14)
Hems et al.[43] 6 or greater	NT	92	61	2.36	0.13	7
Hems et al.[43] 7 or greater	NT	82	67	2.48	0.27	7
Hems et al.[43] 8 or greater	NT	70	72	2.5	0.42	7
Hems et al.[43] 6 or greater symptoms	NT	71	61	1.82	0.48	7
Comments: Points are recorded as follows: (1) 2 pts.—Below 60 years old; (2) 2 pts.—Night pain; (3) 2 pts.—Paresthesia median nerve distribution; (4) 2 pts.—Relief of pain by hand shaking; (5) 1 pt.—Relief of pain by splint; (6) 1 pt.—Clumsiness; (7) 2 pts.—Positive Tinel's sign; (8) 1 pt.—Positive Phalen's test; (9) 2 pts.—Alteration in sensation in distribution of median nerve; (10) 2 pts.—Wasting thenar eminence.						

Purdue Pegboard Test

1) The patient is instructed to sit in front of a Purdue Pegboard, which consists of 50 holes arranged in two rows, with pegs, washers, and collars located across the top.

2) The patient has 30 seconds to fill the holes with pegs; first with their dominant hand, second with their non-dominant hand, and finally with both hands simultaneously.

3) The patient then has 1 minute to assemble in sequence a peg, washer, a collar, and another washer with alternating hands starting with the dominant hand first.

4) Each of the four subsets is completed three times each, and an average for each is obtained.

UTILITY SCORE ?

Study	Reliability	Sensitivity	Specificity	LR+	LR−	QUADAS Score (0–14)
Amirjani et al.[5]	ICC 0.97	NT	NT	NA	NA	6
Comments: There are currently no standards for a positive test result. Amirjani et al.[5] list several averages and common scores for those with and without CTS.						

Subjective Swelling

1) The patient is asked by the examiner if there is a feeling of swelling in the region of the carpal tunnel.

2) A positive test is the patient reporting symptoms of swelling in the region of the carpal tunnel.

UTILITY SCORE

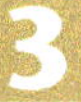

Study	Reliability	Sensitivity	Specificity	LR+	LR−	QUADAS Score (0–14)
Burke et al.[16]	NT	49	32	0.8	1.3	6
Comments: No studies have been performed to replicate this clinical diagnostic test.						

Key Points

1. Carpal tunnel syndrome has numerous diagnostic accuracy studies, in part due to the high incidence and prevalence in the general and industrial population.
2. Very few clinical tests for the wrist and hand have been assessed for reliability.
3. A gap in the literature of diagnostic accuracy appears to be the low number of studies to determine diagnostic accuracy of clinical testing of wrist instability.
4. There exists a significant range of sensitivity and specificity with traditional testing of CTS, which may be indicative of procedural biases that are present.
5. A true reference standard for classifying CTS does not exist. Nerve conduction studies are considered the reference standard for having a moderate sensitivity. However, studies have demonstrated as much as 18% of the control group having positive NCS.

References

1. Ahn DS. Hand elevation: a new test for carpal tunnel syndrome. *Ann Plast Surg.* 2001;46:120–124.
2. Alexander RD, Catalano LW, Barron OA, et al. The extensor pollicis brevis entrapment test in the treatment of de Quervain's disease. *J Hand Surg [Am].* 2002;27:813–816.
3. Amirfeyz R, Gozzard C, Leslie IJ. Hand elevation test for assessment of carpal tunnel syndrome. *J Hand Surg [Br].* 2005;30:361–364.
4. Amirfeyz R, Clark D, Parsons B, et al. Clinical tests for carpal tunnel syndrome in contemporary practice. *Arch Orthop Trauma Surg.* 2010:e-pub ahead of print.
5. Amirjani N, Ashworth NL, Olson JL, et al. Validity and reliability of the Purdue Pegboard test in carpal tunnel syndrome. *Muscle Nerve.* 2010;43:171–177.
6. Ansari NN, Adelmanesh F, Naghdi S, et al. The relationship between symptoms, clinical tests and nerve conduction study findings in carpal tunnel syndrome. *Electromyogr Clin Neurophysiol.* 2009;49:53–57.
7. Atroshi I, Breidenbach WC, McCabe SJ. Assessment of the carpal tunnel outcome instrument in patients with nerve-compression symptoms. *J Hand Surg [Am].* 1997;22:222–227.
8. Beighton PH, Solomon L, Soskolone CL. Articular mobility in an African population. *Am Rheum Dis.* 1973;32:413–418.
9. Bland JD. The value of the history in the diagnosis of carpal tunnel syndrome. *J Hand Surg [Br].* 2000; 25:445–450.
10. Boland RA, Kiernan MC. Assessing the accuracy of a combination of clinical tests for identifying

carpal tunnel syndrome. *J Clinical Neuroscience.* 2008;16:929–933.

11. Borg K, Lindblom U. Diagnostic value of quantitative sensory testing (QST) in carpal tunnel syndrome. *Acta Neurol Scand.* 1988;78:537–541.
12. Borg K, Lindblom U. Increase of vibration threshold during wrist flexion in patients with carpal tunnel syndrome. *Pain.* 1986;26:211–219.
13. Bruske J, Bednarski M, Grzelec H, et al. The usefulness of the Phalen test and the Hoffman-Tinel sign in the diagnosis of carpal tunnel syndrome. *Acta Ortho Belg.* 2002;68:141–144.
14. Buch-Jaeger N, Foucher G. Correlation of clinical signs with nerve conduction tests in the diagnosis of carpal tunnel syndrome. *J Hand Surg [Br].* 1994;19:720–724.
15. Buehler MJ, Thayer DT. The elbow flexion test. A clinical test for the cubital tunnel syndrome. *Clin Orthop Relat Res.* 1988:213–216.
16. Burke DT, Burke MA, Bell R, et al. Subjective swelling: a new sign for carpal tunnel syndrome. *Am J Phys Med Rehabil.* 1999;78:504–508.
17. Buterbaugh GA, Brown TR, Horn PC. Ulnar-sided wrist pain in athletes. *Clin Sports Med.* 1998;17:567–583.
18. Cannon J. Performing Tinel's test and Phalen's test. *Nursing.* 2009;39:16.
19. Cheng CJ, Mackinnon-Patterson B, Beck JL, et al. Scratch collapse test for evaluation of carpal and cubital tunnel syndrome. *J Hand Surg [Am].* 2008;33:1518–1524.
20. Cherniack MG, Moalli D, Viscolli C. A comparison of traditional electrodiagnostic studies, electroneurometry, and vibrometry in the diagnosis of carpal tunnel syndrome. *J Hand Surg [Am].* 1996;21:122–131.
21. Dawson C, Mudgal CS. Staged description of the Finkelstein test. *J Hand Surg.* 2010;35:1513–1515.
22. de Krom MC, Knipschild PG, Kester AD, et al. Efficacy of provocative tests for diagnosis of carpal tunnel syndrome. *Lancet.* 1990;335:393–395.
23. Durkan JA. The carpal-compression test: an instrumented device for diagnosing carpal tunnel syndrome. *Orthop Rev.* 1994;23:522–525.
24. Durkan JA. A new diagnostic test for carpal tunnel syndrome. *J Bone Joint Surg Am.* 1991;73:535–538.
25. Easterling KJ, Wolfe SW. Scaphoid shift in the uninjured wrist. *J Hand Surg [Am].* 1994;19:604–606.
26. Edwards A. Phalen's test with carpal compression: testing in diabetics for the diagnosis of carpal tunnel syndrome. *Orthopedics.* 2002;25:519–520.
27. Elson RA. Rupture of the central slip of the extensor hood of the finger: a test for early diagnosis. *J Bone Joint Surg Br.* 1986;68:229–231.
28. Esberger DA. What value the scaphoid compression test? *J Hand Surg [Br].* 1994;19:748–749.
29. Fertl E, Wober C, Zeitlhofer J. The serial use of two provocative tests in the clinical diagnosis of carpal tunnel syndrome. *Acta Neurol Scand.* 1998;98:328–332.
30. Finkelstein H. Stenosing tenovaginitis at the radial styloid process. *J Bone Joint Surg.* 1930; 12:509–540.
31. Freeland P. Scaphoid tubercle tenderness: a better indicator of scaphoid fractures? *Arch Emerg Med.* 1989;6:46–50.
32. Forman TA, Forman SK, Rose NE. A clinical approach to diagnosing wrist pain. *Am Fam Physician.* 2005;72: 1753–1758.
33. Gellman H, Gelberman RH, Tan AM, et al. Carpal tunnel syndrome: an evaluation of the provocative diagnostic tests. *J Bone Joint Surg Am.* 1986;68:735–737.
34. Gelmers HJ. The significance of Tinel's sign in the diagnosis of carpal tunnel syndrome. *Acta Neurochir (Wien).* 1979;49:255–258.
35. Gerr F, Letz R. The sensitivity and specificity of tests for carpal tunnel syndrome vary with the comparison subjects. *J Hand Surg [Br].* 1998;23:151–155.
36. Gerr F, Letz R, Harris-Abbott D, et al. Sensitivity and specificity of vibrometry for detection of carpal tunnel syndrome. *J Occup Environ Med.* 1995;37:1108–1115.
37. Golding DN, Rose DM, Selvarajah K. Clinical tests for carpal tunnel syndrome: an evaluation. *Br J Rheumatol.* 1986;25:388–390.
38. Gonzalez del Pino J, Delgado-Martinez AD, Gonzalez I, Lovic A. Value of the carpal compression test in the diagnosis of carpal tunnel syndrome. *J Hand Surg [Br].* 1997;22:38–41.
39. Gunnarsson LG, Amilon A, Hellstrand P, et al. The diagnosis of carpal tunnel syndrome: sensitivity and specificity of some clinical and electrophysiological tests. *J Hand Surg [Br].* 1997;22:34–37.
40. Gupta SK, Benstead TJ. Symptoms experienced by patients with carpal tunnel syndrome. *Can J Neurol Sci.* 1997;24:338–342.
41. Hansen PA, Micklesen P, Robinson LR. Clinical utility of the flick maneuver in diagnosing carpal tunnel syndrome. *Am J Phys Med Rehabil.* 2004;83:363–367.
42. Heller L, Ring H, Costeff H, et al. Evaluation of Tinel's and Phalen's signs in diagnosis of the carpal tunnel syndrome. *Eur Neurol.* 1986;25:40–42.
43. Hems TEJ, Miller R, Massraf A, et al. Assessment of a diagnostic questionnaire and protocol for management of carpal tunnel syndrome. *J Hand Surg [Br].* 2009;34:665–670.
44. Heyman P, Gelberman RH, Duncan K, et al. Injuries of the ulnar collateral ligament of the thumb metacarpal-phalangeal joint. Biomechanical and prospective clinical studies on the usefulness of valgus stress testing. *Clin Orthop Relat Res.* 1993:165–171.
45. Johnson RP, Carrera GF. Chronic capitolunate instability. *J Bone Joint Surg Am.* 1986;68:1164–1176.
46. Karl AI, Carney ML, Kaul MP. The lumbrical provocation test in subjects with median inclusive paresthesia. *Arch Phys Med Rehabil.* 2001;82:935–937.
47. Katz JN, Larson MG, Sabra A, et al. The carpal tunnel syndrome: diagnostic utility of the history and

physical examination findings. *Ann Intern Med.* 1990;112:321–327.

48. Katz JN, Stirrat CR. A self-administered hand diagram for the diagnosis of carpal tunnel syndrome. *J Hand Surg [Am].* 1990;15:360–363.

49. Kaul MP, Pagel KJ, Dryden JD. Lack of predictive power of the "tethered" median stress test in suspected carpal tunnel syndrome. *Arch Phys Med Rehabil.* 2000;81:348–350.

50. Kaul MP, Pagel KJ, Wheatley MJ, et al. Carpal compression test and pressure provocative test in veterans with median-distribution paresthesias. *Muscle Nerve.* 2001;24:107–111.

51. Kim JP, Park MJ. Assessment of distal radioulnar joint instability after distal radius fracture: comparison of computed tomography and clinical examination results. *J Hand Surg [Am].* 2008;33:1486–1492.

52. Koris M, Gelberman RH, Duncan K, et al. Carpal tunnel syndrome. Evaluation of a quantitative provocational diagnostic test. *Clin Orthop Relat Res.* 1990:157–161.

53. Kuhlman KA, Hennessey WJ. Sensitivity and specificity of carpal tunnel syndrome signs. *Am J Phys Med Rehabil.* 1997;76:451–457.

54. LaBan MM, Friedman NA, Zemenick GA. "Tethered" median nerve stress test in chronic carpal tunnel syndrome. *Arch Phys Med Rehabil.* 1986;67:803–804.

55. LaJoie AS, McCabe SJ, Thomas B, et al. Determining the sensitivity and specificity of common diagnostic tests for carpal tunnel syndrome using latent class analysis. *Plast Reconstr Surg.* 2005;116:502–507.

56. Lane LB. The scaphoid shift test. *J Hand Surg [Am].* 1993;18:366–368.

57. LaStayo P, Howell J. Clinical provocative tests used in evaluating wrist pain: a descriptive study. *J Hand Ther.* 1995;8:10–17.

58. Lester B, Halbrecht J, Levy IM, et al. "Press test" for office diagnosis of triangular fibrocartilage complex tears of the wrist. *Ann Plast Surg.* 1995;35:41–45.

59. Lim PG, Tan S, Sara Ahmad T. The role of wrist anthropometric measurement in idiopathic carpal tunnel syndrome. *J Hand Surg [Br].* 2008;33:645–647.

60. MacDermid JC, Kramer JF, Roth JH. Decision making in detecting abnormal Semmes-Weinstein monofilament thresholds in carpal tunnel syndrome. *J Hand Ther.* 1994;7:158–162.

61. Meek MF, Dellon AL. Modification of Phalen's wrist-flexion test. *J Neuro Methods.* 2008;170:156–157.

62. Miedany YE, Samia A, Youssef S, et al. Clinical diagnosis of carpal tunnel syndrome: old tests—new concepts. *Joint Bone Spine.* 2008;75:451–457.

63. Molitor PJ. A diagnostic test for carpal tunnel syndrome using ultrasound. *J Hand Surg [Br].* 1988;13:40–41.

64. Mondelli M, Passero S, Giannini F. Provocative tests in different stages of carpal tunnel syndrome. *Clin Neurol Neurosurg.* 2001;103:178–183.

65. Moriya T, Aoki M, Iba K, et al. Effects of triangular ligament tears on distal radioulnar joint instability and evaluation of three clinical tests: a biomechanical study. *J Hand Surg [Br].* 2009;34:219–223.

66. Mossman SS, Blau JN. Tinel's sign and the carpal tunnel syndrome. *Br Med J (Clin Res Ed).* 1987;294:680.

67. O'Gradaigh D, Merry P. A diagnostic algorithm for carpal tunnel syndrome based on Bayes's theorem. *Rheumatology (Oxford).* 2000;39:1040–1041.

68. Pagel KJ, Kaul MP, Dryden JD. Lack of utility of Semmes-Weinstein monofilament testing in suspected carpal tunnel syndrome. *Am J Phys Med Rehabil.* 2002;81:597–600.

69. Paley D, McMurtry R. Median nerve compression test in carpal tunnel syndrome diagnosis: reproduces signs and symptoms in affected wrist. *Orthop Rev.* 1985;14:41–45.

70. Patel MR, Bassini L. A comparison of five tests for determining hand sensibility. *J Reconstr Microsurg.* 1999;15:523–526.

71. Phalen GS. The carpal-tunnel syndrome: seventeen years' experience in diagnosis and treatment of six hundred fifty-four hands. *J Bone Joint Surg Am.* 1966;48:211–228.

72. Phillips GT, Reibach AM, Slomiany WP. Diagnosis and management of scaphoid fractures. *Am Fam Physician.* 2004;70:879–884.

73. Priganc VW, Henry SM. The relationship among five common carpal tunnel syndrome tests and the severity of carpal tunnel syndrome. *J Hand Ther.* 2003;16:225–236.

74. Pryse-Phillips WE. Validation of a diagnostic sign in carpal tunnel syndrome. *J Neurol Neurosurg Psychiatry.* 1984;47:870–872.

75. Radecki P. A gender specific wrist ratio and the likelihood of a median nerve abnormality at the carpal tunnel. *Am J Phys Med Rehabil.* 1994;73:157–162.

76. Reagan DS, Linscheid RL, Dobyns JH. Lunotriquetral sprains. *J Hand Surg [Am].* 1984;9:502–514.

77. Ruland RT, Dunbar RP, Bowen JD. The biceps squeeze test for diagnosis of distal biceps tendon ruptures. *Clin Orthop Relat Res.* 2005:128–131.

78. Sawaya RA, Sakr C. When is the Phalen's test of diagnostic value: An electrophysiologic analysis. *J Clin Neurophys.* 2009;26:132–133.

79. Seror P. Phalen's test in the diagnosis of carpal tunnel syndrome. *J Hand Surg [Br].* 1988;13:383–385.

80. Seror P. Tinel's sign in the diagnosis of carpal tunnel syndrome. *J Hand Surg [Br].* 1987;12:364–365.

81. Spindler HA, Dellon AL. Nerve conduction studies and sensibility testing in carpal tunnel syndrome. *J Hand Surg [Am].* 1982;7:260–263.

82. Stewart JD, Eisen A. Tinel's sign and the carpal tunnel syndrome. *Br Med J.* 1978;2:1125–1126.

83. Szabo RM, Gelberman RH, Dimick MP. Sensibility testing in patients with carpal tunnel syndrome. *J Bone Joint Surg Am.* 1984;66:60–64.

84. Szabo RM, Slater RR, Jr., Farver TB, et al. The value of diagnostic testing in carpal tunnel syndrome. *J Hand Surg [Am]*. 1999;24:704–714.

85. Tekeoglu I, Dogan A, Demir G, et al. The pneumatic compression test and modified pneumatic compression test in the diagnosis of carpal tunnel syndrome. *J Hand Surg [Br]*. 2007;32:697–699.

86. Tetro AM, Evanoff BA, Hollstien SB, et al. A new provocative test for carpal tunnel syndrome: assessment of wrist flexion and nerve compression. *J Bone Joint Surg Br.* 1998;80:493–498.

87. Truong NP, Mann FA, Gilula LA, et al. Wrist instability series: increased yield with clinical-radiologic screening criteria. *Radiology.* 1994;192:481–484.

88. Unay K, Gokcen B, Ozkan K, et al. Examination tests predictive of bone injury in patients with clinically suspected occult scaphoid fracture. *Injury.* 2009; 40:1265–1268.

89. van Andel CJ, Roescher WBM, Tromp MF, et al. Quantification of wrist joint laxity. *J Hand Surg [Am]*. 2008;33: 667–674.

90. Wainner RS, Boninger ML, Balu G, et al. Durkan gauge and carpal compression test: accuracy and diagnostic test properties. *J Orthop Sports Phys Ther.* 2000; 30:676–682.

91. Wainner RS, Fritz JM, Irrgang JJ, et al. Development of a clinical prediction rule for the diagnosis of carpal tunnel syndrome. *Arch Phys Med Rehabil.* 2005;86:609–618.

92. Walters C, Rice V. An evaluation of provocative testing in the diagnosis of carpal tunnel syndrome. *Mil Med.* 2002;167:647–652.

93. Werner RA, Franzblau A, Johnston E. Comparison of multiple frequency vibrometry testing and sensory nerve conduction measures in screening for carpal tunnel syndrome in an industrial setting. *Am J Phys Med Rehabil.* 1995;74:101–106.

94. Werner RA, Franzblau A, Johnston E. Quantitative vibrometry and electrophysiological assessment in screening for carpal tunnel syndrome among industrial workers: a comparison. *Arch Phys Med Rehabil.* 1994;75:1228–1232.

95. Williams TM, Mackinnon SE, Novak CB, et al. Verification of the pressure provocative test in carpal tunnel syndrome. *Ann Plast Surg.* 1992;29:8–11.

96. Yii NW, Elliot D. A study of the dynamic relationship of the lumbrical muscles and the carpal tunnel. *J Hand Surg [Br]*. 1994;19:439–443.

PEARSON **myhealthprofessionskit**™

Use this address to access the Companion Website created for this textbook. Simply select "Physical Therapy" from the choice of disciplines. Find this book and log in using your username and password to access video clips of selected tests.

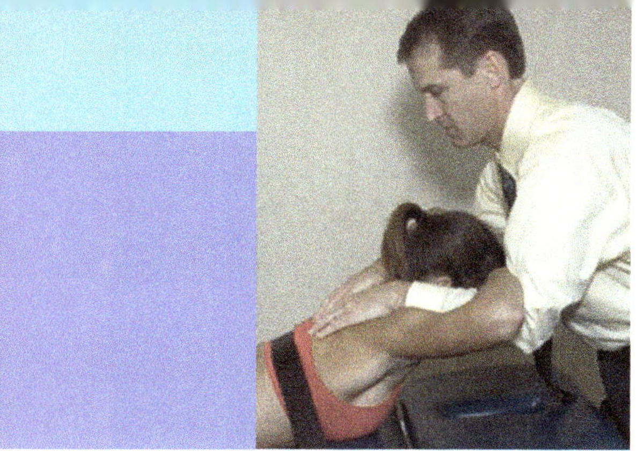

Physical Examination Tests for the Thoracic Spine

Chad E. Cook

Please refer to the chapter "Introduction to Diagnostic Accuracy" before reading this chapter.

Index of Tests

Tests for Thoracic Outlet Syndrome

Hyperabduction Test
Roos Test
Wright Test
Morley's Sign
Supraclavicular Pressure Test
Adson's Test
Cyriax Release Test
Tinel's Sign
Costoclavicular Maneuver
Gillard's Cluster for Thoracic Outlet Syndrome

Tests for Restricted First Rib

Cervical Rotation Lateral Flexion Test (Associated with Brachialgia)
First Rib Spring Test

Test for Scoliosis

Adam's Forward Flexion Test

Test to Identify a Thoracic Compression Fracture

Historical Height Loss Assessment

Test to Determine Potential of Mobility Change in the Thoracic Spine

Structural versus Flexible Kyphosis Test

Test to Determine Disc Involvement or Sympathetic Nervous System Involvement

Thoracic Slump Test (Sympathetic Slump Test)

TESTS FOR THORACIC OUTLET SYNDROME

Hyperabduction Test

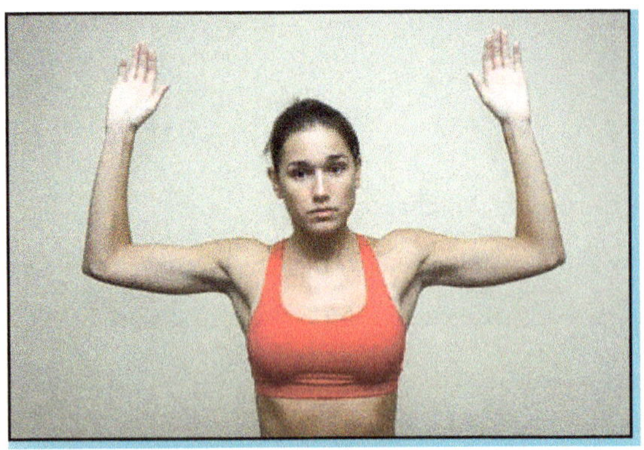

1. The patient sits very straight. Both arms are placed at the sides. The examiner assesses the radial pulse in this position.

2. The patient is instructed to place the arms above 90 degrees of abduction and in full external rotation. The head maintains a neutral position. The arms are held in this position for a full minute.

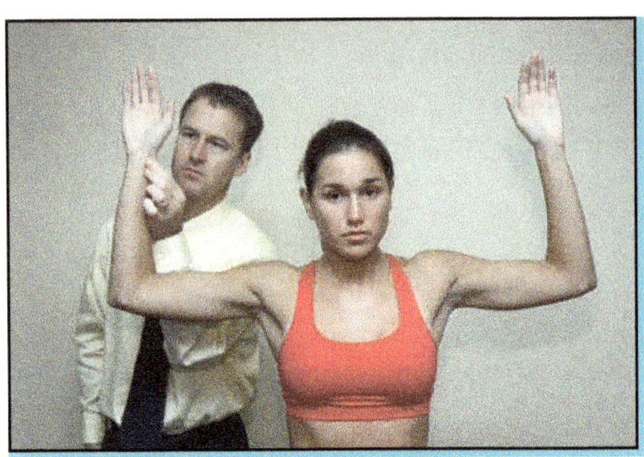

3. The examiner palpates the radial pulse in the hyper-abducted position.

4. The radial pulse is recorded as no change, diminished, or occluded. The patient is also queried for paresthesia.

5. A positive test is change in radial pulse and patient report of paresthesia.

UTILITY SCORE 

Study	Reliability	Sensitivity	Specificity	LR+	LR−	QUADAS Score (0–14)
Rayan & Jensen[12] (Vascular Changes)	NT	NT	43	NA	NA	3
Rayan & Jensen[12] (Paresthesia)	NT	NT	90	NA	NA	3
Plewa & Delinger[11] (Vascular Changes)	NT	NT	38	NA	NA	9
Plewa & Delinger[11] (Pain)	NT	NT	79	NA	NA	9
Plewa & Delinger[11] (Paresthesia)	NT	NT	64	NA	NA	9
Gillard et al.[4] (Pulse Abolition)	NT	52	90	5.2	0.53	8
Gillard et al.[4] (Symptom Reproduction)	NT	84	40	1.4	0.4	8

Comments: The test is also known as the elevated arm stress test (ESRT). Some texts have promoted the use of 2-minute holds. Because thoracic outlet syndrome is a controversial diagnosis, most tests examine specificity only.

TESTS FOR THORACIC OUTLET SYNDROME

Roos Test

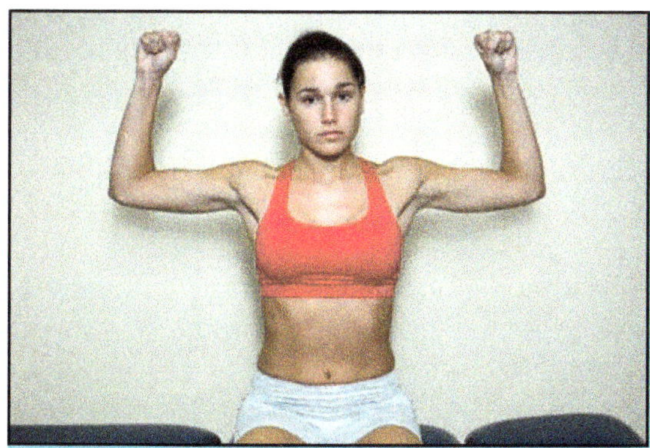

1. The patient sits straight with the arms at the side of his or her body.
2. The patient is instructed to abduct his or her arms and externally rotate to 90 degrees. The patient is then instructed to rapidly open and close his or her hands.
3. The activity is performed for a full minute.
4. A positive test is reproduction of concordant symptoms during opening and closing the fists.

UTILITY SCORE 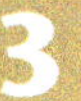

Study	Reliability	Sensitivity	Specificity	LR+	LR−	QUADAS Score (0–14)
Howard et al.[5]	NT	82	100	NA	NA	5
Nord et al.[10]	NT	NT	47	NA	NA	6
Gillard et al.[4]	NT	84	30	1.2	0.53	8

Comments: Some have suggested pumping the hands for 2 minutes. It is likely that this test leads to a high amount of false positives. Note the very poor QUADAS score, suggesting bias.

Wright Test

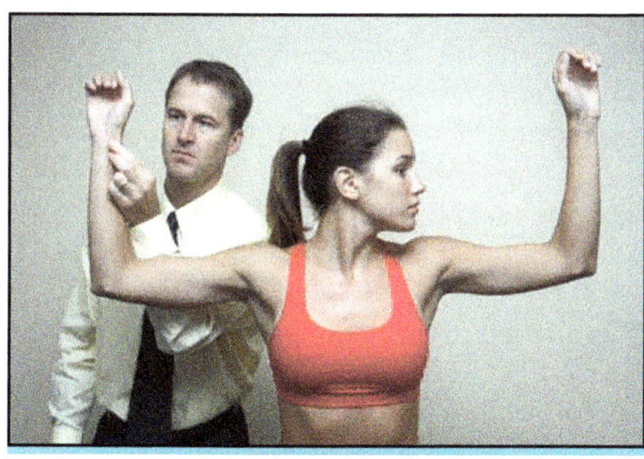

1. The patient assumes a sitting position. The examiner palpates the radial pulse.
2. The patient is instructed to hyperabduct his or her shoulders and flex his or her elbows to 90 degrees. The head should be turned toward the unaffected side.
3. The position is held for 1 to 2 minutes.
4. A positive test includes reproduction of paresthesia or a decrease in the radial pulse.

UTILITY SCORE 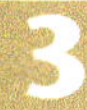

Study	Reliability	Sensitivity	Specificity	LR+	LR−	QUADAS Score (0–14)
Gillard et al.[4] (pulse abolition)	NT	70	53	1.5	0.56	8
Gillard et al.[4] (symptom reproduction)	NT	90	29	1.3	0.34	8

Comments: The study was fairly well designed. There does not seem to be overwhelming value in the use of Wright's test.

TESTS FOR THORACIC OUTLET SYNDROME

Morley's Sign

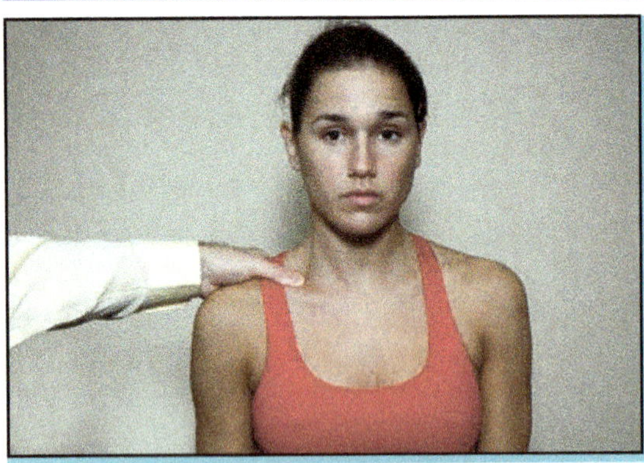

1) The patient sits straight with the arms at the side of his or her body.

2) The examiner palpates the supraclavicular fossa with his or her thumb.

3) Tenderness in the supraclavicular fossa is considered a positive finding for thoracic outlet syndrome.

UTILITY SCORE 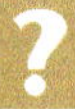

Study	Reliability	Sensitivity	Specificity	LR+	LR−	QUADAS Score (0–14)
Matsuyama et al.[9]	NT	NT	NT	NA	NA	NT
Comments: This test will likely also be painful for patients with cervical radiculopathy. To increase the specificity, referral of symptoms along the lower brachial plexus should be targeted.						

Supraclavicular Pressure Test

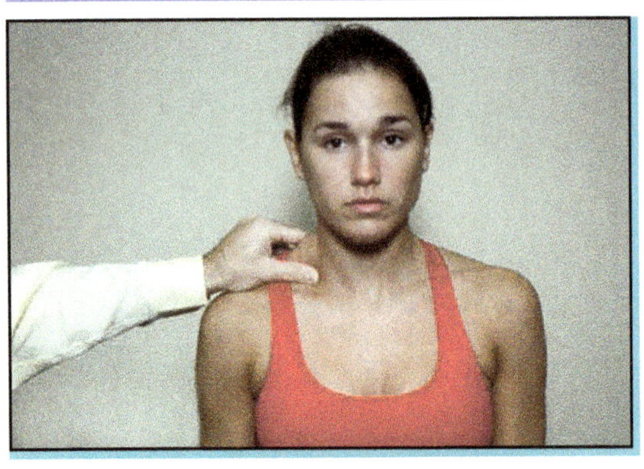

1) The patient sits straight with the arms at the sides.

2) The examiner places his or her fingers on the upper trapezius and the thumbs contacting the lowest portion of the anterior scalene muscle near the first ribs.

3) The examiner squeezes the fingers and thumbs together for 30 seconds.

4) The patient is queried for changes in paresthesia.

5) A positive test is a report of paresthesia by the patient.

TESTS FOR THORACIC OUTLET SYNDROME

UTILITY SCORE 

Study	Reliability	Sensitivity	Specificity	LR+	LR−	QUADAS Score (0–14)
Plewa & Delinger[11] (vascular changes)	NT	NT	79	NA	NA	9
Plewa & Delinger[11] (pain)	NT	NT	98	NA	NA	9
Plewa & Delinger[11] (paresthesia)	NT	NT	85	NA	NA	9
Nord et al.[10]	NT	NT	56	NA	NA	6
Comments: The test differs from Morley's sign only in the compression of both thumb and forefinger. This test will likely also be painful for patients with cervical radiculopathy.						

Adson's Test

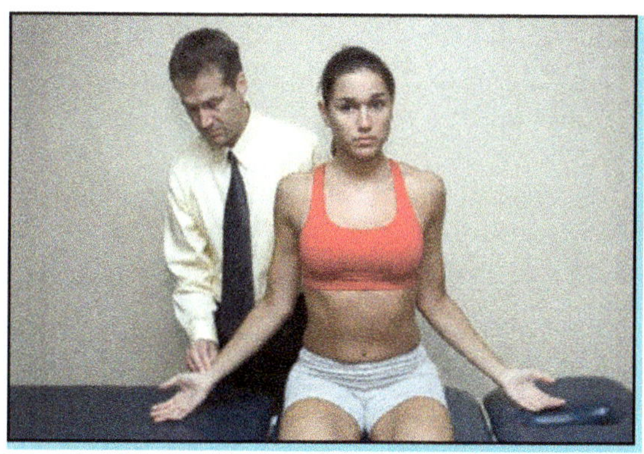

1) The patient sits straight with the arms placed at 15 degrees of abduction. The radial pulse is palpated.

2) The patient is instructed to inhale deeply, hold his or her breath, tilt the head back, and rotate the head, so that the chin is elevated and pointed toward the examined side.

3) The examiner records the radial pulse as diminished or occluded and queries the patient for paresthesia.

4) A positive test is a change in radial pulse and patient report of paresthesia.

UTILITY SCORE 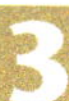

Study	Reliability	Sensitivity	Specificity	LR+	LR−	QUADAS Score (0–14)
Rayan & Jensen[12] (vascular changes)	NT	NT	87	NA	NA	3
Rayan & Jensen[12] (paresthesia)	NT	NT	74	NA	NA	3
Plewa & Delinger[11] (vascular changes)	NT	NT	89	NA	NA	9
Plewa & Delinger[11] (pain)	NT	NT	100	NA	NA	9
Plewa & Delinger[11] (paresthesia)	NT	NT	89	NA	NA	9
Lee et al.[6]	NT	50	NT	NA	NA	4
Gillard et al.[4]	NT	79	76	3.3	0.27	8
Nord et al.[10]	NT	NT	16–20	NA	NA	6
Comments: Lee et al.[6] used Doppler imaging to classify a positive test. Because vascular problems associated with thoracic outlet are less prevalent, it is likely that neurological changes will be missed using this test.						

TESTS FOR THORACIC OUTLET SYNDROME

Cyriax Release Test

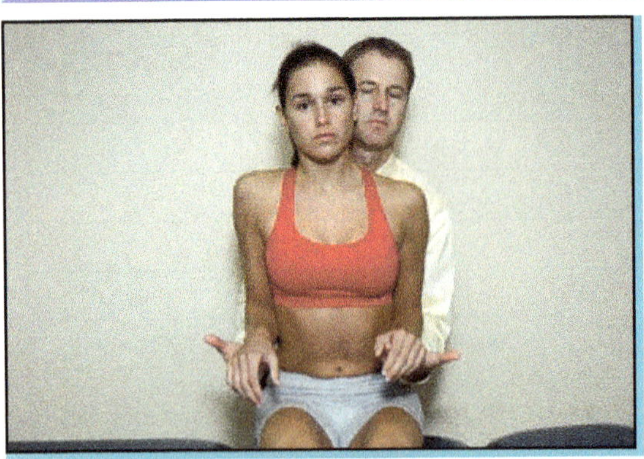

1. The patient assumes either a sitting or standing position.
2. The examiner stands behind the patient and grasps under the forearms holding the elbows at approximately 80–90 degrees while maintaining the forearms, wrists, and hands in neutral.

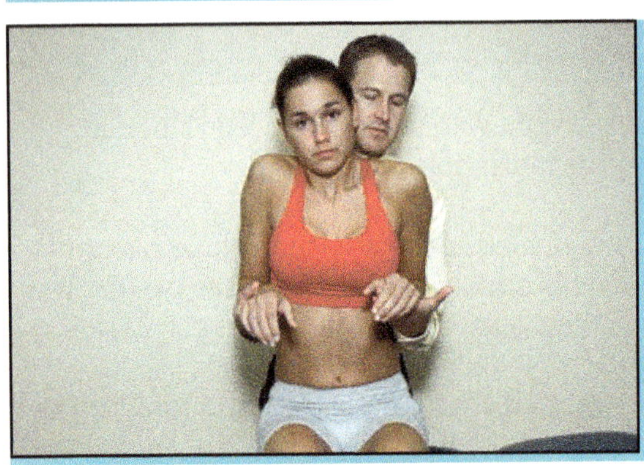

3. The examiner should lean the patient's trunk posteriorly, approximately 15 degrees from vertical, and elevate the patient's shoulder girdle close to end-range (lifted).
4. This position is held up to 3 minutes.
5. The patient is queried for reproduction of the patient's symptoms or a release phenomenon.

UTILITY SCORE

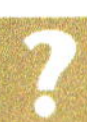

Study	Reliability	Sensitivity	Specificity	LR+	LR−	QUADAS Score (0–14)
Brismee et al.[2] (1-minute hold)	NT	NT	97	NA	NA	7
Brismee et al.[2] (15-minute hold)	NT	NT	77	NA	NA	7
Comments: Hold times have varied between 1 minute and several minutes. The examiner may use a chair to "prop" the arms in position if a longer hold time is selected. A release phenomenon occurs when symptoms abate with positioning. True test value is questionable.						

TESTS FOR THORACIC OUTLET SYNDROME

Tinel's Sign

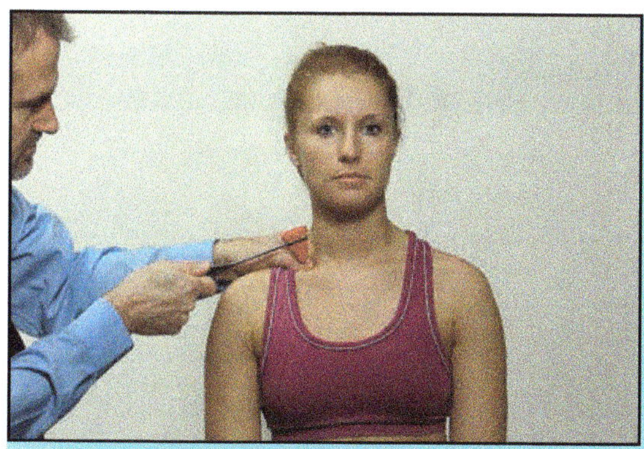

1) The patient sits straight with the arms at the side of his or her body.

2) The examiner taps the supraclavicular fossa with a reflex hammer.

3) Tenderness in the supraclavicular fossa is considered a positive finding for thoracic outlet syndrome.

UTILITY SCORE 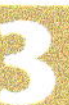

Study	Reliability	Sensitivity	Specificity	LR+	LR−	QUADAS Score (0–14)
Gillard et al.[4]	NT	46	56	1.04	0.96	8
Comments: Limited value in the use of Tinel's sign as a stand-alone test for TOS.						

Costoclavicular Maneuver

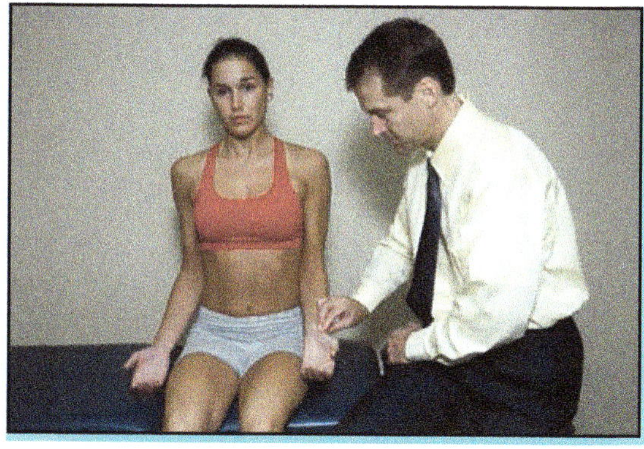

1) The patient sits straight (exaggerated military position). Both arms are placed at the sides. The examiner assesses the radial pulse in this position.

2) The patient is instructed to retract and depress the shoulders while protruding the chest.

3) The position is held for one full minute.

4) The examiner assesses changes in the radial pulse. Patients are also queried for paresthesia.

UTILITY SCORE 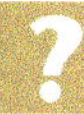

Study	Reliability	Sensitivity	Specificity	LR+	LR−	QUADAS Score (0–14)
Rayan & Jensen[12] (vascular changes)	NT	NT	53	NA	NA	3
Rayan & Jensen[12] (paresthesia)	NT	NT	98	NA	NA	3
Plewa & Delinger[11] (vascular changes)	NT	NT	89	NA	NA	9
Plewa & Delinger[11] (pain)	NT	NT	100	NA	NA	9
Plewa & Delinger[11] (paresthesia)	NT	NT	85	NA	NA	9
Comments: The test appears to be specific, although study design is lacking on both reported findings and nearly all tests have methodological biases.						

TESTS FOR THORACIC OUTLET SYNDROME

Gillard's Cluster for Thoracic Outlet Syndrome

UTILITY SCORE 

Study	Reliability	Sensitivity	Specificity	LR+	LR−	QUADAS Score (0–14)
Gillard et al.[4] (2 of 5 positive findings)	NT	90	6	0.95	1.7	8
Gillard et al.[4] (3 of 5 positive findings)	NT	90	29	1.3	0.34	8
Gillard et al.[4] (4 of 5 positive findings)	NT	87	38	1.4	0.34	8
Gillard et al.[4] (5 of 5 positive findings)	NT	84	84	5.3	0.19	8
Comments: I question the math in calculating the sensitivity for 5 of 5 positive tests. Routinely, the sensitivity declines with so many positive tests. If the values are correct, then the best combination for screening and ruling in involve 5 of 5 positive tests of: Wright, Adson's, hyperabduction, Roos, and Tinel's.						

TESTS FOR RESTRICTED FIRST RIB

Cervical Rotation Lateral Flexion Test (Associated with Brachialgia)

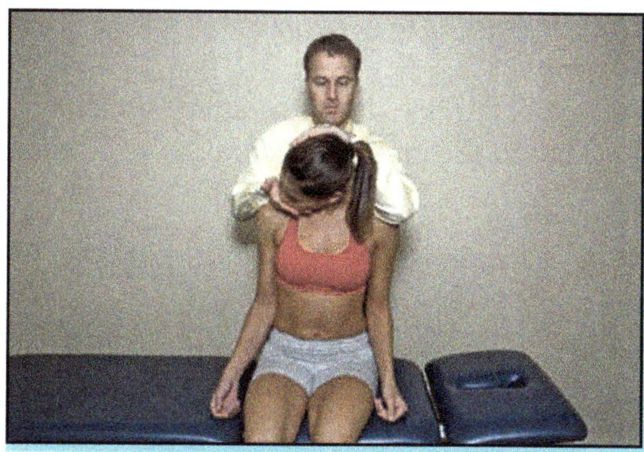

1) The patient assumes a seated position.

2) The examiner passively rotates the patient's head away from the affected side.

3) The examiner gently side flexes the head (ear to chest) passively. The side flexion should be opposite of rotation.

4) The test is considered positive if a bony restriction blocks the lateral flexion.

UTILITY SCORE

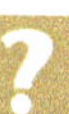

Study	Reliability	Sensitivity	Specificity	LR+	LR−	QUADAS Score (0–14)
Lindgren et al.[7]	1.0 Kappa	NT	NT	NA	NA	NA
Comments: A number of additional factors may influence the finding, including thoracic outlet syndrome, cervical radiculopathy, and upper thoracic pain. Lindgren did show validity with radiographic measures of first rib elevation.						

First Rib Spring Test

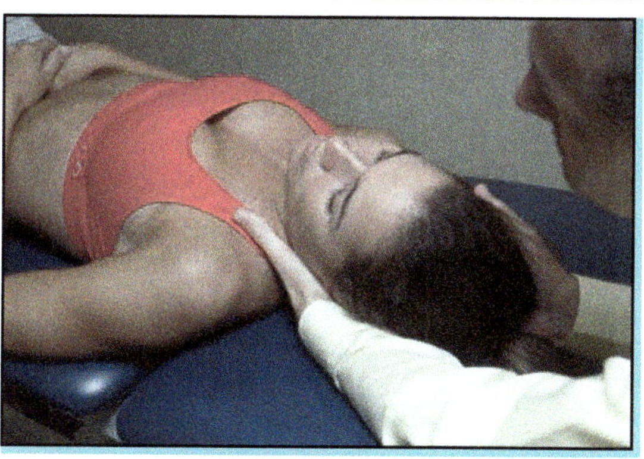

1) The patient lies in a supine position.

2) The examiner passively rotates the patient's head toward the rib that is assessed.

3) The examiner places his or her hand posterior to the first rib. The examiner presses downward in a ventral and caudal direction (toward the opposite hip or opposite shoulder).

4) The opposite side is assessed for comparison. The test is considered positive if the rib is considered stiff as compared with the other side.

UTILITY SCORE

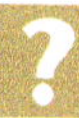

Study	Reliability	Sensitivity	Specificity	LR+	LR−	QUADAS Score (0–14)
Smedmark et al.[14] (C2–3 rotation)	.43 kappa	NT	NT	NA	NA	NA
Comments: By pushing toward the opposite hip or shoulder, the examiner targets the movement of the first rib.						

TEST FOR SCOLIOSIS

Adam's Forward Flexion Test

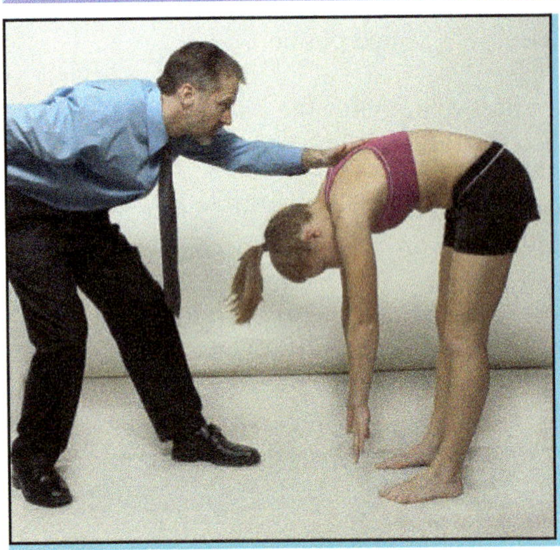

1) The patient assumes a standing position.

2) The examiner instructs the patient to stand with feet shoulder width apart, place their arms together, and bend forward slowly.

3) A positive test is trunk asymmetry (specifically the presence of a rib hump).

UTILITY SCORE 2

Study	Reliability	Sensitivity	Specificity	LR+	LR−	QUADAS Score (0–14)
Coté et al.[3]	0.61 ICC	92	60	2.3	0.13	9
Comments: This was a large trial that was adequately performed.						

TEST TO IDENTIFY A THORACIC COMPRESSION FRACTURE

Historical Height Loss Assessment

1) The patient's height is measured.

2) The patient is queried about their maximal historical height.

3) The clinician subtracts the maximum historical height by the current patient height.

4) The final value is used to determine likelihood of a thoracic compression fracture.

UTILITY SCORE 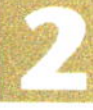

Study	Reliability	Sensitivity	Specificity	LR+	LR−	QUADAS Score (0–14)
Bennani et al.[1] (1.5 cm and greater)	NT	58	61	1.49	0.69	10
Siminoski et al.[13] (no loss)	NT	100	0	1	0	10
Siminoski et al.[13] (0.1 to 2 cm)	NT	87	17	1.04	0.76	10
Siminoski et al.[13] (2.1 to 4 cm)	NT	68	60	1.7	0.53	10
Siminoski et al.[13] (4.1 to 6 cm)	NT	42	79	2	0.73	10
Siminoski et al.[13] (6.1 to 8 cm)	NT	30	94	5	0.74	10
Siminoski et al.[13] (> – 8 cm)	NT	16	98	8	0.85	10
Comments: The test values increase for diagnosis with larger values of loss. Use caution in assuming small amounts of height loss are associated with compression fractures.						

TEST TO DETERMINE POTENTIAL OF MOBILITY CHANGE IN THE THORACIC SPINE

Structural versus Flexible Kyphosis Test

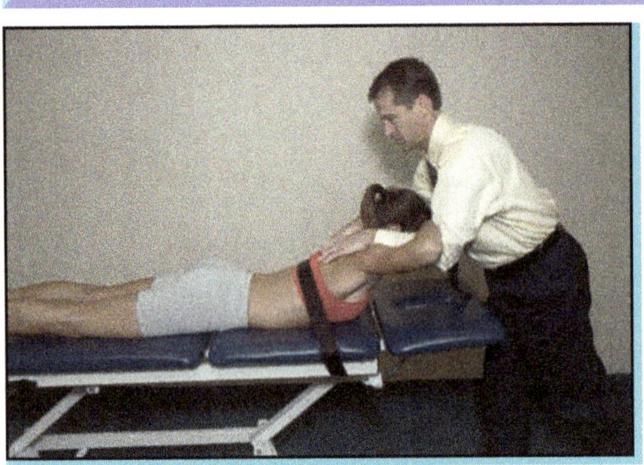

1. The patient assumes a prone position.
2. The examiner uses a stabilization belt to block the patient near T8 or the thoracic apex of kyphosis.
3. The patient either actively or is passively lifted into extension of the thoracic spine by either pulling the patient from the shoulder girdle while standing caudally, or by looping the arms through the patient's hands (pictured).
4. Failure to progress toward thoracic extension is considered a structural kyphosis.

UTILITY SCORE 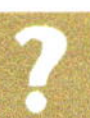

Study	Reliability	Sensitivity	Specificity	LR+	LR−	QUADAS Score (0–14)
Not tested	NT	NT	NT	NA	NA	NA
Comments: The test is considered useful during assessment of postural deformities and to determine if an extension-based program for the thoracic spine may be useful.						

TEST TO DETERMINE DISC INVOLVEMENT OR SYMPATHETIC NERVOUS SYSTEM INVOLVEMENT

Thoracic Slump Test (Sympathetic Slump Test)

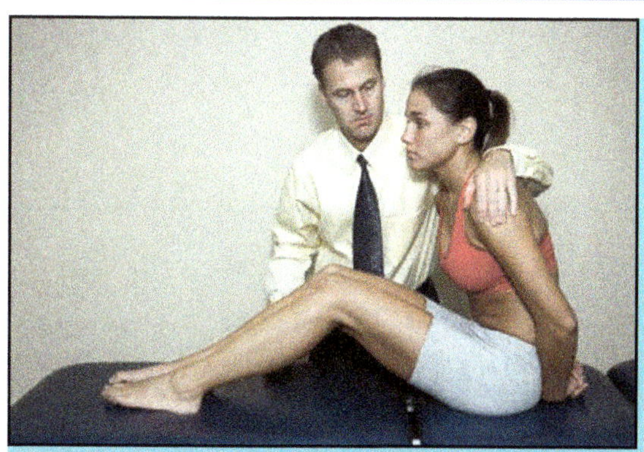

1) The patient assumes a long sitting position with the knees bent approximately 45 degrees. The hands are placed behind the back to allow examiner maneuvering. Resting symptoms are assessed.

2) The examiner loads the patient over the shoulders. Resting symptoms are assessed.

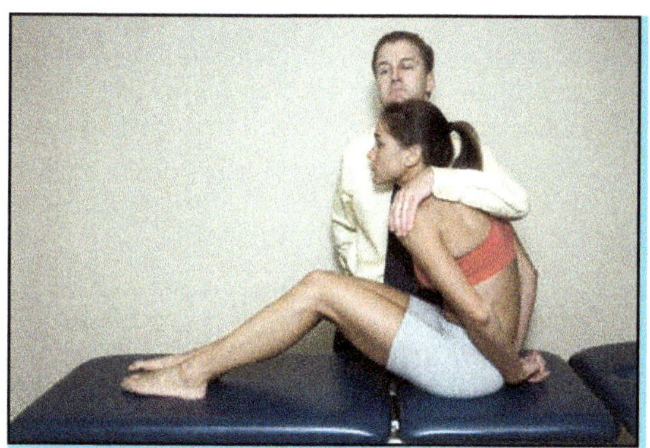

3) The patient is instructed to flex the lower cervical spine and extend the upper cervical spine. The examiner may add overpressure to the movement. Resting symptoms are assessed.

4) The examiner can then add side flexion to the right or left and/or rotation to the right or left to further engage the dural tissue (not pictured). Symptoms are further assessed to determine the concordant nature.

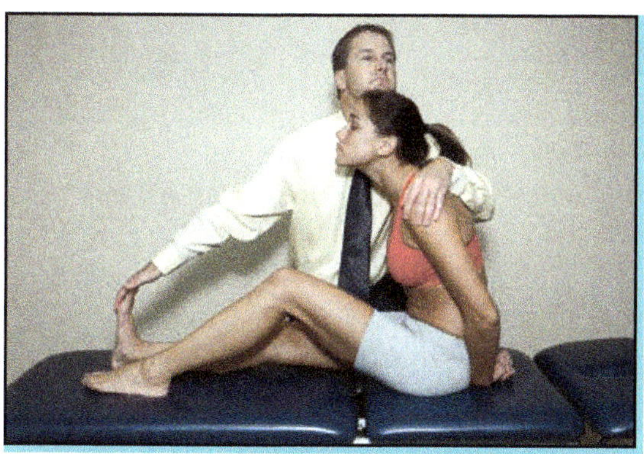

5) The examiner then passively moves the lower extremity on the concordant side into extension and the ankle into dorsiflexion. Resting symptoms are again assessed.

6) In addition, the patient may extend both knees or perform upper limb tension movements during this examination.

7) A positive test is characterized by (1) asymmetry, (2) reproduction of the concordant pain, and (3) sensitization. All three must be present for a positive test.

UTILITY SCORE 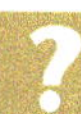

Study	Reliability	Sensitivity	Specificity	LR+	LR−	QUADAS Score (0–14)
Maitland[8]	NT	NT	NT	NA	NA	NA
Comments: The test is unexamined for diagnostic accuracy. Furthermore, if a patient exhibits low back symptoms, the position of the slump sit will be too painful to examine the thoracic spine separately. Some may describe the examination with initiation of the knee movements followed by thoracic movements.						

Key Points

1. Nearly all of the thoracic clinical special tests exhibit high levels of procedural bias.
2. Thoracic clinical special tests are significantly understudied.
3. The lack of a common accepted reference standard has resulted in few studies that have investigated the sensitivity of clinical special tests of thoracic outlet syndrome.
4. The majority of thoracic outlet syndrome special tests demonstrate moderate to poor specificity, indicating that the tests are likely to be positive for patients with conditions outside TOS. Nearly all have not been measured for sensitivity.

References

1. Bennani L, Allali F, Rostom S, et al. Relationship between historical height loss and vertebral fractures in postmenopausal women. *Clin Rheumatol.* 2009;28:1283–1289.
2. Brismee JM, Gilbert K, Isom K, Hall R, Leathers B, Sheppard N, Sawyer S, Sizer P. Rate of false positive using the Cyriax Release test for thoracic outlet syndrome in an asymptomatic population. *J Man Manipulative Ther.* 2004;12:73–81.
3. Coté P, Kreitz BG, Cassidy JD, Dzus AK, Martel J. A study of the diagnostic accuracy and reliability of the Scoliometer and Adam's forward bend test. *Spine* (Philadelphia, PA 1976). 1998;23:796–802; discussion 803.
4. Gillard J, Pérez-Cousin M, Hachulla E, Remy J, Hurtevent JF, Vinckier L, Thévenon A, Duquesnoy B. Diagnosing thoracic outlet syndrome: contribution of provocative tests, ultrasonography, electrophysiology, and helical computed tomography in 48 patients. *Joint Bone Spine.* 2001;68:416–424.
5. Howard M, Lee C, Dellon AL. Documentation of brachial plexus compression (in the thoracic inlet) utilizing provocative neurosensory and muscular testing. *J Reconstr Microsurg.* 2003;19:303–312.
6. Lee AD, Agarwal S, Sadhu D. Doppler Adson's test: predictor of outcome of surgery in non-specific thoracic outlet syndrome. *World J Surg.* 2006;30:291–292.
7. Lindgren KA, Leino E, Manninen H. Cervical rotation lateral flexion test in brachialgia. *Arch Phys Med Rehabil.* 1992;73:735–737.
8. Maitland GD. *Maitland's Vertebral Manipulation.* 6th ed. London; Butterworth-Heinemann: 2001.
9. Matsuyama T, Okuchi K, Goda K. Upper plexus thoracic outlet syndrome—case report. *Neurol Med Chir (Tokyo).* 2002;42:237–241.
10. Nord KM, Kapoor P, Fisher J, et al. False positive rate of thoracic outlet syndrome diagnostic maneuvers. *Electromyogr Clin Neurophysiol.* 2008;48:67–74.
11. Plewa MC, Delinger M. The false-positive rate of thoracic outlet syndrome shoulder maneuvers in healthy patients. *Acad Emerg Med.* 1998;5:337–342.
12. Rayan GM, Jensen C. Thoracic outlet syndrome: provocative examination maneuvers in a typical population. *J Shoulder Elbow Surg.* 1995;4:113–117.
13. Siminoski K, Warshawski RS, Jen H, Lee K. The accuracy of historical height loss for the detection of vertebral fractures in postmenopausal women. *Osteoporos Int.* 2006;17:290–296.
14. Smedmark V, Wallin M, Arvidsson I. Inter-examiner reliability in assessing passive intervertebral motion of the cervical spine. *Man Ther.* 2000;5:97–101.

PEARSON **myhealthprofessionskit**™

Use this address to access the Companion Website created for this textbook. Simply select "Physical Therapy" from the choice of disciplines. Find this book and log in using your username and password to access video clips of selected tests.

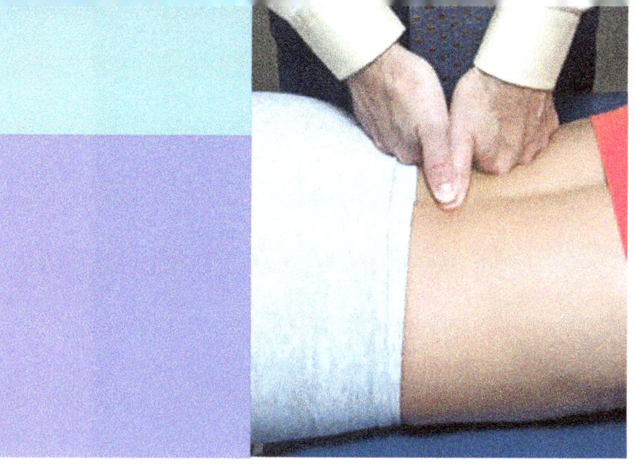

Physical Examination Tests for the Lumbar Spine

Chad E. Cook and Eric J. Hegedus

Please refer to the chapter "Introduction to Diagnostic Accuracy" before reading this chapter.

Index of Tests

Tests for Radiographic Instability of the Spine

Passive Physiological Intervertebral Movements (PPIVMs) Extension

Passive Physiological Intervertebral Movements (PPIVMs) Flexion

The Passive Lumbar Extension Test

The Instability Catch Sign

The Painful Catch Sign

The Stork Standing Test

Prone Instability Test

Specific Spine Torsion Test

Prone Torsion Instability Test

Tests for Lumbar Spinal Stenosis

Two Stage Treadmill Test

Pain Relief upon Sitting

Cook's Clinical Prediction Rule for Lumbar Stenosis

Test for Degenerative Changes in the Spine

Extension Quadrant Test

Tests for Compression Fractures

Percussion Test

Supine Test

Henschke's Clinical Prediction Rule for Compression Fracture

Roman's Clinical Prediction Rule for Compression Fracture

Test for Lumbar Flexion Dysfunction

Flexion Quadrant Test

TESTS FOR LOW BACK PAIN

Sorenson Test

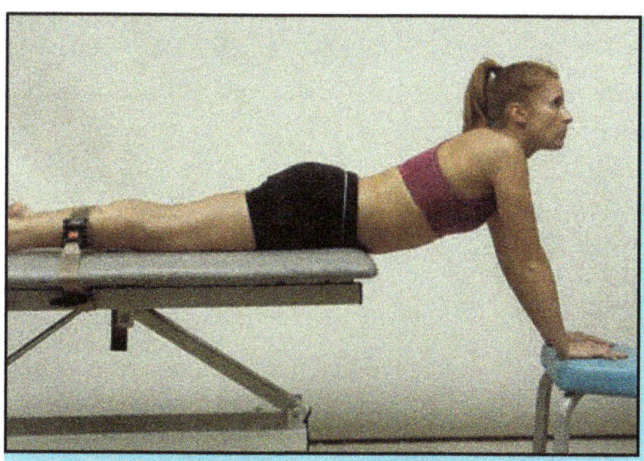

1) The patient lies prone on the examining table with the upper edge of the iliac crests aligned with the edge of the table.

2) The lower extremities are affixed to the table using straps. A chair is placed at the end of the plinth to allow the patient to stabilize their upper body until the test initiates.

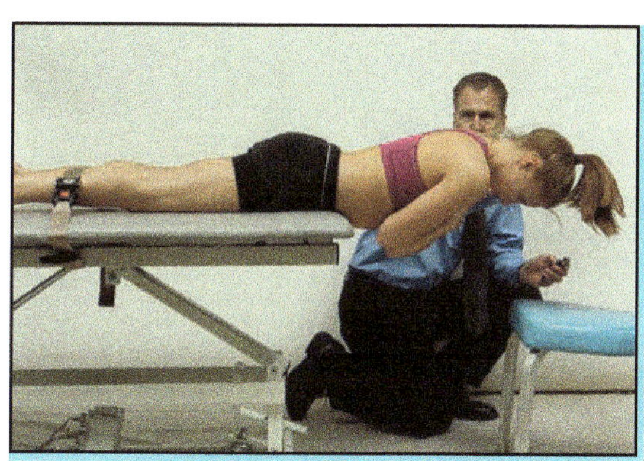

3) The arms are folded across the chest and the patient is asked to maintain the unsupported upper body position in a horizontal plane as long as they can.

4) The event is timed.

UTILITY SCORE

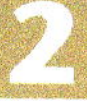

Study	Reliability	Sensitivity	Specificity	LR+	LR−	QUADAS Score (0–14)
Arab et al.[3] (men) > 28 seconds	0.78 ICC	92.3	94	15.4	0.08	9
Arab et al.[3] (women) > 29 seconds	0.78 ICC	84.3	84.6	5.47	0.18	9
Comments: Arab and colleagues defined 28/29 seconds as the cut off for patients who did and did not have pain.						

TESTS FOR LOW BACK PAIN

Prone Isometric Chest Raise Test

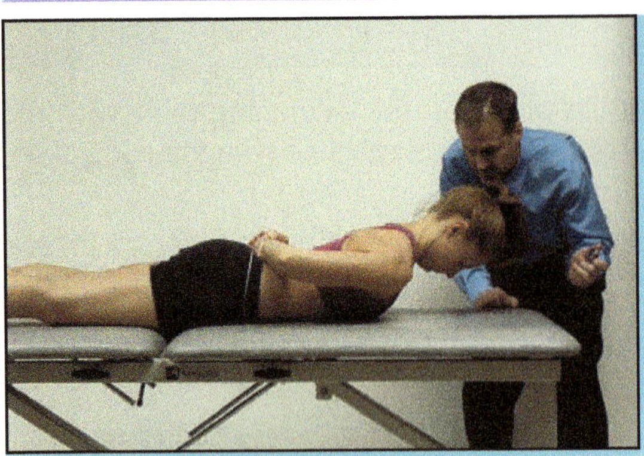

1) The patient lies fully on a plinth in a prone position.

2) The patient is instructed to lift their upper trunk (so that their sternum is off the plinth) and hold this position as long as possible.

3) The patient is instructed to also hold the neck in flexion during the process.

4) The event is timed.

UTILITY SCORE 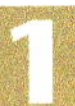 1

Study	Reliability	Sensitivity	Specificity	LR+	LR−	QUADAS Score (0–14)
Arab et al.[3] (men) > 31 seconds	0.90 ICC	80.8	80	15.3	0.08	9
Arab et al.[3] (women) > 33 seconds	0.90 ICC	98	84.6	5.5	0.18	9
Comments: Use caution to make sure the patient doesn't hyperextend their back during the testing process or move beyond 30 degrees to gain a mechanical advantage.						

Supine Isometric Chest Raise Test

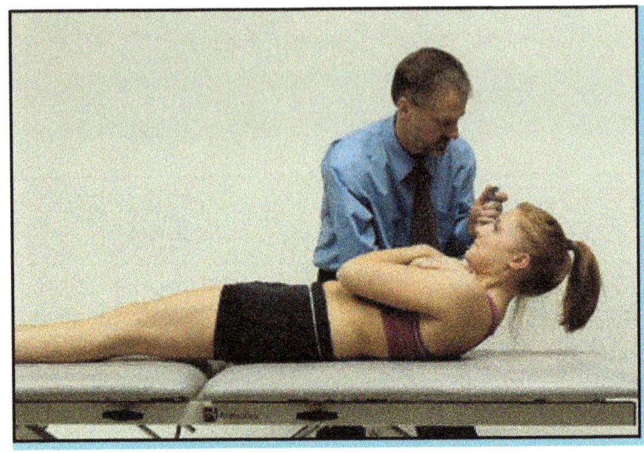

1) The patient lies supine on a plinth. Their hands are crossed at their chest and their knees and hips are flexed to 90 degrees. An alternative version (pictured) involves keeping the hips and knees straight.

2) The patient is instructed to slightly raise their upper trunk off the table and hold this position as long as possible.

3) The neck should be held in a neutral position.

4) The event is timed.

UTILITY SCORE 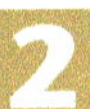 2

Study	Reliability	Sensitivity	Specificity	LR+	LR−	QUADAS Score (0–14)
Arab et al.[3] (men) > 34 seconds	0.92 ICC	96.2	72.0	4.0	0.24	9
Arab et al.[3] (women) > 24 seconds	0.92 ICC	99.4	32.7	6.4	0.02	9
Comments: Use caution to assure that the patient does not flex beyond a few inches from the table.						

TESTS FOR DISCOGENIC SYMPTOMS

Centralization

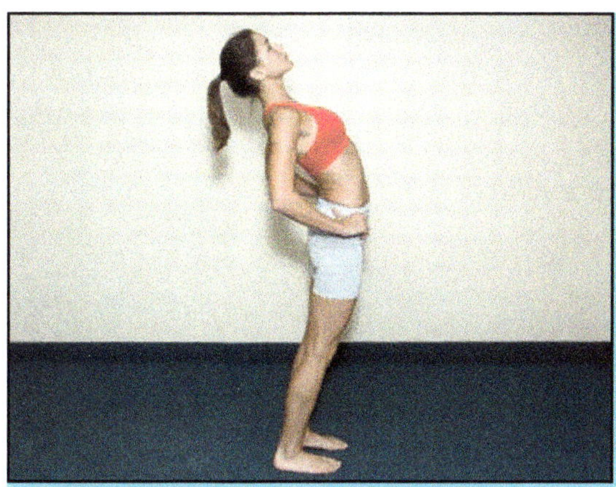

1. The patient either stands or lies prone depending on the intent of a loaded or unloaded assessment.
2. Multiple directions of repeated end-range lumbar testing are targeted. Movements may include extension, flexion, or side flexion.
3. Movements are repeated generally for 5–20 attempts until a definite centralization or peripheralization occurs.
4. Centralization of symptoms is considered a positive finding.

UTILITY SCORE 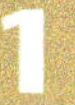

Study	Reliability	Sensitivity	Specificity	LR+	LR−	QUADAS Score (0–14)
Laslett et al.[24]	NT	40	94	6.7	0.63	13
Donelson et al.[10]	NT	92	64	2.6	0.12	12
Comments: Centralization is defined as the progressive retreat of referred pain toward the midline of the back in response to standardized movement testing during evaluation of the effect of repeated movements on pain location and intensity. Centralization is commonly associated with discogenic symptoms.						

Extension Loss

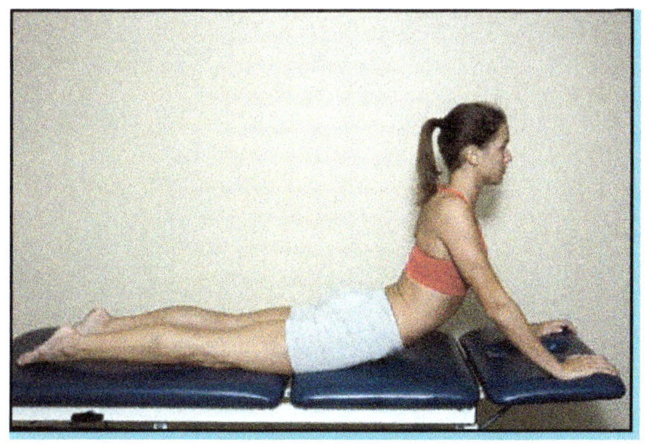

1. The patient is instructed to lie prone.
2. The patient is instructed to extend his or her lumbar spine while keeping pelvis in contact with the plinth.
3. A positive test is moderate or major loss of extension.

UTILITY SCORE 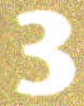

Study	Reliability	Sensitivity	Specificity	LR+	LR−	QUADAS Score (0–14)
Laslett et al.[23]	NT	27	87	2.01	0.84	10
Comments: The test is scored using visual observation only.						

TESTS FOR DISCOGENIC SYMPTOMS

Vulnerability in the Neutral Zone

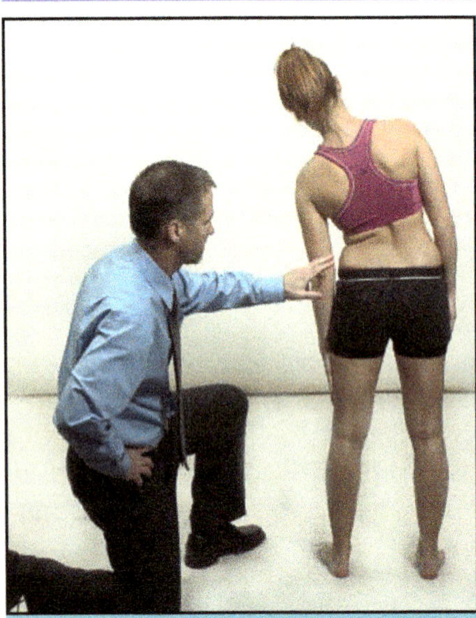

1) The patient is instructed to move into a slightly flexed, slightly extended, or slightly laterally flexed position.

2) The patient is queried whether symptoms are worsened in the neutral zone positions of slight flexion, lateral flexion, or extension.

3) A positive test is worsening of symptoms at neutral ranges.

ULITITY SCORE 

Study	Reliability	Sensitivity	Specificity	LR+	LR−	QUADAS Score (0–14)
Laslett et al.[23]	NT	41	83	2.47	0.71	10
Donelson[10] (1997) (herniated disk)	NT	64	70	2.13	0.51	10
Donelson[10] (herniated disk and annulus disruption)	NT	31	82	1.72	084	10
Comments: A positive test is typically associated with worsening symptoms at mid-range versus end-range.						

TESTS FOR HERNIATED NUCLEUS PULPOSIS OR LUMBAR RADICULOPATHY

Well Leg Raise

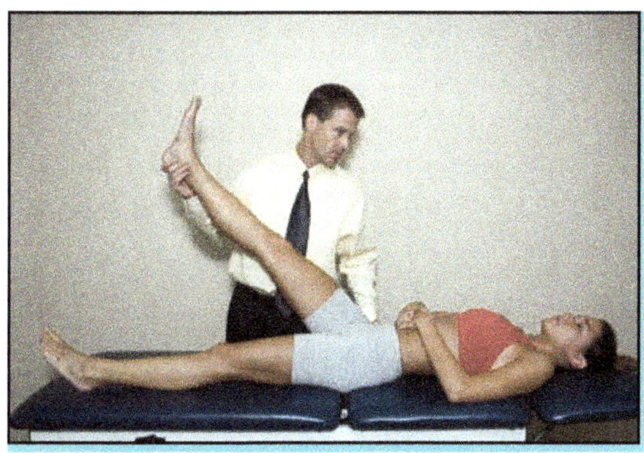

1) The patient should lie on a firm but comfortable surface, the neck and head in the neutral position.

2) The patient's trunk and hips should remain neutral; avoid internal or external rotation, and excessive adduction or abduction.

3) The examiner then supports the patient's noninvolved leg at the heel, maintaining knee extension and neutral dorsiflexion at the ankle.

4) Raise to the point of symptom reproduction of the opposite, comparable leg.

5) A positive test is identified by reproduction of the patient's concordant pain during the raising of the opposite extremity.

UTILITY SCORE 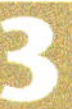

Study	Reliability	Sensitivity	Specificity	LR+	LR−	QUADAS Score (0–14)
Knuttson[18]	NT	25	95	5	0.79	3
Hakelius & Hindmarsh[14]	NT	28	88	2.33	0.82	3
Spangfort[34]	NT	23	88	1.91	0.86	5
Kosteljanetz et al.[20]	NT	24	100	NA	NA	7
Kerr et al.[17]	NT	43	97	14.3	0.59	7
Comments: The test is highly specific and is not sensitive. The test is inappropriate for use as a screen and best functions as a diagnostic test.						

TESTS FOR HERNIATED NUCLEUS PULPOSIS OR LUMBAR RADICULOPATHY

Slump Sit Test

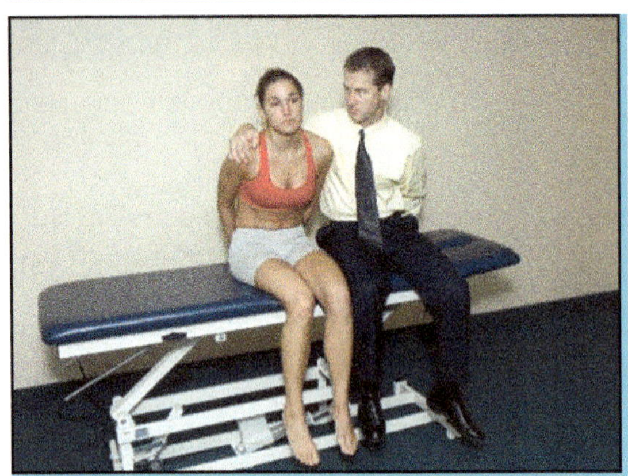

1) The patient sits straight with the arms behind the back, the legs together, and the posterior aspect of the knees against the edge of the treatment table.

2) The patient slumps as far as possible, producing full trunk flexion; the examiner applies firm overpressure into flexion to the patient's back, being careful to keep the sacrum vertical.

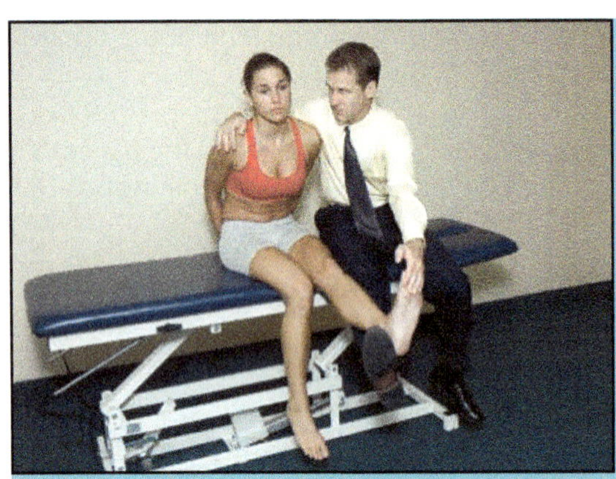

3) While maintaining full spinal flexion with overpressure, the examiner asks the patient to extend the knee, or passively extends the knee.

4) The examiner then moves the foot into dorsiflexion while maintaining knee extension.

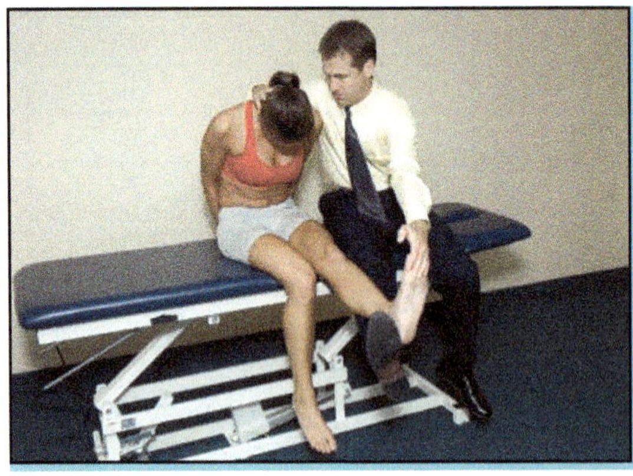

5) Neck flexion is then added to assess symptoms. Neck flexion is released to see if symptoms abate.

6) A positive test is concordant reproduction of symptoms, sensitization, and asymmetry findings.

UTILITY SCORE 

Study	Reliability	Sensitivity	Specificity	LR+	LR−	QUADAS Score (0–14)
Stankovic et al.[36]	NT	83	55	1.82	0.32	11
Majilesi et al.[28]	NT	84	83	4.94	0.19	7
Rabin et al.[32]	NT	41	NT	NT	NT	10
Comments: The slump has been described as distal and proximal initiation. At present, no studies have examined the differences in diagnostic values of each.						

TESTS FOR HERNIATED NUCLEUS PULPOSIS OR LUMBAR RADICULOPATHY

Straight Leg Raise

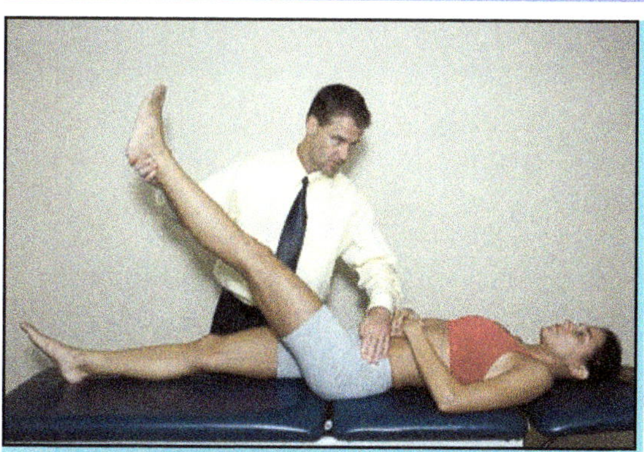

1) The patient should lie on a firm but comfortable surface, the neck and head in the neutral position.

2) The examiner then supports the patient's leg at the heel, maintaining knee extension and neutral dorsiflexion at the ankle. The clinician raises the leg to the point of symptom reproduction.

3) The patient's trunk and hips should remain neutral, avoiding internal or external rotation of the leg or adduction or abduction of the hip.

4) A positive test is concordant reproduction of symptoms, sensitization, and asymmetry findings.

UTILITY SCORE 

Study	Reliability	Sensitivity	Specificity	LR+	LR−	QUADAS Score (0–14)
Bertilson et al.[4]	0.92 kappa	NT	NT	NA	NA	NA
Charnley[6]	NT	78	64	2.16	0.34	5
Knuttson[18]	NT	96	10	1.06	0.40	3
Hakelius & Hindmarsh[14]	NT	96	17	1.15	0.24	3
Spangfort[34]	NT	97	11	1.08	0.27	5
Kosteljanetz et al.[20]	NT	76	45	1.38	0.53	9
Kosteljanetz et al.[20]	NT	89	14	1.03	0.78	7
Lauder et al.[25] (used EMG as reference standard)	NT	19	84	1.61	0.90	6
Albeck[2]	NT	82	21	1.03	0.86	7
Gurdijan et al.[13]	NT	81	52	1.68	0.36	4
Kerr et al.[17]	NT	98	44	1.75	0.05	7
Vroomen et al.[37]	NT	97	57	2.23	0.05	10
Lyle et al.[26] (for degenerative spine)	NT	16	NT	NT	NT	9
Porchet et al.[31] (extreme lateral disk herniation)	NT	83	NT	NT	NT	5
Rabin et al.[32]	NT	67	NT	NT	NT	10
Majilesi et al.[28]	NT	52	89	4.72	0.53	7
Comments: In many cases, the procedure and the reference for a positive test was variable. Traditionally, the foot should be held in neutral dorsiflexion for testing.						

TEST FOR LOW BACK RELATED LEG PAIN

Manual Palpation of the Sciatic, Tibial, and Common Peroneal Nerves

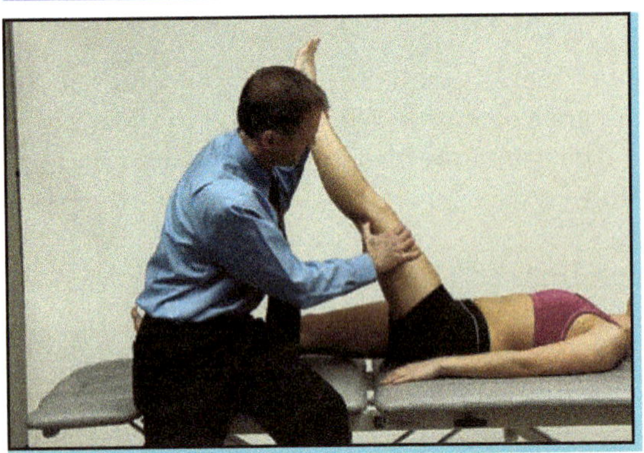

1) The patient is instructed to lie supine for the common peroneal nerve testing, and prone for sciatic and tibial nerve testing.

2) The clinician applies gentle pressure behind the head of the fibula (for peroneal nerve testing), at the midway point of the line from the ischial tuberosity to the greater trochanter of the femur (for the sciatic nerve), and where the tibial nerve bisects the popliteal fossa at the midpoint of the popliteal crease (for the tibial nerve).

3) A positive test is pain or discomfort on one side versus the other.

UTILITY SCORE 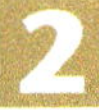

Study	Reliability	Sensitivity	Specificity	LR+	LR−	QUADAS Score (0–14)
Walsh & Hall[38] (sciatic)	0.96 kappa	85	60	2.12	0.25	11
Walsh & Hall[38] (tibial)	0.66 kappa	65	72	2.32	0.48	11
Walsh & Hall[38] (peroneal)	0.78 kappa	65	56	1.48	0.63	11
Walsh & Hall[38] (1 or more positive)	NT	90	36	1.40	0.27	11
Walsh & Hall[38] (2 or more positive)	NT	83	73	3.07	0.23	11
Walsh & Hall[38] (3 of 3 positive)	NT	40	84	2.50	0.71	11
Comments: One well performed study that shows some value in clustering findings toward low back related leg pain.						

TEST FOR FAR LATERAL LUMBAR DISK HERNIATION

Femoral Nerve Tension Test

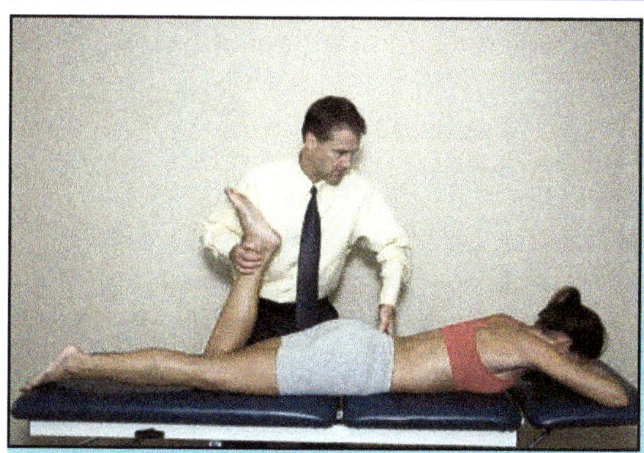

1) The patient lies prone in a symmetric pain-free posture.

2) The examiner places one hand on the PSIS, the same side of the knee that the examiner will bend into flexion.

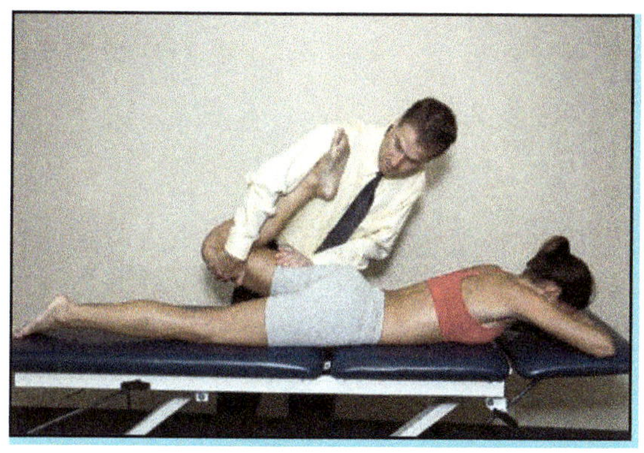

3) The examiner then gently moves the lower extremity into knee flexion, bending the knee until the onset of symptoms.

4) Once symptoms are engaged, the examiner slightly backs the leg out of the painful position.

5) At this point, the examiner may use plantarflexion, dorsiflexion, or head movements to sensitize the findings.

6) Further sensitization can be elicited by implementing hip extension. The examiner can repeat on the opposite side if desired.

7) A positive test is reproduction of pain in the affected extremity.

UTILITY SCORE 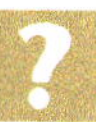

Study	Reliability	Sensitivity	Specificity	LR+	LR−	QUADAS Score (0–14)
Porchet et al.[31]	NT	84	NT	NA	NA	5

Comments: All cases in the Porchet et al.[31] study were associated with extreme lateral disk herniations. The test is sometimes described as an upper lumbar disk assessment and frequently as a femoral nerve tension test. Only the far lateral disk herniation patient pool has been investigated.

TEST FOR UPPER LUMBAR HERNIATION

Crossed Femoral Nerve Tension Test

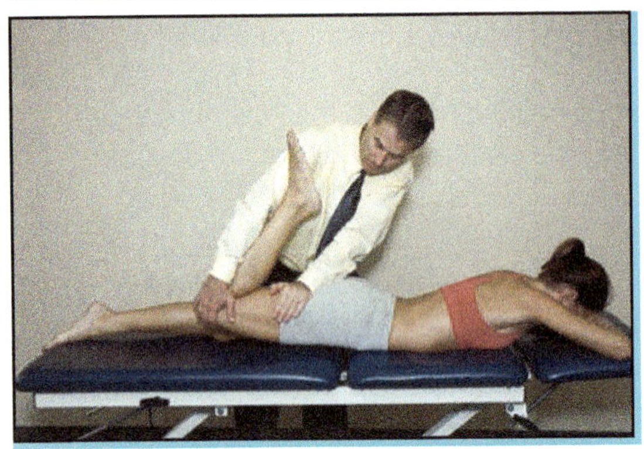

1) The patient lies prone in a symmetric pain-free posture.

2) The examiner places one hand on the PSIS, the same side of the knee that the examiner will bend into flexion.

3) The examiner then gently moves the noninvolved lower extremity into knee flexion, bending the knee until the onset of symptoms.

4) Once symptoms are engaged, the examiner slightly backs out of the painful position. At this point, the examiner may use plantarflexion, dorsiflexion, or head movements to sensitize the findings.

5) Further sensitization can be elicited by implementing hip extension.

6) A positive test is reproduction of concordant pain in the opposite extremity.

UTILITY SCORE 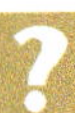

Study	Reliability	Sensitivity	Specificity	LR+	LR−	QUADAS Score (0–14)
Kreitz et al.[21]	NT	NT	NT	NA	NA	NT
Comments: The test is sometimes described as a far lateral disk herniation assessment and frequently as a femoral nerve tension test when performed unilaterally on the affected side.						

TEST FOR ZYGAPOPHYSEAL JOINT PAIN

Extension-Rotation Test

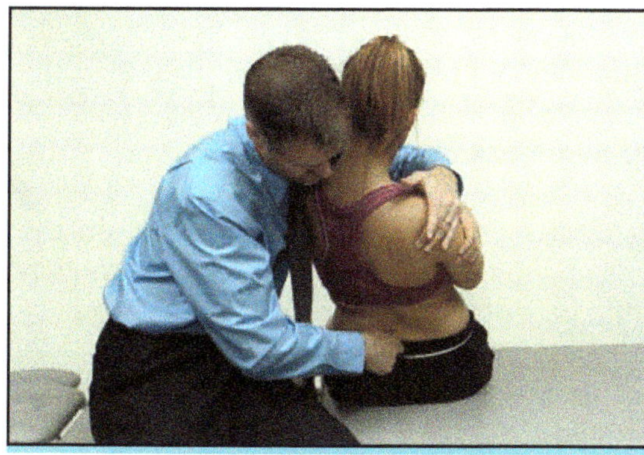

1) The patient is placed in a sitting position and the knees are blocked.

2) The patient is passively pushed into full extension.

3) The patient is taken into full rotation on both left and right sides; while maintaining full extension.

4) A positive finding is pain at end-range extension and rotation.

UTILITY SCORE 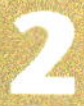

Study	Reliability	Sensitivity	Specificity	LR+	LR−	QUADAS Score (0–14)
Laslett et al.[23]	NT	100	22	1.28	0.00	10
Schwarzer et al.[35]	NT	100	12	1.13	0.00	10
Comments: This highly sensitive test is most useful in ruling out a zygapophyseal joint dysfunction.						

TEST FOR LEVEL OF PATHOLOGY OR RADIOGRAPHIC INSTABILITY OF THE SPINE

Posterior-Anterior (PA)

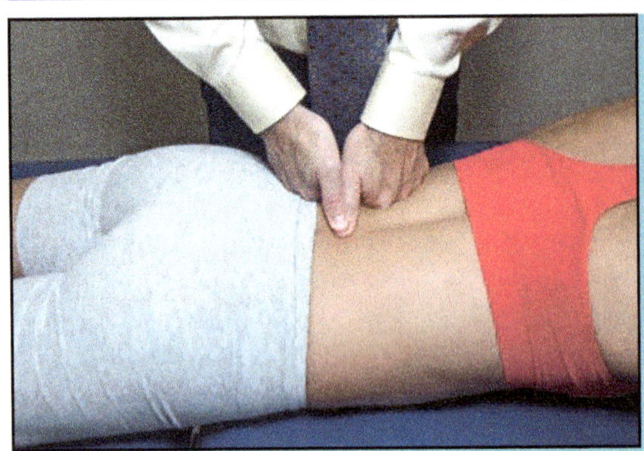

1) The patient is placed in prone. Using a thumb pad to thumb pad grip, apply gentle force perpendicular to the spinous process of the lumbar spine. The force should be about 4 kg or thumbnail blanching.

2) The examiner starts proximal and moves distal on the patient's spine, asking for the reproduction of the concordant sign of the patient.

3) A joint is cleared if a significant amount of PA force is applied and no pain is present.

4) A dysfunctional joint will elicit the concordant sign during the mobilization, and may reproduce radicular or referred symptoms. Repeated movement or sustained holds help determine the appropriateness of the technique.

5) A positive test is identified by reproduction of the patient's concordant pain or presence of linear displacement during assessment.

UTILITY SCORE 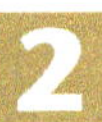

Study	Reliability	Sensitivity	Specificity	LR+	LR−	QUADAS Score (0–14)
Bertilson et al.[4] (for identification of pain)	.44 kappa	NT	NT	NA	NA	NA
Matyas & Bach[29]	0.09–0.46*r*	NT	NT	NA	NA	NA
Maher & Adams[27] (L1–5) (for identification of pain)	.67–.73 ICC	NT	NT	NA	NA	NA
Maher & Adams[27] (L1–5) (for identification of stiffness)	.03–.37 ICC	NT	NT	NA	NA	NA
Binkley et al.[5] (identification of proper level to treat)	.30 kappa	NT	NT	NA	NA	NA
Binkley et al.[5] (assessment of mobility)	.09 kappa	NT	NT	NA	NA	NA
Chiradejnant et al.[7]	.78 ICC	NT	NT	NA	NA	9
Phillips & Twomey[30] (tissue response agreement for transverse glides [TG], central PAs [CPA], and unilateral PAs [UPA])	− 0.16–0.22 (TG) − 0.15–0.19 (CPA) − 0.09–0.28 (UPA)	NT	NT	NA	NA	9

TEST FOR LEVEL OF PATHOLOGY OR RADIOGRAPHIC INSTABILITY OF THE SPINE

Study	Reliability	Sensitivity	Specificity	LR+	LR−	QUADAS Score (0–14)
Phillips & Twomey[30] (verbal response combined to identify the painful segment)	NA	75	90	7.5	0.27	9
Phillips & Twomey[30] (nonverbal response combined to identify the painful segment)	NA	50	78	2.24	0.64	9
Abbott et al.[1] (rotational PAs to diagnose radiographic instability)	NT	33	88	2.75	0.75	11
Abbott et al.[1] (transitional PAs to diagnose radiographic instability)	NT	29	89	2.63	0.79	11
Fritz et al.[12] (lack of hypomobility to diagnose radiographic instability)	NT	43	95	8.6	0.60	12
Fritz et al.[12] (presence of hypermobility to diagnose radiographic instability)	.48 kappa	46	81	2.42	0.66	12
Fritz et al.[12] (presence of pain to diagnose radiographic instability)	.57 kappa	43	81	2.26	0.70	12
Comments: Unfortunately, the procedure and positive identifier for each study was variable. The test is likely not diagnostic, but is a useful tool to identify the impaired segment.						

TESTS FOR RADIOGRAPHIC INSTABILITY OF THE SPINE

Passive Physiological Intervertebral Movements (PPIVMs) Extension

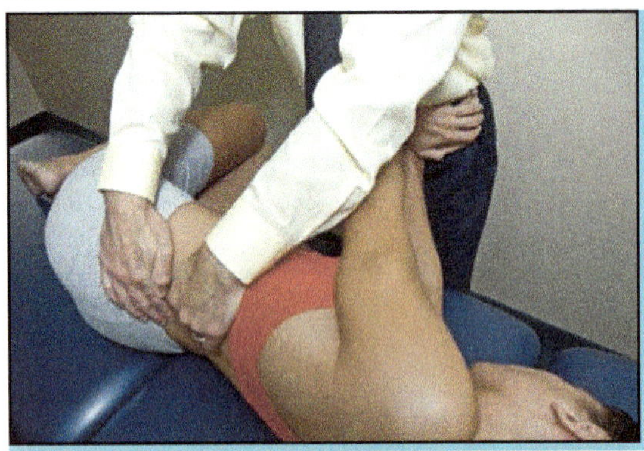

1) The patient is placed in a sidelying position. The patient's elbows are locked in extension and his or her hands are placed on the ASIS of the assessing examiner.

2) The examiner applies a posterior to anterior (PA) force at the caudal level (i.e., at L5 when assessing L4–L5 mobility).

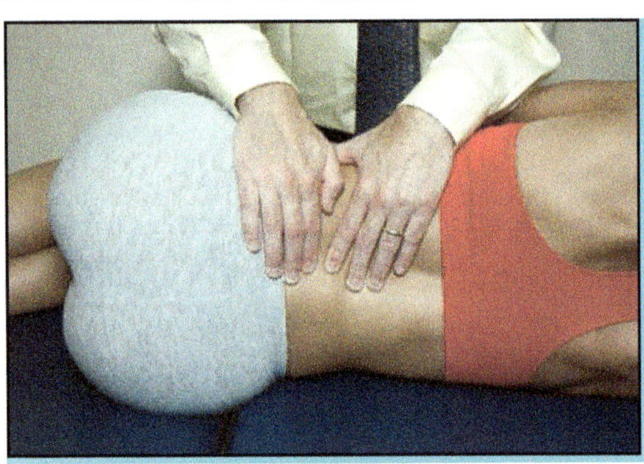

3) The cephalic segment is palpated just inferior at the interspinous space (i.e., during L4–L5 assessment, the interspinous space is palpated to assess movement). One may repeat on the other side, although most likely results are similar.

4) A positive test is identified by detection of excessive movement during examination.

UTILITY SCORE 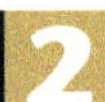

Study	Reliability	Sensitivity	Specificity	LR+	LR−	QUADAS Score (0–14)
Abbott et al.[1] (extension rotational PPIVMs)	NT	22	97	7.3	0.80	11
Abbott et al.[1] (extension transitional PPIVMs)	NT	16	98	8	0.85	11
Comments: Abbott et al.[1] used very specific criteria in identifying a positive finding, which explains the low sensitivity values.						

TESTS FOR RADIOGRAPHIC INSTABILITY OF THE SPINE

Passive Physiological Intervertebral Movements (PPIVMs) Flexion

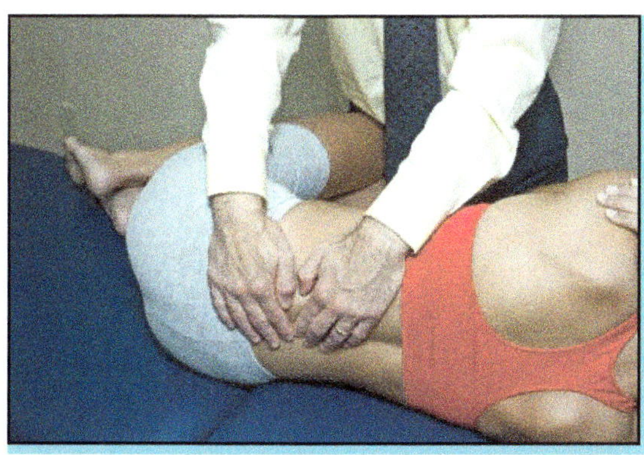

1) The patient is placed in a sidelying position. The hips of the patient are flexed to 90 degrees and the patient's knees are placed against the ASIS of the examiner.

2) The examiner stabilizes the superior segments by pulling posterior to anterior on the patient's spine. The examiner applies an anterior to posterior force at the caudal level (i.e., at L5 when assessing L4–L5 mobility) by applying a force through the flexed femurs.

3) The cephalic segment is palpated just inferior at the interspinous space (i.e., during L4–L5 assessment, the interspinous space is palpated to assess movement).

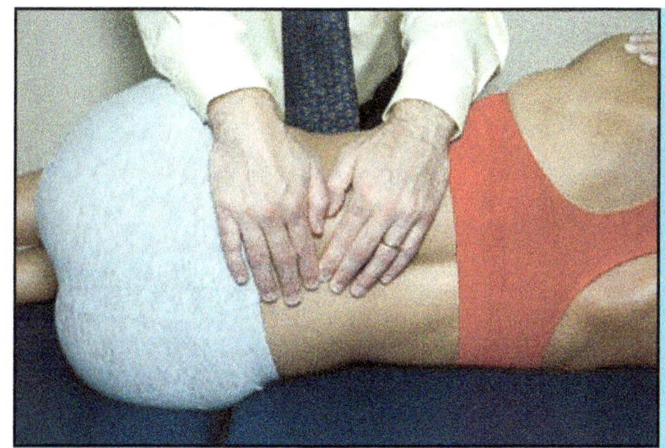

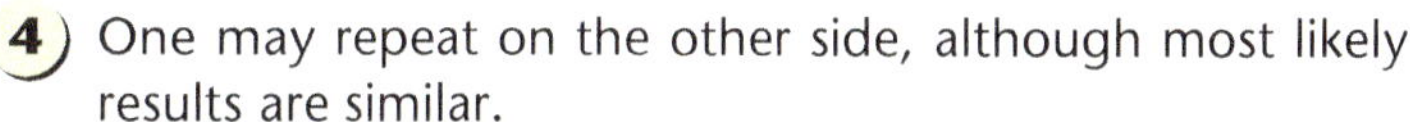

4) One may repeat on the other side, although most likely results are similar.

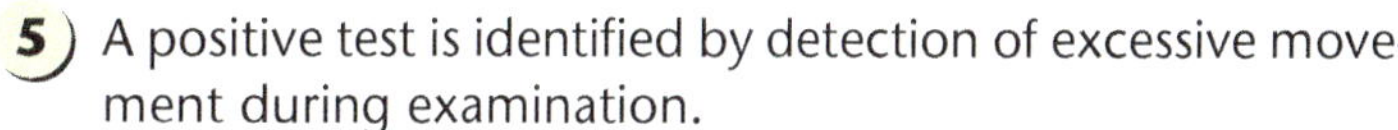

5) A positive test is identified by detection of excessive movement during examination.

UTILITY SCORE

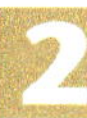

Study	Reliability	Sensitivity	Specificity	LR+	LR−	QUADAS Score (0–14)
Abbott et al.[1] (Flexion Rotational PPIVMs)	NT	05	99	5	0.96	11
Abbott et al.[1] (Flexion Transitional PPVIMs)	NT	05	99	10	0.95	11
Comments: Abbott et al.[1] used very specific criteria in identifying a positive finding, which explains the low sensitivity values.						

TESTS FOR RADIOGRAPHIC INSTABILITY OF THE SPINE

The Passive Lumbar Extension Test

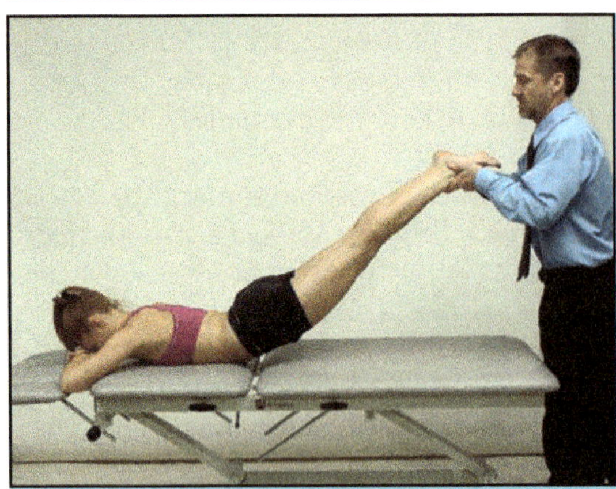

1) The patient is instructed to lie prone.

2) The clinician lifts the legs of the patient off the plinth (about 30 cm, while keeping the knees extended) and queries the patient regarding pain in the low back.

3) A positive test is a patient complaint of strong pain, heavy feeling in the low back, or a feeling that the back is "coming off."

UTILITY SCORE 

Study	Reliability	Sensitivity	Specificity	LR+	LR−	QUADAS Score (0–14)
Kasai et al.[16]	NT	84.2	90.4	8.78	0.17	12
Comments: This is a striking finding that needs replication.						

The Instability Catch Sign

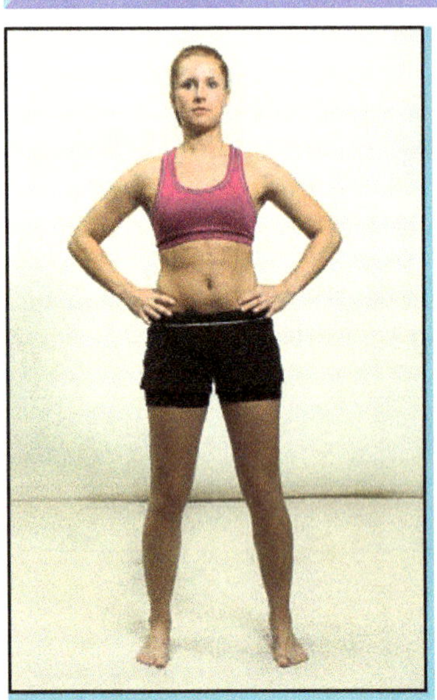

1) The patient is examined in standing.

2) The patient is asked to bend his or her bodys forward as much as possible then return to an erect position.

3) A positive test is an inability to return to a full erect position.

UTILITY SCORE 

Study	Reliability	Sensitivity	Specificity	LR+	LR−	QUADAS Score (0–14)
Kasai et al.[16]	NT	85.7	45.5	1.57	0.31	12
Comments: A useful finding to rule out instability.						

TESTS FOR RADIOGRAPHIC INSTABILITY OF THE SPINE

The Painful Catch Sign

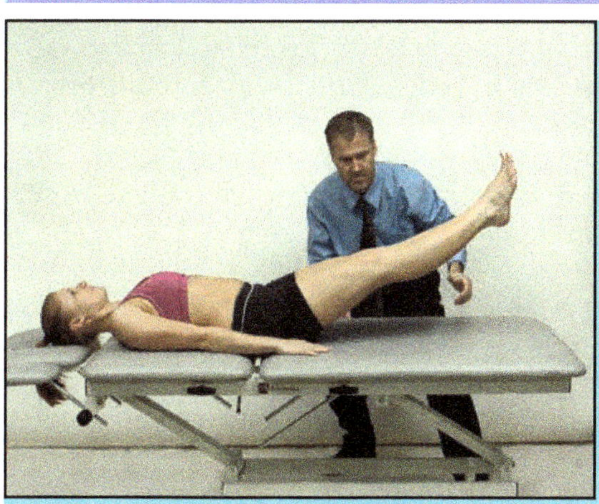

1) The patient is examined in a supine position.

2) The patient is asked to lift his or her legs (while maintaining knee extension) about 30 cm high. They are then asked to lower their legs back to the table.

3) A positive test is when the legs are rapidly dropped during the return phase.

UTILITY SCORE 3

Study	Reliability	Sensitivity	Specificity	LR+	LR−	QUADAS Score (0–14)
Kasai et al.[16]	NT	36.8	72.6	1.34	0.87	12
Comments: A well done study. The finding is not compelling to diagnosis instability.						

The Stork Standing Test

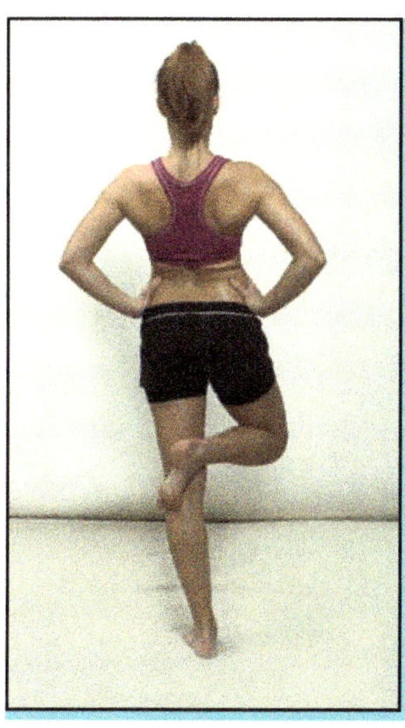

1) The patient is placed in a standing position with hands on the hips.

2) The patient is asked to stand on one leg (the other is propped against the weight bearing leg) and extend backward.

3) A positive test is pain during extension.

UTILITY SCORE 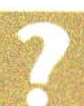

Study	Reliability	Sensitivity	Specificity	LR+	LR−	QUADAS Score (0–14)
None	NT	NT	NT	NA	NA	NA
Comments: Pain in the low back during extension is thought to be associated with a compromised pars interarticularis on the loaded side.						

TESTS FOR RADIOGRAPHIC INSTABILITY OF THE SPINE

Prone Instability Test

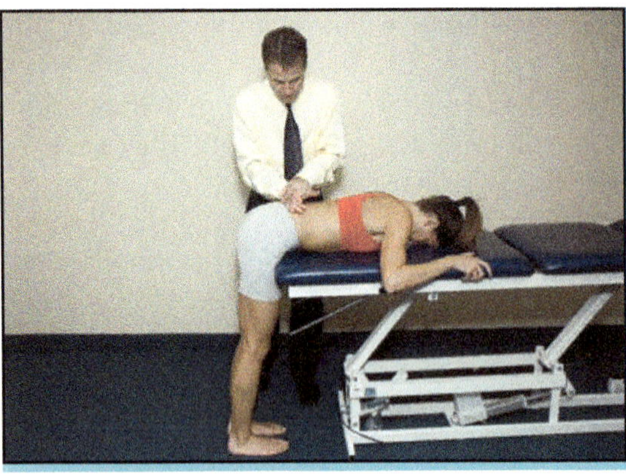

1) The patient is prone with the torso on the examining table and the legs over the edge of the plinth and the feet resting on the floor.

2) The examiner performs a PA spring on the low back to elicit back pain using the pisiform grip.

3) The patient is requested to lift his or her legs off the floor by using a back contraction.

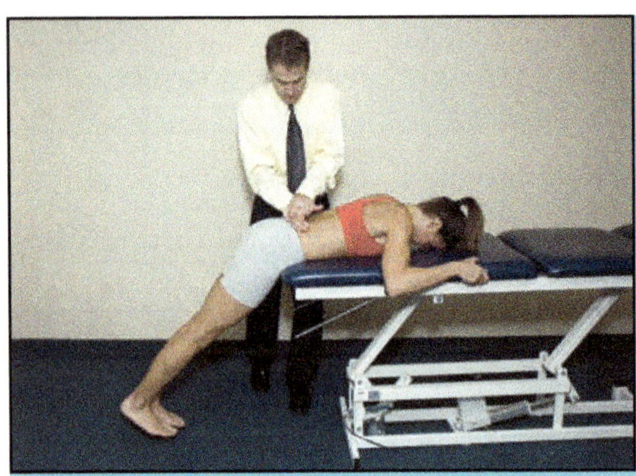

4) The examiner maintains the PA force to the low back.

5) A positive test is reduction of painful symptoms (as applied during the PA) during raising of the patient's legs.

UTILITY SCORE 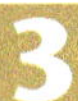

Study	Reliability	Sensitivity	Specificity	LR+	LR−	QUADAS Score (0–14)
Fritz et al.[12]	.69 kappa	61	57	1.41	0.69	12
Comments: The test has poor diagnostic value but has been used in a clinical prediction rule for detecting lumbar instability.						

TESTS FOR RADIOGRAPHIC INSTABILITY OF THE SPINE

Specific Spine Torsion Test

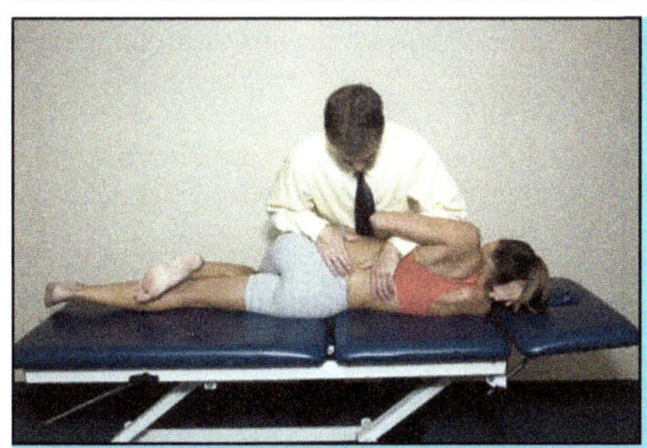

1. The patient is asked to lie on his or her side and is positioned at 60 degrees of hip flexion and approximately 90 degrees of knee flexion (top leg).
2. The examiner uses his or her forearm to take up the slack in the hip and his or her finger to loop underneath the spinous process of S1.

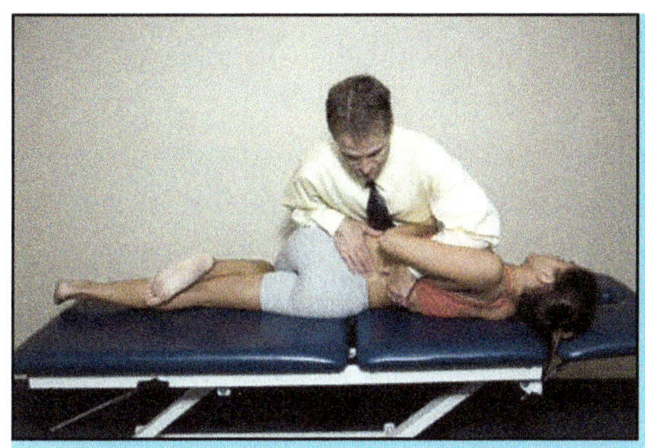

3. Using the force of the examiner's forearm placed on the side of the rib cage and gently applying a force on L5 toward the treatment table with his or her thumb, the examiner applies a distraction moment at the L5–S1 facet.
4. The force is in a diagonal to emphasize the direction of the facets.
5. Excessive movement, pain, or gapping should be noted as, ideally, rotation is minimal in nature.
6. Progress cephalically and perform the same procedure for L4–L5.
7. A positive test is reproduction of the patient's pain and/or hypermobility during torsion testing.

UTILITY SCORE 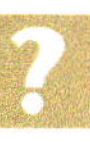

Study	Reliability	Sensitivity	Specificity	LR+	LR−	QUADAS Score (0–14)
Cook et al.[8]	NT	NT	NT	NA	NA	NT
Comments: The Specific Spine Torsion test is untested.						

TESTS FOR RADIOGRAPHIC INSTABILITY OF THE SPINE

Prone Torsion Instability Test

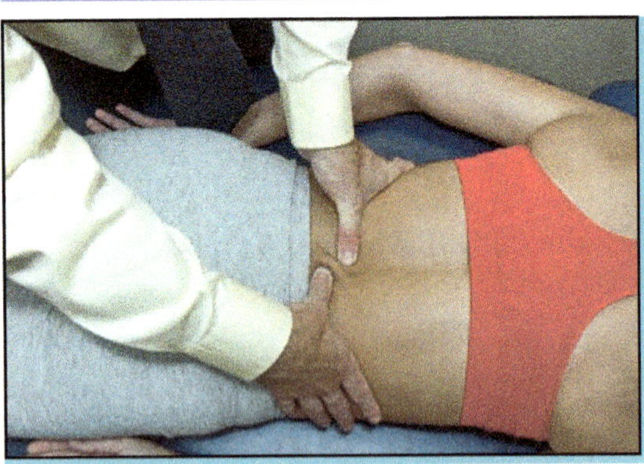

1) The patient should lie prone on a firm but comfortable surface.

2) The examiner uses his or her thumbs to palpate at either side of the spinous processes: one level above, one below.

3) Concurrently, the examiner applies a medial force to both spinous processes.

4) The examiner assesses multiple levels, feeling for movement and pain provocation.

5) A positive test is reproduction of the patient's pain and/or hypermobility during torsion testing.

UTILITY SCORE

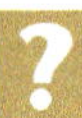

Study	Reliability	Sensitivity	Specificity	LR+	LR−	QUADAS Score (0–14)
None	NT	NT	NT	NA	NA	NT
Comments: The Prone Torsion test is untested. Because so little rotation is available at the lumbar spine, one should feel very little movement during testing.						

TESTS FOR LUMBAR SPINAL STENOSIS

Two Stage Treadmill Test

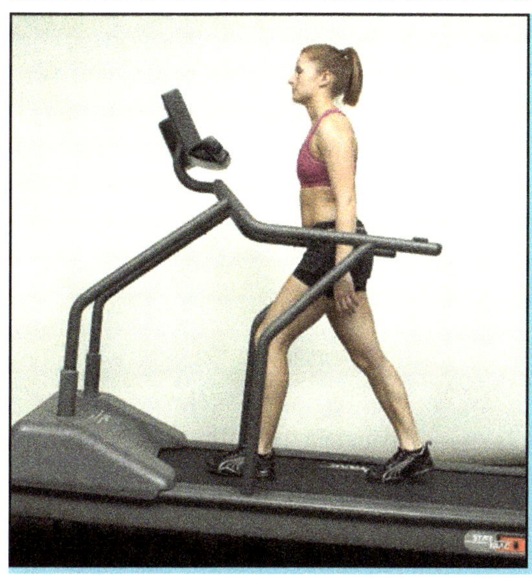

1) The patient is instructed to walk on a treadmill on a level plane for 10 minutes.

2) A 10 minute rest period is implemented. The patient is then instructed to walk on a treadmill at a 15 degree plane for 10 minutes.

3) In both cases, patients are asked to report their symptoms after each bout. Worsening after walking at a 15 degree plane is considered a positive finding.

UTILITY SCORE 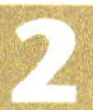

Study	Reliability	Sensitivity	Specificity	LR+	LR−	QUADAS Score (0–14)
Fritz et al.[11]	NT	50	92.3	6.49	0.54	8
Comments: The study also looked at patient history and found items such as pain relieved during sitting, better when walking with a shopping cart, and postural positions to be small predictors of change. Use caution, the study used imaging as the reference standard whereas stenosis is a clinical diagnosis.						

TESTS FOR LUMBAR SPINAL STENOSIS

Pain Relief upon Sitting

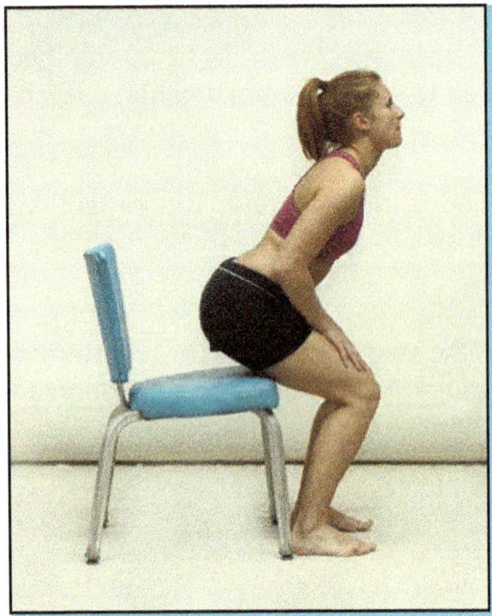

1. The patient is queried about leg pain during walking versus sitting.
2. Pain lessened during sitting is considered a positive finding for stenosis.

UTILITY SCORE 3

Study	Reliability	Sensitivity	Specificity	LR+	LR−	QUADAS Score (0–14)
Fritz et al.[11]	NT	88.5	38.9	1.5	0.29	8
Cook et al.[9]	NT	26	86	1.9	0.86	7

Comments: The Fritz et al.[11] study actually looked at a sitting position versus walking or standing, for one's "best" position. The Cook et al.[9] study actually investigated if sitting "relieved" symptoms.

Cook's Clinical Prediction Rule for Lumbar Stenosis

UTILITY SCORE 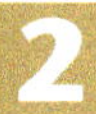

Study	Reliability	Sensitivity	Specificity	LR+	LR−	QUADAS Score (0–14)
Cook et al.[9] (less than 1 of 5 positive findings)	NT	96	20	1.2	0.19	7
Cook et al.[9] (4 of 5 positive findings)	NT	6	98	4.6	0.95	7

Comments: The five tests included in the cluster are: (1) bilateral symptoms, (2) leg pain more than back pain, (3) pain during walking/standing, (4) pain relief upon sitting, and (5) age >48 years. The low QUADAS score reflects the potential bias associated with an imaging-confirmed clinical diagnosis of lumbar stenosis. The study was retrospective and did involve nearly 1500 subjects.

TEST FOR DEGENERATIVE CHANGES IN THE SPINE

Extension Quadrant Test

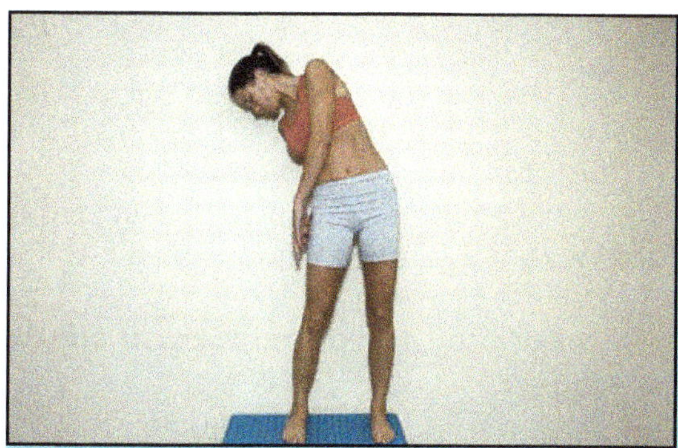

1) The patient stands with equal dispersion of weight on both legs.

2) The patient is instructed to lean back, rotate, and side-flex toward one side.

3) The movement is a combined motion of extension, rotation, and side flexion.

4) The movement is repeated to the opposite side.

5) A positive test is identified by reproduction of the patient's concordant pain.

UTILITY SCORE 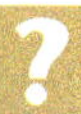

Study	Reliability	Sensitivity	Specificity	LR+	LR−	QUADAS Score (0–14)
Lyle et al.[26]	NT	70	NT	NA	NA	9
Comments: The test is commonly used to rule out the lumbar spine when differentiating between hip and lumbar spine. It is questionable whether this test is appropriate as a screen.						

TESTS FOR COMPRESSION FRACTURES

Percussion Test

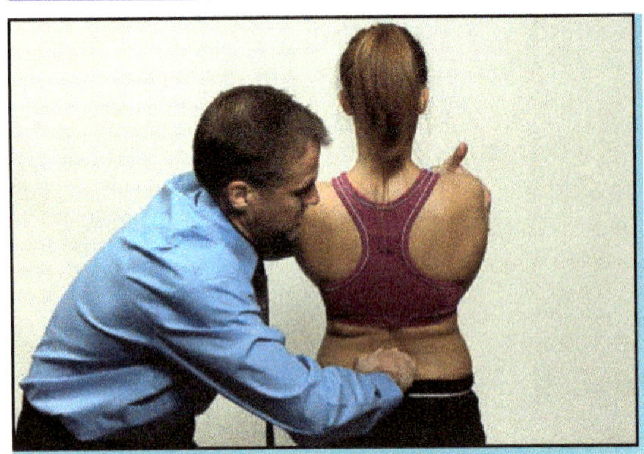

1) The patient is placed in a standing position.

2) The instructor typically stands behind the patient and uses a mirror to gauge the patient's reaction to the test (not pictured). The entire length of the spine is examined by placing a force at each level using a firm, closed fist.

3) A positive test is when the patient complains of a sharp, sudden, "fracture" pain.

UTILITY SCORE 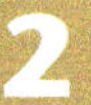

Study	Reliability	Sensitivity	Specificity	LR+	LR−	QUADAS Score (0–14)
Langdon et al.[22]	NT	87.5	90	8.8	0.14	10
Comments: One may question the specificity of this finding. The test was poorly described in the study.						

Supine Test

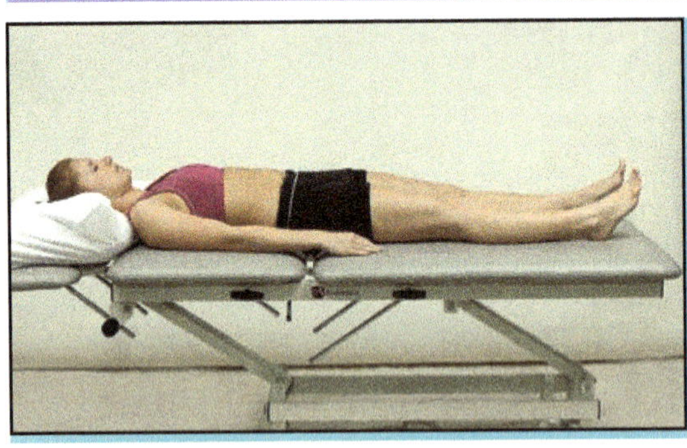

1) The patient is instructed to lie supine with only one pillow.

2) The test is positive when a patient is unable to lie supine due to severe pain in their spine.

UTILITY SCORE 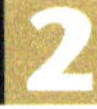

Study	Reliability	Sensitivity	Specificity	LR+	LR−	QUADAS Score (0–14)
Langdon et al.[22]	NT	81	93	11.6	0.20	10
Comments: This test also has questionable specificity.						

TESTS FOR COMPRESSION FRACTURES

Henschke's Clinical Prediction Rule for Compression Fracture

UTILITY SCORE 3

Study	Reliability	Sensitivity	Specificity	LR+	LR−	QUADAS Score (0–14)
Henschke et al.[15]	NT	38	100	218	0.62	4
Comments: A combination of findings including age > 70, significant trauma, and prolonged use of corticosteroids was used in the model. The study involved over 1000 subjects and not all individuals received the reference standard in the study.						

Roman's Clinical Prediction Rule for Compression Fracture

UTILITY SCORE 2

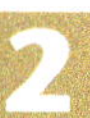

Study	Reliability	Sensitivity	Specificity	LR+	LR−	QUADAS Score (0–14)
Roman et al.[33] (1 of 5 or lower)	NT	95	34	1.4	0.16	8
Roman et al.[33] (4 of 5 or greater)	NT	37	96	9.6	0.65	8
Comments: The five items of the test involve: (1) age > 52 years, (2) no presence of leg pain, (3) body mass index < 22, (4) does not regularly exercise, and (5) female gender. The study was retrospective but involved over 1400 subjects.						

TEST FOR LUMBAR FLEXION DYSFUNCTION

Flexion Quadrant Test

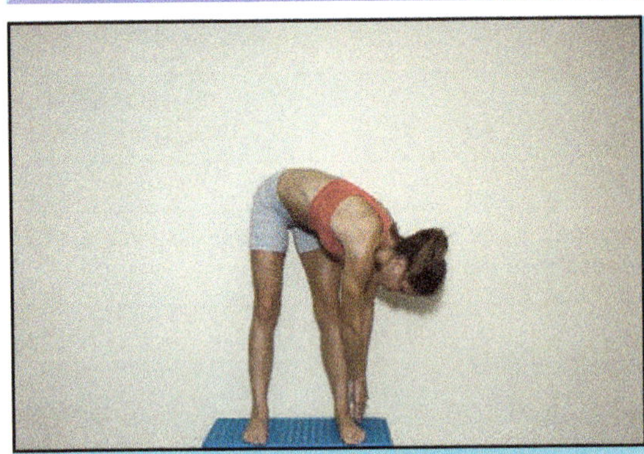

1. The patient stands with equal dispersion of weight on both legs.
2. The patient is instructed to reach forward and touch one foot with both hands.
3. The movement is a combined motion of flexion, rotation, and side flexion to one side.
4. The movement is repeated to the opposite side.
5. A positive test is identified by reproduction of the patient's concordant pain.

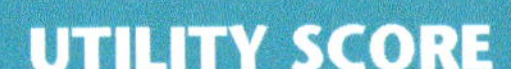

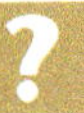

Study	Reliability	Sensitivity	Specificity	LR+	LR−	QUADAS Score (0–14)
None	NT	NT	NT	NA	NA	NA
Comments: The test is often used to rule out a disk herniation.						

Key Points

1. The majority of clinical special tests of the lumbar spine have demonstrated poor diagnostic value.
2. Tests such as the SLR and slump are somewhat sensitive but lack specificity. They are not conclusive tests for herniation of the lumbar spine.
3. Centralization is a moderately strong predictor of discogenic dysfunction.
4. Clinical special tests designed to measure instability are understudied and often lack a common reference for instability.
5. Posterior-anterior and passive physiological tests lack a common procedural standard for the index test, resulting in a variety of potential outcomes for these tests.
6. Clustering tests and measures typically improve the diagnostic capacity of the tools.

References

1. Abbott JH, McCane B, Herbison P, Moginie G, Chapple C, Hogarty T. Lumbar segmental instability: a criterion-related validity study of manual therapy assessment. *BMC Musculoskelet Disord.* 2005;6:56.
2. Albeck M. A critical assessment of clinical diagnosis of disc herniation in patients with monoradicular sciatica. *Acta Neurochir.* 1996;138:40.
3. Arab AM, Abdollahi I, Joghataei MT, Golafshani Z, Kazemnejad A. Inter- and intra-examiner reliability of single and composites of selected motion palpation and pain provocation tests for sacroiliac joint. *Man Ther.* 2009;14:213–221.
4. Bertilson BC, Bring J, Sjoblom A, Sundell K, Strender LE. Inter-examiner reliability in the assessment of low back

pain (LBP) using the Kirkaldy-Willis classification (KWC). *Eur Spine J.* 2006;1–9.

5. Binkley J, Stratford PW, Gill C. Interrater reliability of lumbar accessory motion mobility testing. *Phys Ther.* 1995;75(9):786–792.
6. Charnley J. Orthopaedic signs in the diagnosis of disc protrusion with special reference to the straight-leg raising test. *Lancet.* 1951;1:186–192.
7. Chiradejnant A, Maher CG, Latimer J. Objective manual assessment of lumbar posteroanterior stiffness is now possible. *J Manipulative Physiol Ther.* 2003;26(1):34–39.
8. Cook C, Cook A, Fleming R. Rehabilitation for clinical lumbar instability in an adolescent diver with spondylolisthesis. *J Man Manipulative Ther.* 2004;12(2):91–99.
9. Cook C, Brown C, Michael K, et al. The clinical value of a cluster of patient history and observational findings as a diagnostic support tool for lumbar spine stenosis. *Physiother Res Int.* 2010 Nov 11. doi: 10.1002/pri.500.
10. Donelson R, Aprill C, Medcalf R, Grant W. A prospective study of centralization of lumbar and referred pain. A predictor of symptomatic discs and anular competence. *Spine.* 1997;22 (10):1115–1122.
11. Fritz JM, Erhard RE, Delitto A, Welch WC, Nowakowski PE. Preliminary results of the use of a two-stage treadmill test as a clinical diagnostic tool in the differential diagnosis of lumbar spinal stenosis. *J Spinal Disord.* 1997;10:410–416.
12. Fritz JM, Piva S, Childs J. Accuracy of the clinical examination to predict radiographic instability of the lumbar spine. *Eur Spine J.* 2005;14(8):743–750.
13. Gurdijan E, Webster J, Ostrowski AZ, Hardy W, Lindner D, Thomas L. Herniated lumbar intervertebral discs: an analysis of 1176 operated cases. *J Trauma.* 1961;1:158–176.
14. Hakelius A, Hindmarsh J. The comparative reliability of preoperative diagnostic methods in lumbar disc surgery. *Acta Orthop Scand.* 1972;43:234–238.
15. Henschke N, Maher CG, Refshauge KM, Herbert RD, et al. Prevalence of and screening for serious spinal pathology in patients presenting to primary care settings with acute low back pain. *Arthritis Rheum.* 2009;60:3072–3080.
16. Kasai Y, Morishita K, Kawakita E, Kondo T, Uchida A. A new evaluation method for lumbar spinal instability: passive lumbar extension test. *Phys Ther.* 2006;86:1661–1667.
17. Kerr RSC, Cadoux-Hudson TA, Adams CBT. The value of accurate clinical assessment in the surgical management of the lumbar disc protrusion. *J Neurol Neurosurg Psychiatr.* 1988;51:169–173.
18. Knuttson B. Comparative value of electromyographic, myelographic, and clinical-neurological examinations in diagnosis of lumbar root compression syndrome. *Acta Ortho Scand.* 1961;(Suppl 49):19–49.
19. Kosteljanetz M, Bang F, Schmidt-Olsen S. The clinical significance of straight leg raising (Lasegue's sign) in the diagnosis of prolapsed lumbar disc. *Spine.* 1988;13:393–395.
20. Kosteljanetz M, Espersen O, Halaburt H, Miletic T. Predictive value of clinical and surgical findings in patients with lumbago-sciatica: a prospective study (part 1). *Acta Neurochirugica.* 1984;73:67–76.
21. Kreitz BG, Cote P, Yong-Hing K. Crossed femoral stretching test: a case report. *Spine.* 1996;21(13):1584–1586.
22. Langdon J, Way A, Heaton S, Bernard J, Molloy S. Vertebral compression fractures—new clinical signs to aid diagnosis. *Ann R Coll Surg Engl.* 2010;92:163–166.
23. Laslett M, Aprill CN, McDonald B, Oberg B. Clinical predictors of lumbar provocation discography: a study of clinical predictors of lumbar provocation discography. *Eur Spine J.* 2006;1–12.
24. Laslett M, Oberg B, Aprill CN, McDonald B. Centralization as a predictor of provocation discography results in chronic low back pain, and the influence of disability and distress on diagnostic power. *Spine J.* 2005;5(4):370–380.
25. Lauder TD, Dillingham TR, Andary MT, Kumar S, Pezzin LE, Stephens RT. Effect of history and exam in predicting electrodiagnostic outcome among patients with suspected lumbosacral radiculopathy. *Am J Phys Med Rehabil.* 2000;79:60–68.
26. Lyle MA, Manes S, McGuinness M, Ziaei S, Iversen MD. Relationship of physical examination findings and self-reported symptom severity and physical function in patients with degenerative lumbar conditions. *Phys Ther.* 2005;85(2):120–133.
27. Maher C, Adams R. Reliability of pain and stiffness assessments in clinical manual lumbar spine examination. *Phys Ther.* 1994;74(9):801–809.
28. Majlesi J, Togay H, Unalan H, Toprak S. The sensitivity and specificity of the Slump and the Straight Leg Raising tests in patients with lumbar disc herniation. *J Clin Rheumatol.* 2008;14:87–91.
29. Matyas T, Bach T. The reliability of selected techniques in clinical arthrometrics. *Aust J Physio.* 1985;31:175–199.
30. Phillips DR, Twomey LT. A comparison of manual diagnosis with a diagnosis established by a uni-level lumbar spinal block procedure. *Man Ther.* 1996;1(2):82–87.
31. Porchet F, Fankhauser H, de Tribolet N. Extreme lateral lumbar disc herniation: clinical presentation in 178 patients. *Acta Neurochir (Wien).* 1994; 127(3–4):203–209.
32. Rabin A, Gerszten PC, Karausky P, Bunker CH, Potter DM, Welch WC. The sensitivity of the seated straight-leg raise test compared with the supine straight-leg raise test in patients presenting with magnetic resonance imaging evidence of lumbar nerve root compression. *Arch Phys Med Rehabil.* 2007;88:840–843.
33. Roman M, Brown C, Richardson W, Isaacs R, Howes C, Cook C. The development of a clinical decision making algorithm for detection of osteoporotic vertebral compression fracture or wedge deformity. *J Man Manip Ther.* 2010;18:44–49.
34. Spangfort EV. The lumbar disc herniation: a computer aided analysis of 2504 operations. *Acta Orthop Scand.* 1972;11(Supl 142):1–93.

35. Schwarzer AC, Derby R, Aprill CN, Fortin J, Kine G, Bogduk N. Pain from the lumbar zygapophyseal joints: a test of two models. *J Spinal Disord.* 1994; 7:331–336.

36. Stankovic R, Johnell O, Maly P, Willner S. Use of lumbar extension, slump test, physical and neurological examination in the evaluation of patients with suspected herniated nucleus pulposus: a prospective clinical study. *Man Ther.* 1999;4(1):25–32.

37. Vroomen PC, de Krom MC, Wilmink JT, Kester AD, Knottnerus JA. Diagnostic value of history and physical examination in patients suspected of lumbosacral nerve root compression. *J Neurol Neurosurg Psychiatry.* 2002;72(5):630–634.

38. Walsh J, Hall T. Reliability, validity and diagnostic accuracy of palpation of the sciatic, tibial and common peroneal nerves in the examination of low back related leg pain. *Man Ther.* 2009;14:623–629.

PEARSON
myhealthprofessionskit™

Use this address to access the Companion Website created for this textbook. Simply select "Physical Therapy" from the choice of disciplines. Find this book and log in using your username and password to access video clips of selected tests.

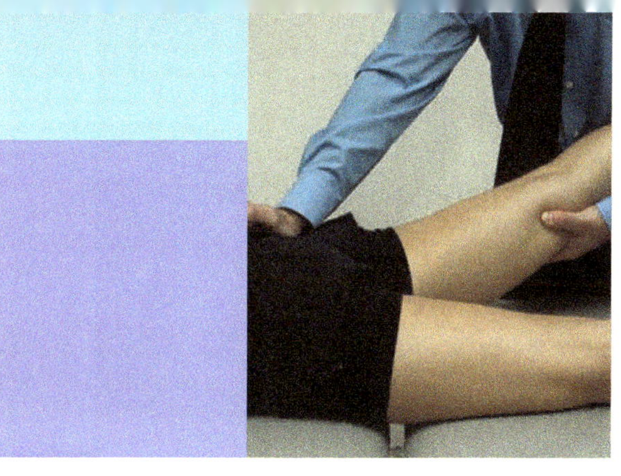

Physical Examination Tests for the Sacroiliac Joint and Pelvis

Chad E. Cook

Please refer to the chapter "Introduction to Diagnostic Accuracy" before reading this chapter.

Index of Tests

Tests for Sacroiliac Pain Origin

Thigh Thrust (also known as the Ostagaard Test, 4P Test, Sacrotuberous Stress Test, and POSH Test)
Pain Mapping
Groin Pain
Distraction Test (Gapping Test)
Compression Test
Gaenslen's Test
Sacral Thrust
Patrick's Test (also known as the FABER Test)
Mennell's Test
Resisted Hip Abduction
Fortin Finger Test
Centralization
Sacroiliac Joint Palpation
Laguere's Sign
Mazion's Pelvic Maneuver (Standing Lunge Test)
Prone Distraction Test
Torsion Stress Test
Squish Test
Passive Physiological Counternutation
Passive Physiological Nutation
Maitland Test
Cranial Shear Test
Combinations of Pain Provocation Tests
Laslett's Cluster Number One
Van der Wurff's Cluster
Laslett's Cluster Number Two
Ozgocmen's Cluster

Tests for Sacroiliac Dysfunction

Piedallus Test
Standing ASIS Asymmetry
Seated ASIS Asymmetry
Standing PSIS Asymmetry
Seated PSIS Asymmetry
Standing or Unilateral Standing
Gillet Test (Marching Test)
Sitting Bend Over Test (Sitting Forward Flexion Test)
Standing Bend Over Test (Standing Flexion Test)
Long Sit Test (Leg Length Test)
Sacral Base Position
Sacral Sulci Position
Inferior Lateral Angle Position
Medial Malleoli Position
Combinations of Palpatory Tests
Cibulka & Koldehoff's Cluster
Riddle and Freburger's Cluster
Kokmeyer et al.'s Cluster
Arab's Palpation Cluster
Arab's Pain Provocation Cluster

Tests for Sacroiliac Pain Associated with Pregnancy-Related Posterior Pelvic Pain

Active Straight Leg Raise
Prone Active Straight Leg Raise
Self-Test P4
Bridging Test
Four Point Kneeling Test
Thumb-PSIS Test (Click-Clack Test)
Heel Bank Test
Abduction Test
Long Dorsal Ligament Palpation
The Lunge
Sit to Stand
Deep Squat
Step Up Test
Cook's Cluster Number 1
Cook's Cluster Number 2
Cook's Cluster Number 3
Cook's Cluster Number 4
Cook's Cluster Number 5

Test for Motor Control Dysfunction

Stork Test

Test for Symphysiolysis

Pubic Symphysis Palpation
Resisted Hip Adduction

Tests for Pelvic Ring Fracture

Posterior Pelvic Palpation
Hip Flexion Test
Pubic Compression Test
AP and Lateral Compression Test
Active Hip Range of Motion

Test for Bursitis, Tumor, or Abscess of the Buttock Region

Sign of the Buttock

TESTS FOR SACROILIAC PAIN ORIGIN

Thigh Thrust (also known as the Ostagaard Test, 4P Test, Sacrotuberous Stress Test, and POSH Test)

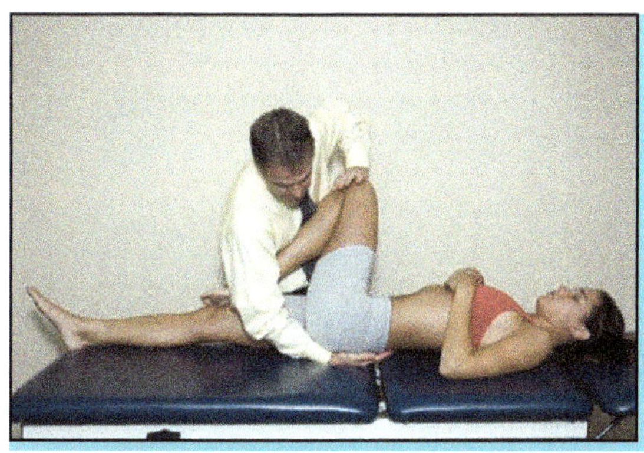

1) The patient is positioned in supine. Resting symptoms are assessed.
2) The examiner stands opposite the painful side of the patient.
3) The hip on the painful side is flexed to 90 degrees.

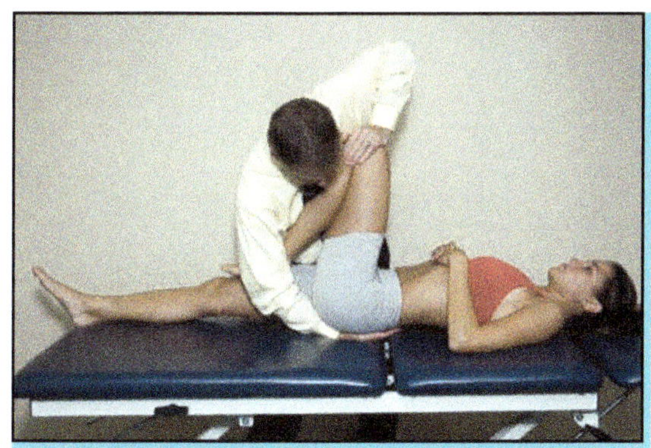

4) The examiner places his or her hand under the sacrum to form a stable "bridge" for the sacrum.
5) A downward pressure is applied through the femur to force a posterior translation of the innominate. The patient's symptoms are assessed to determine if they are concordant.
6) A positive test is concordant pain that is posterior to the hip or near the sacroiliac joint. A positive test requires reproduction of pain on the thrust side (the side of the loaded femur).

UTILITY SCORE 2

Study	Reliability	Sensitivity	Specificity	LR+	LR−	QUADAS Score (0–14)
Laslett & Williams[25]	0.82	NT	NT	NA	NA	NA
Dreyfuss et al.[13]	0.64	36	50	0.72	1.28	10
Kokmeyer et al.[23]	0.67	NT	NT	NA	NA	NA
Damen et al.[11]	NT	62	72	2.2	0.53	8
Ostagaard & Andersson[36]	NT	80	81	4.21	0.25	5
Broadhurst & Bond[6]	NT	80	100	NA	NA	9
Albert et al.[1]	0.70	84–93*	98	46.5	0.07–0.16	7
Laslett et al.[24]	NT	88	69	2.8	0.17	12
Arab et al.[2]	0.60 right 0.40 left	NT	NT	NA	NA	NA
Ozgocmen et al.[37*] (Right)	NT	55	70	1.91	0.62	10
Ozgocmen et al.[37*] (Left)	NT	45	86	3.29	0.63	10
Gutke et al.[18]	NT	88	89	8.0	0.13	7

Comments: One of the few sacroiliac tests that exhibits fair sensitivity. To accurately perform the test make sure the thigh is held in neutral adduction and at 90 degrees of flexion.

*Ozgocmen et al.[37] assessed patients with acute sacroilitis.

TESTS FOR SACROILIAC PAIN ORIGIN

Pain Mapping

1) During the patient history, the patient identifies a specific pain referral pattern.

2) A positive test is representative of pain in the "sacroiliac pain pattern" of unilateral buttock pain below the level of L5, in the absence of midline pain.

UTILITY SCORE 2

Study	Reliability	Sensitivity	Specificity	LR+	LR−	QUADAS Score (0–14)
Slipman et al.[42] (Lower Lumbar and Buttock	NT	30	NT	NA	NA	6
Slipman et al.[42] (Buttock Alone)	NT	12	NT	NA	NA	6
Slipman et al.[42] (Lower Lumbar, Buttock, and Thigh)	NT	10	NT	NA	NA	6
Slipman et al.[42] (Lower Lumbar, Buttock, Thigh, and Leg)	NT	10	NT	NA	NA	6
Slipman et al.[42] (Lower Lumbar Alone)	NT	6	NT	NA	NA	6
Slipman et al.[42] (Buttock and Thigh)	NT	4	NT	NA	NA	6
Slipman et al.[42] (Buttock, Groin, and Thigh)	NT	4	NT	NA	NA	6
Slipman et al.[42] (Buttock, Thigh, Leg, Ankle, and Foot)	NT	4	NT	NA	NA	6
Slipman et al.[42] (Buttock and Leg)	NT	2	NT	NA	NA	6
Slipman et al.[42] (Lower Lumbar, Buttock, and Groin)	NT	2	NT	NA	NA	6
Comments: It appears the referral pattern of sacroiliac pain is variable and lacks sensitivity (primarily if targeting only one location) and should never be used in isolation. However, it's worth noting that there are a number of locations in which SIJ pain can refer.						

Groin Pain

1) During the patient interview, the patient identifies a referred pain pattern that includes the groin.

2) A positive test is identified by pain reported in the groin.

UTILITY SCORE 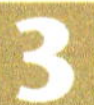

Study	Reliability	Sensitivity	Specificity	LR+	LR−	QUADAS Score (0–14)
Dreyfuss et al.[13]	.70	19	63	.09	1.3	10
Slipman et al.[42] (Any Variation of Groin Pain)	NT	14	NT	NA	NA	6
Comments: This finding appears to be neither sensitive nor specific for sacroiliac pain.						

TESTS FOR SACROILIAC PAIN ORIGIN

Distraction Test (Gapping Test)

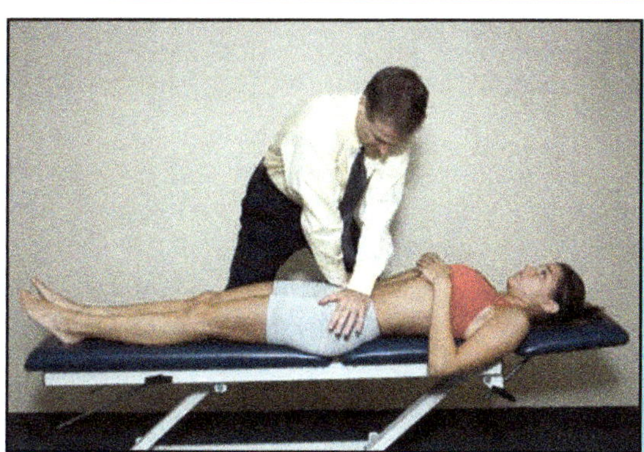

1) The patient assumes a supine position. Resting symptoms are assessed.

2) The medial aspect of both anterior superior iliac spines are palpated by the examiner. The examiner crosses his or her arms, creating an X at the forearms, and a force is applied in a lateral-posterior direction. For comfort, it is often required that the examiner relocate his or her hands on the anterior superior iliac spine (ASIS) several times.

3) The examiner holds the position for 30 seconds, then applies a vigorous force repeatedly in an attempt to reproduce the concordant sign of the patient.

4) A positive test is reproduction of the concordant sign of the patient.

UTILITY SCORE 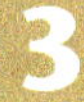

Study	Reliability	Sensitivity	Specificity	LR+	LR−	QUADAS Score (0–14)
Blower & Griffin[4]	63% agreement	NT	89	NA	NA	5
Russell et al.[41]	NT	11	90	1.1	0.98	5
Laslett & Williams[25]	0.69	NT	NT	NA	NA	NA
McCombe et al.[31]	0.36	NT	NT	NA	NA	NA
Kokmeyer et al.[23]	0.46	NT	NT	NA	NA	NA
Albert et al.[1]	0.84	04–14	100	NA	NA	7
Laslett et al.[24]	NT	60	81	3.2	0.5	12
Ham et al.[19*]	NT	50	74	1.9	0.67	10
Potter & Rothstein[38]	94% agreement	NT	NT	NA	NA	NA
Ozgocmen et al.[37**]	NT	23	81	1.24	0.94	10

Comments: Of the many sacroiliac tests, the Distraction test is considered to have fair reliability and moderate specificity. Does not appear to be a strong test when used alone.

*Ham et al.[19] used the Distraction test as a measure for pelvis fracture.

**Ozgocmen et al.[37] assessed patients with acute sacroilitis.

TESTS FOR SACROILIAC PAIN ORIGIN

Compression Test

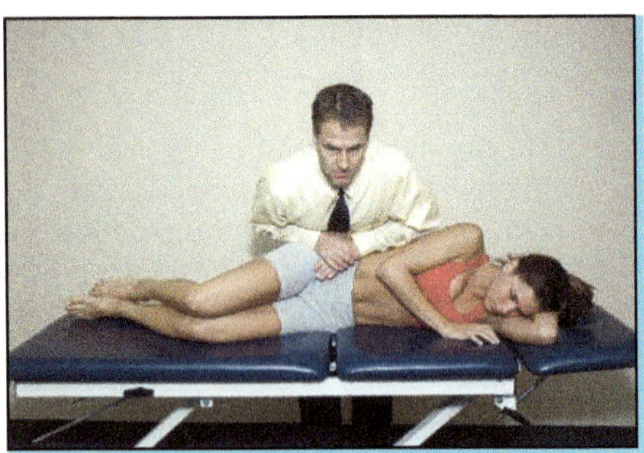

1. The patient assumes a sidelying position with his or her painful side up superior to the plinth. Resting symptoms are assessed.
2. The examiner then cups the iliac crest of the painful side and applies a downward force through the ilium. This position is held for 30 seconds. As with the other sacroiliac tests, considerable vigor is required to reproduce the symptoms; in some cases, repeated force is necessary.
3. A positive test is reproduction of the concordant sign of the patient.

UTILITY SCORE 

Study	Reliability	Sensitivity	Specificity	LR+	LR−	QUADAS Score (0–14)
Blower & Griffin[4]	64% agreement	NT	100	NA	NA	5
Russell et al.[41]	NT	7	90	0.7	1.03	5
Kokmeyer et al.[23]	0.57	NT	NT	NA	NA	NA
Strender et al.[43]	0.26	NT	NT	NA	NA	NA
Laslett & Williams[25]	0.77	NT	NT	NA	NA	NA
McCombe et al.[31]	0.16	NT	NT	NA	NA	NA
Albert et al.[1]	0.79	25–38	100	NA	NA	7
Laslett et al.[24]	NT	69	69	2.2	0.4	12
Ham et al.[19*]	NT	60	63	1.6	.63	10
Potter & Rothstein[38]	76% agreement	NT	NT	NA	NA	NA
Ozgocmen et al.[37**] (Right)	NT	22	83	1.37	0.92	10
Ozgocmen et al.[37] (Left)	NT	27	93	3.95	0.78	10

Comments: The test has fair reliability and fair specificity. However, the sensitivity is low to fair and the test should not be considered a screen. Does not appear to be a strong test when used alone.
*Ham et al.[19] used the test as a measure of pelvis fracture.
**Ozgocmen et al.[37] assessed patients with acute sacroilitis.

TESTS FOR SACROILIAC PAIN ORIGIN

Gaenslen's Test

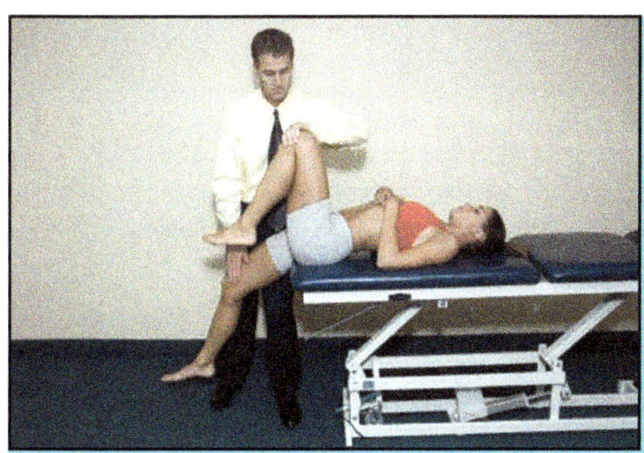

1) The patient is positioned in supine with the painful leg resting very near the end of the treatment table. Resting symptoms are assessed.

2) The examiner sagitally raises the nonpainful side of the hip (with the knee bent) up to 90 degrees. Test both sides if the patient complains of pain bilaterally.

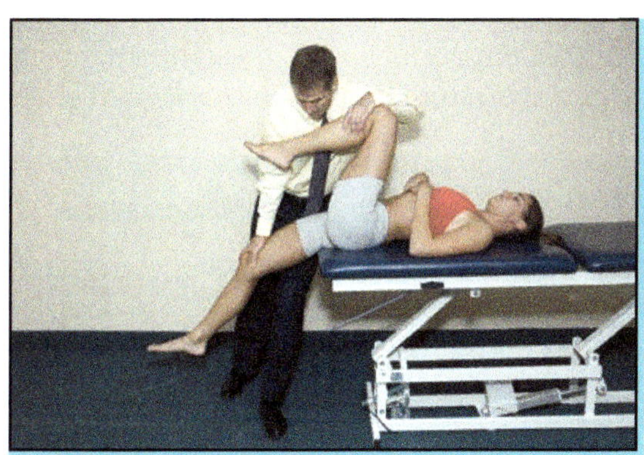

3) A downward force (up to 6 bouts) is applied to the lower leg (painful side) while a flexion-based counterforce is applied to the flexed leg (pushing the leg in the opposite direction). The effect causes a torque to the pelvis. Concordant symptoms are assessed.

4) The test is positive if the torque reproduces pain of the concordant sign.

UTILITY SCORE 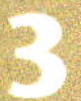

Study	Reliability	Sensitivity	Specificity	LR+	LR−	QUADAS Score (0–14)
Laslett & Williams[25]	0.72	NT	NT	NA	NA	NA
Dreyfuss et al.[13]	0.61	71	26	1.02	1.11	10
Kokmeyer et al.[23]	0.60	NT	NT	NA	NA	NA
Laslett et al.[24] (Right)	NT	53	71	1.8	0.66	12
Laslett et al.[24] (Left)	NT	50	77	2.2	0.65	12
Ozgocmen et al.[37*] (Right)	NT	44	80	2.29	0.68	10
Ozgocmen et al.[37*] (Left)	NT	36	75	1.5	0.83	10

Comments: Occasionally, the test is required on both sides to determine pain. This test demonstrates poor diagnostic value secondary to poor to fair specificity. It should not be used as a stand-alone test.
*Ozgocmen et al.[37] assessed patients with acute sacroilitis.

TESTS FOR SACROILIAC PAIN ORIGIN

Sacral Thrust

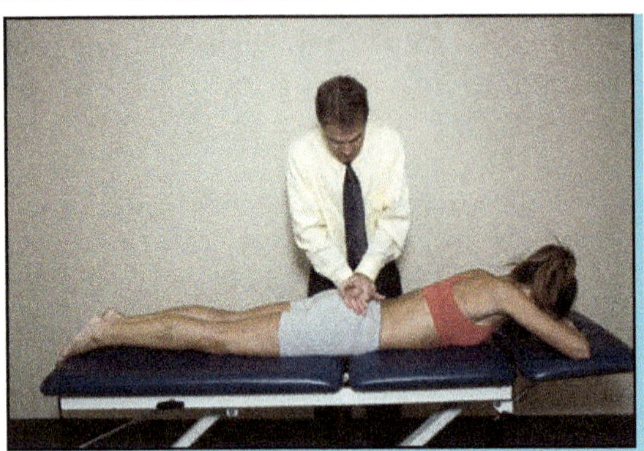

1. The patient lies in a prone position. Resting symptoms are assessed.
2. The examiner palpates the second or third spinous process of the sacrum. Using the pisiform the examiner places a downward pressure on the sacrum at S3. By targeting the midpoint of the sacrum, the examiner is less likely to force the lumbar spine into hyperextension.
3. Vigorously and repeatedly (up to 6 thrusts), the examiner applies a strong downward force to the sacrum in an attempt to reproduce the concordant sign of the patient.
4. A positive test is a reproduction of the concordant sign during downward pressure.

UTILITY SCORE 2

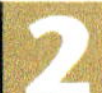

Study	Reliability	Sensitivity	Specificity	LR+	LR−	QUADAS Score (0–14)
Laslett & Williams[25]	0.32	NT	NT	NA	NA	NA
Dreyfuss et al.[13]	0.30	53	29	0.74	1.62	10
Laslett et al.[24]	NT	63	75	2.5	.49	12
Blower & Griffin[4]	64% agreement	NT	86	NA	NA	5
Ozgocmen et al.[37*] (Right)	NT	33	74	1.29	0.89	10
Ozgocmen et al.[37*] (Left)	NT	45	89	4.39	0.60	10

Comments: It is imperative not to push the lumbar spine into extension; otherwise, the test specificity will be artificially reduced. In isolation, the test provides only marginal diagnostic value. The test demonstrates a wide range of values.

*Ozgocmen et al.[37] assessed patients with acute sacroilitis.

TESTS FOR SACROILIAC PAIN ORIGIN

Patrick's Test (also known as the FABER Test)

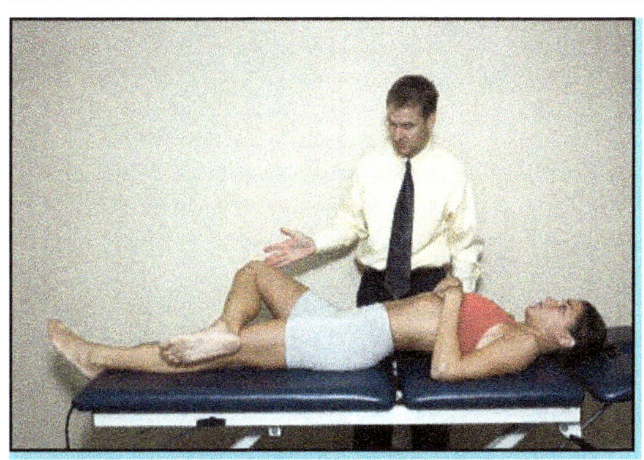

1) The patient is positioned in supine. Resting symptoms are assessed.

2) The painful side leg is placed in a "figure four" position. The ankle is placed just above the knee of the other leg.

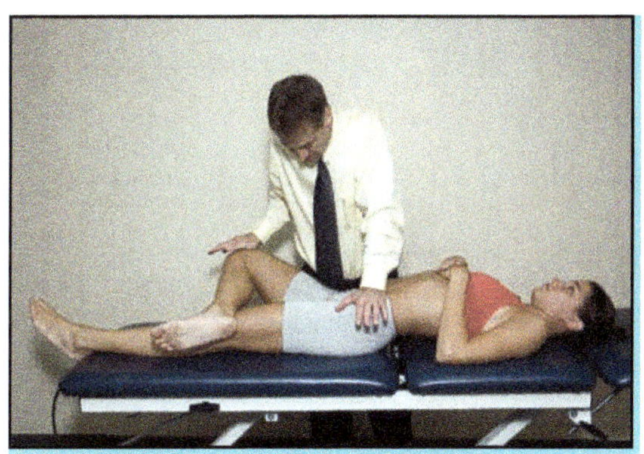

3) The examiner provides a gentle downward pressure on both the knee of the painful side and the ASIS of the non-painful side.

4) Concordant pain is assessed, specifically the location and type of pain.

UTILITY SCORE 

Study	Reliability	Sensitivity	Specificity	LR+	LR−	QUADAS Score (0–14)
Dreyfuss et al.[13]	0.62	69	16	0.82	1.94	10
Van Deursen et al.[46]	0.38	NT	NT	NA	NA	NA
Broadhurst & Bond[6]	NT	77	100	NA	NA	9
Albert et al.[1]	0.54	40–70	99	41	0.58–0.60	7
Hansen et al.[20] (Piriformis)	NT	48	77	2.1	0.68	7
Rost et al.[40] (One-Side Positive) (PPPP)	NT	36	NT	NA	NA	7
Rost et al.[40] (Two-Sides Positive) (PPPP)	NT	36	NT	NA	NA	7
Arab et al.[2]	0.44 right 0.49 left	NT	NT	NA	NA	NA
Ozgocmen et al.[37*] (Right)	NT	66	51	1.37	0.64	10
Ozgocmen et al.[37*] (Left)	NT	54	62	1.43	0.73	10

Comments: The wide range of values are likely reflective of the variety of patients used in each study and the bias that results. For sacroiliac pain, the chief complaint is typically posterior. The test is also used to assess hip dysfunction, although the location of pain is different between sacroiliac dysfunction and hip pain.

*Ozgocmen et al.[37] assessed patients with acute sacroilitis.

TESTS FOR SACROILIAC PAIN ORIGIN

Mennell's Test

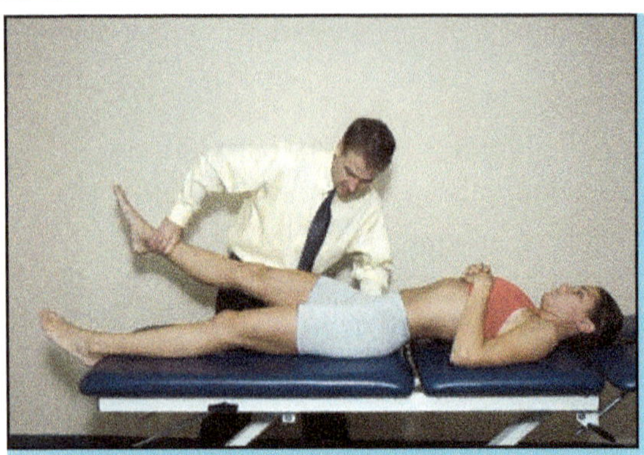

1) The patient is supine.

2) The patient moves one leg into 30 degrees abduction and 10 degrees of flexion of the hip joint.

3) The examiner pushes the lower leg into and then away from the pelvis in a sagittal motion (extension then flexion).

4) A positive test is reproduction of concordant symptoms.

UTILITY SCORE 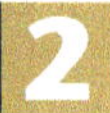

Study	Reliability	Sensitivity	Specificity	LR+	LR−	QUADAS Score (0–14)
Albert et al.[1]	.87	.54–.70	100	Inf	NA	7
Ozgocmen et al.[37*] (Right)	NT	66	80	3.44	0.41	10
Ozgocmen et al.[37*] (Left)	NT	45	86	3.29	0.63	10

Comments: Weakness is not considered a positive finding.
*Ozgocmen et al.[37] assessed patients with acute sacroilitis.

Resisted Hip Abduction

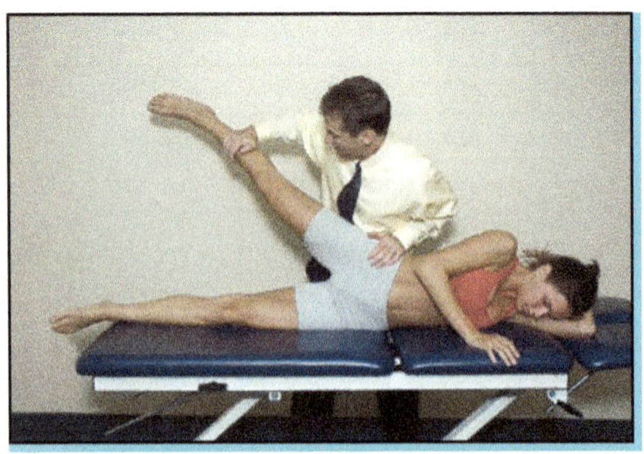

1) The patient is placed in a sidelying position.

2) The examiner fully extends the hip and places the hip at 30 degrees of abduction.

3) The examiner applies a force medially while the patient counters the force by lateral pressure (movement into abduction).

4) Reproduction of pain in the cephalic aspect of the sacro-iliac joint is considered positive.

TESTS FOR SACROILIAC PAIN ORIGIN

UTILITY SCORE 2

Study	Reliability	Sensitivity	Specificity	LR+	LR−	QUADAS Score (0–14)
Broadhurst & Bond[6]	NT	87	100	Inf	NA	9
Arab et al.[2]	0.78 right 0.50 left	NT	NT	NA	NA	NA
Cook et al.[10]	NT	33	83	2.0	0.80	11
Comments: Weakness is not considered a positive finding. There appears to be some value in this test.						

Fortin Finger Test

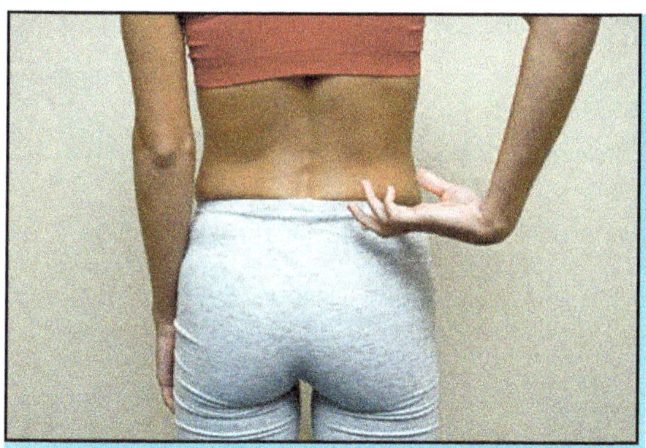

1) The patient completes a pain diagram.

2) The patient is instructed to point to the region of pain with one finger.

3) The examiner reviews the area of pain and the pain diagram for consistency.

4) The patient is requested to repeat the procedure of pointing to his or her pain.

5) A positive test is identified by (1) the patient could localize the pain with one finger, (2) the area pointed to was within 1 cm of, and immediately inferomedial to, the posterior superior iliac spine, and (3) the patient consistently pointed to the same area over at least two trials.

UTILITY SCORE 2

Study	Reliability	Sensitivity	Specificity	LR+	LR−	QUADAS Score (0–14)
Fortin & Falco[16]	NT	100	NT	NA	NA	5
Dreyfuss et al.[13]	.81% agreement	76	47	.09	1.3	10
Comments: This test was poorly performed by Fortin & Falco[16], and no mention of referred pain is made for the Fortin Finger Test. This test may be useful in ruling out SIJ pain.						

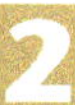

TESTS FOR SACROILIAC PAIN ORIGIN

Centralization

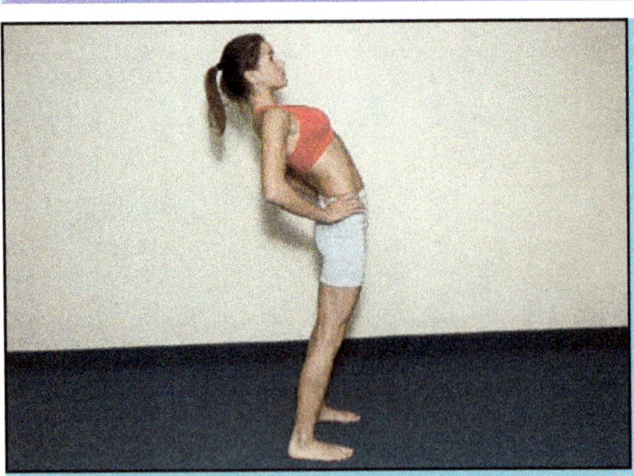

1) The patient either stands or lies prone depending on the intent of a loaded or unloaded assessment.

2) Multiple directions of repeated end-range lumbar testing is targeted. Movements may include extension, flexion, or side flexion.

3) Movements are repeated for 5 to 20 attempts until a definite centralization or peripheralization occurs.

4) A positive finding is centralization of symptoms and is generally considered a low back dysfunction.

UTILITY SCORE 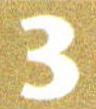

Study	Reliability	Sensitivity	Specificity	LR+	LR−	QUADAS Score (0–14)
Young et al.[50]	NT	9	79	.42	1.2	10
Comments: Centralization is defined as the progressive retreat of referred pain toward the midline of the back in response to standardized movement testing during evaluation of the effect of repeated movements on pain location and intensity. The test is sometimes used to rule out the presence of SIJ dysfunction, as the test exhibits strong diagnostic value for lumbar spine dysfunction.						

Sacroiliac Joint Palpation

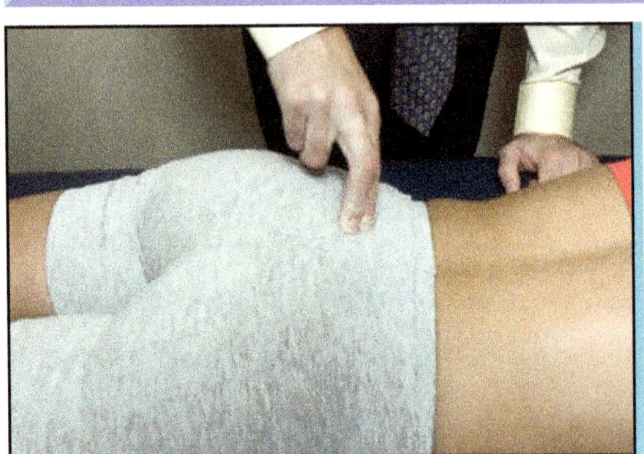

1) The patient is placed in a prone position.

2) The examiner carefully palpates the sacrum, bilateral sacroiliac joints, and surrounding ligaments and muscles.

3) A positive test is associated with local tenderness with moderately deep palpation.

TESTS FOR SACROILIAC PAIN ORIGIN

UTILITY SCORE 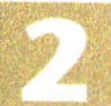

Study	Reliability	Sensitivity	Specificity	LR+	LR−	QUADAS Score (0–14)
Hansen et al.[20] (Sacroiliac Joint)	NT	86	92	10.8	0.15	7
Hansen et al.[20] (Sacrotuberous Ligament)	NT	33	86	2.4	0.78	7
Hansen et al.[20] (Piriformis)	NT	62	97	20.7	0.39	7
Hansen et al.[20] (Paravertebral Muscles)	NT	43	84	2.7	0.68	7
Hansen et al.[20] (Glutei Muscles)	NT	33	97	11	0.69	7
Hansen et al.[20] (Iliopsoas)	NT	43	81	2.26	0.7	7
Albert et al.[1] (Long Dorsal Ligament)	.34 kappa	11 to 49	100	NA	NA	7
Dreyfuss et al.[12]	NT	95	9	1.04	0.55	10

Comments: A positive test is identified by reproduction of the patient's concordant pain during palpation of the long dorsal ligament, surrounding sacroiliac ligaments, or other related structures. Regarding Dreyfuss et al.'s[12] findings, the test may be useful as an initial screen. This test deserves further study and better designs.

Laguere's Sign

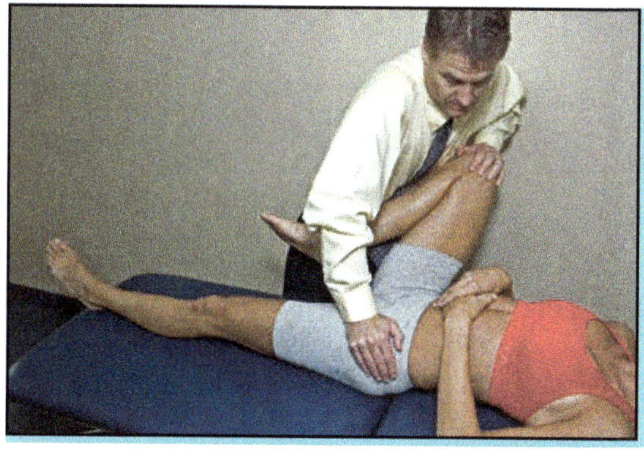

1) The patient is placed in a supine position.

2) The examiner applies a passive force into flexion, abduction, and external rotation at the hip. Overpressure is applied in this position.

3) The examiner stabilizes the opposite side by applying a downward force on the pelvis.

4) A positive test was replication of concordant symptoms during the testing.

UTILITY SCORE 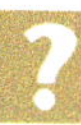

Study	Reliability	Sensitivity	Specificity	LR+	LR−	QUADAS Score (0–14)
Magee[30]	NT	NT	NT	NA	NA	NA

Comments: Expect to see many false positives in patients with hip pathology.

TESTS FOR SACROILIAC PAIN ORIGIN

Mazion's Pelvic Maneuver (Standing Lunge Test)

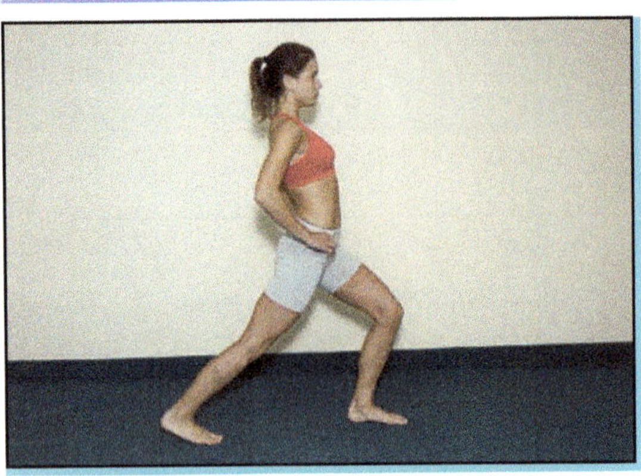

1) The patient stands in a straddle position with the unaffected side forward. The feet need to be 2–3 feet apart (pictured).

2) The patient bends forward in an attempt to touch the floor until the heel of the rear foot rises.

3) If pain is reproduced on the affected side, the test is considered positive.

UTILITY SCORE 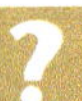

Study	Reliability	Sensitivity	Specificity	LR+	LR−	QUADAS Score (0–14)
Evans[14]	NT	NT	NT	NA	NA	NA
Comments: Essentially, this is a test of torque on the affected (rear) side.						

Prone Distraction Test

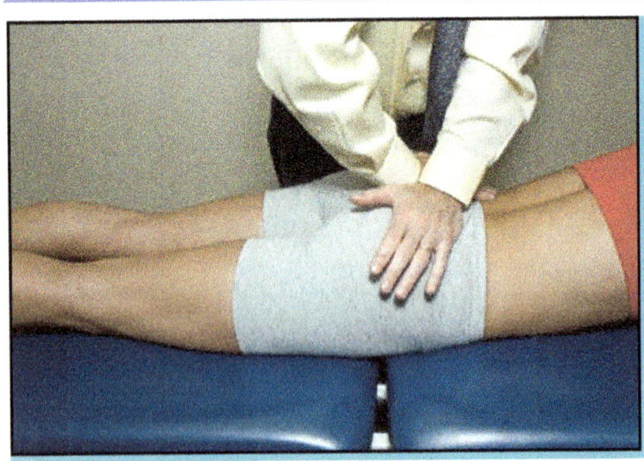

1) The patient assumes a prone position.

2) The examiner applies a compressive force over the PSIS of the patient.

3) Reproduction of concordant symptoms is considered a positive test.

UTILITY SCORE 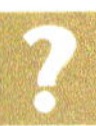

Study	Reliability	Sensitivity	Specificity	LR+	LR−	QUADAS Score (0–14)
Not tested	NT	NT	NT	NA	NA	NA
Comments: An uninvestigated test.						

TESTS FOR SACROILIAC PAIN ORIGIN

Torsion Stress Test

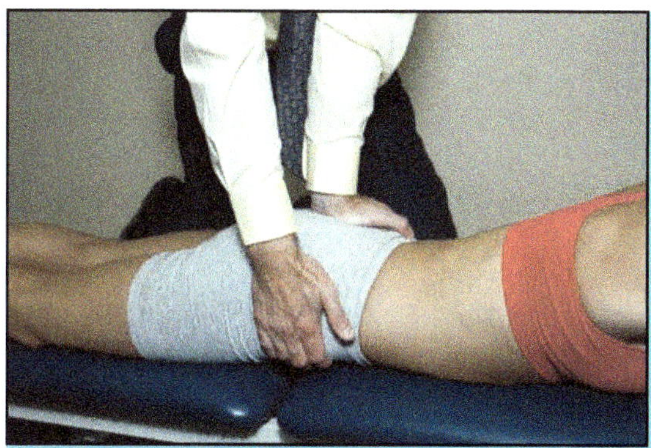

1) The patient assumes a prone position.

2) The examiner applies a downward force on the sacrum and pulls upward on the ASIS.

3) A positive test is pain reproduction during the torsion movement.

UTILITY SCORE 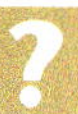

Study	Reliability	Sensitivity	Specificity	LR+	LR−	QUADAS Score (0–14)
Not tested	NT	NT	NT	NA	NA	NA
Comments: The position is sometimes used for manipulation of the sacroiliac joint.						

Squish Test

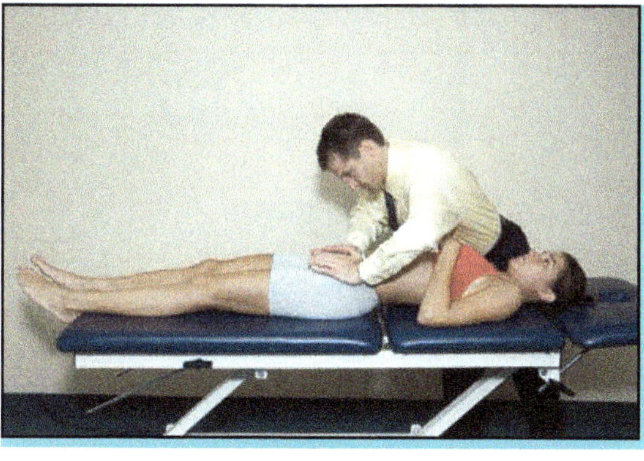

1) The patient assumes a supine position.

2) The examiner places both hands on the ASIS.

3) The examiner applies a downward and medial force on the ASIS.

4) Reproduction of concordant pain is considered a positive sign.

UTILITY SCORE 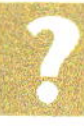

Study	Reliability	Sensitivity	Specificity	LR+	LR−	QUADAS Score (0–14)
Magee[30]	NT	NT	NT	NA	NA	NA
Comments: The test position is sometimes used during mobilization of the ilium on the sacrum.						

TESTS FOR SACROILIAC PAIN ORIGIN

Passive Physiological Counternutation

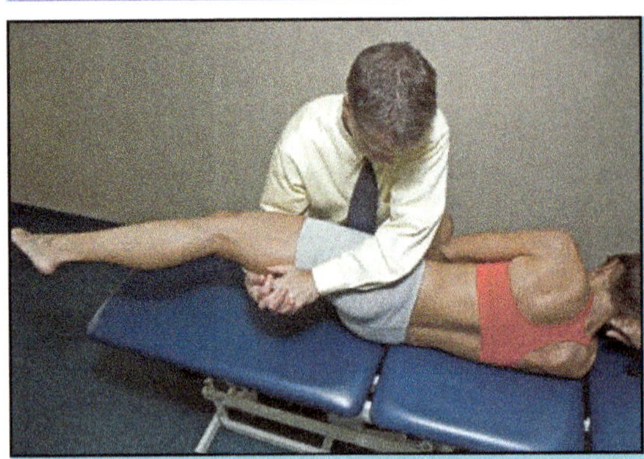

1) The patient assumes a sidelying position, the painful side up. Resting symptoms are assessed.

2) The painful sided leg is extended and the plinth side leg is flexed to 90 degrees. The motion is the mirror image of passive physiological nutation.

3) The examiner cradles the leg with the caudal side hand and encourages further movement into hip extension. The cranial side arm is placed on the PSIS and promotes anterior rotation of the innominate.

4) The patient's pelvis is passively moved to the first sign of concordant pain.

5) The examiner then moves the patient beyond the first point of pain toward end-range. The patient's symptoms are reassessed for concordance.

6) If concordant pain is bilateral, the process is repeated on the opposite side.

UTILITY SCORE 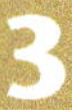

Study	Reliability	Sensitivity	Specificity	LR+	LR−	QUADAS Score (0–14)
Cook et al.[10]	NT	27	83	1.6	0.88	12
Comments: The test position is also sometimes used as a treatment if pain recedes during movement. For Cook et al.'s[10] study, both nutation and counternutation movements were combined.						

TESTS FOR SACROILIAC PAIN ORIGIN

Passive Physiological Nutation

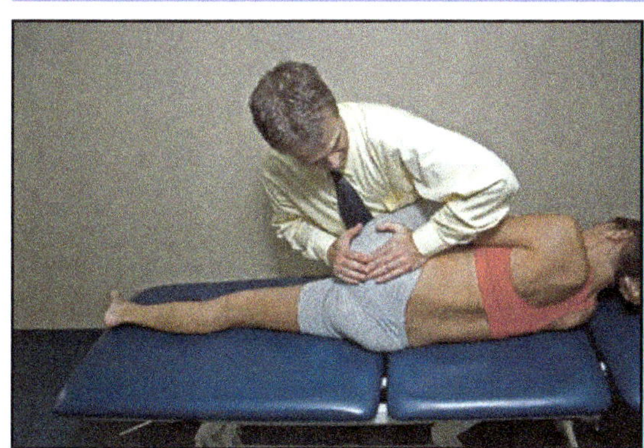

1) The patient assumes a sidelying position, the painful side up. Resting symptoms are assessed.

2) The painful-sided leg is flexed beyond 90 degrees to engage the pelvis and to promote passive physiological flexion.

3) The examiner then situates his or her body into the popliteal fold of the painful-sided leg to "snug up" the position. The plinth-sided leg remains in an extended position.

4) The examiner then places his or her hands on the ischial tuberosity and the ASIS to promote further physiological rotation. The patient's pelvis is passively moved to the first sign of concordant pain.

5) The examiner then moves the patient beyond the first point of pain toward end-range. The patient's symptoms are reassessed for concordance.

6) If concordant pain is bilateral, the process is repeated on the opposite side.

UTILITY SCORE 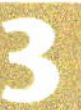

Study	Reliability	Sensitivity	Specificity	LR+	LR−	QUADAS Score (0–14)
Cook et al.[10]	27	83	1.6	0.88	NA	NT
Comments: The test position is also sometimes used as a treatment if pain recedes during movement. For Cook et al.'s[10] study, both nutation and counternutation movements were combined.						

TESTS FOR SACROILIAC PAIN ORIGIN

Maitland Test

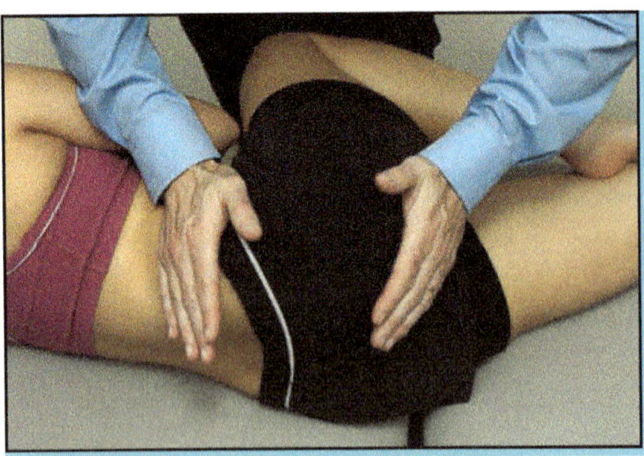

1) The patient assumes a sidelying position. The clinician rotates the targeted innominate posteriorly, passively.

2) A positive test is identified by pain reported during the rotation.

UTILITY SCORE 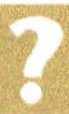

Study	Reliability	Sensitivity	Specificity	LR+	LR−	QUADAS Score (0–14)
None	NT	NT	NT	NA	NA	NA
Comments: It is highly unlikely that the vigor necessary to provoke pain will be substantial enough using this test.						

Cranial Shear Test

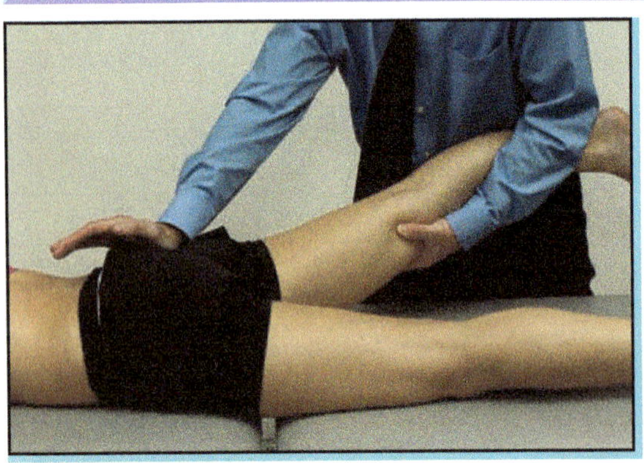

1) The patient assumes a prone position.

2) The examiner applies a pressure to the sacrum near the coccygeal end, directed cranially.

3) The examiner applies a counter force in the form of a traction to the leg.

4) A positive test involves pain.

UTILITY SCORE 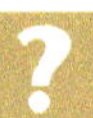

Study	Reliability	Sensitivity	Specificity	LR+	LR−	QUADAS Score (0–14)
Cattley et al.[8]	NT	NT	NT	NA	NA	NA
Comments: This test has been mentioned a number of times in texts but to our knowledge has not been studied.						

TESTS FOR SACROILIAC PAIN ORIGIN

Combinations of Pain Provocation Tests

Laslett's Cluster Number One

Thigh Thrust, Distraction Test, Sacral Thrust, and Compression Test

UTILITY SCORE 

Study	Reliability	Sensitivity	Specificity	LR+	LR−	QUADAS Score (0–14)
Laslett et al.[24] (2 of 4)	NT	88	78	4.00	0.16	12
Comments: Well designed study in which patients with low back pain were removed from the sample. One should consider using the Thigh Thrust and the Distraction tests first.						

Van der Wurff's Cluster

Distraction Test, Compression Test, Thigh Thrust, Patrick Sign, Gaenslen's Test

UTILITY SCORE 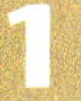

Study	Reliability	Sensitivity	Specificity	LR+	LR−	QUADAS Score (0–14)
Van der Wurff et al.[45] (3 of 5)	NT	85	79	4.02	0.19	12
Comments: Another well designed study in which the FABER test (Patrick sign) can substitute for the sacral thrust.						

Laslett's Cluster Number Two

Distraction Test, Thigh Thrust, Gaenslen's Test, Compression Test, and Sacral Thrust

UTILITY SCORE 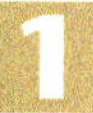

Study	Reliability	Sensitivity	Specificity	LR+	LR−	QUADAS Score (0–14)
Laslett et al.[26] (3 of 5)	NT	91	87	4.16	0.11	13
Comments: Original study using 3 of 5 tests. Well designed.						

TESTS FOR SACROILIAC PAIN ORIGIN

Ozgocmen's Cluster

Combination of Gaenslen, FABER, Mennell, Compression Thigh Thrust, or Sacral Thrust, Distraction for Active Sacroilitis

Study	Reliability	Sensitivity	Specificity	LR+	LR−	QUADAS Score (0–14)
Ozgocmen et al.[37*] (2 of 3)	NT	55	83	3.44	0.52	10
Ozgocmen et al.[37*] (3 of 5)	NT	43	83	2.75	0.66	10
Ozgocmen et al.[37*] (4 of 5)	NT	45	84	2.75	0.66	10

Comments: The five-test composite was the Gaenslen, FABER, Mennell, Thigh Thrust, and Sacral thrust. The three-test combination was the Gaenslen, Mennell, and Thigh Thrust.

*Ozgocmen et al.[37] assessed patients with acute sacroilitis.

TESTS FOR SACROILIAC DYSFUNCTION

Piedallus Test

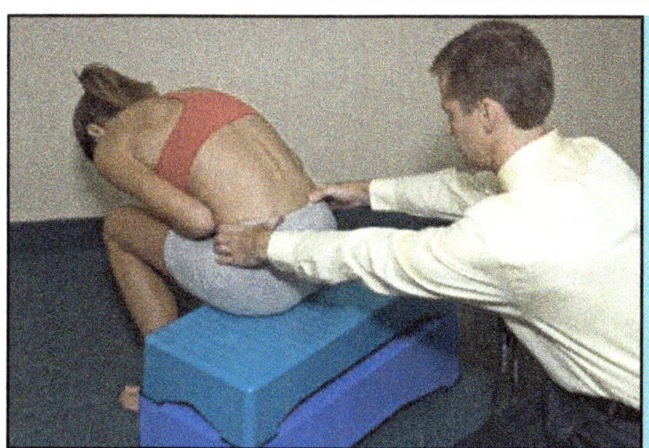

1) The patient sits on a hard surface.
2) The examiner palpates the levels of the PSIS.
3) The patient is instructed to flex forward.
4) Asymmetry in the PSIS is considered a positive finding.

UTILITY SCORE 

Study	Reliability	Sensitivity	Specificity	LR+	LR−	QUADAS Score (0–14)
Albert et al.[1]	0.0 kappa	14–69	98	35	0.9–0.87	7
Comments: This test differs from the Sitting Bend Over Test in that the surface used for sitting is hard instead of soft. Like other palpatory tests, this examination lacks reliability.						

Standing ASIS Asymmetry

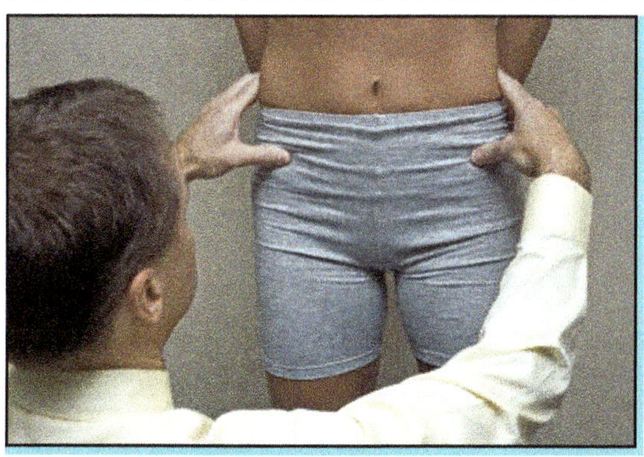

1) The patient is placed in standing.
2) Using the iliac crests as a guide, the examiner measures the symmetry of the iliac crests then the ASIS.
3) A positive test is characterized by asymmetry.

UTILITY SCORE 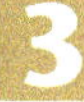

Study	Reliability	Sensitivity	Specificity	LR+	LR−	QUADAS Score (0–14)
Levangie[28]	.75	74	21	.94	1.24	11
Potter & Rothstein[38]	37.5% agreement	NT	NT	NA	NA	NA
Tong et al.[44]	0.15 kappa	NT	NT	NA	NA	NA
Comments: Based on Levangie's[28] findings, this test actually provides bias and no value during the examination. There is poor reliability.						

TESTS FOR SACROILIAC DYSFUNCTION

Seated ASIS Asymmetry

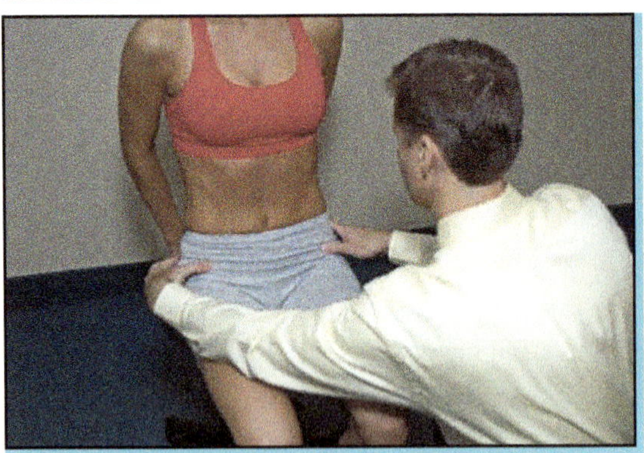

1) The patient sits in front of the examiner.
2) Using the iliac crests as a guide, the examiner evaluates the symmetry of the ASIS.
3) A positive test is characterized by asymmetry.

UTILITY SCORE 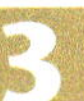

Study	Reliability	Sensitivity	Specificity	LR+	LR−	QUADAS Score (0–14)
Potter & Rothstein[38]	43.7% agreement	NT	NT	NA	NA	NA
Comments: The test appears to lack reliability. Agreement is not chance corrected, meaning that the findings could be related to luck versus skill of the examination.						

Standing PSIS Asymmetry

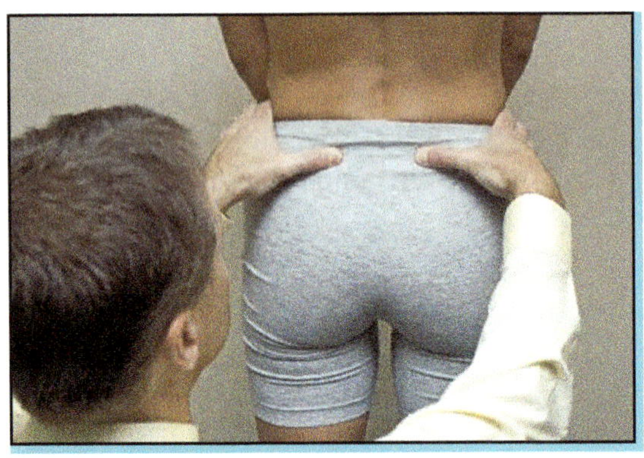

1) The patient is placed in standing.
2) Using the iliac crests as a guide, the examiner measures the symmetry of the iliac crests, then the PSIS.
3) A positive test is characterized by asymmetry.

UTILITY SCORE 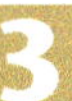

Study	Reliability	Sensitivity	Specificity	LR+	LR−	QUADAS Score (0–14)
Levangie[29]	.70	79	29	1.11	0.72	11
Rost et al.[40]	NT	55.8	NT	NA	NA	7
Potter & Rothstein[38]	35.2% agreement	NT	NT	NA	NA	NA
Comments: Based on Levangie's[29] findings, this test actually provides little value during the examination and certainly does not qualify as a screening tool.						

TESTS FOR SACROILIAC DYSFUNCTION

Seated PSIS Asymmetry

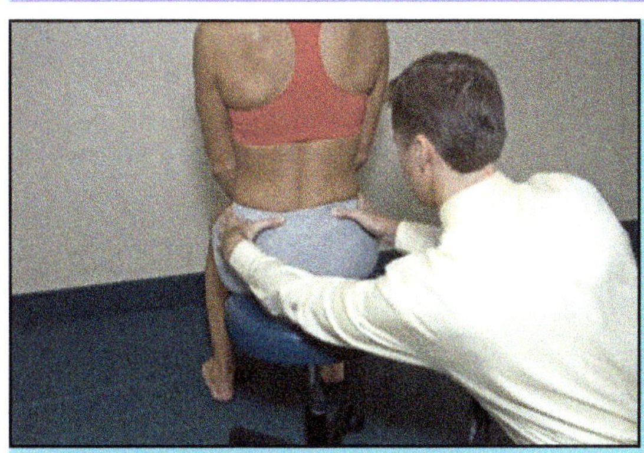

1) The patient sits in front of the examiner.
2) Using the iliac crests as a guide, the examiner evaluates the symmetry of the PSIS.
3) A positive test is characterized by asymmetry.

UTILITY SCORE 

Study	Reliability	Sensitivity	Specificity	LR+	LR−	QUADAS Score (0–14)
Levangie[28]	.63	69	22	.88	1.4	11
Potter & Rothstein[38]	35.2% agreement	NT	NT	NA	NA	NA

Comments: Based on Levangie's[28] findings, this test actually provides little value during the examination and certainly does not qualify as a screening tool.

Standing or Unilateral Standing

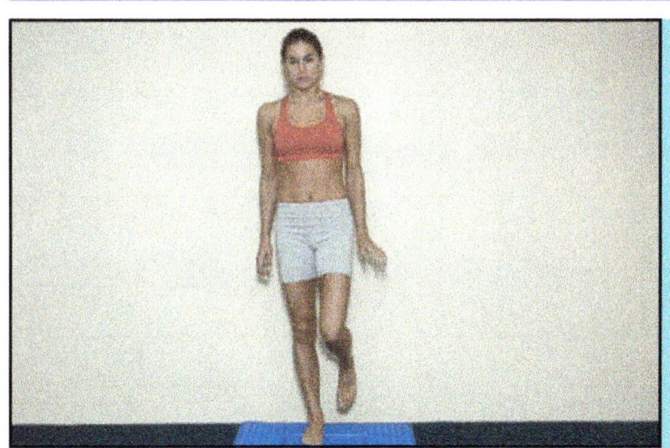

1) The patient assumes a standing position.
2) The patient is instructed to stand unilaterally on one leg.
3) Reproduction of pain at the pubis symphysis or the sacro-iliac joint is considered a positive test.

UTILITY SCORE 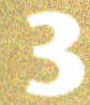

Study	Reliability	Sensitivity	Specificity	LR+	LR−	QUADAS Score (0–14)
Hansen et al.[20] (Unilateral Standing)	NT	19	100	Inf	NA	7
Dreyfuss et al.[12] (Bilateral Standing)	NT	7	98	3.5	.95	10

Comments: Unilateral standing as a measure of sacroiliac pain lacks sensitivity and should not be used during screening.

TESTS FOR SACROILIAC DYSFUNCTION

Gillet Test (Marching Test)

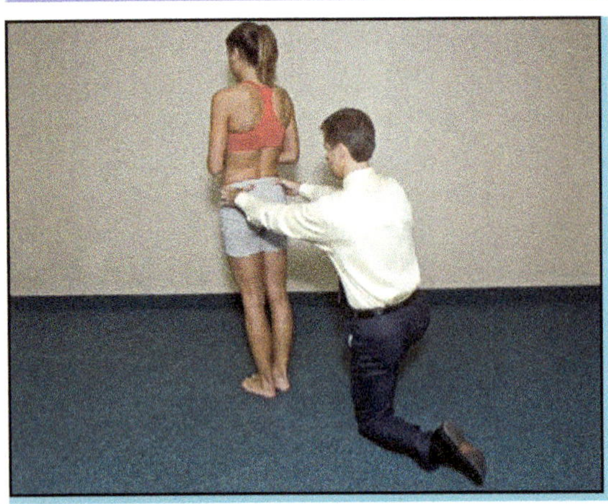

1) The patient stands in front of the examiners with his or her back to the examiner.

2) The patient is instructed to elevate his or her hip to 90 degrees, while maintaining stance on one leg.

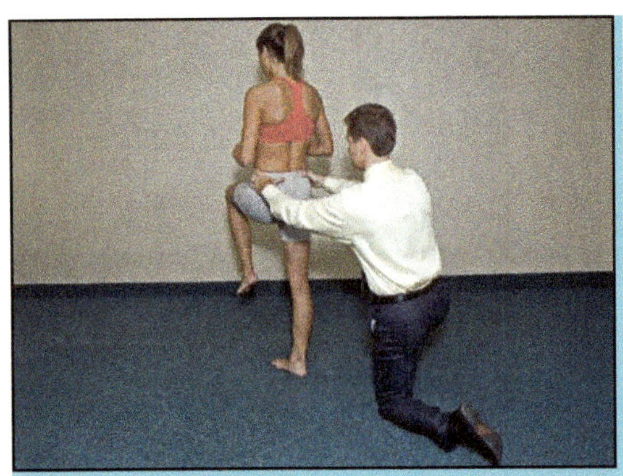

3) The examiner palpates both PSIS and evaluates whether the same-sided PSIS drops during hip flexion (a normal response) or rotates anteriorly (or superior in respect to the weight-bearing side).

4) If the PSIS does not drop or slides superiorly, the test is considered positive for that side.

UTILITY SCORE 

Study	Reliability	Sensitivity	Specificity	LR+	LR−	QUADAS Score (0–14)
Dreyfuss et al.[13]	.22	43	68	1.34	0.84	10
Carmichael[7]	0.02	NT	NT	NA	NA	NA
Levangie[29]	NT	8	93	1.07	0.99	10
Dreyfuss et al.[12]	NT	NT	84	NA	NA	7
Meijne et al.[33]	0.08 kappa	NT	NT	NA	NA	NA
Potter & Rothstein[38]	46.7% agreement	NT	NT	NA	NA	NA
Arab et al.[2]	0.41 right 0.34 left	NT	NT	NA	NA	NA
Tong et al.[44]	0.27 kappa	NT	NT	NA	NA	NA

Comments: This test is purported to be a screen for sacroiliac dysfunction, but demonstrates poor reliability and has a very poor sensitivity.

TESTS FOR SACROILIAC DYSFUNCTION

Sitting Bend Over Test (Sitting Forward Flexion Test)

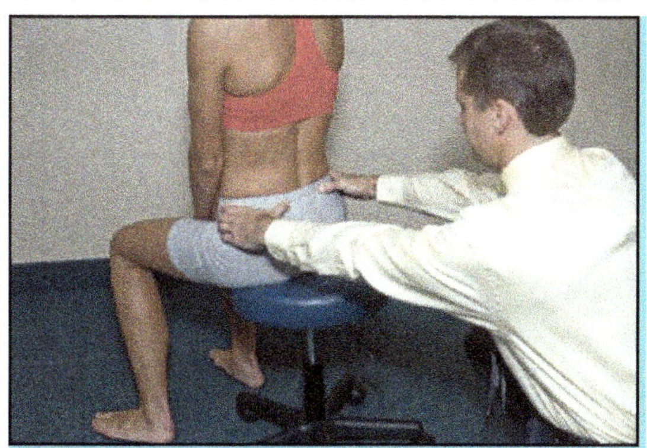

1) The patient assumes a sitting position on a soft surface.

2) The examiner palpates both PSIS (inferiorly) of the patient.

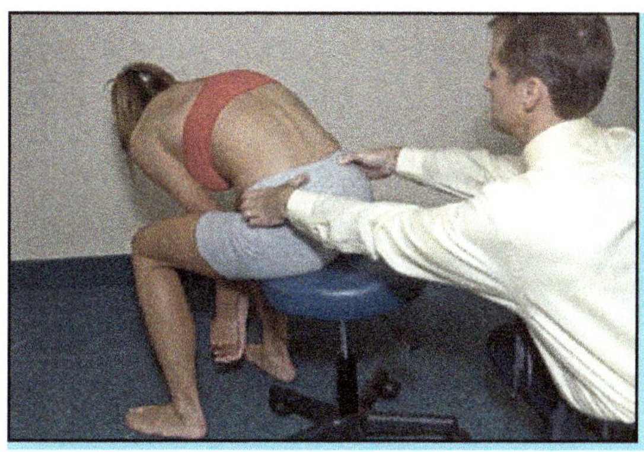

3) The patient is instructed to bend forward toward the midline. Midline movement ensures equity of movement on the left and right.

4) The examiner palpates both PSIS and evaluates whether movements are symmetrical (a normal response) or asymmetrical. The test is repeated during palpation of the inferior lateral angle of the sacrum.

5) A positive finding is asymmetry or palpable differences between PSIS and sacral movements.

UTILITY SCORE 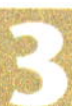

Study	Reliability	Sensitivity	Specificity	LR+	LR−	QUADAS Score (0–14)
Riddle & Freburger[39]	.37	NT	NT	NA	NA	NA
Dreyfuss et al.[12]	.22	3	90	0.3	1.08	10
Levangie[29]	NT	9	93	1.01	0.98	11
Dreyfuss et al.[12]	NT	NT	92	NA	NA	7
Potter & Rothstein[38]	50% agreement	NT	NT	NA	NA	NA
Arab et al.[2]	0.75 right 0.64 left	NT	NT	NA	NA	NA
Tong et al.[44]	0.06 kappa	NT	NT	NA	NA	NA

Comments: This test is purported to be a screen for sacroiliac dysfunction, but demonstrates poor sensitivity, poor reliability, and has a very poor diagnostic value. The test differs from the Piedallus test based on surface selection.

TESTS FOR SACROILIAC DYSFUNCTION

Standing Bend Over Test (Standing Flexion Test)

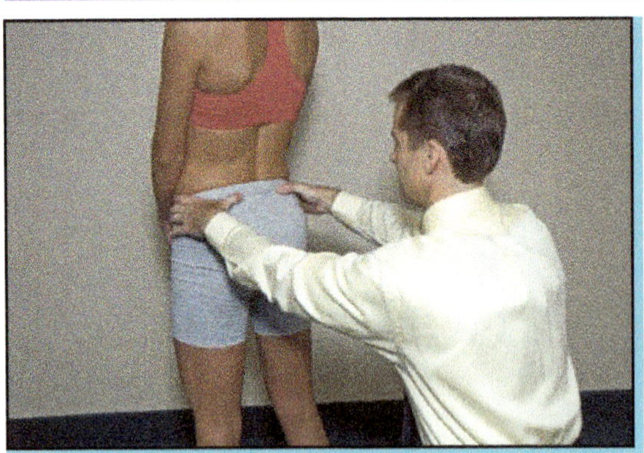

1) The patient assumes a standing position.

2) The examiner palpates both PSIS of the patient.

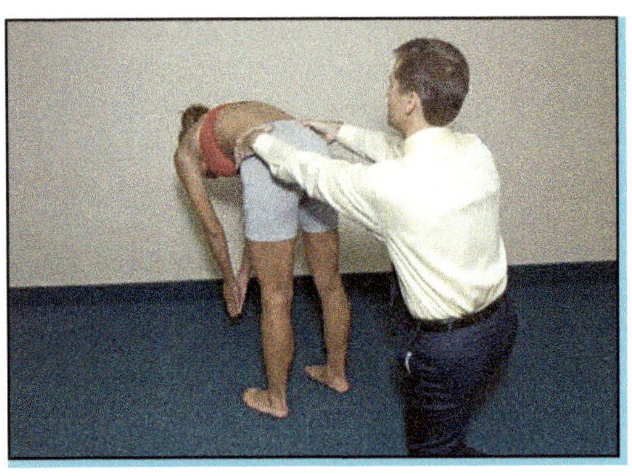

3) The patient is instructed to bend forward toward the midline. Midline movement ensures equity of movement on the left and right.

4) The examiner palpates both PSIS and evaluates whether movements are symmetrical (a normal response) or asymmetrical. The test is repeated during palpation of the inferior lateral angle of the sacrum.

UTILITY SCORE 

Study	Reliability	Sensitivity	Specificity	LR+	LR−	QUADAS Score (0–14)
Vincent-Smith & Gibbons[48]	0.05 kappa	NT	NT	NA	NA	NA
Bowman & Gribbe[5]	0.23 kappa	NT	NT	NA	NA	NA
Riddle & Freburger[39]	0.32 kappa	NT	NT	NA	NA	NT
Levangie[29]	NT	17	79	0.81	1.05	11
Dreyfuss et al.[12]	NT	NT	87	NA	NA	7
Potter & Rothstein[38]	43.7% agreement	NT	NT	NA	NA	NA
Arab et al.[2]	0.51 right 0.55 left	NT	NT	NA	NA	NA
Tong et al.[44]	0.14 kappa	NT	NT	NA	NA	NA

Comments: This test is purported to be a screen for sacroiliac dysfunction, but demonstrates poor sensitivity and reliability, and has a very poor diagnostic value.

TESTS FOR SACROILIAC DYSFUNCTION

Long Sit Test (Leg Length Test)

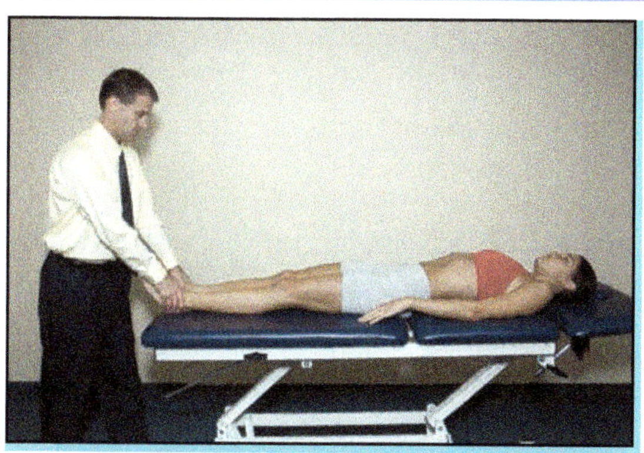

1) The patient is instructed to lie supine in a hooklying position.

2) The patient is instructed to bridge and return to hooklying. The examiner passively moves the knees into extension.

3) The examiner evaluates the leg length differences by assessing the comparative levels of the medial malleoli.

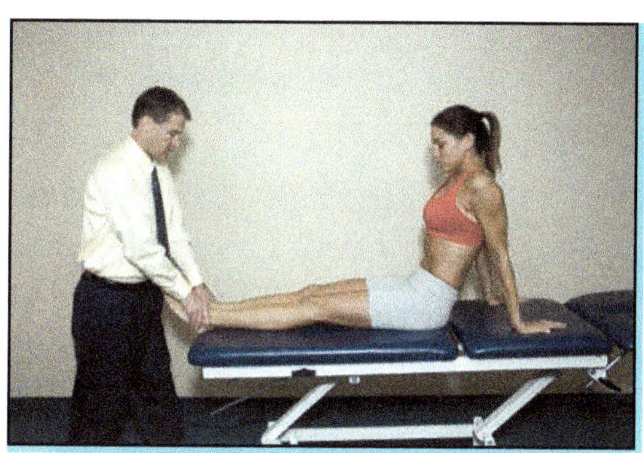

4) The patient is directed to sit up and the examiner again measures the comparative length of the malleoli.

5) If one leg moves further than the other, the patient is considered to have a pelvic rotation.

UTILITY SCORE 

Study	Reliability	Sensitivity	Specificity	LR+	LR−	QUADAS Score (0–14)
Riddle & Freburger[39]	0.19	NT	NT	NA	NA	NA
Albert et al.[1]	0.06	NT	NT	NA	NA	7
Levangie[29] (LS)	NT	44	64	1.37	0.88	10
Potter & Rothstein[38]	40% agreement	NT	NT	NA	NA	NA
Bemis & Daniel[3]	NT	62	83	3.6	0.46	7
Tong et al.[44]	0.21 kappa	NT	NT	NA	NA	NA

Comments: Supine to sit of one malleolus from short to long is indicative of a posterior rotation of the innominate. Supine to sit of one malleolus from long to short is indicative of an anterior rotation of the innominate. Nonetheless, the test demonstrates poor reliability, questionable validity, and may not yield useful results. Bemis & Daniel[3] used a reference standard that does not reflect sacroiliac dysfunction.

TESTS FOR SACROILIAC DYSFUNCTION

Sacral Base Position

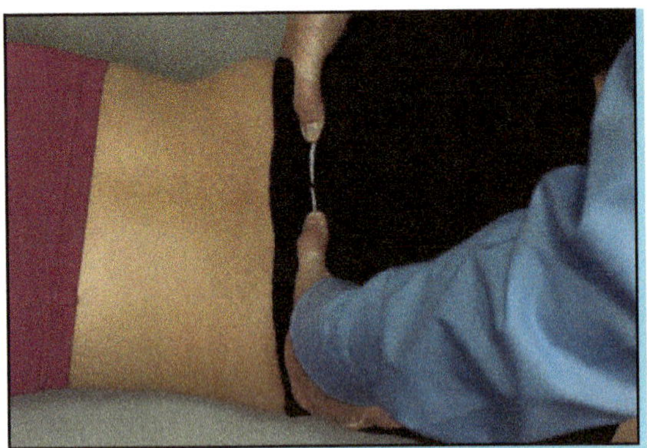

1. The patient assumes a prone position.
2. The examiner palpates the location of the base of the sacrum.
3. An asymmetry associated with one side being more prominent than the other is considered a positive finding.

UTILITY SCORE 3

Study	Reliability	Sensitivity	Specificity	LR+	LR−	QUADAS Score (0–14)
Tong et al.[44]	0.08 kappa	NT	NT	NA	NA	NA
Comments: Very poor reliability.						

Sacral Sulci Position

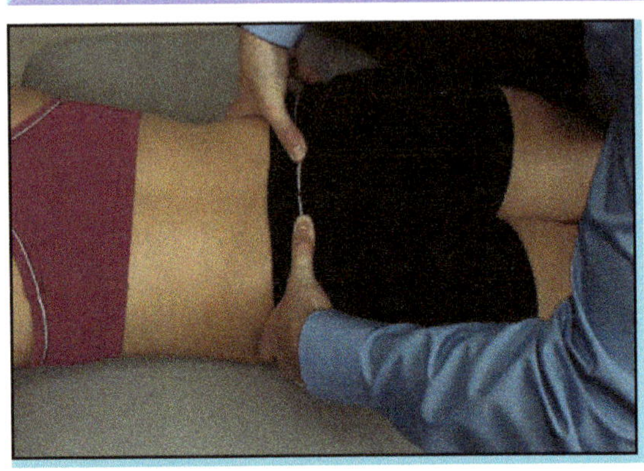

1. The patient is placed in a prone position.
2. The clinician palpates the location of the sacral sulci, looking for asymmetry (by placing the thumbs on the PSIS).
3. A positive finding is asymmetry.

UTILITY SCORE 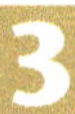

Study	Reliability	Sensitivity	Specificity	LR+	LR−	QUADAS Score (0–14)
Holmgren & Waling[21]	0.11 kappa	NT	NT	NA	NA	NA
Comments: This is another study that suggests poor reliability.						

TESTS FOR SACROILIAC DYSFUNCTION

Inferior Lateral Angle Position

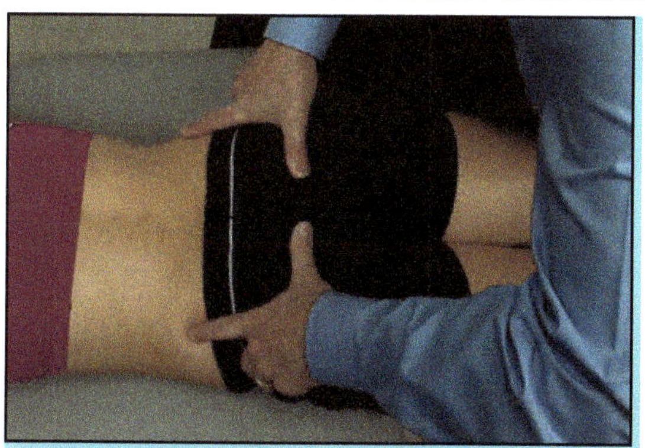

1) The patient is placed in a prone position.
2) The clinician palpates the location of the inferior lateral angles, looking for asymmetry (specifically if one side appeared more posterior than the other).
3) A positive finding is asymmetry.

UTILITY SCORE 3

Study	Reliability	Sensitivity	Specificity	LR+	LR−	QUADAS Score (0–14)
Holmgren & Waling[21]	0.11 kappa	NT	NT	NA	NA	NA
Comments: Yet another study that suggests poor reliability.						

Medial Malleoli Position

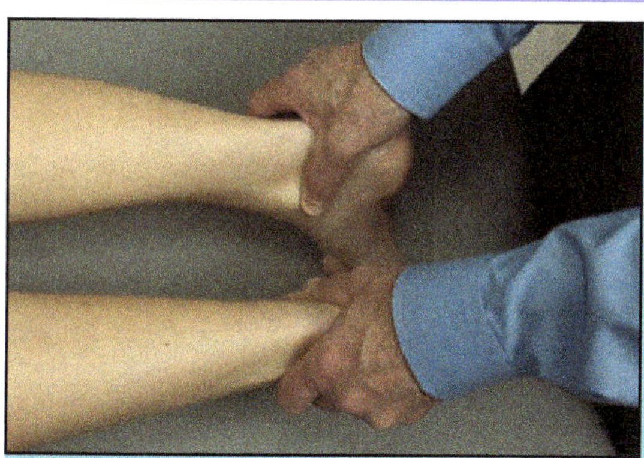

1) The patient is instructed to lie in a prone position.
2) The clinician places his or her thumbs at the medial border of the medial malleoli.
3) A positive test finding is asymmetry.

UTILITY SCORE 3

Study	Reliability	Sensitivity	Specificity	LR+	LR−	QUADAS Score (0–14)
Holmgren & Waling[21]	0.28 kappa	NT	NT	NA	NA	NA
Comments: Very similar to the long sit test only performed in prone. Poor to fair reliability.						

TESTS FOR SACROILIAC DYSFUNCTION

Combinations of Palpatory Tests

Cibulka & Koldehoff's Cluster

Standing Flexion, Sitting Posterior Superior Iliac Spine (PSIS) Palpation, Supine to Sit Test, Prone Knee Flexion Test

UTILITY SCORE 3

Study	Reliability	Sensitivity	Specificity	LR+	LR−	QUADAS Score (0–14)
Cibulka & Koldehoff[9] (4 of 4)	NT	82	88	6.83	0.20	5
Comments: Unfortunately, this study was highly biased. Use caution when interpreting the results.						

Riddle and Freburger's Cluster

Standing Flexion, Prone Knee Flexion, Supine Long Sitting Test, Sitting PSIS Test

UTILITY SCORE 3

Study	Reliability	Sensitivity	Specificity	LR+	LR−	QUADAS Score (0–14)
Riddle & Freburger[39] (3 of 4)	0.11–0.23	NT	NT	NA	NA	NA
Comments: Poor reliability.						

Kokmeyer et al.'s Cluster

Gapping, Compression Test, Gaenslen's Test, Thigh Thrust, and Patrick's Test

UTILITY SCORE 3

Study	Reliability	Sensitivity	Specificity	LR+	LR−	QUADAS Score (0–14)
Kokmeyer et al.[23] (3 of 5)	0.71	NT	NT	NA	NA	NA
Comments: Improved reliability but the tests used lack validity.						

Arab's Palpation Cluster

Gillet, Standing Flexion, Sitting Flexion, and Prone Knee Flexion

UTILITY SCORE 3

Study	Reliability	Sensitivity	Specificity	LR+	LR−	QUADAS Score (0–14)
Arab et al.[2] (4 of 4)	0.77 right 0.33 left	NT	NT	NA	NA	NA
Comments: The patients in the study were actually patients with low back pain.						

Arab's Pain Provocation Cluster

Thigh Thrust, Hip Abduction, and FABER

UTILITY SCORE 

Study	Reliability	Sensitivity	Specificity	LR+	LR−	QUADAS Score (0–14)
Arab et al.[2] (3 of 3)	0.88 right 1.0 left	NT	NT	NA	NA	NA
Comments: The patients in the study were actually patients with low back pain.						

TESTS FOR SACROILIAC PAIN ASSOCIATED WITH PREGNANCY-RELATED POSTERIOR PELVIC PAIN

Active Straight Leg Raise

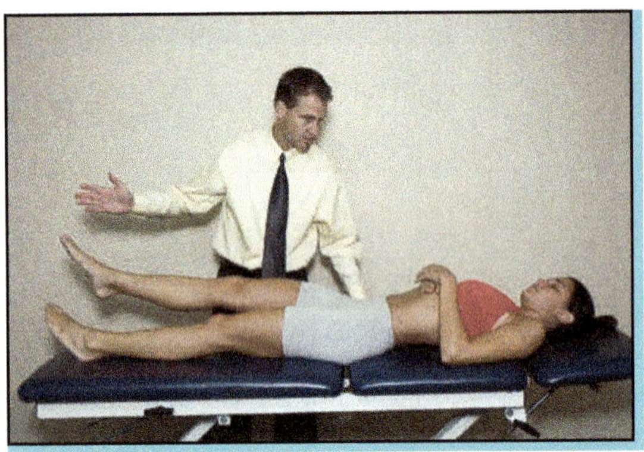

1) The patient is positioned in supine. Resting symptoms are assessed.

2) The patient is asked to raise the affected leg approximately 6 inches. Pain is queried.

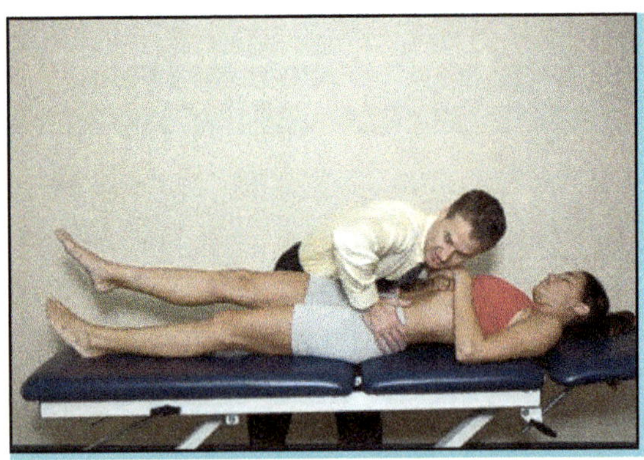

3) If the previous request was painful, the examiner stabilizes the pelvis by compressing the ASIS medially, or by placing a sacroiliac belt around the pelvis.

4) The patient is again asked to raise the affected leg approximately 6 inches. If the movement is no longer painful, the test is considered positive.

UTILITY SCORE 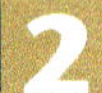

Study	Reliability	Sensitivity	Specificity	LR+	LR−	QUADAS Score (0–14)
Mens et al.[34]	0.82 ICC	87	94	14.5	0.13	8
Damen et al.[11]	NT	77	55	1.7	0.42	8
Rost et al.[40] (PPPP) (One-Sided Positive)	NT	51	NT	NA	NA	7
Rost et al.[40] (PPPP) (Two-Sided Positive)	NT	15	NT	NA	NA	7

Comments: PPPP is pregnancy-related posterior pelvic pain. The test appears to be useful with PPPP and is often graded in degrees of impairment. Past studies have shown that higher degrees of impairment (inability to perform) are associated with higher disability scores. As a whole, the studies that have examined this test are mediocre. To be honest, it's probably a better test for treatment decision making than for diagnosis.

TESTS FOR SACROILIAC PAIN ASSOCIATED WITH PREGNANCY-RELATED POSTERIOR PELVIC PAIN

Prone Active Straight Leg Raise

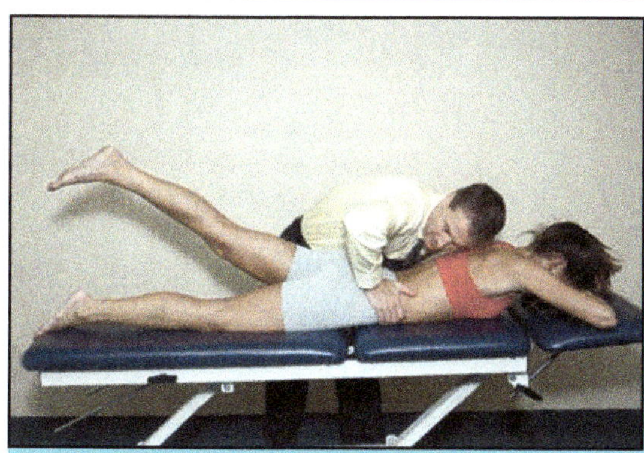

1) The patient assumes a prone position.

2) The patient performs hip extension and is queried for pain provocation.

3) The examiner compresses the innominates with his or her hands or a belt and instructs the patient to repeat hip extension. If pain subsides, the test is considered positive.

4) The examiner may repeat the test by adding resistance to hip extension.

5) A positive test is pain during hip extension that decreases with stabilization of the innominate.

UTILITY SCORE 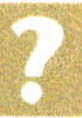

Study	Reliability	Sensitivity	Specificity	LR+	LR−	QUADAS Score (0–14)
Lee[27]	NT	NT	NT	NA	NA	NA
Comments: Although described by Lee,[27] the examination procedure is untested.						

Self-Test P4

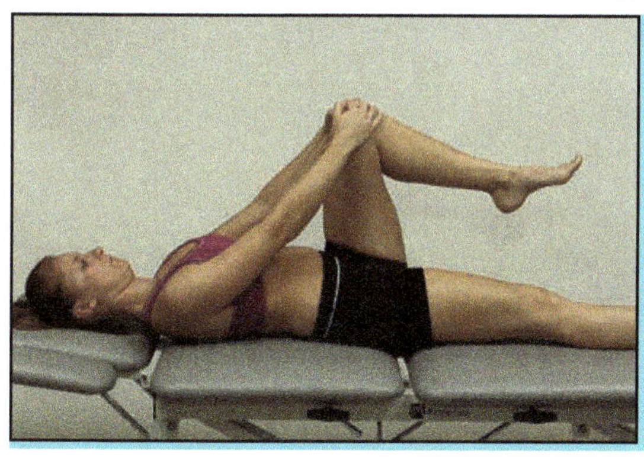

1) The patient lies supine on the plinth with the hip flexed to 90 degrees.

2) The patient self applies a downward force through his or her own hip.

3) A positive test is pain during the downward force.

UTILITY SCORE 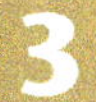

Study	Reliability	Sensitivity	Specificity	LR+	LR−	QUADAS Score (0–14)
Fagevik-Olsén et al.[15]	NT	90	92	11.3	0.11	4
Comments: The sensitivity of the test increases if the patient also has a positive Active Straight Leg test and a positive 4P test.						

TESTS FOR SACROILIAC PAIN ASSOCIATED WITH PREGNANCY-RELATED POSTERIOR PELVIC PAIN

Bridging Test

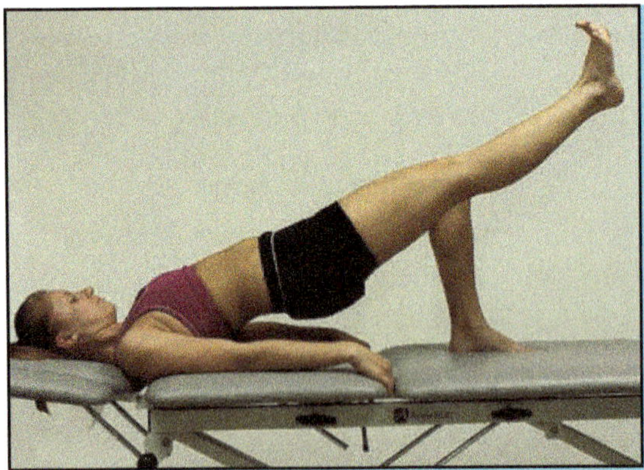

1) The patient assumes a supine position.
2) The patient bridges while extending one leg.
3) A positive test is pain during the bridging activity.

UTILITY SCORE 3

Study	Reliability	Sensitivity	Specificity	LR+	LR−	QUADAS Score (0–14)
Fagevik-Olsén et al.[15]	NT	97	87	7.5	0.03	4
Comments: The sensitivity of the test increases if the patient also has a positive Active Straight Leg test and a positive 4P test.						

Four Point Kneeling Test

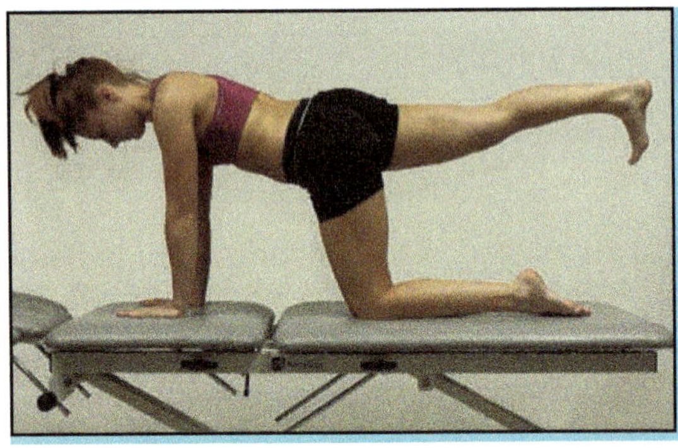

1) The patient assumes a four point kneeling position.
2) The patient extends one leg at a time.
3) A positive test is pain during hip extension.

UTILITY SCORE

Study	Reliability	Sensitivity	Specificity	LR+	LR−	QUADAS Score (0–14)
Fagevik-Olsen et al.[15]	NT	46	88	3.8	0.61	4
Comments: The sensitivity of the test increases if the patient also has a positive Active Straight Leg test and a positive 4P test.						

TESTS FOR SACROILIAC PAIN ASSOCIATED WITH PREGNANCY-RELATED POSTERIOR PELVIC PAIN

Thumb-PSIS Test (Click-Clack Test)

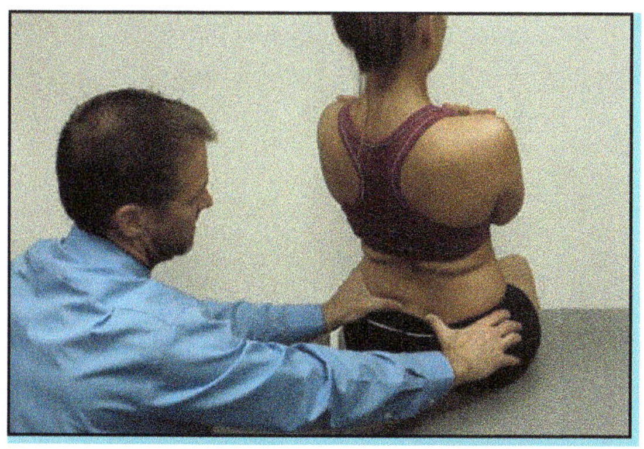

1) The patient assumes a sitting position. The patient sits upright with his or her arms crossed.

2) The clinician places his or her thumbs in the PSIS and measures how level each are to the horizon.

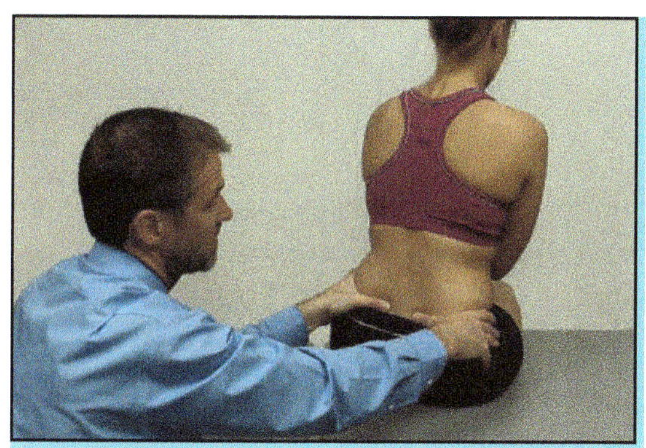

3) The patient moves the pelvis into lordosis and kyphosis. A positive test is a "click clack" sound during movement.

UTILITY SCORE 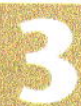

Study	Reliability	Sensitivity	Specificity	LR+	LR−	QUADAS Score (0–14)
Van Kessel-Cobelens et al.[47]	0.00 kappa	NT	NT	NA	NA	NA
Comments: Palpation has low reliability and adding a click clack assessment does not help.						

TESTS FOR SACROILIAC PAIN ASSOCIATED WITH PREGNANCY-RELATED POSTERIOR PELVIC PAIN

Heel Bank Test

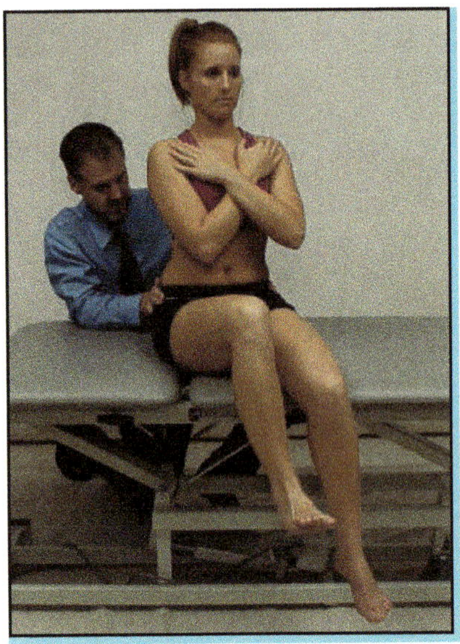

1) The patient assumes a sitting position and the clinician places his or her thumbs in the sacral sulci.

2) The patient is asked to raise his or her knee from the targeted affected side and to lower the knee down to the plinth.

3) If the patient is able to accomplish this with no effort the findings are negative. Any effort (difficulty) seen by the clinician is considered positive.

UTILITY SCORE 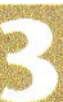 3

Study	Reliability	Sensitivity	Specificity	LR+	LR−	QUADAS Score (0–14)
Van Kessel-Cobelens et al.[47]	0.39 κ (left) 0.06 κ (right)	NT	NT	NA	NA	NA
Comments: I wouldn't consider using this test. The reliability is very poor.						

Abduction Test

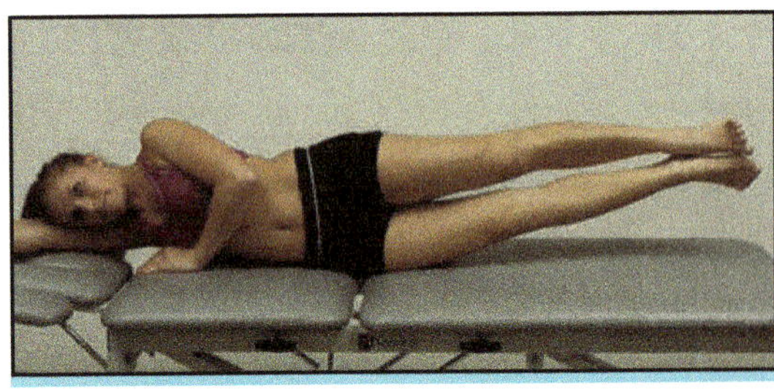

1) The patient assumes a sidelying position. Both sides are tested and a comparison between the two sides is the objective.

2) The patient is requested to lift both knees (while in contact with one another) up 20 cm. The process is repeated on the opposite side.

3) If the patient is able to accomplish this symmetrically with no effort the findings are negative. Any effort (difficulty) seen from one side to the other by the clinician is considered positive.

UTILITY SCORE  3

Study	Reliability	Sensitivity	Specificity	LR+	LR−	QUADAS Score (0–14)
Van Kessel-Cobelens et al.[47]	0.50 left 0.37 right	NT	NT	NA	NA	NA
Comments: Fair reliability, unknown validity.						

TESTS FOR SACROILIAC PAIN ASSOCIATED WITH PREGNANCY-RELATED POSTERIOR PELVIC PAIN

Long Dorsal Ligament Palpation

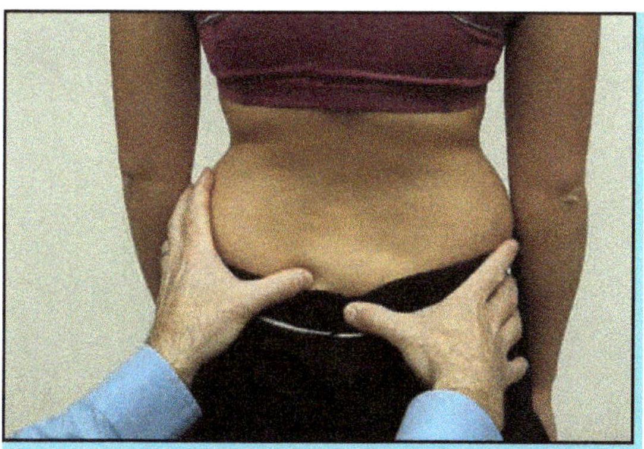

1) The patient assumes a standing or sitting position.
2) The clinician palpates the long dorsal ligament.
3) A positive test is pain during palpation.

UTILITY SCORE 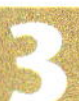

Study	Reliability	Sensitivity	Specificity	LR+	LR−	QUADAS Score (0–14)
Vleeming et al.[49]	NT	76	NT	NA	NA	NA
Comments: The sensitivity of the test increases if the patient also has a positive Active Straight Leg test and a positive 4P test. By itself it has limited value; with other findings, it may be useful.						

The Lunge

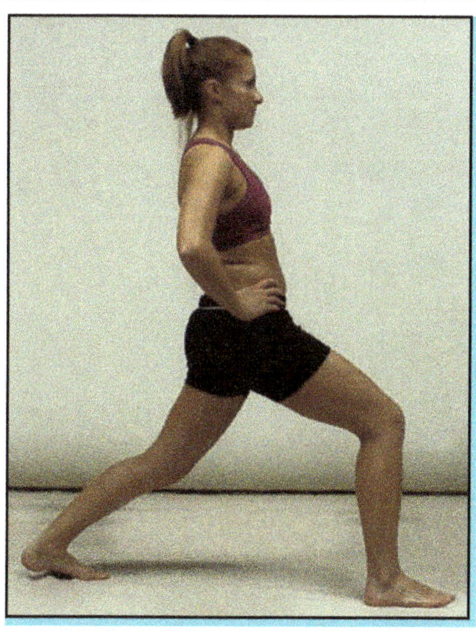

1) The patient is placed in a standing position.
2) The patient is requested to lunge forward, first on the right then the left.
3) A positive finding is pain during the lunge.

UTILITY SCORE 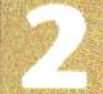

Study	Reliability	Sensitivity	Specificity	LR+	LR−	QUADAS Score (0–14)
Cook et al.[10]	NT	44	83	2.6	0.68	12
Comments: Use caution, there were 21 individuals in the study. May be useful in combination with other tests.						

TESTS FOR SACROILIAC PAIN ASSOCIATED WITH PREGNANCY-RELATED POSTERIOR PELVIC PAIN

Sit to Stand

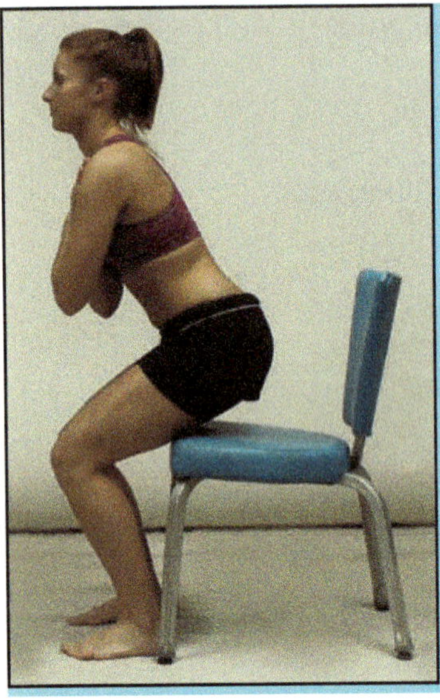

1) The patient initiates the test in a sitting position.
2) Without using his or her arms, the patient stands at request.
3) A positive finding is pain during the transition of sit to stand.

UTILITY SCORE 3

Study	Reliability	Sensitivity	Specificity	LR+	LR−	QUADAS Score (0–14)
Cook et al.[10]	NT	13	100	Inf	0.88	12
Comments: Use caution, there were 21 individuals in the study. It appears to be a very specific finding.						

Deep Squat

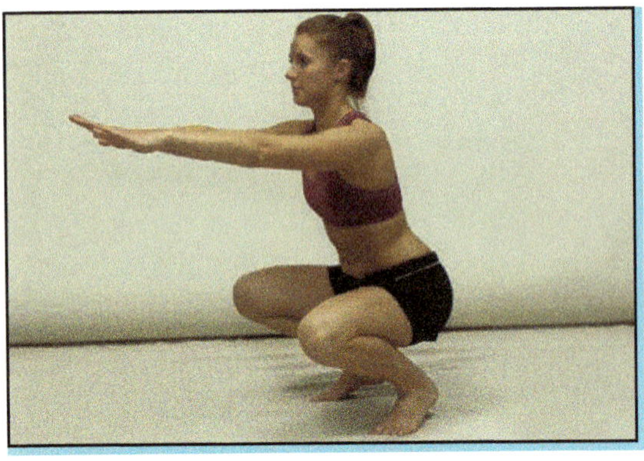

1) The test is initiated in a standing position.
2) The patient is asked to squat to the deepest level they feel safe in doing.
3) A positive finding is pain during a squat.

UTILITY SCORE 2

Study	Reliability	Sensitivity	Specificity	LR+	LR−	QUADAS Score (0–14)
Cook et al.[10]	NT	24	100	Inf	0.76	12
Comments: Use caution, there were 21 individuals in the study.						

TESTS FOR SACROILIAC PAIN ASSOCIATED WITH PREGNANCY-RELATED POSTERIOR PELVIC PAIN

Step Up Test

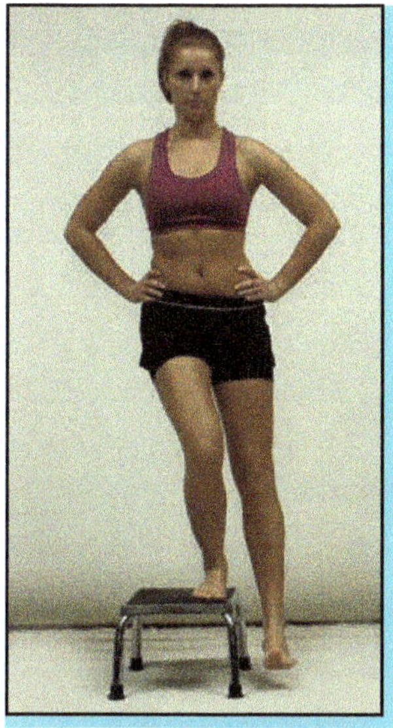

1) The patient is placed in a standing position with a step (~6 inches) in front of them.

2) The patient is asked to step up onto the step with the affected side.

3) A positive finding is pain during the step up.

UTILITY SCORE 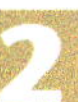

Study	Reliability	Sensitivity	Specificity	LR+	LR−	QUADAS Score (0–14)
Cook et al.[10]	NT	29	100	Inf	0.71	12
Comments: Use caution, there were 21 individuals in the study.						

Cook's Cluster Number 1

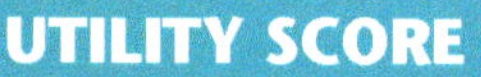 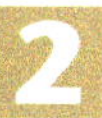

Study	Reliability	Sensitivity	Specificity	LR+	LR−	QUADAS Score (0–14)
Cook et al.[10]	NT	70	83	4.2	0.36	12
Comments: The cluster consisted of a Lunge, Manual Muscle Testing, and Hip Range of Motion (any 1 of 3). Use caution, there were 21 individuals in the study.						

Cook's Cluster Number 2

UTILITY SCORE 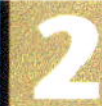

Study	Reliability	Sensitivity	Specificity	LR+	LR−	QUADAS Score (0–14)
Cook et al.[10]	NT	35	83	2.2	0.78	12
Comments: The cluster consisted of a Lunge, Manual Muscle Testing, and Hip Range of Motion (2 of 3 findings). Use caution, there were 21 individuals in the study.						

TESTS FOR SACROILIAC PAIN ASSOCIATED WITH PREGNANCY-RELATED POSTERIOR PELVIC PAIN

Cook's Cluster Number 3

UTILITY SCORE 2

Study	Reliability	Sensitivity	Specificity	LR+	LR−	QUADAS Score (0–14)
Cook et al.[10]	NT	88	66	2.6	0.18	12
Comments: Active Straight Leg Raise test, Gaenslen's test, and the Thigh Thrust (1 of 3 tests). Use caution, there were 21 individuals in the study.						

Cook's Cluster Number 4

UTILITY SCORE 2

Study	Reliability	Sensitivity	Specificity	LR+	LR−	QUADAS Score (0–14)
Cook et al.[10]	NT	58	83	3.5	0.50	12
Comments: Active Straight Leg Raise test, Gaenslen's test, and the Thigh Thrust (2 of 3 tests). Use caution, there were 21 individuals in the study.						

Cook's Cluster Number 5

UTILITY SCORE 2

Study	Reliability	Sensitivity	Specificity	LR+	LR−	QUADAS Score (0–14)
Cook et al. [10]	NT	94	66	2.8	0.09	12
Comments: Active Straight Leg Raise test, Lunge, and Thigh Thrust (1 of 3). Use caution, there were 21 individuals in the study. This is a useful combination to rule out PGP.						

TEST FOR MOTOR CONTROL DYSFUNCTION

Stork Test

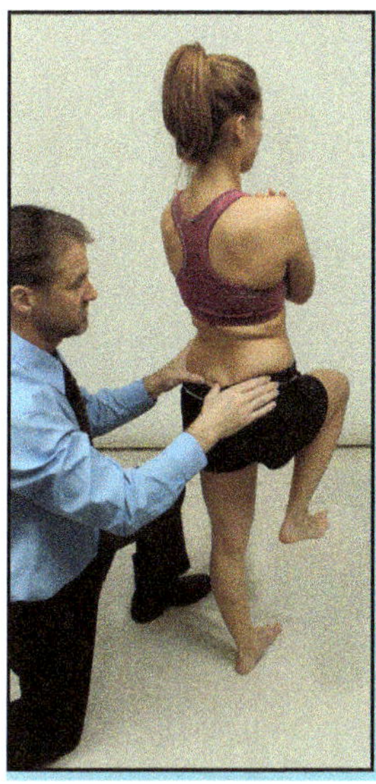

1. The patient is placed in a standing position with feet shoulder width apart.
2. The clinician places one finger on the PSIS (for the weight bearing side) and one finger on the sacrum (S2 spinous process).
3. The patient is instructed to lift the contralateral leg up to 90 degrees at the hip. The movement is tested 3 times.
4. A positive test is when the palpated aspect of the PSIS moved cephaled with respect to the sacrum.

UTILITY SCORE 

Study	Reliability	Sensitivity	Specificity	LR+	LR−	QUADAS Score (0–14)
Hungerford et al.[22]	0.59 κ	NT	NT	NT	NT	NA
Comments: Reasonable reliability, no known validity.						

TEST FOR SYMPHYSIOLYSIS

Pubic Symphysis Palpation

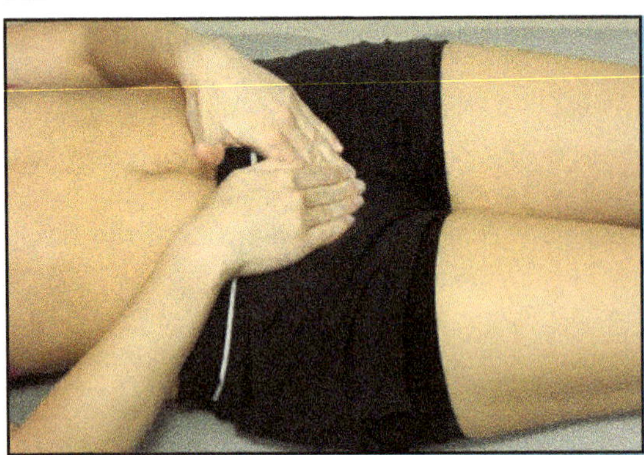

1) The patient is placed in a supine position.
2) The examiner palpates the pubic symphysis near midline.
3) An alternative involves a pubic shear force to the superior and inferior pubis bones (pictured).
4) A positive test is identified by reproduction of the patient's concordant pain.

UTILITY SCORE 2

Study	Reliability	Sensitivity	Specificity	LR+	LR−	QUADAS Score (0–14)
Albert et al.[1]	.89	81	99	4.68	0.19	7
Hansen et al.[20]	NT	76	94	12.7	0.26	7
Comments: This test appears useful in the diagnosis of symphysiolysis.						

Resisted Hip Adduction

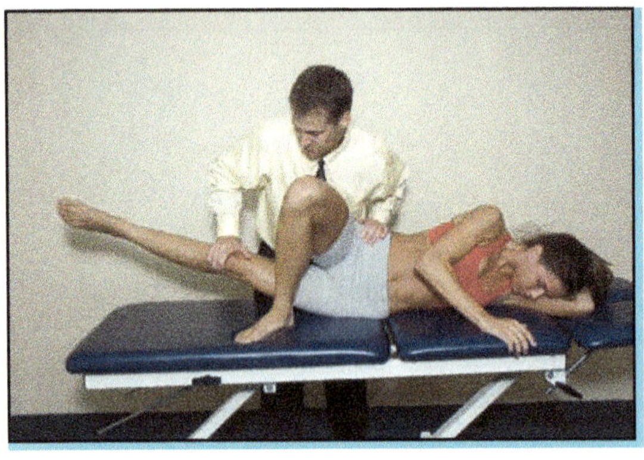

1) The patient is placed in a sidelying position.
2) The patient is instructed to lift the lower leg.
3) The patient is instructed to push medially with his or her knee while the instructor applies a lateral force.
4) Weakness of the hip adductors secondary to pain during the test is considered a positive finding.

UTILITY SCORE 3

Study	Reliability	Sensitivity	Specificity	LR+	LR−	QUADAS Score (0–14)
Mens et al.[35]	0.79 ICC	NT	NT	NA	NA	NA
Rost et al.[40] (PPPP) (for pain reproduction)	NT	54	NT	NA	NA	7
Blower & Griffin[4]	53% agreement	NT	92	NA	NA	5
Comments: PPPP is pregnancy-related posterior pelvic pain. This test suffers from poor designs.						

TESTS FOR PELVIC RING FRACTURE

Posterior Pelvic Palpation

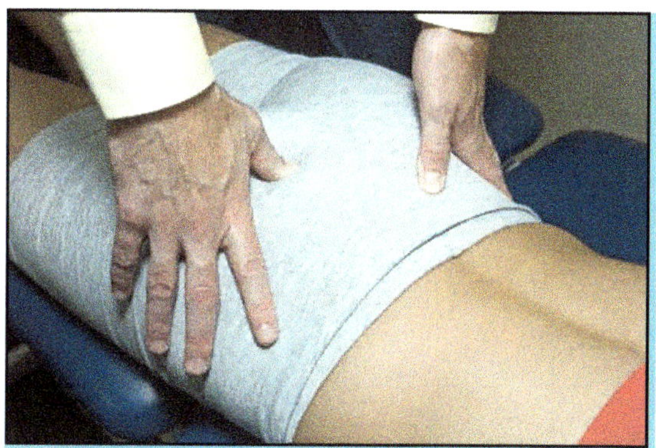

1) The patient is placed in a sitting or prone position.

2) The examiner carefully palpates the sacrum and bilateral sacroiliac joints.

3) A positive test is associated with local tenderness with moderately deep palpation.

UTILITY SCORE 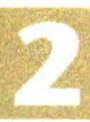

Study	Reliability	Sensitivity	Specificity	LR+	LR−	QUADAS Score (0–14)
McCormick et al.[32]	NT	98	94	16.3	0.02	7
Comments: The test should only be considered positive if pain is concordant and if the patient exhibits historical information synonymous with a pelvis fracture. This finding is more compelling if swelling is also present.						

Hip Flexion Test

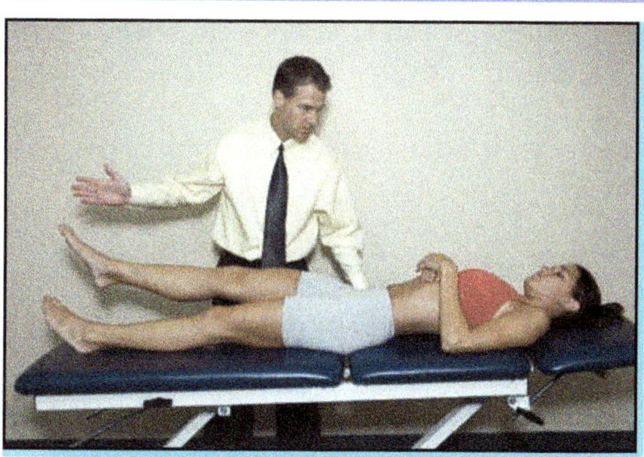

1) The patient is placed in a supine position.

2) The examiner instructs the patient to raise his or her leg actively (straight leg raise).

3) A positive test is associated with reproduction of pain during active movement or inability to raise the leg.

UTILITY SCORE 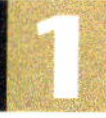

Study	Reliability	Sensitivity	Specificity	LR+	LR−	QUADAS Score (0–14)
Ham et al.[19]	NT	90	95	18	0.10	10
Comments: The test may be useful if the patient history suggests a pelvis fracture.						

TESTS FOR PELVIC RING FRACTURE

Pubic Compression Test

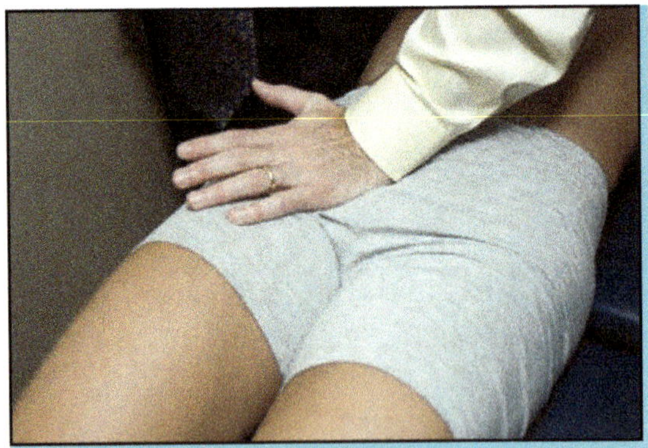

1) The patient is placed in a supine position.
2) The examiner applies a downward pressure on the pubic bones.
3) A positive test is associated with reproduction of pain during compression.

UTILITY SCORE 2

Study	Reliability	Sensitivity	Specificity	LR+	LR−	QUADAS Score (0–14)
Ham et al.[19]	NT	55	84	3.4	0.53	10
Comments: The test value was significantly associated with diagnosis. This test may be useful if patient history suggests a fracture.						

AP and Lateral Compression Test

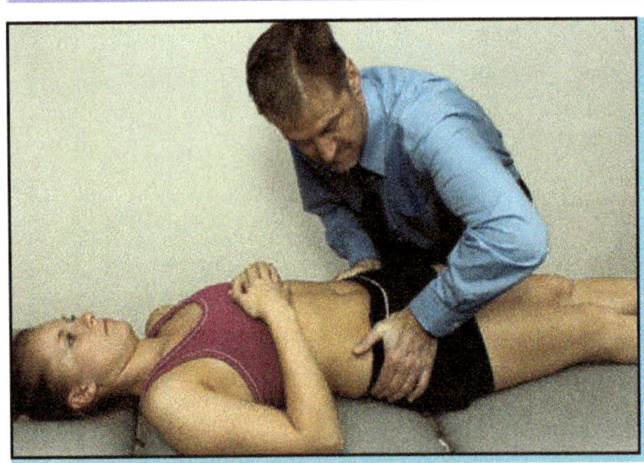

1) The patient is placed in a supine position.
2) The examiner applies an anterior to posterior compression force and a lateral compression force to the iliac wings.
3) A positive test is associated with reproduction of pain during compression.

UTILITY SCORE 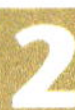

Study	Reliability	Sensitivity	Specificity	LR+	LR−	QUADAS Score (0–14)
McCormick et al.[32]	NT	98	24	1.3	0.08	7
Comments: The test value was significantly associated with diagnosis. This test may be useful if patient history suggests a fracture. It also may be useful as a screen.						

TESTS FOR PELVIC RING FRACTURE

Active Hip Range of Motion

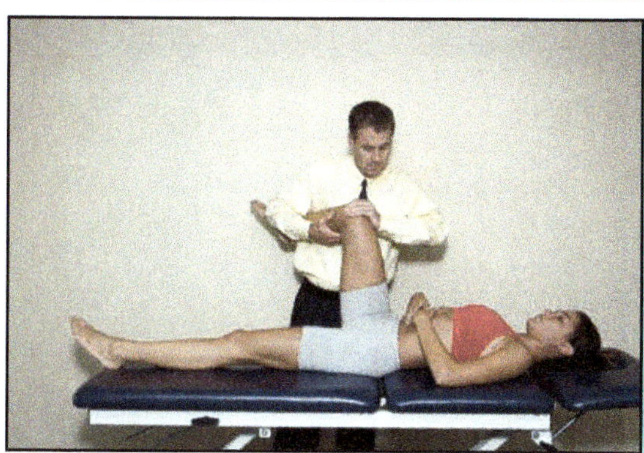

1) The patient is placed in a supine position.

2) The examiner performs a straight leg raise on each side, followed by passive hip flexion, abduction, adduction, internal rotation (pictured), and external rotation.

3) A positive test is associated with reproduction of pain during passive movement.

UTILITY SCORE 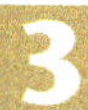

Study	Reliability	Sensitivity	Specificity	LR+	LR−	QUADAS Score (0–14)
McCormick et al.[32]	NT	53	76	2.2	0.62	7
Comments: The test value was significantly associated with diagnosis.						

TEST FOR BURSITIS, TUMOR, OR ABSCESS OF THE BUTTOCK REGION

Sign of the Buttock

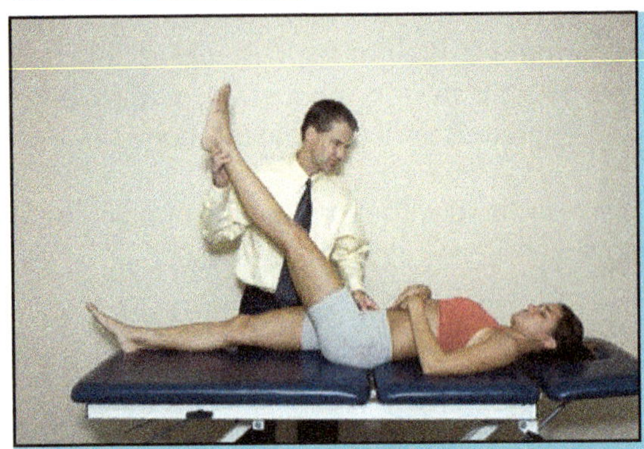

1) The patient lies supine.

2) The examiner passively performs a straight leg raise to the point of pain or restriction.

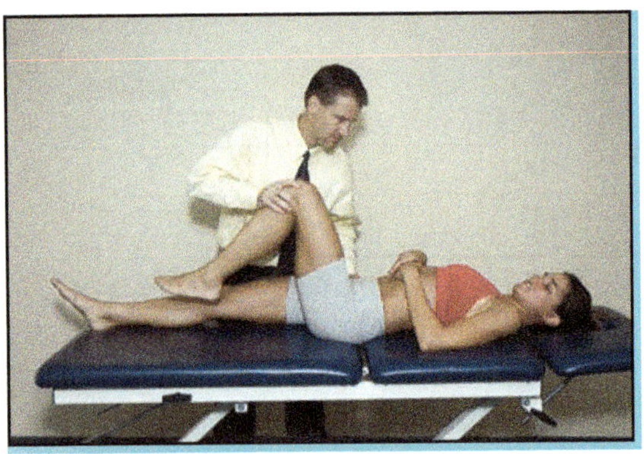

3) The examiner flexes the knee while holding the thigh in the same angle at the hip.

4) The examiner then applies further flexion to the hip.

5) If hip flexion is still restricted or results in the same pain as with the SLR, the finding is positive.

UTILITY SCORE 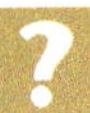

Study	Reliability	Sensitivity	Specificity	LR+	LR−	QUADAS Score (0–14)
Greenwood et al.[17]	NT	NT	NT	NA	NA	NT
Comments: A positive finding is a red flag that suggests further workup is essential.						

Key Points

1. Clinical special tests of the sacroiliac joint as a whole demonstrate poor diagnostic accuracy and poor reliability.
2. Movement-based clinical special tests suffer from very poor reliability.
3. The movement-based clinical special tests that have demonstrated good diagnostic value were performed poorly.
4. Clusters of tests, once low back pain and other contributing disorders have been ruled out, appear to be more accurate than performing tests in singular fashion.
5. Almost all of the sacroiliac tests demonstrate poor sensitivity.
6. Tests that have not used double-blinded double injections as the reference standard have questionable validity. However, it is likely that extraarticular disorders of SIJ are missed with injections.
7. Pain provocation–based clinical special tests have the best diagnostic accuracy.

8. Even after measures are taken to improve the diagnostic value of clusters of tests, the overall LR+ for diagnosing SIJ disorders is only fair to moderate.
9. Tests to determine fractures of the pelvis are more accurate compared to those designed to measure pain of SIJ origin. Patient history should always be considered.
10. Pregnancy-related pelvic girdle pain is often diagnosed by using index tests, thus reducing the validity of the reference standard.

References

1. Albert H, Godskesen M, Westergaard J. Evaluation of clinical tests used in classification procedures in pregnancy-related pelvic joint pain. *Eur Spine J.* 2000;9(2):161–166.
2. Arab AM, Abdollahi I, Joghataei MT, Golafshani Z, Kazemnejad A. Inter- and intra-examiner reliability of single and composites of selected motion palpation and pain provocation tests for sacroiliac joint. *Man Ther.* 2009;14:213–221.
3. Bemis T, Daniel M. Validation of the long sitting test on patients with iliosacral dysfunction. *J Orthop Sports Phys Ther.* 1987;8:336–343.
4. Blower P, Griffin A. (abstract). Clinical sacroiliac tests in ankylosing spondylitis and other causes of low back pain—2 studies. *Annales Rheumatic Disorders.* 1984;43:192–195.
5. Bowman C, Gribbe R. The value of the forward flexion test and three tests of leg length changes in the clinical assessment of the movement of the sacroiliac joint. *J Orthopaedic Med.* 1995;17:66–67.
6. Broadhurst NA, Bond MJ. Pain provocation tests for the assessment of sacroiliac joint dysfunction. *J Spinal Disord.* 1998;11(4):341–345.
7. Carmichael J. Inter- and intra-examiner reliability of palpation for sacroiliac joint dysfunction. *J Manipulative Physiol Therapeutics.* 1987;10:164–171.
8. Cattley P, Winyard J, Trevaskis J, Eaton S. Validity and reliability of clinical tests for the sacroiliac joint. *ACO.* 2002;10:73–80.
9. Cibulka MT, Koldehoff R. Clinical usefulness of a cluster of sacroiliac joint tests in patients with and without low back pain. *J Orthop Sports Phys Ther.* 1999; 29(2):83–89.
10. Cook C, Massa L, Harm-Emandes I, et al. Interrater reliability and diagnostic accuracy of pelvic girdle pain classification. *J Manipulative Physiol Therpeutics.* 2007;30:252–258.
11. Damen L, Buyruk HM, Guler-Uysal F, Lotgering FK, Snijders CJ, Stam HJ. The prognostic value of asymmetric laxity of the sacroiliac joints in pregnancy-related pelvic pain. *Spine.* 2002;27(24):2820–2824.
12. Dreyfuss P, Dreyer S, Griffin J, Hoffman J, Walsh N. Positive sacroiliac screening tests in asymptomatic adults. *Spine.* 1994;19(10):1138–1143.
13. Dreyfuss P, Michaelsen M, Pauza K, McLarty J, Bogduk N. The value of medical history and physical examination in diagnosing sacroiliac joint pain. *Spine.* 1996;21(22):2594–2602.
14. Evans RC. *Illustrated Essentials in Orthopedic Physical Assessment.* St. Louis, MO: Mosby Publishing; 1994.
15. Fagevik-Olsén M, Gutke A, Elden H, et al. Self-administered tests as a screening procedure for pregnancy-related pelvic girdle pain. *Eur Spine J.* 2009;18:1121–1129.
16. Fortin FJ, Falco JD. The Fortin finger test: an indicator of sacroiliac pain. *Am J Orthop.* 1997; 26(7):477–480.
17. Greenwood MJ, Erhard RE, Jones DL. Differential diagnosis of the hip vs. lumbar spine: five case reports. *J Orthop Sports Phys Ther.* 1998;27(4):308–315.
18. Gutke A, Hansson ER, Zetherstrom G, Ostgaard HC. Posterior pelvic pain provocation test is negative in patients with lumbar herniated discs. *Eur Spine J.* 2009;18:1008–1012.
19. Ham SJ, van Walsum DP, Vierhout PAM. Predictive value of the hip flexion test for fractures of the pelvis. *Injury.* 1996;27:543–544.
20. Hansen A, Jensen DV, Larsen EC, Wilken-Jensen C, Kaae BE, Frolich S, Thomsen JS, Hansen TM. Postpartum pelvic pain—the "pelvic joint syndrome": a follow-up study with special reference to diagnostic methods. *Acta Obstet Gynecol Scand.* 2005;84(2):170–176.
21. Holmgren U, Waling K. Inter-examiner reliability of four static palpation tests used for assessing pelvic dysfunction. *Man Ther.* 2008;13:50–56.
22. Hungerford B, Gilleard W, Moran M, Emmerson C. Evaluation of the ability of physical therapists to palpate intrapelvic motion with the Stork Test on the support side. *Phys Ther.* 2007;87:879–887.
23. Kokmeyer DJ, Van der Wurff P, Aufdemkampe G, Fickenscher TC. The reliability of multitest regimens with sacroiliac pain provocation tests. *J Manipulative Physiol Ther.* 2002;25(1):42–48.
24. Laslett M, Aprill C, McDonald B, Young S. Diagnosis of sacroiliac joint pain: validity of individual provocation tests and composites of tests. *Man Ther.* 2005;10:207–218.
25. Laslett M, Williams M. The reliability of selected pain provocation tests for sacroiliac joint pathology. *Spine.* 1994;19(11):1243–1249.
26. Laslett M, Young SB, Aprill CN, McDonald B. Diagnosing painful sacroiliac joints: A validity study of a McKenzie evaluation and sacroiliac provocation tests. *Aust J Physiotherapy.* 2003;49:89–97.
27. Lee D. *The Pelvic Girdle.* 2nd ed. Edinburgh, UK: Churchill Livingston; 1999.

28. Levangie PK. The association between static pelvic asymmetry and low back pain. *Spine.* 1999;24:1234–1242.

29. Levangie PK. Four clinical tests of sacroiliac joint dysfunction: the association of test results with innominate torsion among patients with and without low back pain. *Phys Ther.* 1999;79:1043–1057.

30. Magee D. *Orthopedic physical assessment.* 4th edition. Philadelphia: Saunders; 2002.

31. McCombe P, Fairbank J, Cockersole B, Pynesent P. Reproducibility of physical signs in low back pain. *Spine.* 1989;14:908–917.

32. McCormick JP, Morgan SJ, Smith WR. Clinical effectiveness of the physical examination in diagnosis of posterior pelvic ring injuries. *J Orthop Trauma.* 2003;17(4):257–261.

33. Meijne W, van Neerbos K, Aufdemkampe G, van der Wurff P. Intraexaminer and interexaminer reliability of the Gillet test. *J Manipulative Physiol Ther.* 1999;22:4–9.

34. Mens JM, Vleeming A, Snijders CJ, Koes BW, Stam HJ. Validity of the active straight leg raise test for measuring disease severity in patients with posterior pelvic pain after pregnancy. *Spine.* 2002a;27(2):196–200.

35. Mens JM, Vleeming A, Snijders CJ, Ronchetti I, Stam HJ. Reliability and validity of hip adduction strength to measure disease severity in posterior pelvic pain since pregnancy. *Spine.* 2002b;27(15):1674–1679.

36. Ostagaard H, Andersson G. Previous back pain and risk of developing back pain in future pregnancy. *Spine.* 1991;16:432–436.

37. Ozgocmen S, Bozgeyik Z, Kalcik M, Yildirim A. The value of sacroiliac pain provocation tests in early active sacroilitis. *Clin Rheumatol.* 2008;27:1275–1282.

38. Potter NA, Rothstein JM. Intertester reliability for selected clinical tests of the sacroiliac joint. *Phys Ther.* 1985;65(11):1671–1675.

39. Riddle DL, Freburger JK. Evaluation of the presence of sacroiliac joint region dysfunction using a combination of tests: a multicenter intertester reliability study. *Phys Ther.* 2002;82(8):772–781.

40. Rost CC, Jacqueline J, Kaiser A, Verhagen AP, Koes BW. Pelvic pain during pregnancy: a descriptive study of signs and symptoms of 870 patients in primary care. *Spine.* 2004;29(22):2567–2572.

41. Russell A, Maksymovich W, LeClerq S. Clinical examination of the sacroiliac joints: a prospective study. *Arthritis Rheumatism.* 1981;24:1575–1577.

42. Slipman C, Jackson H, Lipetz J. Sacroiliac joint pain referral zones. *Arch Phys Med Rehab.* 2000;81:334–338.

43. Strender L, Sjoblom A, Sundell K, Ludwig R, Taube A. Interexaminer reliability in physical examination of patients with low back pain. *Spine.* 1997;22:814–820.

44. Tong HC, Heyman OG, Lada D, Isser MM. Interexaminer reliability of three methods of combining test results to determine side of sacral restriction, sacral base position, and innominate bone position. *JAOA.* 2006;106:464–468.

45. van der Wurff P, Buijs EJ, Groen GJ. A multitest regimen of pain provocation tests as an aid to reduce unnecessary minimally invasive sacroiliac joint procedures. *Arch Phys Med Rehabil.* 2006;87(1):10–14.

46. van Deursen L, Oatijn J, Ockhuysen A, Vortman B. The value of some clinical tests of the sacroiliac joint. *Man Med.* 1990;5:96–99.

47. van Kessel-Cobelens A, Verhagen A, Mens J, Snijders C, Koes BW. Pregnancy-related pelvic girdle pain: Intertester reliability of 3 tests to determine asymmetric mobility of the sacroiliac joint. *J Manipulative Physiol Ther.* 2008;31:130–136.

48. Vincent-Smith B, Gibbons P. Inter-examiner and intra-examiner reliability of the standing flexion test. *Man Ther.* 1999;4(2):87–93.

49. Vleeming A, de Vries H, Mens J, van Wingerden JP. Possible role of the long dorsal sacroiliac ligament in women with peripartum pelvic pain. *Acta Obstet Gynecol Scand.* 2002;81:430–436.

50. Young S, Aprill C, Laslett M. Correlation of clinical examination characteristics with three sources of chronic low back pain. *Spine J.* 2003; 3(6):460–465.

PEARSON myhealthprofessionskit™

Use this address to access the Companion Website created for this textbook. Simply select "Physical Therapy" from the choice of disciplines. Find this book and log in using your username and password to access video clips of selected tests.

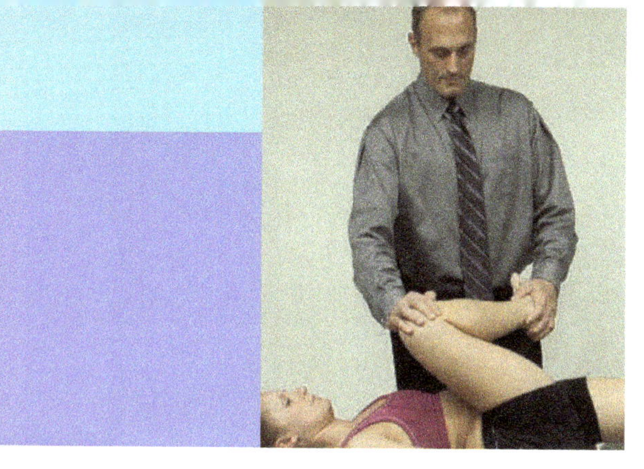

Physical Examination Tests for the Hip

Michael Reiman and Chad E. Cook

Please refer to the chapter "Introduction to Diagnostic Accuracy" before reading this chapter.

Index of Tests

From Chapter 12 of *Orthopedic Physical Examination Tests: An Evidence-Based Approach*, Second Edition. Chad Cook, Eric Hegedus.

Tests for Generalized Capsular Laxity

Dial Test
Log Roll Test
Abduction-Extension-External Rotation Test
Long Axis Femoral Distraction Test
Individualized Clinical Examination

Tests for Capsular or Muscular Dysfunction

Thomas Test
Prone Hip Extension Test

Test for Iliotibial Band Restriction

Ober Test

Tests for a Tear of the Gluteus Medius of the Hip

Trendelenburg's Sign
Resisted Hip Abduction
Passive Internal Rotation

Tests for Greater Trochanter Pain Syndrome

Single-Leg Stance Held for 30 Seconds
Resisted External Derotation Test
Composite Examination for Gluteal Tendon Pathology

Tests for Piriformis Syndrome

Flexion-Adduction-Internal Rotation (FAIR) Test
Pace Test
Freiberg Sign
Beatty Maneuver
Forceful Internal Rotation

Test for Avascular Necrosis

Combined Results

Tests for Early Signs of Hip Dysplasia

Passive Hip Abduction Test
Flexion Adduction Test

Tests for Fracture of the Hip or Femur

Patellar-Pubic Percussion Test
Stress Fracture (Fulcrum) Test

TEST FOR ALIGNMENT OF THE HIP JOINT

Craig's Test

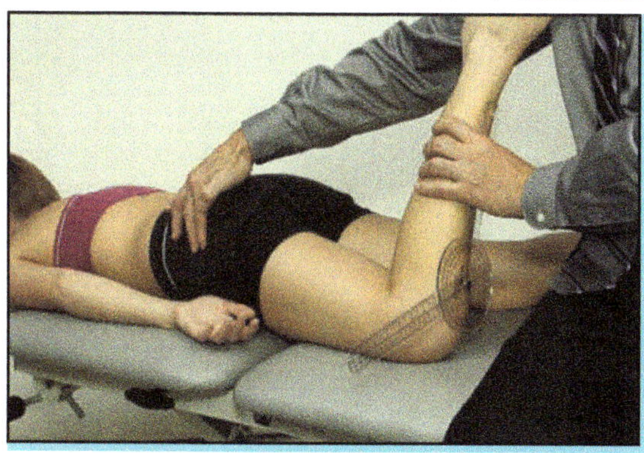

1) The patient lies prone with bilateral lower extremities in a neutral position.

2) The examiner prepositions the involved knee into approximately 90 degrees of flexion and palpates the greater trochanter of the ipsilateral side.

3) The examiner then passively rotates the hip (via the tibia) internally and externally until the greater trochanter is parallel with the plinth, or it reaches its most lateral position.

4) The examiner then aligns a standard (stationary arm horizontal and parallel to the plinth, moving arm along the tibia through the midpoint of the anterior ankle) or bubble goniometer.

5) A comparison of both sides is warranted.

6) Ten to 15 degrees of anterior torsion is normal. Anteversion is any angle greater and retroversion is any angle less than this normal.

UTILITY SCORE

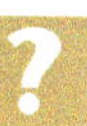

Study	Reliability	Sensitivity	Specificity	LR+	LR−	QUADAS Score (0–14)
Chung et al.[12]	0.81 (inter-tester) ICC Agreement (R) = 0.86 (CT scan)	NT	NT	NA	NA	NA
Hudson[25]	0.90 (intra-tester) ICC Agreement (β) = 0.58 (ultrasound)	NT	NT	NA	NA	NA
Lesher et al.[36]	0.47 (inter-tester) ICC	NT	NT	NA	NA	NA
Piva et al.[490]	0.45 (inter-tester) ICC	NT	NT	NA	NA	NA
Ruwe et al.[52]	Agreement (R) = .88 to .93 (intra-operative investigation)	NT	NT	NA	NA	NA
Shultz et al.[54]	0.90–0.95 (intra-tester), and 0.80–0.99 (inter-tester) ICC	NT	NT	NA	NA	NA
Shultz et al.[55]	0.77–0.97 (intra-tester), and 0.48–0.74 (inter-tester) ICC	NT	NT	NA	NA	NA
Souza & Powers[58]	0.88–0.90 (intra-tester), and 0.83 (inter-tester) ICC Agreement (ICC) 0.67 and 0.69 (MRI)	NT	NT	NA	NA	NA
Sutlive et al.[60]	0.17 (inter-tester) ICC	NT	NT	NA	NA	NA
Comments: The clinical utility of this test should be carefully considered due to variable levels of reliability and agreement with standard measures. An additional consideration is the various patient populations investigated (normals, patellofemoral pain, etc).						

TESTS FOR OSTEOARTHRITIS

Range of Motion Planes

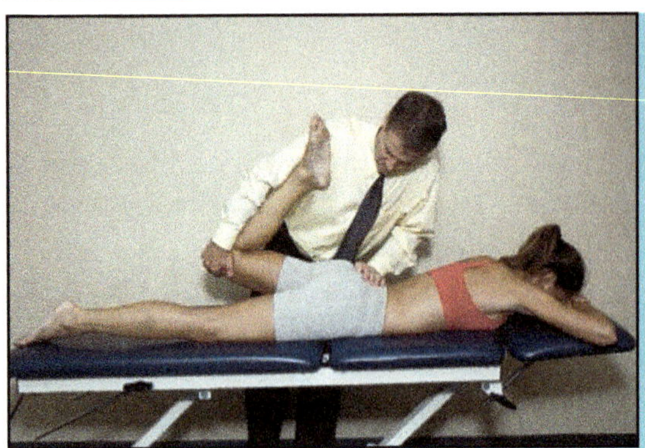

Hip Extension

1) The patient lies in a prone position.
2) The examiner passively moves the hip into extension.

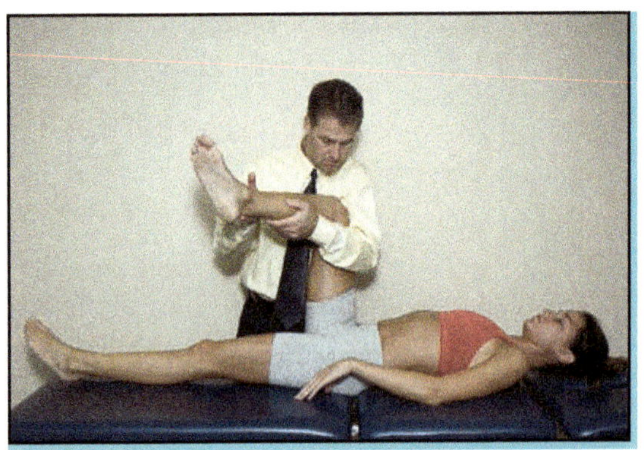

Hip External Rotation

1) The patient lies in a supine position.
2) The hip is passively flexed to 90 degrees.
3) The examiner passively moves the hip into external rotation.

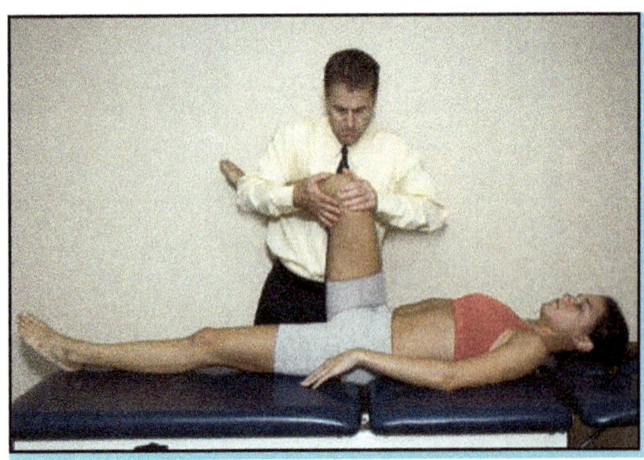

Hip Internal Rotation

1) The patient lies in a supine position.
2) The hip is passively flexed to 90 degrees.
3) The examiner passively moves the hip into internal rotation.

TESTS FOR OSTEOARTHRITIS

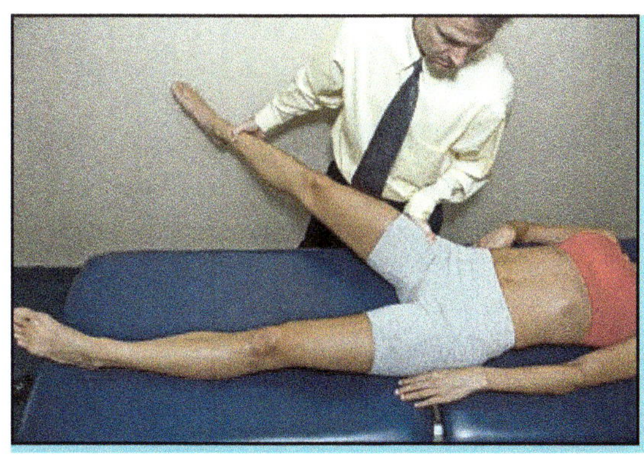

Hip Abduction

1) The patient lies in a supine position.

2) The examiner passively moves the hip into abduction.

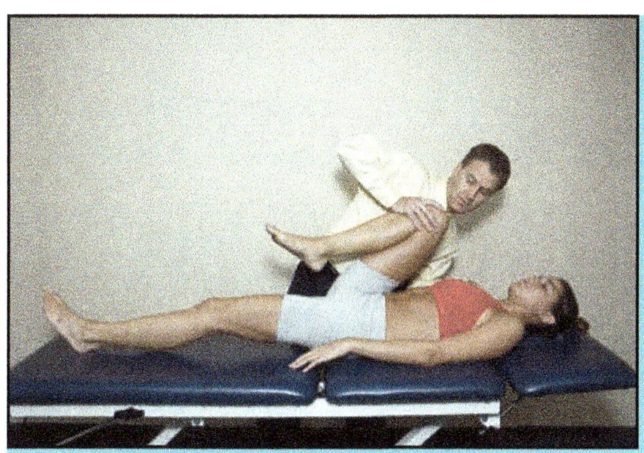

Hip Flexion

1) The patient lies in a supine position.

2) The examiner passively moves the hip into flexion.

3) A positive test is identified by reproduction of the patient's concordant pain concurrently during documented range of motion loss in comparison to the opposite extremity.

UTILITY SCORE 2

Study	Reliability	Sensitivity	Specificity	LR+	LR−	QUADAS Score (0–14)
Birrell et al.[7] (0 planes)	NT	100	0	1.0	NA	8
Birrell et al.[7] (1 plane)	NT	86	54	1.87	0.26	8
Birrell et al.[7] (2 planes)	NT	57	77	2.48	0.56	8
Birrell et al.[7] (3 planes)	NT	33	93	4.71	0.72	8

Comments: This association is between the numbers of planes with restricted movement and mild to moderate hip OA (Croft grade ≥ 2). Specificity only increases to a good value if three planes or more are restricted. Note that a capsular pattern is not used as it has not shown predictability in patients with osteoarthritis.

TESTS FOR OSTEOARTHRITIS

UTILITY SCORE 2

Study	Reliability	Sensitivity	Specificity	LR+	LR−	QUADAS Score (0–14)
Birrell et al.[7] (0 planes)	NT	100	0	1.0	NA	8
Birrell et al.[7] (1 plane)	NT	100	42	1.72	NA	8
Birrell et al.[7] (2 planes)	NT	81	69	2.61	0.28	8
Birrell et al.[7] (3 planes)	NT	54	88	4.5	0.52	8
Comments: This association is between the numbers of planes with restricted movement and severe hip OA (minimum joint space ≤ 1.5 mm). Specificity only increases to a good value if three planes or more are restricted. Note that a capsular pattern is again not used as it has not shown predictability in patients with osteoarthritis.						

UTILITY SCORE 3

Study	Reliability	Sensitivity	Specificity	LR+	LR−	QUADAS Score (0–14)
Altman et al.[2] (flexion)	NT	80	40	1.33	0.50	8
Altman et al.[2] (extension)	NT	64	50	1.28	0.72	8
Altman et al.[2] (abduction)	NT	76	44	1.36	0.54	8
Altman et al.[2] (adduction)	NT	68	54	1.48	0.59	8
Altman et al.[2] (internal rotation)	NT	82	39	1.34	0.46	8
Altman et al.[2] (external rotation)	NT	79	37	1.25	0.57	8
Comments: As shown below and in combined results from Altman et al.[2] the most sensitive values were for flexion and internal rotation, although these values alone are poor screening tests.						

UTILITY SCORE 

Study	Reliability	Sensitivity	Specificity	LR+	LR−	QUADAS Score (0–14)
Altman et al.[2] (flexion ≤ 115 degrees)	NT	96	18	1.17	0.22	8
Altman et al.[2] (internal rotation < 15 degrees)	NT	66	72	2.35	0.47	8
Comments: These criteria alone had lower diagnostic/screening value than the combined results listed below.						

TESTS FOR OSTEOARTHRITIS

Combined Results

UTILITY SCORE 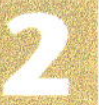

Study	Reliability	Sensitivity	Specificity	LR+	LR−	QUADAS Score (0–14)
Altman et al.[2]	NT	86	75	3.4	0.19	8

Comments: Clinical diagnosis was used, which included the following index testing methods. Signs and symptoms involve (1) hip pain, (2) IR < 15 degrees, (3) pain with IR, (4) morning stiffness ≤ 60 minutes, and (5) age > 50 years.

Other Combined Results

UTILITY SCORE 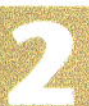

Study	Reliability	Sensitivity	Specificity	LR+	LR−	QUADAS Score (0–14)
Youdas et al.[67] (resisted hip abduction)	0.97 and 0.98 (intra-tester) ICC	35	90	3.5	0.72	10
Youdas et al.[67] (Trendelenburg test)	0.63 and 0.69 (intra-tester) ICC	55	70	1.83	0.82	10

Comments: Youdas et al.[67] utilized these tests in attempts to identify patients with hip osteoarthritis. Resisted manual muscle test (MMT) was performed with a supine "make" test against a dynamometer. Detailed description of the Trendelenburg test is listed under gluteus medius dysfunction.

UTILITY SCORE 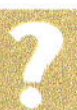

Study	Reliability	Sensitivity	Specificity	LR+	LR−	QUADAS Score (0–14)
Cibere et al.[13] (Trendelenburg test)	0.06	NT	NT	NA	NA	NA
Cibere et al.[13] (hip pain with log roll test)	0.88	NT	NT	NA	NA	NA
Cibere et al.[13] (FABER test)	0.80	NT	NT	NA	NA	NA
Cibere et al.[13] (Thomas test)	0.88	NT	NT	NA	NA	NA
Cibere et al.[13] (Ober test)	0.80	NT	NT	NA	NA	NA

Comments: All measures were inter-rater amongst orthopedic surgeons and rheumatologists on patients with mild to moderate hip osteoarthritis. Each value was listed as post-standardization prevalence-adjusted bias-adjusted kappa values. Each test is explained later in this chapter.

Clinical Prediction Rule for Diagnosing Hip Osteoarthritis

UTILITY SCORE 

Study	Reliability	Sensitivity	Specificity	LR+	LR−	QUADAS Score (0–14)
Sutlive et al.[60] (5 predictors present)	0.52 (inter-rater) kappa for end-feel assessment (Scour test) 0.90 (inter-rater) ICC for motion assessment; 0.47 (inter-rater) kappa for end-feel assessment (FABER test)	14	98	7.3	0.87	13
Sutlive et al.[60] (≥ 4 predictors present)		0.48	0.98	24.3	0.53	13
Sutlive et al.[60] (≥ 3 predictors present)		0.71	0.86	5.2	0.33	13
Sutlive et al.[60] (≥ 2 predictors present)		0.81	0.61	2.1	0.31	13
Sutlive et al.[60] (≥ 1 predictor present)		0.95	0.18	1.2	0.27	13

Comments: Low subject number in the study and a lack of a validation study should caution the clinician regarding the implementation of this clinical prediction rule for routine clinical practice, despite the high QUADAS score.
Predictor variables included: self-report of squatting as aggravating factor, active hip flexion causing lateral pain, passive internal rotation ≤ 25 degrees, active hip extension causing hip pain. Detailed descriptions of Scour and FABER tests are later in the chapter.

TESTS FOR INTRA-ARTICULAR PATHOLOGY

Hip Scour

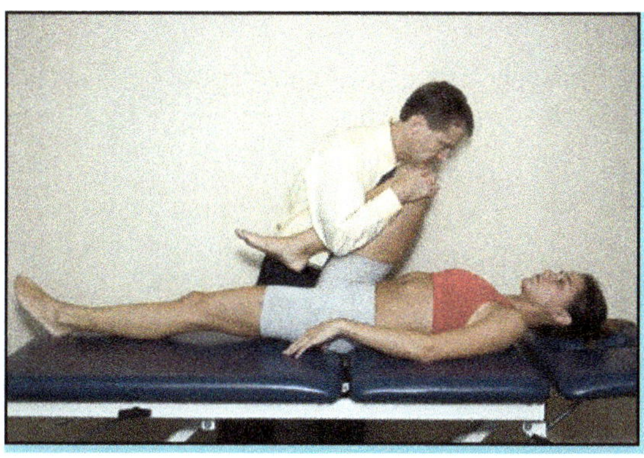

1) The patient assumes a supine position.

2) The examiner flexes the patient's knee and provides an axial load through the femur.

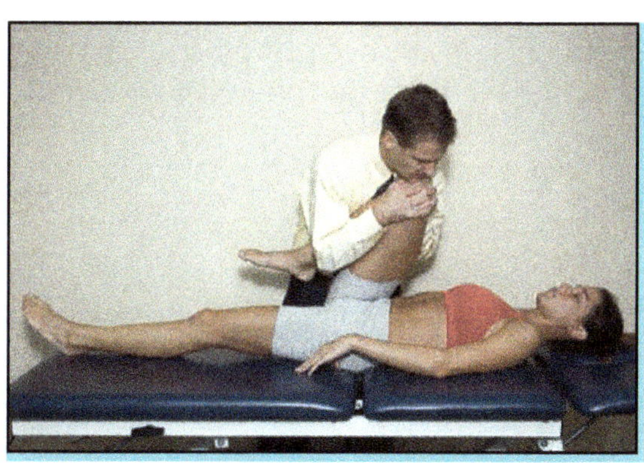

3) The examiner performs a sweeping compression and rotation movement from external rotation to internal rotation.

4) A positive test is pain or apprehension at a given point during the examination.

UTILITY SCORE 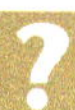

Study	Reliability	Sensitivity	Specificity	LR+	LR−	QUADAS Score (0–14)
Cliborne et al.[14]	0.87 (intra-rater) ICC	NT	NT	NT	NA	NA

Comments: Other tests have similar components, but variability in title and performance of these tests required their description as per original author's title and performance descriptions. These tests are all listed later in the chapter under impingement/labral tear testing.
Cliborne et al.[14] measurements were administered on patients with knee osteoarthritis.

TESTS FOR INTRA-ARTICULAR PATHOLOGY

Hip Quadrant

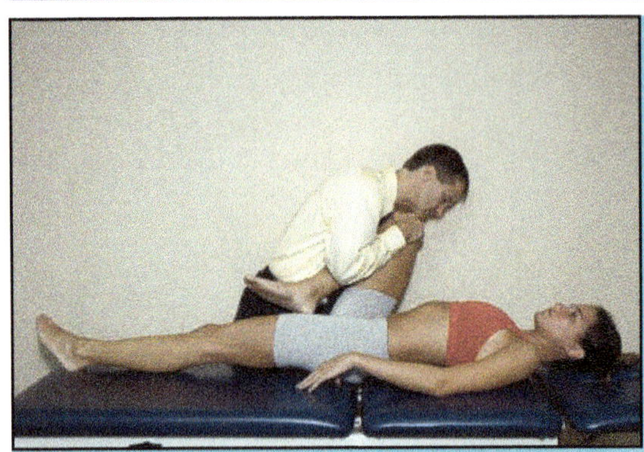

1) The patient assumes a supine position.

2) The examiner passively moves the hip through the combined motions of flexion, abduction, and internal rotation.

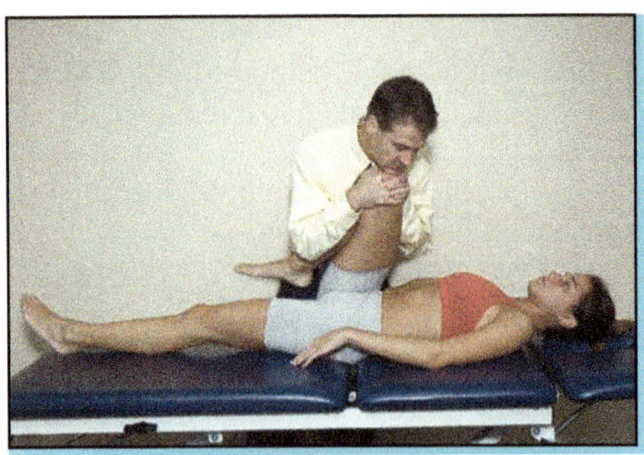

3) The passive combined movements of flexion, abduction, and external rotation have also been described as components of this test after the above motions were completed.

4) A positive test is reproduction of the hip symptoms.

UTILITY SCORE 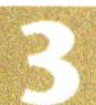

Study	Reliability	Sensitivity	Specificity	LR+	LR−	QUADAS Score (0–14)
Mitchell et al.[44]	NT	NT	NT	NA	NA	7
Comments: No investigation has been performed on this test as described.						

TESTS FOR INTRA-ARTICULAR PATHOLOGY

Flexion Abduction External Rotation (FABER) Test (Patrick Test)

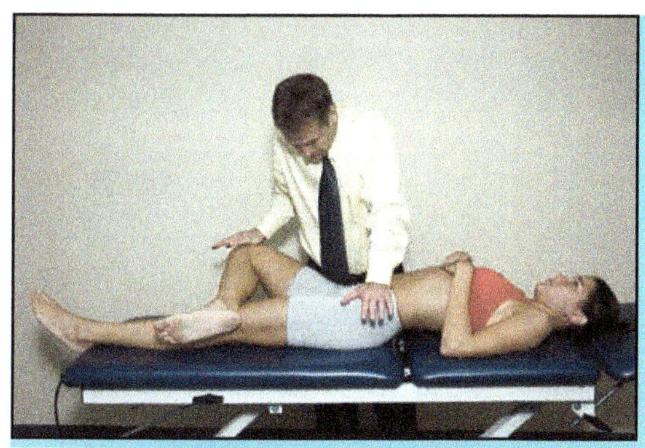

1) The patient is positioned in supine. Resting symptoms are assessed.

2) The painful side leg is placed in a "figure four" position. The ankle is placed just above the knee of the other leg.

3) The examiner provides a gentle downward pressure on both the knee of the painful side and the ASIS of the non-painful side. Concordant pain is assessed, specifically the location and type of pain.

4) A positive test is concordant pain near the anterior or lateral capsule of the hip.

UTILITY SCORE 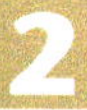 2

Study	Reliability	Sensitivity	Specificity	LR+	LR−	QUADAS Score (0–14)
Cliborne et al.[14] (gravity inclinometer)	0.87 (inter-rater) ICC	NT	NT	NA	NA	NA
Clohisy et al.[15]	NT	99	NT	NA	NA	9
Martin & Sekiya[40]	0.63 (inter-rater) kappa	NT	NT	NA	NA	NA
Mitchell et al.[44]	NT	88	NT	NA	NA	7
Philippon et al.[48]	NT	97	NT	NA	NA	7
Ross et al.[51]	0.93 (intra-tester) ICC	NT	NT	NA	NA	NA
Sutlive et al.[60]	0.90 (inter-rater) ICC for motion assessment; 0.47 (inter-rater) kappa for end-feel assessment	57	71	1.9	0.61	13
Theiler et al.[62] (tape measure)	0.66 and .74 (inter-rater) ICC	NT	NT	NA	NA	NA
Troelsen et al.[64]	NT	41	100	Inf	0.59	9

Comments: The FABER test is also a test for sacroiliac pain. Pain posteriorly is associated with sacroiliac dysfunction. The high sensitivity and specificity (in different studies) are indicative of the potential for both a screening and diagnostic tool respectively, although study designs were poor. Most studies only investigated patients with known pathology, therefore specificity is unknown. Clohisy et al.[15] utilized this test for hip anterior impingement pathology. Philippon et al.[48] criteria for a positive test was any loss of distance between knee and table compared to the other side, potentially resulting in false positive results as compared to a positive result of pain and limited motion. Troelsen et al.[64] only investigated subjects with previous periacetabular osteotomies due to symptomatic, acetabular dysplasia.

TESTS FOR INTRA-ARTICULAR PATHOLOGY

Composite Examination

UTILITY SCORE 3

Study	Reliability	Sensitivity	Specificity	LR+	LR−	QUADAS Score (0–14)
Symptoms (Martin et al.[39])						
(+) Groin pain	NT	59	14	0.67	3	10
(+) Catching	NT	63	54	1.39	0.68	10
(+) Pinching pain sitting	NT	48	54	1.1	0.95	10
(–) Lateral thigh pain	NT	78	36	1.2	0.61	10
Signs (Martin et al.[39])						
(+) FABER	NT	60	18	0.73	2.2	10
(+) Impingement	NT	78	10	0.86	2.3	10
(–) Trochanteric tenderness	NT	57	45	1.1	0.93	10
Comments: The clinical utility of these signs and symptoms to consistently identify subjects with primary intra-articular pain sources was poor. The reference standard utilized in this study was greater than 50% relief with intra-articular anesthetic-steroid injection.						

Flexion-Adduction-Internal Rotation (Click) Test

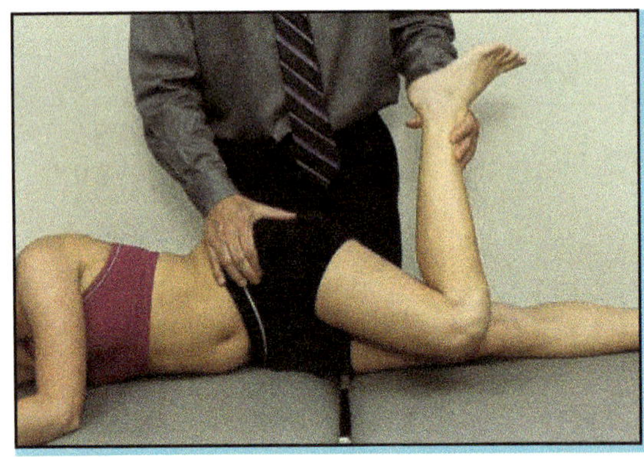

1. The patient is sidelying. The symptomatic lower extremity is placed upward; the asymptomatic lower extremity is placed on the plinth side.
2. The examiner prepositions the knee into flexion.
3. The examiner stabilizes the pelvis at the iliac crest.
4. The examiner then guides the lower extremity passively from 50 to 100 degrees of hip flexion and adduction while internally rotating the hip.
5. A comparison of both sides is warranted.
6. A positive test is indicated with the presence of a click or reproduction of symptoms (indicative of some form of intra-articular pathology, including femoroacetabular impingement [FAI]).

UTILITY SCORE 

Study	Reliability	Sensitivity	Specificity	LR+	LR−	QUADAS Score (0–14)
None	NT	NT	NT	NA	NA	NT
Comments: Although this test is purported for intra-articular pathology, similar testing is suggestive for other pathologies like piriformis syndrome.						

Heel Strike Test

1) The patient lies supine, with bilateral lower extremities in neutral.
2) The examiner lifts the lower extremity to be assessed.
3) The examiner, keeping the knee straight, strikes the heel of the lower extremity.
4) A comparison of both sides is warranted.
5) A positive test is indicated by the reproduction of pain or patient's symptoms, specifically deep hip pain.

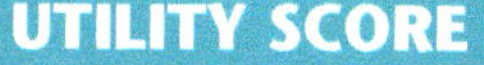

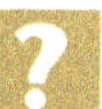

Study	Reliability	Sensitivity	Specificity	LR+	LR−	QUADAS Score (0–14)
None	NT	NT	NT	NA	NA	NA
Comments: This type of testing has also been utilized to implicate fracture/stress fracture in the lower extremity, and therefore is likely not specific to intra-articular hip pathology.						

TESTS FOR INTRA-ARTICULAR PATHOLOGY

Resisted Straight Leg Raise Test

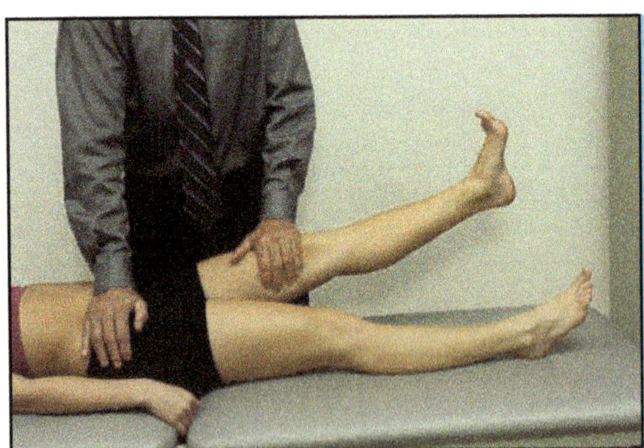

1) The patient is supine with bilateral lower extremities in neutral position.

2) The examiner places their hand on the thigh of the painful lower extremity.

3) The patient raises the painful lower extremity 30 cm off the plinth.

4) The examiner applies a downward force at the distal thigh as the patient resists this force.

5) A comparison of both sides is warranted.

6) A positive test involves reproduction of pain in the lower quadrant, indicating possible peritoneal inflammation, appendicitis, or inflammation of the iliopsoas.

UTILITY SCORE 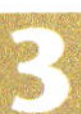

Study	Reliability	Sensitivity	Specificity	LR+	LR−	QUADAS Score (0–14)
Clohisy et al.[15]	NT	56	NT	NA	NA	9
Troelsen et al.[64]	NT	5	NT	NA	NA	9

Comments: There are other names (Iliopsoas, Stitchfield's test) and variable descriptions of this test. Troelsen et al.[64] implemented this test to diagnose hip labral tear. Other descriptions have been purported for differential diagnosis of lower quadrant pain (possible peritoneal inflammation, appendicitis, or inflammation of the iliopsoas muscle). Clohisy et al.[15] utilized this test for hip anterior impingement pathology.

Other Composite Tests

UTILITY SCORE 3

Study	Reliability	Sensitivity	Specificity	LR+	LR−	QUADAS Score (0–14)
Maslowski et al.[41] (FABER test [F])	NT	82	25	1.1	0.72	6
Maslowski et al.[41] (Resisted straight-leg-raise: Stinchfield test [St])	NT	59	32	0.87	1.28	6
Maslowski et al.[41] (Scour test [Sc])	NT	50	29	0.70	1.72	6
Maslowski et al.[41] (Internal rotation overpressure [IROP])	NT	91	18	1.1	0.5	6
Maslowski et al.[41] (F + St)	NT	96	11	1.1	0.36	6
Maslowski et al.[41] (F + St + Sc)	NT	100	11	1.1	0	6
Maslowski et al.[41] (F + St + Sc + IROP)	NT	100	0	1.0	0	6
Comments: Internal rotation overpressure (IROP) is performed in supine with pelvis stabilized, hip and knees flexed to 90 degrees, and passive internal rotation to end-range with gentle overpressure. Composite testing demonstrated improved screening and diagnostic capabilities versus individual testing, although the study has demonstrated poor design.						

TESTS FOR FEMOROACETABULAR IMPINGEMENT AND/OR LABRAL TEAR

Femoral Acetabular Impingement (Flexion-Adduction-Internal Rotation Impingement Test) (FADDIR) Test

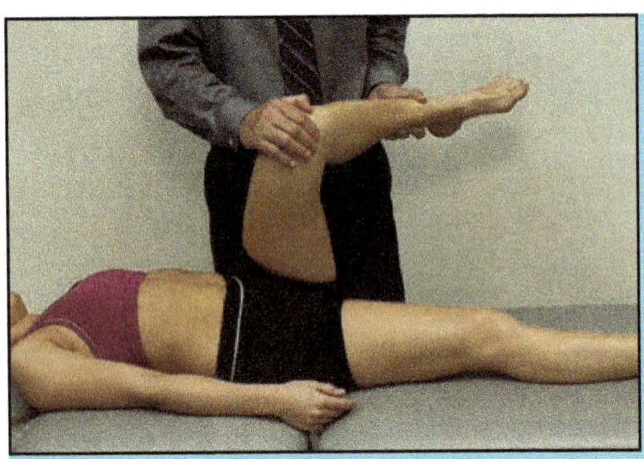

1) The patient lies supine with bilateral lower extremities in neutral position.

2) The examiner prepositions the involved hip into approximately 90 degrees of flexion.

3) The examiner then adducts and internally rotates the involved hip.

4) A comparison of both sides is warranted.

5) A positive test is reproduction of groin pain, indicative of mechanical impingement and/or labral pathology.

UTILITY SCORE 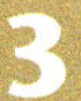

Study	Reliability	Sensitivity	Specificity	LR+	LR−	QUADAS Score (0–14)
Beaule et al.[4]	NT	100	0	1.0	NA	7
Beck et al.[5]	NT	100	NT	NA	NA	7
Burnett et al.[9]	NT	95	NT	NA	NA	8
Clohisy et al.[15]	NT	88	NT	NA	NA	9
Ito et al.[26]	NT	96 (labral tear)	NT	NA	NA	8
Kassarjian et al.[31]	NT	100	NA	NA	NA	6
Keeney et al.[32]	NT	100	NT	1.0	NA	8
Klaue et al.[33]	NT	NT	NT	NA	NA	7
Leunig et al.[34]	NT	91	NT	NA	NA	8
Martin & Sekiya[40]	0.58 (inter-rater) kappa	NT	NT	NA	NA	NA
Philippon et al.[48]	NT	99	NT	NA	NA	7
Sink et al.[56]	NT	100	NT	NA	NA	9
Troelsen et al.[64]	NT	59	100	Inf	0.41	9

Comments: This combined movement engages the femoral head-neck junction into the anterior superior labrum and acetabular rim. Some have described full flexion vs. 90 degrees of flexion. Reproduction of groin pain has been described as an indicator for femoroacetabular impingement and/or labral tear. Most studies only investigated patients with known impingement or labral pathology, therefore specificity is unknown. Additionally, many of the studies were retrospective analyses.

TESTS FOR FEMOROACETABULAR IMPINGEMENT AND/OR LABRAL TEAR

Impingement Provocation Test (Postero-Inferior Labrum)

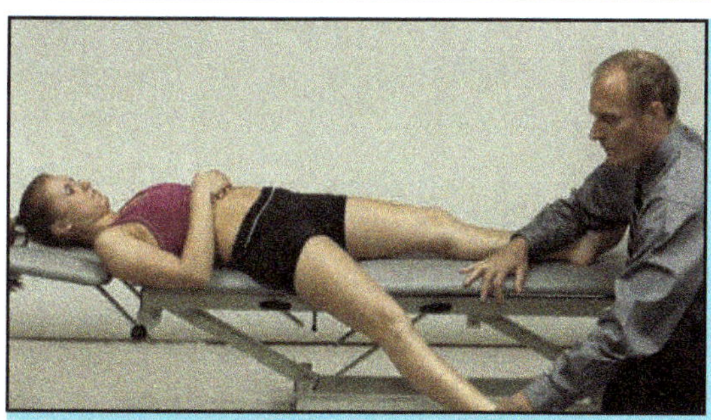

1) The patient is supine, bilateral lower extremities in neutral, and close to the edge of the plinth on the side to be assessed.

2) The examiner guides the involved hip into hyperextension, abduction, and external rotation.

3) A comparison of both sides is warranted.

4) A positive test is reproduction of discomfort and apprehension on the part of the patient.

UTILITY SCORE 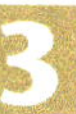

Study	Reliability	Sensitivity	Specificity	LR+	LR−	QUADAS Score (0–14)
Clohisy et al.[15]	NT	21	NT	NA	NA	9
Leunig et al.[34]	NT	100	0	1.0	NA	8

Comments: The authors mention discomfort and apprehension as a positive test, although they did not specifically define a positive test or location of discomfort. It is theorized that this test is impinging the femoral head against the postero-inferior rim of the acetabulum.

Individualized Clinical Examination

1) Examiner performed clinical examination as normal in the clinical practice.

2) A positive test was determined individually by examiner.

UTILITY SCORE 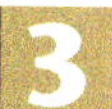

Study	Reliability	Sensitivity	Specificity	LR+	LR−	QUADAS Score (0–14)
Martin et al.[37]	65% agreement	70	56	1.6	0.43	6

Comments: Study utilized eight orthopedic surgeons to perform clinical exams as they normally would. Components of each clinical exam are unknown. Clinical exam results were compared with arthroscopy, and agreement amongst surgeons was investigated.

TESTS FOR FEMOROACETABULAR IMPINGEMENT AND/OR LABRAL TEAR

Patient History—Clicking or Locking

1) The patient is queried regarding pain during sitting.
2) The patient is queried regarding clicking or popping during gait, squatting, or other activities.
3) A positive test is present if a click is present during active or passive motion of the hip.

UTILITY SCORE 3

Study	Reliability	Sensitivity	Specificity	LR+	LR−	QUADAS Score (0–14)
Dorrell & Catterall[17]	NT	50	NT	NA	NA	6
Fitzgerald[21]	NT	79	NT	NA	NA	3
Narvani et al.[45]	NT	100	85	6.67	0.0	7
Comments: Most authors use click and catch synonymously. Essentially, the study designs were so poor one cannot extrapolate the benefits of these findings.						

Posterior Hip Labrum Test

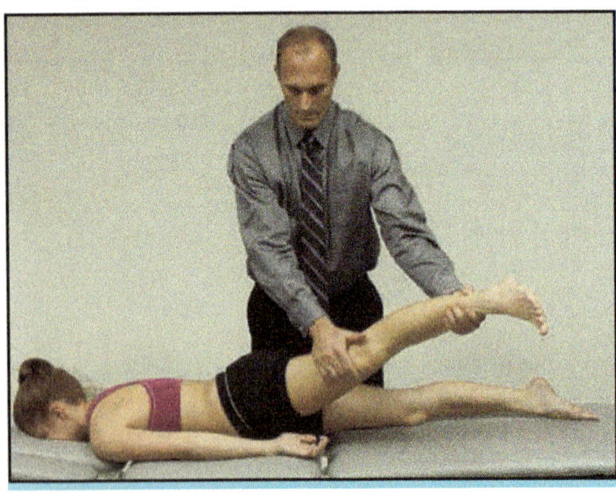

1) The patient lies in a prone position.
2) The examiner slowly moves the hip on the painful side near full extension and moderate abduction.
3) The examiner then applies a concurrent external hip rotation while completing the full extension.
4) A positive test is identified by reproduction of the patient's concordant pain.

UTILITY SCORE 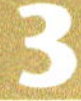

Study	Reliability	Sensitivity	Specificity	LR+	LR−	QUADAS Score (0–14)
Leunig et al.[34]	NT	22	NT	NA	NA	8
Comments: The use of a belt across the patient's buttocks has also been described with the performance of this test.[21] Leunig et al.[34] only investigated patients with known hip labrum tears, thus the specificity of this test is unknown. It is likely that patients with tight anterior hip flexors will experience false positives with this test.						

TESTS FOR FEMOROACETABULAR IMPINGEMENT AND/OR LABRAL TEAR

Palpation Posterior to Greater Trochanter

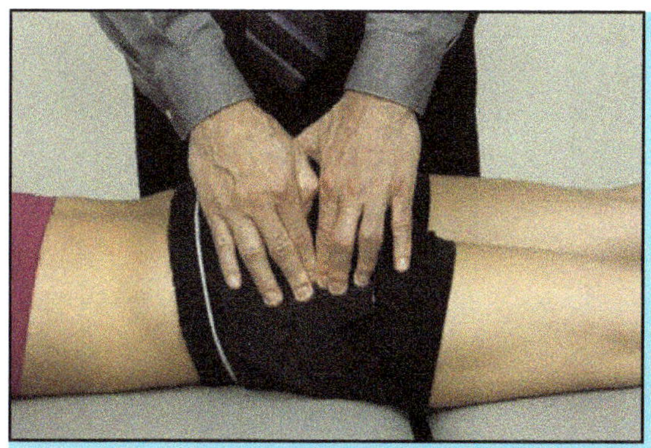

1) The examiner palpates posterior to the greater trochanter on the involved side.

2) A comparison of both sides is warranted.

3) A positive test is reproduction of pain/discomfort.

UTILITY SCORE 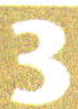

Study	Reliability	Sensitivity	Specificity	LR+	LR−	QUADAS Score (0–14)
Hase & Ueo[24]	NT	80	NT	NA	NA	9
Martin & Sekiya[40]	0.66 (inter-rater) kappa	NT	NT	NA	NA	NA
Comments: Hase & Ueo[24] used positive tenderness as a sign of labral tear. Other studies have suggested negative tenderness here is a screening tool for extra-articular pathology.						

TESTS FOR FEMOROACETABULAR IMPINGEMENT AND/OR LABRAL TEAR

Flexion-Internal Rotation Test

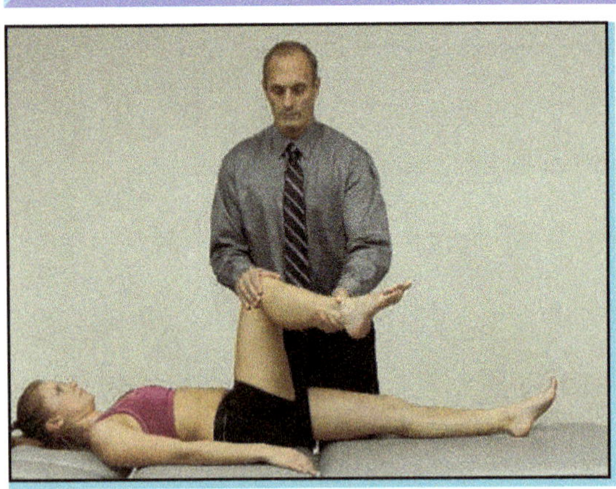

1) The patient lies in a supine position.
2) The examiner passively performs the combined motions of flexion to 90 degrees and internal rotation.
3) A comparison of both sides is warranted.
4) A positive test is reproduction of pain/discomfort in the groin (similar to impingement testing) indicative of labral degeneration, fraying, or tearing.

UTILITY SCORE 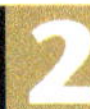

Study	Reliability	Sensitivity	Specificity	LR+	LR−	QUADAS Score (0–14)
Chan et al.[11] (MRI)	NT	100	0	1.0	NA	11
Chan et al.[11] (arthroscopy)	NT	100	0	1.0	NA	11
Hase & Ueo[24]	NT	100	NT	1.0	NA	9
Petersilge et al.[47]	NT	100	0	1.0	NA	9
Santori & Villar[53]	NT	100	NT	NA	NA	10
Comments: These studies were a combination of retrospective and prospective analyses of potential surgical candidates for intra-articular pathology. Petersilge et al.[47] and Hase & Ueo[24] had subject numbers less than 10.						

TESTS FOR FEMOROACETABULAR IMPINGEMENT AND/OR LABRAL TEAR

Flexion-Adduction-Axial Compression Test

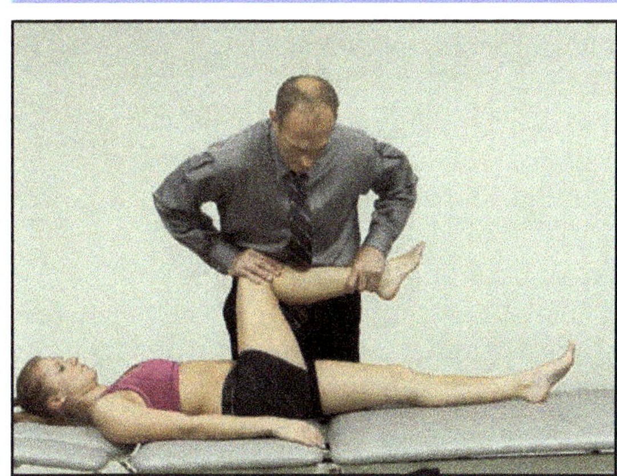

1) The patient lies in a supine position.

2) The examiner passively performs the combined motions of hip flexion, internal rotation, and adduction.

3) A comparison of both sides is warranted.

4) A positive test is reproduction of pain/discomfort in the groin (similar to impingement testing) indicative of labral degeneration, fraying, or tearing.

UTILITY SCORE 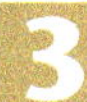

Study	Reliability	Sensitivity	Specificity	LR+	LR−	QUADAS Score (0–14)
Hase & Ueo[24]	NT	100	NT	NA	NA	9
Comments: Again, low subject numbers in this retrospective study of patients with labral tear pathology.						

TESTS FOR FEMOROACETABULAR IMPINGEMENT AND/OR LABRAL TEAR

Internal Rotation-Flexion-Axial Compression Test

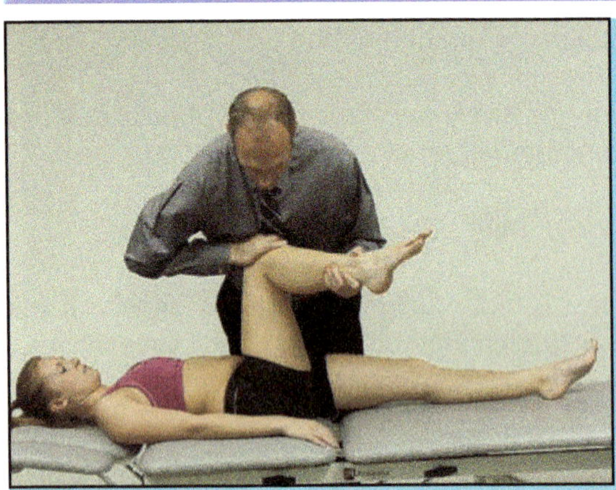

1) The patient lies in a supine position.

2) The examiner passively performs the combined motions of hip flexion, internal rotation, and axial compression (longitudinally through the femur).

3) A comparison of both sides is warranted.

4) A positive test is reproduction of pain/discomfort in the groin (similar to impingement testing) indicative of labral degeneration, fraying, or tearing.

UTILITY SCORE 

Study	Reliability	Sensitivity	Specificity	LR+	LR−	QUADAS Score (0–14)
Narvani et al.[45]	NT	75	43	1.32	0.58	7
Comments: Although similar to the Hip Scour test, the description of the test is per Narvani et al.[45] As with other various impingement/labral testing, the proposed mechanism is mechanical abutment of the femoral head against the acetabular rim (anterior-superior portion in the case of anterior impingement).						

TESTS FOR FEMOROACETABULAR IMPINGEMENT AND/OR LABRAL TEAR

Maximum Flexion-Internal Rotation (MFIR) Test

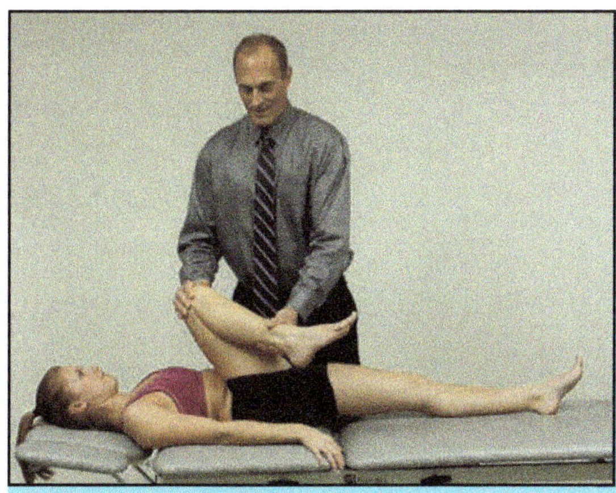

1) The patient lies in a supine position.
2) The examiner passively performs the combined motions of maximum hip flexion, and internal rotation.
3) A comparison of both sides is warranted.
4) A positive test is reproduction of patient's pain.

UTILITY SCORE 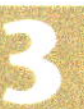

Study	Reliability	Sensitivity	Specificity	LR+	LR−	QUADAS Score (0–14)
Guanche & Sikka[23]	NT	100	NT	NA	NA	6
Suenaga et al.[59] (all types of tears)	Accuracy: 0.77 (intra-tester); 0.78 (inter-tester)	38	NT	NA	NA	6
Suenaga et al.[59] (posterior-superior complete tears)	As above for all tears	79	50	1.6	0.42	6

Comments: Poor study designs limit the applicability of this test as a screening tool. This test has been one of various descriptions for the quadrant test. Suenaga et al.[59] indicated that a partial tear of the labrum was the only positive finding.

TESTS FOR FEMOROACETABULAR IMPINGEMENT AND/OR LABRAL TEAR

Maximum Flexion-External Rotation (MFER) Test

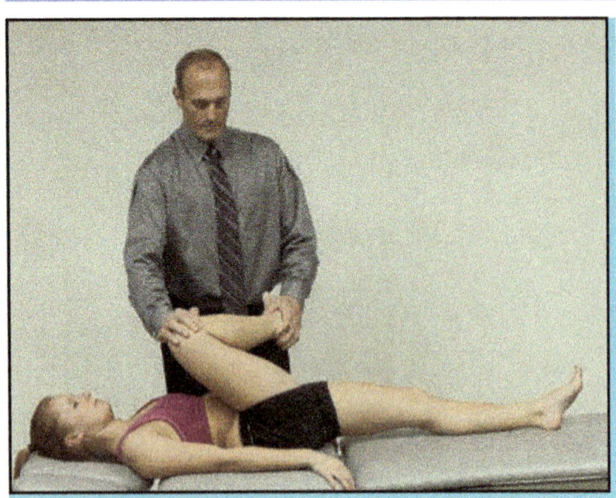

1) The patient lies in a supine position.
2) The examiner passively performs the combined motions of maximum hip flexion and external rotation.
3) A comparison of both sides is warranted.
4) A positive test is reproduction of patient's pain.

UTILITY SCORE 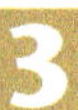

Study	Reliability	Sensitivity	Specificity	LR+	LR−	QUADAS Score (0–14)
Suenaga et al.[59]	Accuracy: 0.68 (intra-tester); 0.65 (inter-tester)	27	NT	NA	NA	6

Comments: Poor study designs limit the applicability of this test as a screening tool.
This test has been one of various descriptions for the quadrant test. Suenaga et al.[59] indicated that a partial tear of the labrum was the only positive finding.

Fitzgerald Test—Anterior Labral Tear

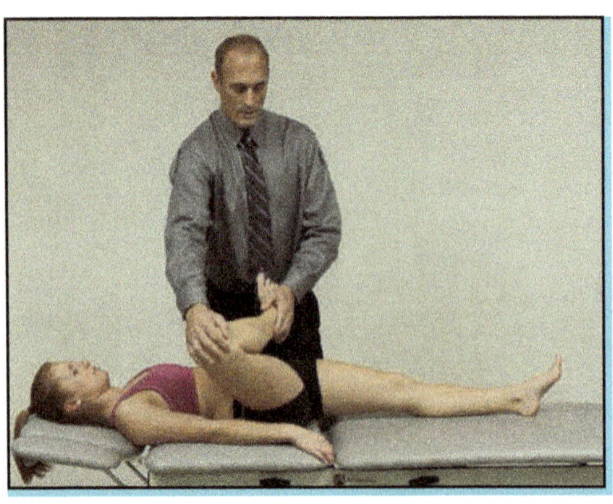

1) The patient lies in a supine position.
2) The examiner passively moves the hip into the combined motions of full flexion, external rotation, and abduction as a starting point.

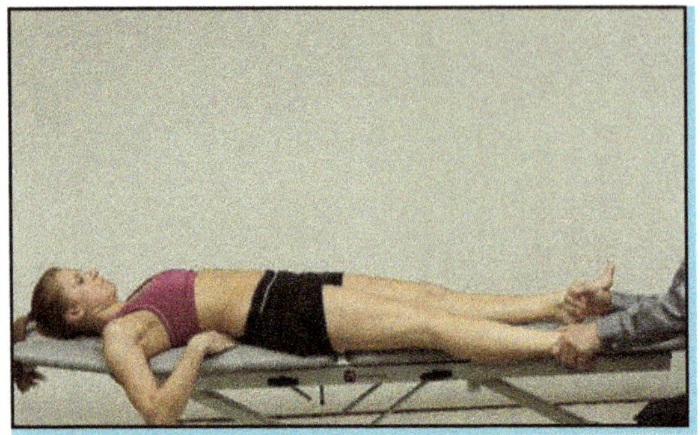

3) The examiner then extends the hip combined with internal rotation and adduction.
4) A comparison of both sides is warranted.
5) A positive test is reproduction of patient's pain with/without a click.

TESTS FOR FEMOROACETABULAR IMPINGEMENT AND/OR LABRAL TEAR

Fitzgerald Test—Posterior Labral Tear

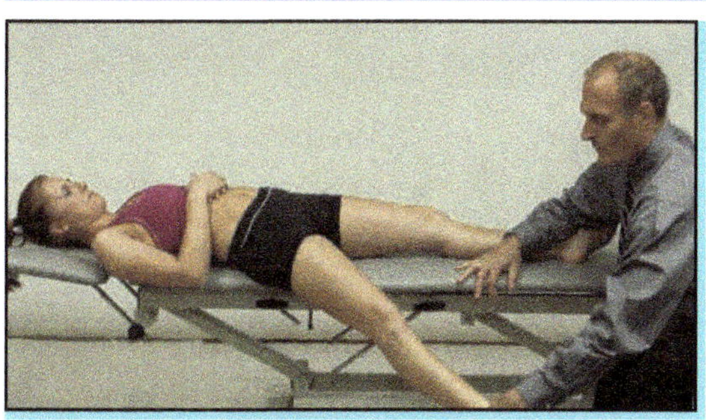

1) The patient lies in a supine position.

2) The examiner passively moves the hip into the combined motions of full extension, external rotation, and abduction as a starting point.

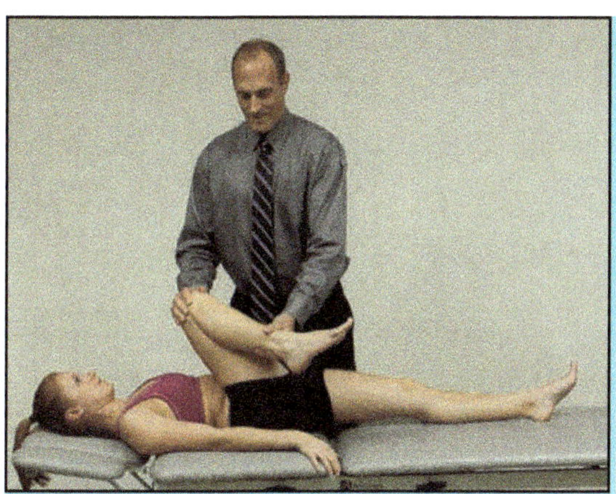

3) The examiner then flexes the hip combined with adduction and internal rotation.

4) A comparison of both sides is warranted.

5) A positive test is reproduction of patient's pain with/without a click.

UTILITY SCORE 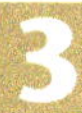

Study	Reliability	Sensitivity	Specificity	LR+	LR−	QUADAS Score (0–14)
Fitzgerald[21]	NT	96	NT	NA	NA	3
Comments: Due to poor research design, the ability of this test to be used as a screening tool should be cautioned despite the high sensitivity. Fitzgerald[21] described two maneuvers, one for anterior and one for posterior labral tear. They did not differentiate positive test findings on this test versus posterior labral tear test.						

TESTS FOR FEMOROACETABULAR IMPINGEMENT AND/OR LABRAL TEAR

McCarthy Test

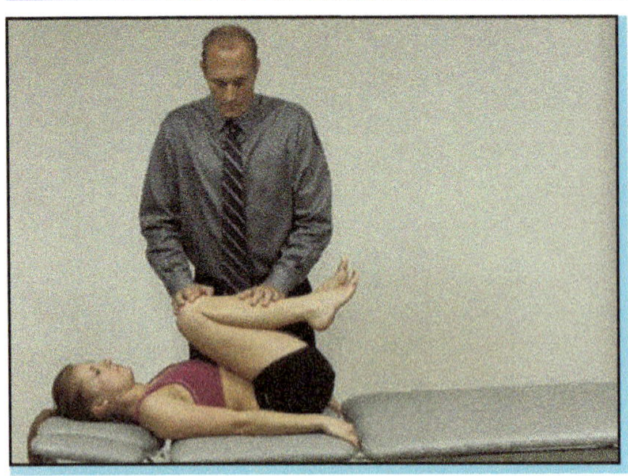

1) The patient lies in a supine position.
2) The examiner passively moves bilateral lower extremities into full flexion.
3) The patient holds non-tested lower extremity in full flexion with bilateral hands.

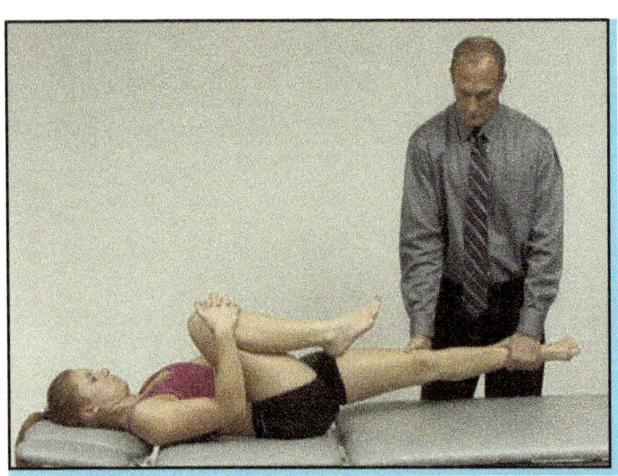

4) The examiner extends the lower extremity to be assessed, first into external rotation, and then into internal rotation.
5) A comparison of both sides is warranted.
6) A positive test is reproduction of patient's pain with/without a click.

UTILITY SCORE 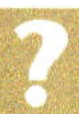

Study	Reliability	Sensitivity	Specificity	LR+	LR−	QUADAS Score (0–14)
None	NT	NT	NT	NA	NA	NA
Comments: This test, although described in multiple articles, has not had any diagnostic values reported. The external rotation with extension component of this maneuver has also been described as the posterior rim impingement test, although no diagnostic studies have been performed.						

TESTS FOR FEMOROACETABULAR IMPINGEMENT AND/OR LABRAL TEAR

Individualized Clinical Examination

1) Examiner performed clinical examination as would normally be done in the clinical practice.

2) A positive test was determined individually by examiner.

UTILITY SCORE 2

Study	Reliability	Sensitivity	Specificity	LR+	LR–	QUADAS Score (0–14)
Martin et al.[40]	63% agreement	53	92	6.63	0.52	6

Comments: Study utilized eight orthopedic surgeons to perform clinical exams as they normally would. Components of each clinical exam are not specifically known. Therefore, the clinical application of this study is unknown. Clinical exam results were compared with arthroscopy, and agreement amongst surgeons was investigated.

UTILITY SCORE 3

Study	Reliability	Sensitivity	Specificity	LR+	LR–	QUADAS Score (0–14)
Springer et al.[57] (PT)	85% (PT); 84% (OS); 80% (OR) agreement to surgical findings	100	0	1.0	0	8
Springer et al.[57] (OS)		100	0	1.0	0	8
Springer et al.[57] (OR)		92	0	1.0	0	8

Comments: Study utilized a physical therapist (PT), orthopedic surgeon (OS), and an orthopedic resident (OR) to compare clinical diagnostic accuracy between clinical examination and surgical findings of a labral tear. Clinical diagnostic accuracy versus surgical findings: 85% (PT), 84% (OS), and 80% (OR).

TESTS FOR GENERALIZED CAPSULAR LAXITY

Dial Test

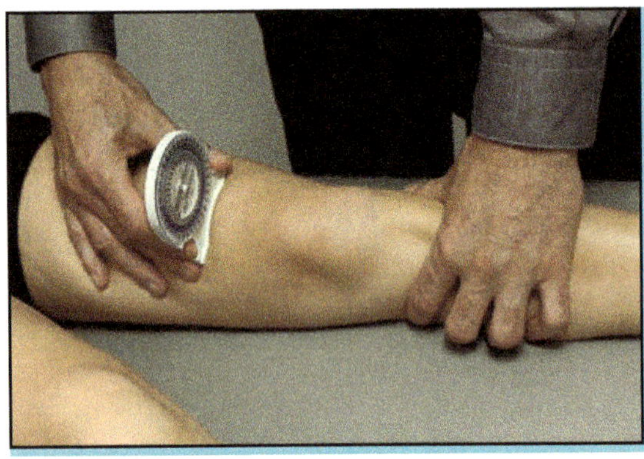

1) The patient lies supine with bilateral lower extremities extended and in a neutral flexion/extension and abduction/adduction position.

2) The examiner grasps the lower extremity to be tested at the distal femur and proximal tibia.

3) The examiner then passively rolls the lower extremity into full internal rotation.

4) The lower extremity is then released and allowed to externally rotate.

5) Using a goniometer or inclinometer, the examiner then measures the degree of passive external rotation at a firm endpoint.

6) A comparison of both sides is warranted.

7) A positive test is passive external rotation greater than 45 degrees (suggestive of capsular laxity) or a clicking sensation.

UTILITY SCORE 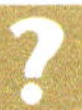

Study	Reliability	Sensitivity	Specificity	LR+	LR−	QUADAS Score (0–14)
None	NT	NT	NT	NA	NA	NT
Comments: The potential for muscle guarding and possible false-negative results must be recognized with this test. A relationship between this test and capsular laxity has been suggested.						

TESTS FOR GENERALIZED CAPSULAR LAXITY

Log Roll Test

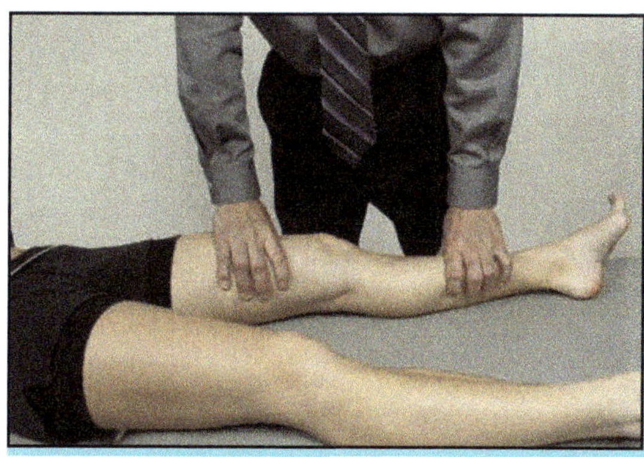

1) The patient lies supine with bilateral lower extremities extended and in a neutral flexion/extension and abduction/adduction position.

2) The examiner grasps the lower extremity to be tested at the distal femur.

3) The examiner then passively rolls the lower extremity into full internal rotation and external rotation (pictured).

4) A comparison of both sides is warranted.

5) A click reproduced during this test is suggestive of labral tear, while increased external rotation range-of-motion may indicate iliofemoral ligament laxity.

UTILITY SCORE 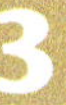

Study	Reliability	Sensitivity	Specificity	LR+	LR−	QUADAS Score (0–14)
Clohisy et al.[15]	NT	30	NT	NA	NA	9
Martin et al.[38]	0.63 ICC	NT	NT	NA	NA	NA
Martin & Sekiya[40]	0.61 (inter-rater) kappa	NT	NT	NA	NA	NA

Comments: The potential for muscle guarding and possible false-negative results must be recognized with this test. Clohisy et al.[15] utilized this test for hip anterior impingement pathology.

TESTS FOR GENERALIZED CAPSULAR LAXITY

Abduction-Extension-External Rotation Test

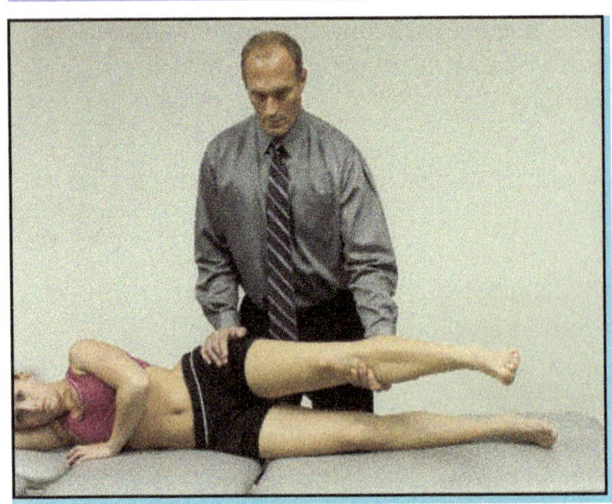

1) The patient assumes a sidelying position. The symptomatic lower extremity is placed upward; the asymptomatic lower extremity is placed on the plinth side.

2) The examiner grasps the lower extremity under the knee.

3) The examiner then places cranial hand just posterior to the greater trochanter.

4) The examiner then abducts the lower extremity about 30 degrees.

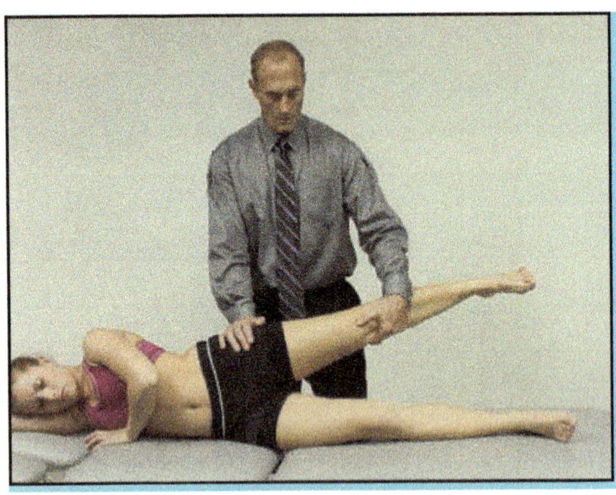

5) The examiner guides the lower extremity from 10 degrees of flexion to terminal extension, while externally rotating the straight leg and pushing forward on the greater trochanter.

6) A comparison of both sides is warranted.

7) A positive test is a reproduction of any complaints of pain or discomfort.

UTILITY SCORE 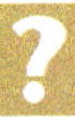

Study	Reliability	Sensitivity	Specificity	LR+	LR−	QUADAS Score (0–14)
None	NT	NT	NT	NA	NA	NA
Comments: No data regarding the reliability or diagnostic accuracy of this test is available.						

TESTS FOR GENERALIZED CAPSULAR LAXITY

Long Axis Femoral Distraction Test

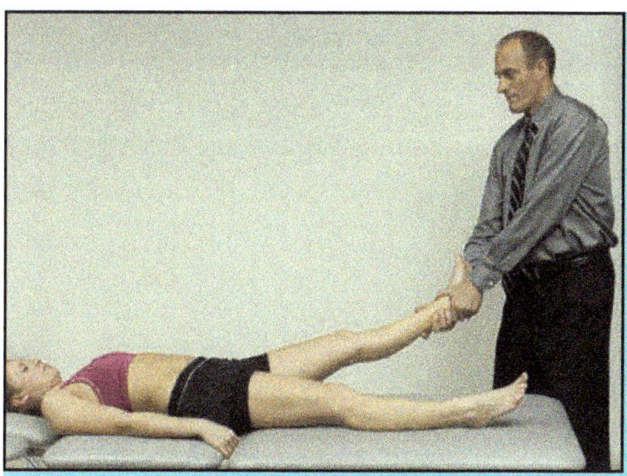

1) The patient lies supine with bilateral lower extremities extended and in a neutral position.

2) The examiner grasps the lower extremity to be tested just above the medial malleolus with the hip in 30 degrees of flexion, 30 degrees of abduction, and 10–15 degrees of external rotation (open packed position of the hip).

3) The examiner then passively distracts the joint by leaning backward while holding the lower extremity.

4) A comparison of both sides is warranted.

5) The patient with capsular laxity may have increased motion and a feeling of apprehension with this maneuver. Comparatively, a patient with hypomobility may have decreased motion and relief of pain.

UTILITY SCORE 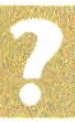

Study	Reliability	Sensitivity	Specificity	LR+	LR−	QUADAS Score (0–14)
Martin et al.[38]	NT	NT	NT	NA	NA	NA
Comment: The potential for muscle guarding and possible false-negative results must be recognized with this test. This movement is often performed under anesthesia for diagnosis of capsular laxity.						

Individualized Clinical Examination

1) Examiner performed clinical examination as normal in the clinical practice to diagnose capsular laxity.

2) A positive test was determined individually by examiner.

UTILITY SCORE 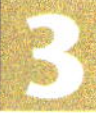

Study	Reliability	Sensitivity	Specificity	LR+	LR−	QUADAS Score (0–14)
Martin et al.[39]	58% agreement	55	61	1.41	0.78	6
Comments: Study utilized eight orthopedic surgeons to perform clinical exams as they normally would. Components of each clinical exam are unknown. Clinical exam results were compared with arthroscopy, and agreement amongst surgeons was investigated.						

TESTS FOR CAPSULAR OR MUSCULAR DYSFUNCTION

Thomas Test

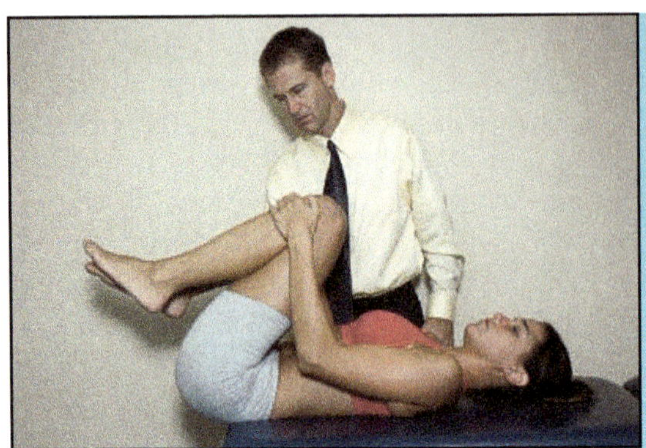

1) The patient sits at the edge of the plinth. The patient is then instructed to lie back, pulling both knees to his or her chest.

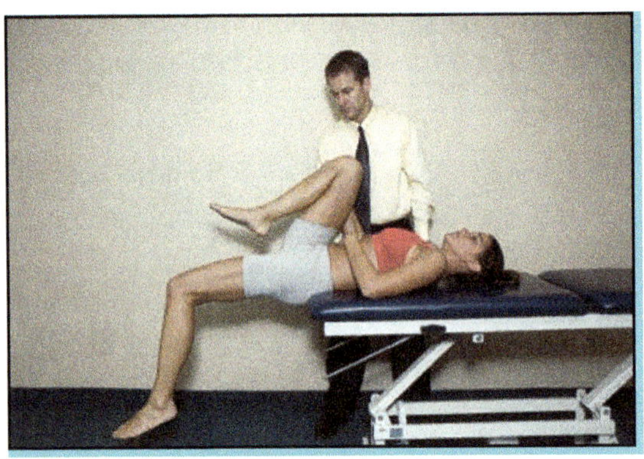

2) One knee (the asymptomatic side) is held to the chest and the other is slowly lowered into extension of the hip. The knee is allowed to extend.

3) The patient is instructed to pull his or her pelvis into posterior rotation.

4) The examiner then uses a goniometer to measure the extension angle of the hip and/or the knee.

5) A positive test is significant tightness of the hip flexors of the extended leg.

UTILITY SCORE 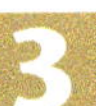

Study	Reliability	Sensitivity	Specificity	LR+	LR−	QUADAS Score (0–14)
Narvani et al.[45]	NT	NT	NT	NA	NA	7
Comments: This popular test is untested for diagnostic value. There are multiple suggested iterations of the test, none of which has been substantiated. No correlation was found between this test and labral tear.[45]						

TESTS FOR CAPSULAR OR MUSCULAR DYSFUNCTION

Prone Hip Extension Test

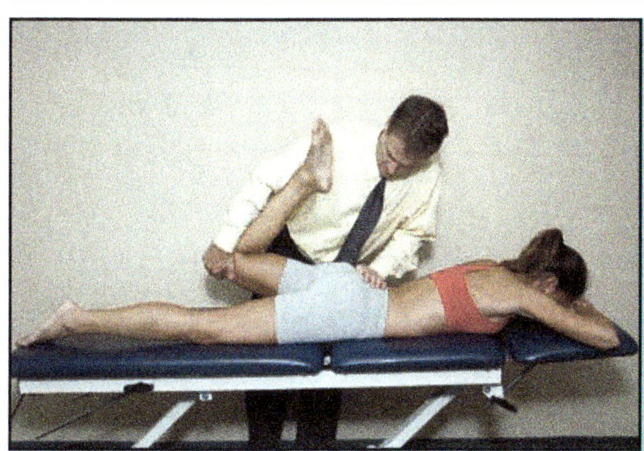

1) The patient is instructed to lie prone.

2) The examiner then places two belts (not pictured) around the patient: one just distal to the PSIS, the other just proximal to the gluteal fold. A special effort to unencumber hip extension should be made.

3) The examiner then passively moves the hip into extension.

4) The extension angle at the hip is measured with a goniometer.

5) A positive test is significant tightness of the hip flexors of the extended hip.

UTILITY SCORE 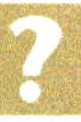

Study	Reliability	Sensitivity	Specificity	LR+	LR−	QUADAS Score (0–14)
None	NT	NT	NT	NA	NA	NA
Comments: It is likely that other conditions (e.g., labral tear) that would also be positive in this position may hamper the test's specificity.						

TEST FOR ILIOTIBIAL BAND RESTRICTION

Ober Test

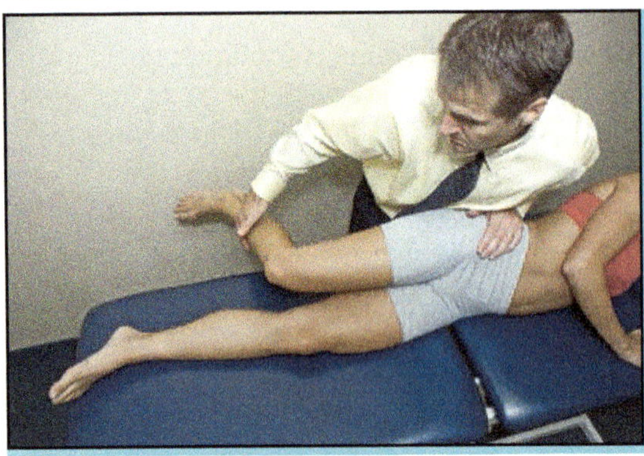

1) The patient assumes a sidelying position. The symptomatic leg is placed upward; the asymptomatic leg is placed on the plinth side.
2) The examiner prepositions the knee into flexion.
3) The examiner stabilizes the pelvis at the iliac crest.
4) The examiner then guides the lower extremity (at the hip) into extension and slight abduction.
5) Using a goniometer or inclinometer, the examiner then measures the degree of abduction or adduction.
6) A comparison of both sides is warranted.
7) A positive test is failure of the knee to drop to the plinth and is indicative of tightness of structures.

UTILITY SCORE 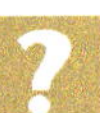

Study	Reliability	Sensitivity	Specificity	LR+	LR−	QUADAS Score (0–14)
Gajdosik et al.[22]	0.82 to 0.92 (goniometer)	NT	NT	NA	NA	NT
Melchione & Sullivan[42]	0.94 ICC (intra-tester); 0.73 (inter-tester) (inclinometer)	NT	NT	NA	NA	NT
Piva et al.[49]	0.97 (inter-tester) kappa	NT	NT	NA	NA	NT
Reese & Bandy[50]	0.90 ICC for Ober's; 0.91 ICC for modified Ober's (inclinometer)	NT	NT	NA	NA	NT

Comments: This extremely common technique is untested for diagnostic value. Melchione & Sullivan[42] improve the reliability by attaching a level to the spine to maintain pelvis position. They used a goniometer to measure the angle at the hip. The test can be repeated with the knee in extension or slight flexion.

TESTS FOR A TEAR OF THE GLUTEUS MEDIUS OF THE HIP

Trendelenburg's Sign

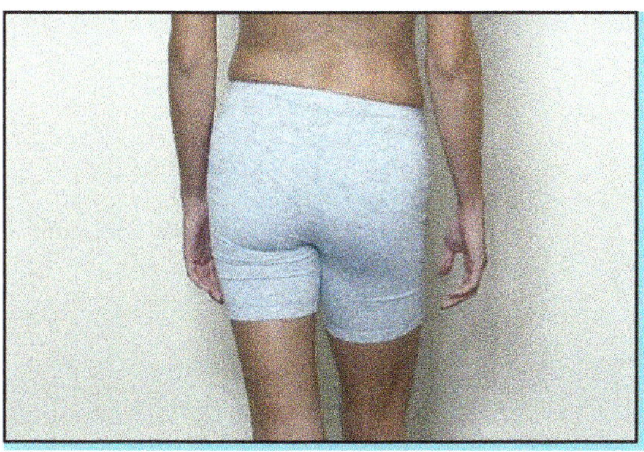

1) The patient stands in front of the examiner.
2) The examiner instructs the patient to stand on one leg.
3) The examiner evaluates the degree of drop of the contralateral pelvis once the leg is lifted.
4) Confirmation of abnormal pelvic drop is required during gait.
5) A positive test is identified by an asymmetric drop of one hip compared to the other during single stance.

UTILITY SCORE 

Study	Reliability	Sensitivity	Specificity	LR+	LR−	QUADAS Score (0–14)
Bird et al.[6]	0.676 (intra-tester) kappa	73	77	3.15	0.35	11
Burnett et al.[9]	NT	38	NT	NA	NA	8
Keeney et al.[32]	NT	40	NT	NA	NA	8

Comments: The test is performed in standing and confirmed during gait observation. In essence, the study is neither sensitive nor specific, although the likelihood ratio is fair. It is likely that significant weakness of the gluteus medius will present similar to a tear. Bird et al.[6] is the only study that investigated gluteal pathology. Burnett et al.[9] investigated this test as a screening tool for labral pathology. Youdas et al.[67] utilized this test in attempts to identify patients with hip osteoarthritis. Consideration of lateral pelvic tilt alone in this test may not be sensitive enough as a screening tool.

Resisted Hip Abduction

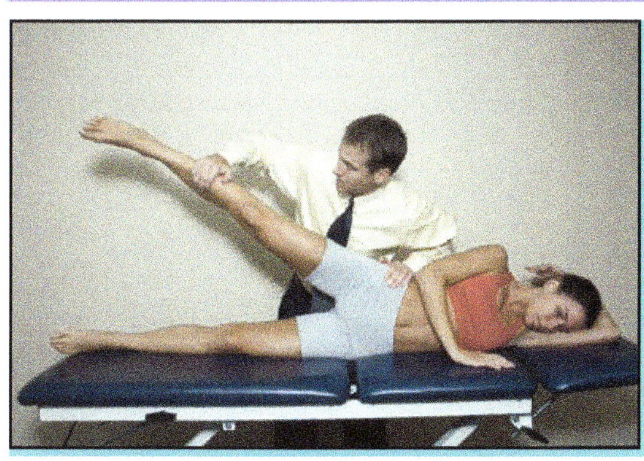

1) The patient is placed in a sidelying position.
2) The examiner instructs the patient to abduct the leg to 45 degrees.
3) The examiner applies force, resisting hip abduction against the leg.
4) A positive test is replication of symptoms during the testing.

(continued)

TESTS FOR A TEAR OF THE GLUTEUS MEDIUS OF THE HIP

UTILITY SCORE 2

Study	Reliability	Sensitivity	Specificity	LR+	LR−	QUADAS Score (0–14)
Bird et al.[6]	0.625 (intra-tester) kappa	73	46	1.35	0.59	11
Youdas et al.[67]	0.97 and 0.98 (intra-tester) ICC	35	90	3.5	0.72	13

Comments: Weakness is not a positive finding for the test. The poor specificity may be related to the myriad of other disorders, such as hip bursitis or abductor tendonitis that would also be painful during this procedure. Youdas et al.[67] utilized this test in attempts to identify patients with hip osteoarthritis. A weak, positive correlation between hip-abduction strength and hip-adduction angle was found during the Trendelenburg test on healthy individuals ($r = 0.22$, $P = 0.13$).[6]

Passive Internal Rotation

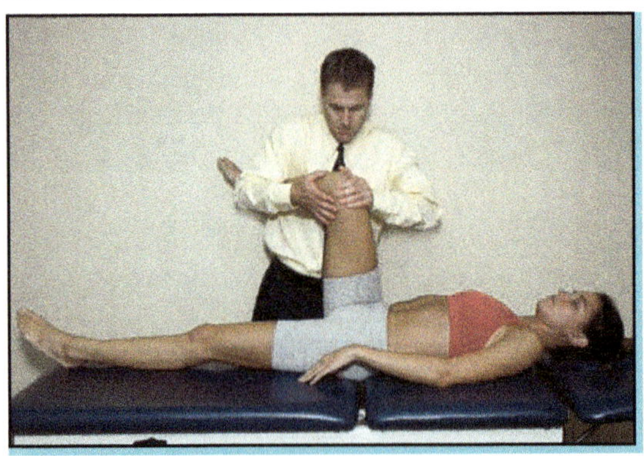

1) The patient lies in a supine position.
2) The hip is passively flexed to 90 degrees.
3) The examiner passively moves the hip into internal rotation.
4) A positive test is identified by reproduction of the patient's concordant pain (for a tear) or substantial limitation of internal rotation (for osteoarthritis).

UTILITY SCORE 3 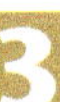

Study	Reliability	Sensitivity	Specificity	LR+	LR−	QUADAS Score (0–14)
Bird et al.[6]	0.027 (intra-tester) kappa	55	69	1.77	0.66	11
Brown et al.[8] (pain during IR)	NT	61	NT	NA	NA	11
Brown et al.[8] (limitation during IR)	NT	72	NT	NA	NA	11

Comments: Note the only fair sensitivity, suggesting that this test is not appropriate as a screen. A tear is typically associated with pain, whereas limitations are associated with osteoarthritis.

TESTS FOR GREATER TROCHANTER PAIN SYNDROME

Single-Leg Stance Held for 30 Seconds

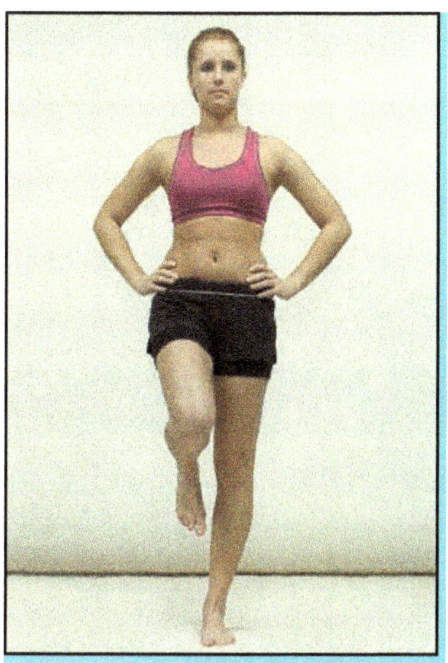

1) The patient starts in the standing position, while gently holding onto examiner.

2) The patient lifts the non-tested lower extremity off the ground and stands on the tested lower extremity for 30 seconds.

3) No lateral deviation of trunk to ipsilateral side is allowed.

4) The patient is asked whether any concordant pain occurred.

5) Pain similar to spontaneous pain is recorded as immediate, early, or late if it occurred after 0–5 seconds, 6–15 seconds, or 16–30 seconds, respectively.

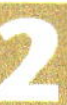

UTILITY SCORE 2

Study	Reliability	Sensitivity	Specificity	LR+	LR−	QUADAS Score (0–14)
Lequesne et al.[35]	NT	100	97.3	37	0.0	10
Comments: Primary difference between this test and Trendelenburg is the pain response consideration for a positive result in this test, versus dropping of pelvis in Trendelenburg test.						

Resisted External Derotation Test

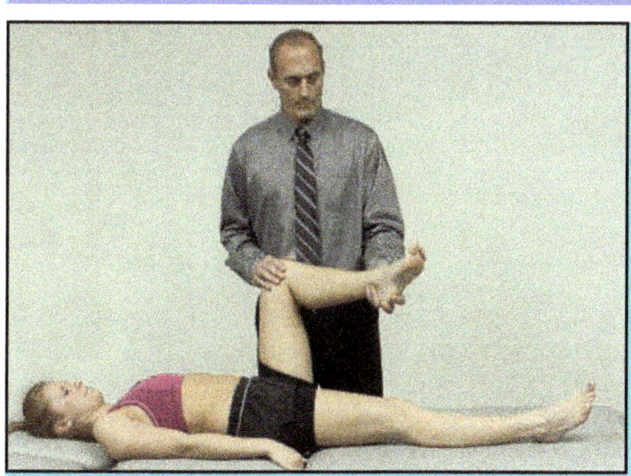

1) The patient lies supine, with hip and knee flexed at 90 degrees, hip in external rotation.

2) The examiner slightly diminishes the external rotation just enough to relieve the pain (if any was present).

3) The patient then actively returns the lower extremity to neutral rotation (place the lower extremity along the axis of the bed) against resistance.

4) The test was considered positive if spontaneous pain was reproduced.

5) If the result was negative, the test was repeated with the patient lying prone, hip extended and knee flexed at 90 degrees.

(continued)

TESTS FOR GREATER TROCHANTER PAIN SYNDROME

UTILITY SCORE 3

Study	Reliability	Sensitivity	Specificity	LR+	LR−	QUADAS Score (0–14)
Lequesne et al.[35]	NT	88	97.3	32.6	0.12	10
Comments: The sensitivity increased to 94% with positive results in the prone position in the case of negative results in the supine position.						

Composite Examination for Gluteal Tendon Pathology

UTILITY SCORE 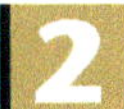

Study	Reliability	Sensitivity	Specificity	LR+	LR−	QUADAS Score (0–14)
Woodley et al.[66] (decreased passive hip IR)	Agreement for diagnosis between radiologist and physical therapy clinical examinations was–0.04 kappa for bursitis, 0.17 kappa for gluteal tendon pathology, and 0.21 kappa for osteoarthritis	43	86	3.0	0.67	11
Woodley et al.[66] (pain with active hip IR)		31	86	2.2	0.81	11
Woodley et al.[66] (pain with AROM hip abduction)		59	93	8.3	0.44	11
Woodley et al.[66] (pain with passive hip IR)		53	86	3.7	0.54	11
Woodley et al.[66] (pain with resisted GMin)		47	86	3.3	0.62	11
Woodley et al.[66] (pain with resisted GMed and GMin)		47	86	3.3	0.62	11
Woodley et al.[66] (decreased strength GMed and GMin)		80	71	2.8	0.28	11
Woodley et al.[66] (decreased strength GMin)		80	57	1.9	0.35	11
Woodley et al.[66] (positive Trendelenberg test)		23	94	3.6	0.82	11
Comments: This study demonstrated large confidence intervals. Little agreement existed between clinical and radiological examination.						

TESTS FOR PIRIFORMIS SYNDROME

Flexion-Adduction-Internal Rotation (FAIR) Test

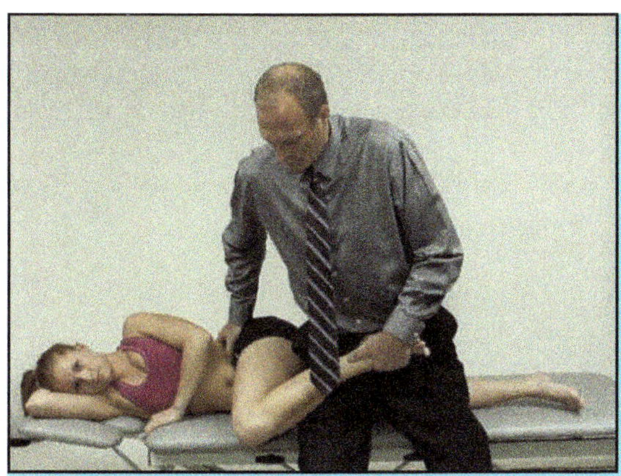

1) The patient starts in the sidelying position.

2) The examiner passively brings the lower extremity to be tested into the combined motions of approximately 90 degrees of hip flexion, maximal adduction, and knee flexion to 90 degrees.

3) The examiner ensures bilateral acetabuli remain vertically oriented.

4) Upward and lateral pressure is then applied to the shin of the lower extremity to be tested, passively internally rotating the thigh to 45 degrees, or as near to 45 degrees as patient can tolerate.

5) Pitain elicited at the intersection of the sciatic nerve and the piriformis is considered a positive test.

UTILITY SCORE 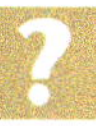

Study	Reliability	Sensitivity	Specificity	LR+	LR−	QUADAS Score (0–14)
Fishman & Zybert[20]	NT	NT	NT	NA	NA	NA

Comments: No data regarding the reliability or diagnostic accuracy of this test is available. The above description is per original Fishman & Zybert,[20] Fishman et al.[19] later describe the addition of simultaneous downward pressure at the flexed knee and passive superolateral movement of shin. Alternative versions of this test have been described with the patient supine or seated, knee and hip flexed, and hip medially rotated; as well as having the patient resist the examiners attempts to externally rotate and abduct the hip from this position. This test has also been referred to by some as the FADIR test, especially when described in supine with passive movement of flexion, adduction, and internal rotation.

TESTS FOR PIRIFORMIS SYNDROME

Pace Test

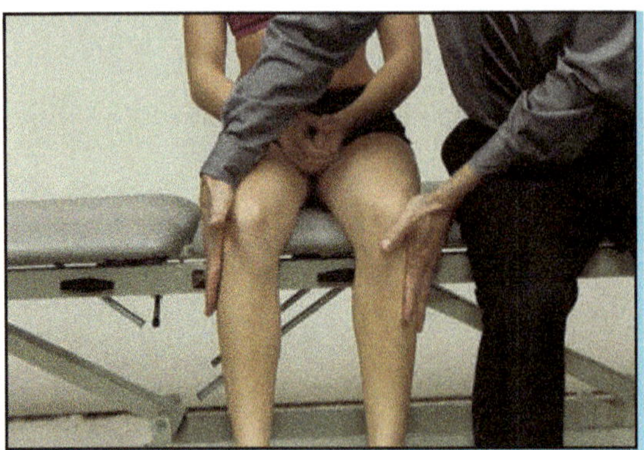

1) The patient is in the sitting position with hips and knees flexed, bilateral shins off the edge of the table.

2) The examiner places his or her hands on the lateral aspects of the knees and asks the patient to push the hands apart.

3) Faltering, pain, and weakness of the involved lower extremity is a positive result.

UTILITY SCORE 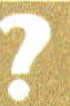

Study	Reliability	Sensitivity	Specificity	LR+	LR−	QUADAS Score (0–14)
Pace & Nagle[46]	NT	NA	NT	NA	NA	NA
Comments: No data regarding the reliability or diagnostic accuracy of this test is available.						

Freiberg Sign

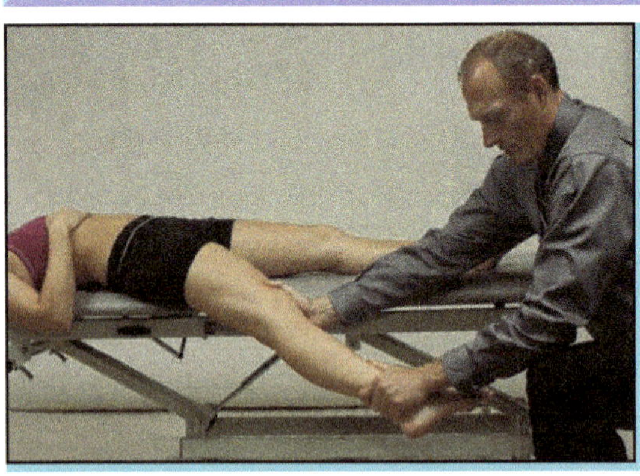

1) The patient starts in the supine position with bilateral lower extremities extended.

2) The examiner passively internally rotates the extended lower extremity forcefully.

3) Reproduction of pain is a positive result, thought to stretch the irritated piriformis and provoke sciatic nerve compression.

UTILITY SCORE 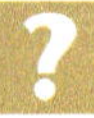

Study	Reliability	Sensitivity	Specificity	LR+	LR−	QUADAS Score (0–14)
Fanucci et al.[18]	NT	NA	NT	NA	NA	NA
Comments: No data regarding the reliability or diagnostic accuracy of this test is available.						

TESTS FOR PIRIFORMIS SYNDROME

Beatty Maneuver

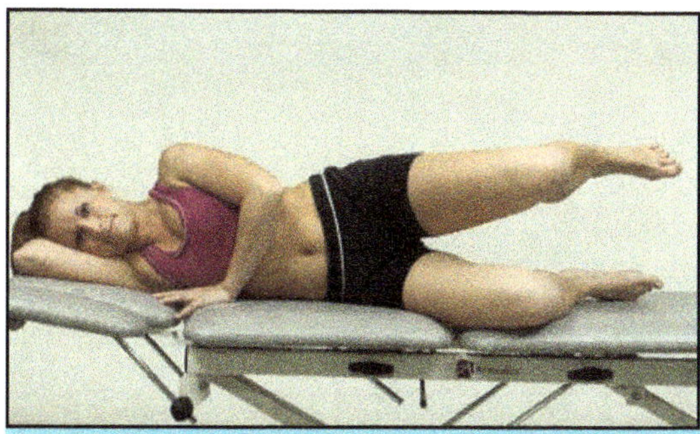

1) The patient is in the sidelying, lateral decubitus position.

2) The patient actively abducts the slightly flexed involved lower extremity.

3) Pain in the buttock, but not the lumbar spine, is a positive result.

UTILITY SCORE 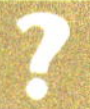

Study	Reliability	Sensitivity	Specificity	LR+	LR−	QUADAS Score (0–14)
None	NT	NT	NT	NA	NA	NA
Comments: No data regarding the reliability or diagnostic accuracy of this test is available.						

Forceful Internal Rotation

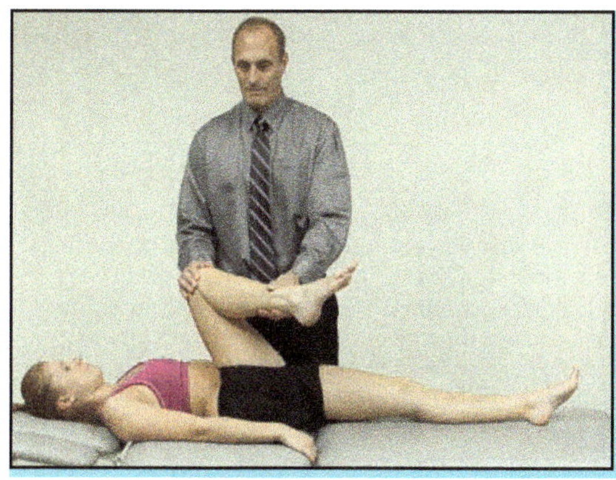

1) The patient starts in the supine position.

2) The examiner passively flexes the hip of the lower extremity to be tested.

3) The examiner then applies forceful internal rotation to the lower extremity to be tested.

4) Reproduction of pain is a positive result.

UTILITY SCORE 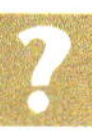

Study	Reliability	Sensitivity	Specificity	LR+	LR−	QUADAS Score (0–14)
None	NT	NA	NT	NA	NA	NA
Comments: This test has also been described as the modified Pace test.						

TEST FOR AVASCULAR NECROSIS

Combined Results

1) The patient's passive range-of-motion was measured for each motion listed below.

2) Range-of-motion criteria are listed for each motion.

UTILITY SCORE 3

Study	Reliability	Sensitivity	Specificity	LR+	LR−	QUADAS Score (0–14)
Joe et al.[28] (extension < 15 degrees)	NT	19	92	2.38	0.88	10
Joe et al.[28] (abduction < 45 degrees)	NT	31	85	2.07	0.81	10
Joe et al.[28] (internal rotation < 15 degrees)	NT	50	67	1.52	0.75	10
Joe et al.[28] (external rotation < 60 degrees)	NT	38	73	0.48	0.85	10
Joe et al.[28] (pain with internal rotation)	NT	13	86	0.93	1.01	10
Joe et al.[28] (pain complex)	NT	25	71	0.86	1.06	10
Joe et al.[28] (passive range-of-motion complex)	NT	69	46	1.28	0.67	10
Joe et al.[28] (exam complex)	NT	88	34	1.33	0.35	10

Comments: This study was conducted on asymptomatic HIV infected subjects. Those considered positive for the pain complex included any patient with pain in the hip or groin with any of the tests or maneuvers listed. Those positive for the test complex included any of the patients with at least one of the provocative tests, i.e. Patrick's, Thomas, Ober's, straight leg raise, axial loading maneuver, femoral head compression and distraction in the supine position with leg extended, single leg stand for two minutes, or single-leg hopping for 10–20 repetitions. Those positive for the exam complex included any hip in which one or more positive test from any complex was identified. No single clinical test identifies patients with MRI findings of avascular necrosis. Passive range-of-motion of internal rotation of the hip was the most effective test. The physical findings are too insensitive to serve as a screening tool for asymptomatic avascular necrosis. Due to the use of multiple provocation tests, and lack of description of the frequency of positive/negative results of each specific test, it is impossible to discern clinical applicability for each test listed.

TESTS FOR EARLY SIGNS OF HIP DYSPLASIA

Passive Hip Abduction Test

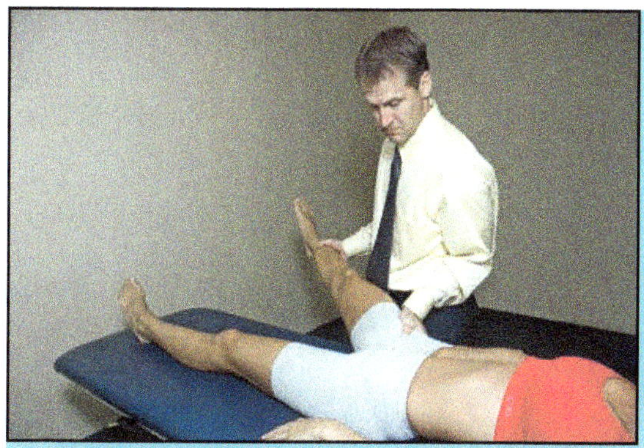

1) The patient assumes a supine position.
2) The examiner passively moves the hip into abduction.
3) A restriction of abduction as compared to the opposite side is considered a positive finding.

UTILITY SCORE 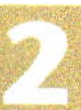

Study	Reliability	Sensitivity	Specificity	LR+	LR−	QUADAS Score (0–14)
Jari et al.[27]	NT	70	90	7.0	0.33	7
Castelein & Korte[10]	NT	69	54	1.5	0.57	5
Comments: Although the test designs were poor, this test does not appear overly sensitive but may be specific. The Jari et al.[27] study was employed on neonates considered "at risk." The clinical assessment was with both hips flexed to 90 degrees and full abduction was attempted. A greater than 20 degree difference compared to the other side was considered a positive result. Positive result for Castelein & Korte[10] (infants older than 90 days of age) was defined as a hip that showed < 60 degrees of abduction in 90 degrees flexion or an asymmetry in abduction of ≥ 20 degrees.						

Flexion Adduction Test

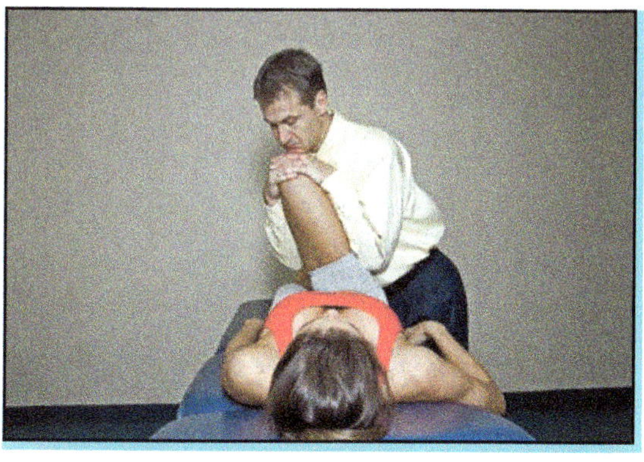

1) The patient assumes a supine position.
2) The examiner flexes the knee to 90 degrees while maintaining the contact of the patient's pelvis to the plinth.
3) The examiner attempts to adduct the thigh of the patient toward the opposite hip. Inability to adduct the hip passively beyond midline is considered a precursor to early hip disease.
4) A positive test is the inability to adduct the flexed hip past midline toward the opposite hip.

UTILITY SCORE 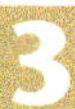

Study	Reliability	Sensitivity	Specificity	LR+	LR−	QUADAS Score (0–14)
Woods & Macnicol[67]	NT	100	NT	NA	NA	3
Comments: The test was performed on adolescents and demonstrated many design flaws.						

TESTS FOR FRACTURE OF THE HIP OR FEMUR

Patellar-Pubic Percussion Test

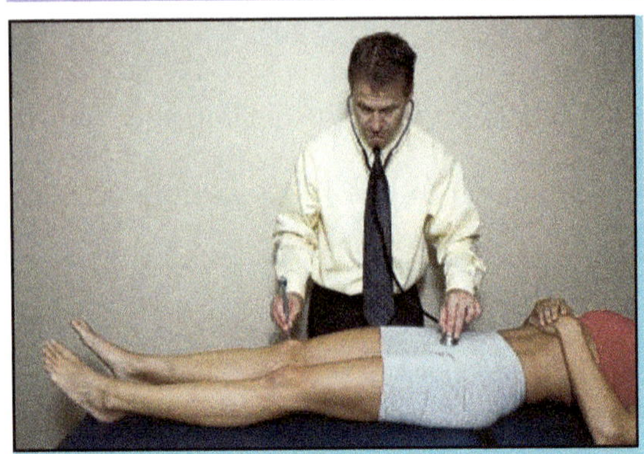

1) The patient assumes a supine position.

2) The examiner places a stethoscope over the pubic symphysis of the patient.

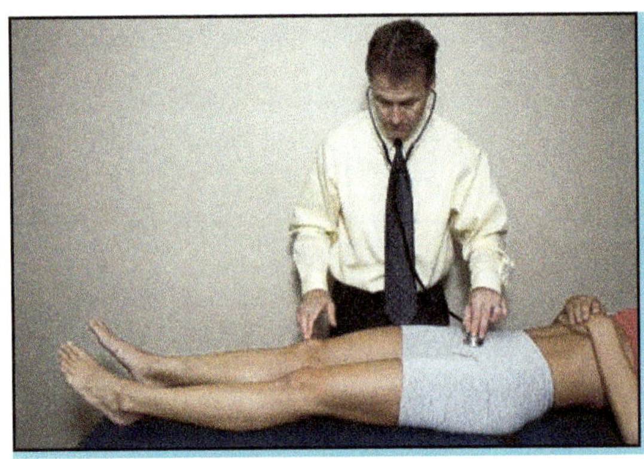

3) The examiner taps the patella of the patient's affected side and qualitatively reports the sound.

4) The examiner repeats the process on the opposite side to determine a difference in auscultation.

5) A positive test is a diminished percussion noted on the side of pain and a negative test is no difference in percussion note. A tuning fork can be used in place of tapping.

UTILITY SCORE 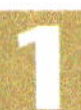

Study	Reliability	Sensitivity	Specificity	LR+	LR−	QUADAS Score (0–14)
Adams & Yarnold[1]	89.2% agreement	94	95	20.4	0.06	9
Bache & Cross[3]	NT	91	82	5.1	0.11	8
Misurya et al.[3]	NT	89	NT	NA	NA	5
Tiru et al.[63]	NT	96	86	6.73	0.75	8

Comments: Although the designs are not superb, this test does appear to have diagnostic value as a screening tool and as a diagnostic tool. The vibration testing appeared to demonstrate better results. Bache & Cross[3] describe the use of the tuning fork only and at either the medial femoral condyle or patella. Additionally, they describe the test for femoral neck fracture only.

TESTS FOR FRACTURE OF THE HIP OR FEMUR

Stress Fracture (Fulcrum) Test

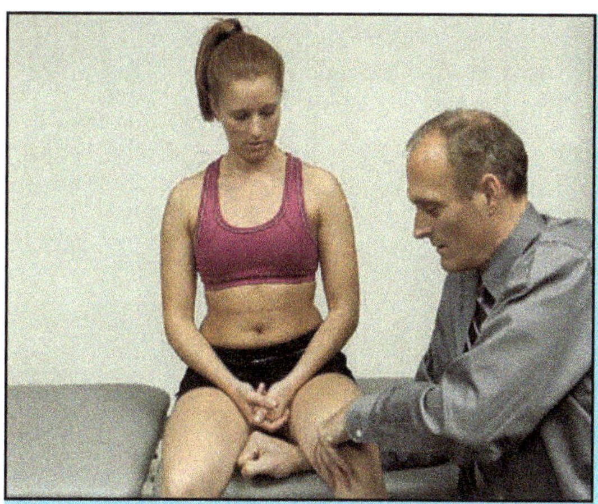

1) The patient sits with bilateral feet over the edge of the table.

2) The examiner places one forearm under the patient's thigh to be tested.

3) The examiner's upper extremity is used as a fulcrum under the thigh and is moved from the distal to proximal thigh as gentle pressure is applied to the dorsum of the knee with the opposite upper extremity.

4) A comparison of both sides is warranted.

5) The test is considered positive if the patient reports increased discomfort/sharp pain, usually accompanied by apprehension.

UTILITY SCORE 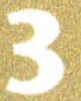

Study	Reliability	Sensitivity	Specificity	LR+	LR−	QUADAS Score (0–14)
Johnson et al.[29]	NT	100	100	Inf	0	6
Kang et al.[30]	NT	100	0	1.0	NA	7
Comment: Confirmation of a stress fracture requires a bone scan, therefore a positive finding warrants physician referral. Poor study designs caution this as a screening or diagnostic tool.						

Key Points

1. Clinical special tests of the hip are exceedingly understudied.
2. Most of the clinical special tests of the hip have been performed poorly and are hampered by internal bias.
3. The patellar-percussion test appears to be an effective screen and diagnostic tool for hip-related fractures.
4. The majority of hip labrum tests lack specificity and only display moderate to good sensitivity.
5. While assessment of loss of range of motion planes is an effective screen for osteoarthritis, the finding is not specific enough in absence of radiographic findings.
6. Clinical special tests, such as the hip scour (quadrant), could potentially be positive for conditions such as hip labrum, capsulitis, osteoarthritis, and femoral acetabular impingement syndrome.
7. Variability in special test description has resulted in multiple combinations of tests, dependent on specific passive movements of the hip for impingement and labral testing.
8. Caution is suggested in interpretation of impingement and labral tear testing due to study designs, variable descriptions, and variable reference standards.

References

1. Adams S, Yarnold P. Clinical use of the patellar-pubic percussion sign in hip trauma. *Am J Emerg Med.* 1997;15:173–175.

2. Altman R, Alarcon G, Appelrouth D, et al. The American College of Rheumatology criteria for the classification and reporting of osteoarthritis of the hip. *Arthritis Rheum.* 1991;34(5):505–514.

3. Bache JB, Cross AB. The Barford test: a useful diagnostic sign in fractures of the femoral neck. *Practitioner.* 1984;228:305–308.

4. Beaule P, Zaragoza E, Motamedi K, Copelan N, Dorey FJ. Three-dimensional computed tomography of the hip in the assessment of femoroacetabular impingement. *J Orthop Res.* 2005;23:1286–1292.

5. Beck M, Parvizi J, Boutier V, Wyss D, Ganz R. Anterior femoracetabular impingement: part II. Midterm results of surgical treatment. *Clin Orthop Relat Res.* 2004;67–73.

6. Bird PA, Oakley SP, Shnier R, Kirham BW. Prospective evaluation of magnetic resonance imaging and physical examination findings in patients with greater trochanteric pain syndrome. *Arthritis Rheumatism.* 2001;44:2138–2145.

7. Birrell F, Croft P, Cooper C, Hosie G, Macfarlane G, Silman A. Predicting radiographic hip osteoarthritis from range of movement. *Rheumatology.* 2001;40:506–512.

8. Brown M, Gomez-Martin O, Brookfield K, Stokes P. Differential diagnosis of hip disease versus spine disease. *Clin Orthop.* 2004;419:280–284.

9. Burnett RSJ, Della Rocca GJ, Prather H, Curry M, Maloney WJ, Clohisy JC. Clinical presentation of patients with tears of the acetabular labrum. *J Bone Joint Surg Am.* 2006;88A:1448–1457.

10. Castelein RM, Korte J. Limited hip abduction in the infant. *J Ped Orthoped.* 2001;21:668–670.

11. Chan YS, Lien LC, Hsu HL, et al. Evaluating hip labral tears using magnetic resonance arthrography: a prospective study comparing hip arthroscopy and magnetic resonance arthrography diagnosis. *Arthroscopy.* 2005;21:1250.el–1250.e8.

12. Chung CY, Lee KM, Park MS, Lee SH, Choi IH, Cho TJ. Validity and reliability of measuring femoral anteversion and neck-shaft angle in patients with cerebral palsy. *J Bone Joint Surg Am.* 2010;92:1195–1205.

13. Cibere J, Thorne A, Bellamy N, et al. Reliability of the hip examination in osteoarthritis: effect of standardization. *Arthritis Rheum.* 2008;59;373–381.

14. Cliborne AV, Wainner RS, Rhon DI, et al. Clinical hip tests and a functional squat test in patients with knee osteoarthritis: reliability, prevalence of positive test findings, and short-term response to hip mobilization. *J Orthop Sports Phys Ther.* 2004;34:676–685.

15. Clohisy JC, Knaus ER, Hunt DM, Lesher JM, Harris-Hayes M, Prather H. Clinical presentation of patients with symptomatic anterior hip impingement. *Clin Orthop Relat Res.* 2009;467:638–644.

16. DiMattia M, Livengood A, Uhl T, Mattaclola C, Malone T. What are the validity of the single-leg-squat test and its relationship to hip-abduction strength? *J Sport Rehabil.* 2005;14:108–123.

17. Dorrell JH, Catterall A. The torn acetabular labrum. *J Bone Joint Surg Br.* 1986;68:400–403.

18. Fanucci E, Massala S, Sodani G, et al. CT-guided injection of botulinic toxin for percutaneous therapy of piriformis muscle syndrome with preliminary MRI results about degenerative process. *Eur Radiol.* 2001; 11:2543–2548.

19. Fishman L, Dombi G, Michaelson C, et al. Piriformis syndrome: diagnosis, treatment, and outcome—a 10 year study. *Arch Phys Med Rehabil.* 2002;83:295–301.

20. Fishman L, Zybert P. Electrophysiologic evidence of piriformis syndrome. *Arch Phys Med Rehabil.* 1992; 84-B:104–107.

21. Fitzgerald RH, Jr. Acetabular labrum tears. Diagnosis and treatment. *Clin Orthop Relat Res.* 1995:60–68.

22. Gajdosik RL, Sandler MM, Marr HL. Influence of knee positions and gender on the Ober test for length of the iliotibial band. *Clin Biomech.* 2003;18:77–79.

23. Guanche CA, Sikka RS. Acetabularlabral tears with underlying chondromalacia: A possible association with high-level running. *Arthroscopy.* 2005;21:580–585.

24. Hase T, Ueo T. Acetabularlabral tears: arthroscopic diagnosis and treatment. *Arthroscopy* 1999;15:138–141.

25. Hudson D. A comparison of ultrasound to goniometric and inclinometer measurements of torsion in the tibia and femur. *Gait Posture.* 2008;28:708–710.

26. Ito K, et al. Histopathologic features of the acetabular labrum in femoroacetabular impingement. *Clin Orthop Relat Res.* 2004;262–271.

27. Jari S, Paton RW, Srinivasan MS. Unilateral limitation of abduction of the hip: a valuable clinical sign for DDH? *J Bone Jnt Surg.* 2002;84:104–107.

28. Joe G, Kovacs J, Miller K, et al. Diagnosis of avascular necrosis of the hip in asymptomatic HIV-infected patients: clinical correlation of physical examination with magnetic resonance imaging. *J Back Musculoskel Rehabil.* 2002;16:135–139.

29. Johnson AW, Weiss CB, Wheeler DL. Stress fractures of the femoral shaft in athletes more common than expected. *Am J Sports Med.* 1994;22:248–256.

30. Kang L, Belcher D, Hulstyn MJ. Stress fractures of the femoral shaft in women's college lacrosse: a report of seven cases and a review of the literature. *Br J Sport Med.* 2005;39:902–906.

31. Kassarjian A, Yoon LS, Belzile E, Connolly SA, Millis MB, Palmer WE. Triad of MR arthrographic findings in patients with cam type femoroacetabular impingement. *Radiology.* 2005;236:588–592.

32. Keeney JA, Peelle MW, Jackson J, Rubin D, Maloney WJ, Clohisy JC. Magnetic resonance arthrography versus

arthroscopy in the evaluation of articular hip pathology. *Clin Orthop* 2004;429:163–169.

33. Klaue K, Durnin CW, Ganz R. The acetabular rim syndrome: a clinical presentation of dysplasia of the hip. *J Bone Jnt Surg.* 1991;73:423–429.

34. Leunig M, Werlen S, Ungersbock A, Ito K, Ganz R. Evaluation of the acetabular labrum by MR arthrography. *J Bone Joint Surg Br.* 1997;79:230–234.

35. Lequesne M, Mathieu P, Vuillemin-Bodaghi V, Bard H, Djian P. Gluteal tendinopathy in refractory greater trochanter pain syndrome: diagnostic value of two clinical tests. *Arthritis Rheum.* 2008;59:241–246.

36. Lesher JD, Sutlive TG, Miller GA, Chine NJ, Garber MB, Wainner RS. Development of a clinical prediction rule for classifying patients with patellofemoral pain syndrome who respond to patellar taping. *J Orthop Sports Phys Ther.* 2006;36:854–866.

37. Martin RL, Kelly BT, Leunig M. Reliability of clinical diagnosis in intraarticular hip diseases. *Knee Surg Sports Traumatol Arthrosc.* 2010;18:685–690.

38. Martin RL, Enseki KR, Draovitch P, Trapuzzano T, Philippon MJ. Acetabular labral tears of the hip: examination and diagnostic challenges. *J Orthop Sports Phys Ther.* 2006;36:503–515.

39. Martin RL, Irrang JJ, Seikya JK. The diagnostic accuracy of a clinical examination in determining intra-articular hip pain for potential hip arthroscopy patients. *Arthroscopy.* 2008;24:1013–1018.

40. Martin RL, Sekiya JK. The interrater reliability of 4 clinical tests used to assess individuals with musculoskeletal hip pain. *J Orthop Sports Phys Ther.* 2008;38:71–77.

41. Maslowski E, Sullivan W, Forster Harwood J, et al. The diagnostic validity of hip provocation maneuvers to detect intra-articular hip pathology.

42. Melchione W, Sullivan S. Reliability of measurements obtained by use of an instrument designed to measure iliotibial band length indirectly. *J Orthop Sports Phys Ther.* 1993;18:511–515.

43. Misurya RK, Khare A, Mallick A, Sural A, Vishwakarma GK. Use of tuning fork in diagnostic auscultation of fractures. *Injury.* 1987;18:63–64.

44. Mitchell B, McCrory P, Burkner P, O'Donnell J, Colson E, Howells R. Hip joint pathology: clinical presentation and correlation between magnetic resonance arthrography, ultrasound, and arthroscopic findings. *Clin J Sport Med.* 2003;13:152–156.

45. Narvani A, Tsiridis E, Kendall S, Chaudhuri R, Thomas P. A preliminary report on prevalence of acetabular labrum tears in sports patients with groin pain. *Knee Surg Traumatol Arthrosc.* 2003;11:403–408.

46. Pace JB, Nagle D. Piriform syndrome. *West J Med.* 1976;124:435–439.

47. Petersilge CA, et al. Acetabularlabral tears: evaluation with MR arthrography. *Radiology.* 1996;200:231–235.

48. Philippon MJ, Maxwell RB, Johnston TL, Schenker M, Briggs KK. Clinical presentation of femoroacetabular impingement. *Knee Surg Sports Traumatol Arthrosc.* 2007;15:1041–1047.

49. Piva SR, Fitzgerald K, Irrgang JJ, et al. Reliability of measures of impairments associated with patellofemoral pain syndrome. *BMC Musculoskel Dis.* 2006;7:33.

50. Reese NB, Bandy WD. Use of an inclinometer to measure flexibility of the iliotibial band using the Ober test and the modified Ober test: differences in magnitude and reliability of measurements. *J Orthop Sports Phys Ther.* 2003;33:326–330.

51. Ross MD, Nordeen MH, Barido M. Test-retest reliability of Patrick's hip range of motion test in healthy college-aged men. *J Strength Cond Res.* 2003;17:156–161.

52. Ruwe PA, Gage JR, Ozonoff MB, DeLuca PA. Clinical determination of femoral anteversion. A comparison with established techniques. *J Bone Joint Surg Am.* 1992;74:820–830.

53. Santori N, Villar R. Acetabular labral tears: Result of arthroscopic partial limbectomy. *Arthroscopy.* 2000;16:11–15.

54. Shultz SJ, Nguyen AD, Schmitz, RJ. Differences in lower extremity anatomical and postural characteristics in males and females between maturation groups. *J Orthop Sports Phys Ther.* 2008;38:137–149.

55. Shultz SJ, Nguyen AD, Windley TC, Kulas AS, Botic TL, Beynnon BD. Intratester and intertester reliability of clinical measures of lower extremity anatomic characteristics: implications for multicenter studies. *Clin J Sport Med.* 2006;16:155–161.

56. Sink EL, Gralla J, Ryba A, Dayton M. Clinical Presentation of Femoroacetabular Impingement in Adolescents. *J Pediatr Orthop.* 2008;28:806–811.

57. Springer BA, Gill NW, Freedman BA, Ross AE, Javernick MA, Murphy KP. Acetabular labral tears: diagnostic accuracy of clinical examination by a physical therapist, orthopaedic surgeon, and orthopaedic residents. *North Am J Sports Phys Ther.* 2009;4:38–45.

58. Souza RB, Powers CM. Concurrent criterion-related validity and reliability of a clinical test to measure femoral anteversion. *J Orthop Sports Phys Ther.* 2009;39:586–592.

59. Suenaga E, Noguchi Y, Jingushi S, et al. Relationship between the maximum flexion internal rotation test and the torn acetabular labrum of a dysplastic hip. *J Orthop Sci* 2002;7:26–32.

60. Sutlive TP, Lopez HP, Schnitker DE, et al. Development of a clinical prediction rule for diagnosing hip osteoarthritis in individuals with unilateral hip pain. *J Orthop Sports Phys Ther.* 2008;38:542–550.

61. Sutlive TG, Mitchell SD, Maxfield SN, et al. Identification of individuals with patellofemoral pain whose symptoms improved after a combined program of foot orthosis use and modified activity: a preliminary investigation. *Phys Ther.* 2004;84:49–61.

62. Theiler R, Stucki G, Schotz R, et al. Parametric and nonparametric measures in the measurement of knee and hip osteoarthritis: interobserver reliability and correlation with radiology. *Osteoarthritis Cartilage.* 1996;4:35–42.

63. Tiru M, Goh S, Low B. Use of percussion as a screening tool in the diagnosis of occult hip fractures. *Singapore Med J.* 2002;43:467–469.

64. Troelsen A, Mechlenburg I, Gelineck J, Bolvig L, Jacobsen S, Sballe K. What is the role of clinical tests and ultrasound in acetabularlabral tear diagnostics? *Acta Orthopaed.* 2009;80:314–318.

65. Woods D, Macnicol M. The flexion-adduction test: an early sign of hip disease. *J Ped Orthop.* 2001: 10:180–185.

66. Woodley SJ, Nicholson HE, Livingstone V, et al. Lateral hip pain: findings from magnetic resonance imaging and clinical examination. *J Orthop Sports Phys Ther.* 2008;38:313–328.

67. Youdas JW, Madson TJ, Hollman JH. Usefulness of the Trendelenburg test for identification of patients with hip joint osteoarthritis. *Phys Theory Pract.* 2010;26:184–194.

PEARSON myhealthprofessionskit™

Use this address to access the Companion Website created for this textbook. Simply select "Physical Therapy" from the choice of disciplines. Find this book and log in using your username and password to access video clips of selected tests.

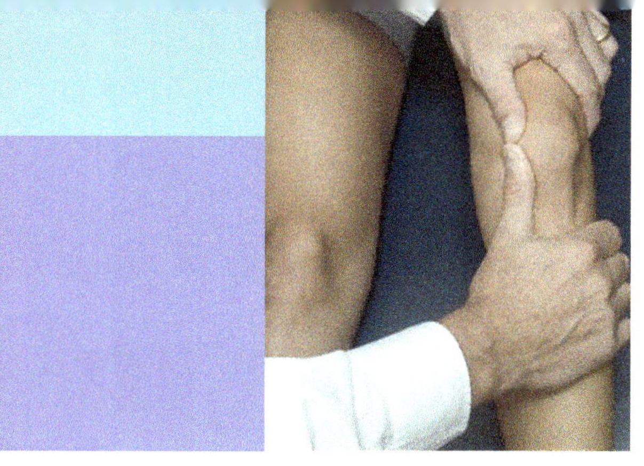

Physical Examination Tests for the Knee

Ben Stern, Eric J. Hegedus, and Dawn Driesner

Please refer to the chapter "Introduction to Diagnostic Accuracy" before reading this chapter.

Index of Tests

From Chapter 13 of *Orthopedic Physical Examination Tests: An Evidence-Based Approach*, Second Edition. Chad Cook, Eric Hegedus.

Quadriceps Active Test (PCL Tear)

Reverse Pivot-Shift Test [PCL Tear, Posterolateral Rotary Instability (PLRI) Tear]

Reverse Lachman's Test or Trillat's Test (PCL Tear)

Varus/Valgus Instability at 0 Degrees (PCL Tear)

External Rotation Recurvatum Test

Anterior Abrasion Sign (PCL Tear)

Fixed Posterior Subluxation (PCL Tear)

Proximal Tibial Percussion Test (PCL Tear)

Posterior Functional Drawer Test (PCL Tear)

Modified Posterolateral Drawer Test or Loomer's Test (PCL Tear/PLRI)

Posterolateral Rotation Test or Dial Test (PCL Tear/PLRI)

Posterolateral Drawer Test (PLRI)

Standing Apprehension Test (PLRI)

Posterior Medial Displacement of the Medial Tibial Plateau with Valgus Stress [Posteromedial Rotatory Instability (PMRI)]

Tests for Torn Collateral Ligament

Composite Physical Exam [Medial Collateral Ligament (MCL) Tear]

Valgus Stress Test (MCL Tear)

Composite Physical Exam [Lateral Collateral Ligament (LCL) Tear]

Varus Stress Test (LCL Tear)

Tests for Patellofemoral Dysfunction

Patellar Apprehension Test or Fairbank's Apprehension Test

Pain During Functional Activity (Patellofemoral Pain Syndrome)

Resisted Knee Extension (Patellofemoral Pain Syndrome)

Waldron Test (Patellofemoral Joint Pathology)

Passive Patellar Tilt Test (Patellofemoral Joint Instability)

Clarke's Sign/Patellar Grind/Patellar Tracking with Compression (Patellofemoral Joint Pathology)

Lateral Pull Test (Patellofemoral Tracking/Instability)

Patella Alta Test

Vastus Medialis Coordination Test (Patellofemoral Tracking)

Eccentric Step Test (Patellofemoral Joint Dysfunction)

McConnell Test for Patellar Orientation (Patellofemoral Joint)

Zohler's Sign (Patellofemoral Joint Dysfunction)

Tubercle Sulcus Test (Patellofemoral Joint Alignment)

Q-Angle (Patellofemoral Joint Alignment)

Lateral Patellar Glide (Patellofemoral Joint Instability)

Medial Patellar Glide (Patellofemoral Joint Instability)

Patella Mobility Testing (Patellofemoral Pain Syndrome)

Palpation (Patellofemoral Pain Syndrome)

Patellar Compression Test (Patellofemoral Pain Syndrome)

Historical Elements (Patellofemoral Dysfunction)

Palpation for Tendinopathy (Jumper's Knee)

Clusters of Findings

Tests for Plica Syndrome

- Composite Examination/Clusters of Findings
- MPP Test (Medial Patellar Plica Syndrome)
- Medial Plica Shelf Test (Medial Patellar Plica Syndrome)
- Medial Plica Test (Medial Patellar Plica Syndrome)
- Rotation Valgus Test (Medial Patellar Plica Syndrome)
- Holding Test (Medial Patellar Plica Syndrome)
- Patellar Stutter Test (Suprapatellar Plica Syndrome)

Tests for Proximal Tibiofibular Joint Instability

- Fibular Head Translation Test
- Radulescu Sign

Tests for Knee Effusion

- Ballottement Test
- Patient Report of Noticed Swelling
- Clusters of Findings for Effusion

Tests for Osteochondral Lesions

- Composite Examination/Clusters of Findings for Osteoarthritis (OA)/ Degenerative Joint Disease (DJD)
- Composite Examination/Clusters of Findings for Loose Bodies
- Composite Examination/Clusters of Findings for Chondral Fracture

TESTS FOR FRACTURE AT THE KNEE

Ottawa Knee Decision Rule

Criteria

1) Age ≥ 55 years.

2) Tenderness at the head of the fibula.

3) Isolated tenderness of the patella.

4) Inability to flex the knee to at least 90 degrees.

5) Inability by the patient to bear weight both immediately and in the emergency department for four steps.

6) A positive test is the presence of any one of the four characteristics and is an indication for referral for an x-ray to confirm fracture.

UTILITY SCORE 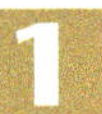

Study	Reliability	Sensitivity	Specificity	LR+	LR−	QUADAS Score (0–14)
Jackson et al.[49]	NT	100	49	1.9	0.11	NA
Richman et al.[104]	NT	85	50	1.7	0.30	12

Comments: The Jackson et al.[49] study reported diagnostic values based on the compilation of seven studies. Richman et al.[104] compared the Bauer et al.[12] criteria with the Ottawa[123,124,125] criteria in two hospitals: a community hospital and a tertiary care center. The Ottawa Knee Rule[123,124,125] is a valuable tool in the primary care setting to rule out a knee fracture.

Pittsburgh Knee Decision Rule

Criteria

1) Patient history of blunt trauma or a fall.

2) Inability by the patient to bear weight both immediately and in the emergency department for four steps.

3) Age younger than 12 or older than 50 years.

4) A positive test is a patient history of blunt trauma or fall and one of either the second or third criterion.

5) A positive test is an indication to refer for an x-ray to confirm a fracture at the knee.

TESTS FOR FRACTURE AT THE KNEE

UTILITY SCORE 1

Study	Reliability	Sensitivity	Specificity	LR+	LR−	QUADAS Score (0–14)
Seaberg & Jackson[111]	NT	100	79	NA	NA	11
Seaberg et al.[112]	NT	99	60	2.5	0.02	11
Comments: The Pittsburgh Knee Rule[111] appears to be a valuable tool in the primary care setting to rule out a knee fracture but more research is needed.						

Knee Decision Rule of Bauer

Criteria

1) Inability by the patient to bear weight both immediately and in the emergency department for four steps.

2) Presence of knee effusion.

3) Presence of ecchymosis.

4) A positive test is the presence of any one of the three characteristics and is an indication for referral for an x-ray to confirm fracture.

UTILITY SCORE 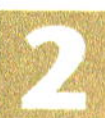

Study	Reliability	Sensitivity	Specificity	LR+	LR−	QUADAS Score (0–14)
Bauer et al.[12]	NT	100	63	NA	NA	11
Richman et al.[104]	NT	85	49	1.7	0.31	12
Comments: Not enough research has been performed to validate the decision rule of Bauer et al.,[12] the values of which are slightly lower than the two more established decision rules.						

TESTS FOR A TORN TIBIAL MENISCUS

Composite Physical Exam/Clusters of Findings

UTILITY SCORE 2

Study	Reliability	Sensitivity	Specificity	LR+	LR−	QUADAS Score (0–14)
Dervin et al.[26] (Fellows) (Orthopedic Staff)	κ = 0.24	87 88	21 20	1.1 1.5	0.62 0.60	11 11
Rose & Gold[105] (Medial) (Lateral)	NT NT	92 67	60 90	2.3 6.7	0.13 0.37	10 10
Kocabey et al.[60] (Medial) (Lateral)	NT NT	87 75	68 95	2.7 15.0	0.19 0.26	10 10
Kocher et al.[61] (Medial) (Lateral)	NT NT	62 50	81 89	3.3 4.5	0.47 0.56	11 11
O'Shea et al.[97] (Medial) (Lateral)	NT NT	88 51	77 90	3.8 5.1	0.16 0.54	9 9
Jackson et al.[49] (Medial) (Lateral)	NT NT	86 88	72 92	3.1 11.0	0.19 0.13	NA NA
Wagemakers et al.[132]	NT	15	97	5.8	0.9	11
Miao et al.[85] (failed meniscus repair) At least 1 of 4 signs At least 2 of 4 signs (swelling, joint-line tenderness, locking, McMurray's test)	NT	58 58	75 96	2.32 14.5	0.56 0.44	11
Muellner et al.[89] 2 of 5 tests (joint-line tenderness, Bohler test, McMurray's, Steinman I test, Apley's test, Payr test)	NT	97	87	7.46	0.03	9
Bonamo & Shulman[15] (expert opinion based on history and effusion, joint-line tenderness, McMurray's, pain with flexion, squat test)	NT	85	84	5.31	0.18	8
Lowery et al[77] 5 tests positive at least 4 tests at least 3 tests (locking, joint-line tenderness, McMurray's, pain with flexion, pain with hyperextension)	NT	11 17 31	99 96 90	11.45 4.29 3.15	0.90 0.86 0.77	8

TESTS FOR A TORN TIBIAL MENISCUS

Study	Reliability	Sensitivity	Specificity	LR+	LR−	QUADAS Score (0–14)
Rayan et al.[103] (Medial) (Lateral) (unspecified history, joint-line tenderness, McMurray's)	NT	86 56	73 95	3.19 11.0	0.19 0.46	8
Butt et al.[18] (Apley's, squat, McMurray's)	NT	83	63	2.2	0.27	7
Loo et al.[71] (locking or decreased motion and McMurray's)	NT	16	94	2.7	0.89	6
Oberlander et al.[98] (Medial) (Lateral)	NT	87 81	93 93	12.43 11.57	0.14 0.20	9
Yoon et al.[138] (Medial) (Lateral)	NT	87 81	93 93	12.43 11.57	0.14 0.20	9
Ryan et al.[107]	NT	77	67	2.33	0.34	8
Esmaili et al.[31] (Medial) (Lateral) (history, joint-line tenderness, McMurray's)	NT	100 85	96 91	25.0 9.44	0 0.16	8

Comments: The study by Dervin et al.[26] combined history, physical findings, special tests, and radiographic findings and although the level of agreement was fair, likelihood ratios would indicate that a composite physical examination is not an accurate predictor of an unstable torn meniscus in those with primary osteoarthritis of the knee. This article can make no conclusions about those with meniscus tears not related to chronic degeneration. The Kocher et al.[61] study would seem to indicate that there is small value in composite physical examination for meniscus tears in athletic children. The O'Shea et al.[97] study was performed only on male military personnel. Apparently, none of the physical examinations were performed in the acute stage of injury. The Jackson et al.[49] study is a meta-analysis and combines the data of 19 studies for the medial meniscus and 17 studies for the lateral meniscus. The data supplied by all authors above would seem to suggest that in nonarthritis-related meniscus injuries, clinicians seem to be able to detect a torn tibial meniscus when history and physical examination findings are combined. With regard to the Wagemakers et al.[132] study, although the use of MRI as a reference standard may bias the results, this is one of the few studies performed outside of an orthopedic specialty care setting. The Miao et al.[85] study was not diagnostic in the classic sense but instead evaluated the ability of clinical findings to determine if a meniscus repair had failed.

TESTS FOR A TORN TIBIAL MENISCUS

McMurray's[84] Test

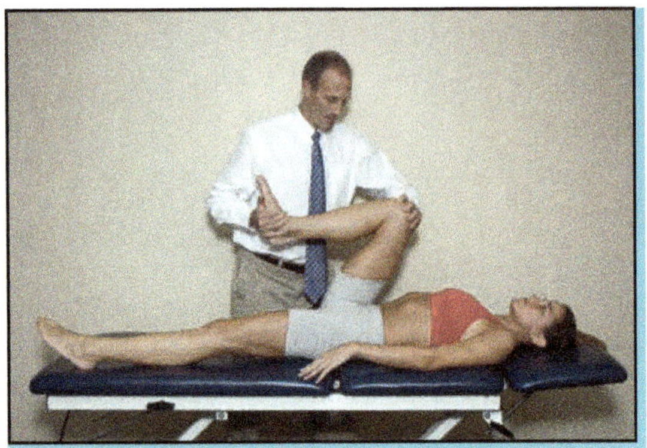

1. The patient assumes a supine position. The examiner stands to the side of the patient's involved knee.

2. The examiner grasps the patient's heel and flexes the knee to end range with one hand while using the thumb and index finger of the other hand to palpate the medial and lateral tibiofemoral joint line.

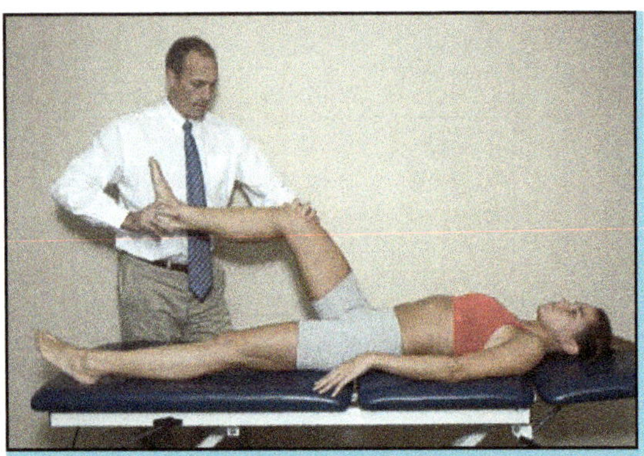

3. To test the medial meniscus, the examiner rotates the tibia into external rotation, then slowly extends the knee.

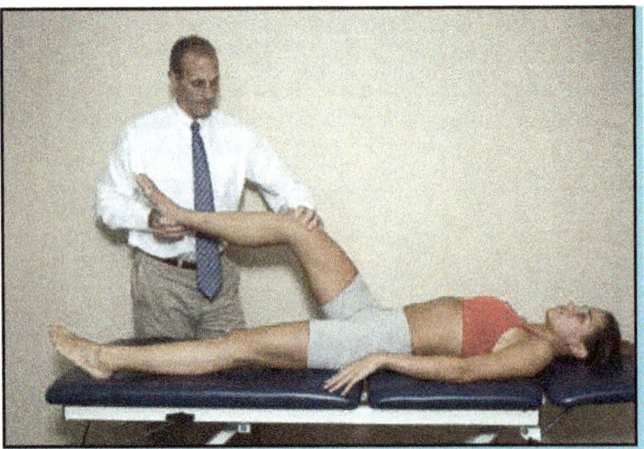

4. To test the lateral meniscus, the examiner reflexes the knee but now internally rotates the patient's tibia and slowly extends the knee.

5. A positive test traditionally is indicated by an audible or palpable "thud" or "click."

UTILITY SCORE 2

Study	Reliability	Sensitivity	Specificity	LR+	LR−	QUADAS Score (0–14)
Karachalios et al.[55] (Medial)	0.95	48	94	8.0	0.55	9
(Lateral)	0.95	65	86	4.6	0.41	9
Akseki et al.[2] (Medial)	NT	67	69	2.2	0.48	11
(Lateral)	NT	53	88	4.4	0.53	11
Kurosaka et al.[64] (Combined)	NT	37	77	1.6	0.86	10

TESTS FOR A TORN TIBIAL MENISCUS

Study	Reliability	Sensitivity	Specificity	LR+	LR−	QUADAS Score (0–14)
Corea et al.[23] (Medial)	NT	65	93	9.3	0.38	7
(Lateral)	NT	52	94	8.7	0.51	7
(Combined)	NT	59	93	8.4	0.44	7
Evans et al.[32] (Medial)	κ = 0.35	16	98	8.0	0.86	10
Dervin et al.[26]	κ = 0.16	NT	NT	NA	NA	NA
Pookarnjanamorakot et al.[101] (Combined)	NT	28	92	3.5	0.78	11
Saengnipanthkul et al.[109] (Medial)	NT	47	94	7.8	0.56	8
Boeree & Ackroyd [13] (Medial)	NT	29	87	2.2	0.82	9
(Lateral)	NT	25	90	2.5	0.83	9
Fowler & Lubliner[36] (Combined)	κ = 0.25	29	96	7.3	0.74	10
Anderson & Lipscomb[6] (Combined)	NT	58	29	0.82	1.45	9
Noble & Erat[94] (Combined)	NT	63	57	1.5	0.65	9
Miao et al.[85]	NT	25	96	6.25	0.78	11
Lowery et al.[77]	NT	20	96	5.0	0.83	8
Mirzatolooei et al.[86]	NT	51	91	6.3	0.53	10
Konan et al.[62] (Medial)	NT	50	77	2.17	0.65	8
(Lateral)		21	94	3.50	0.84	
(Medial + ACL)		25	89	2.27	0.84	
(Lateral + ACL)		14	94	2.33	0.91	
Jain et al.[51] (Medial + ACL)	NA	36	86	2.56	0.74	8
(Lateral + ACL)		22	100	NA	NA	
Jaddue et al.[50] (Medial)	NT	50	78	2.27	0.64	11
Manzotti et al.[79] (Medial)	NT	88	50	1.76	0.24	9
(Lateral)		80	20	0.99	1.03	
Sae-Jung et al.[108] (Combined)	NT	71	82	3.94	0.35	9
(Medial)		70	61	1.79	0.49	
(Lateral)		68	48	1.31	0.67	

Comments: McMurray's Test[84] has changed over the years and many examiners have added varus/valgus stress and used reproduction of joint-line pain as another positive sign of meniscus tear. Generally speaking, whether trying to detect a torn medial meniscus, lateral meniscus, or a tear of either meniscus, McMurray's Test has some value as a specific test where a positive test would rule in the disease. Interobserver agreement in regard to the interpretation of McMurray's Test is generally fair. The Miao et al.[85] study seems to indicate that a positive McMurray's is specific for a failed meniscus repair but only 6 of 81 patients in their study had a positive test.

TESTS FOR A TORN TIBIAL MENISCUS

Apley's Test[8]

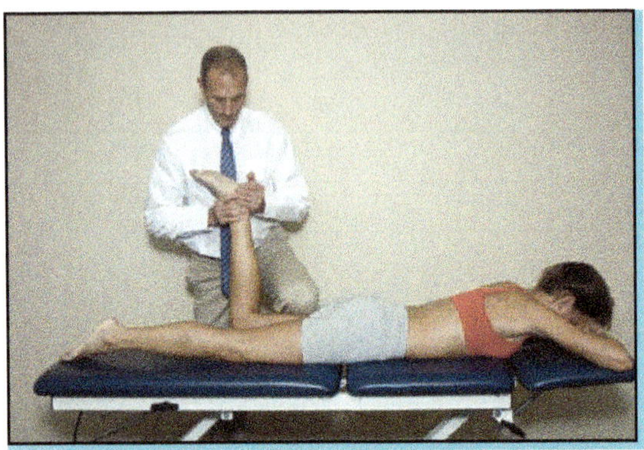

1) The patient lies prone.

2) The examiner half-kneels, placing his or her knee on the hamstring of the patient and flexes the knee to 90 degrees.

3) The examiner grasps the patient's foot with both hands, distracts the tibia, and rotates the tibia, noting whether or not pain is reproduced.

4) A positive test is indicated by worse pain with rotation and is indicative of a "rotation sprain" of soft tissue.

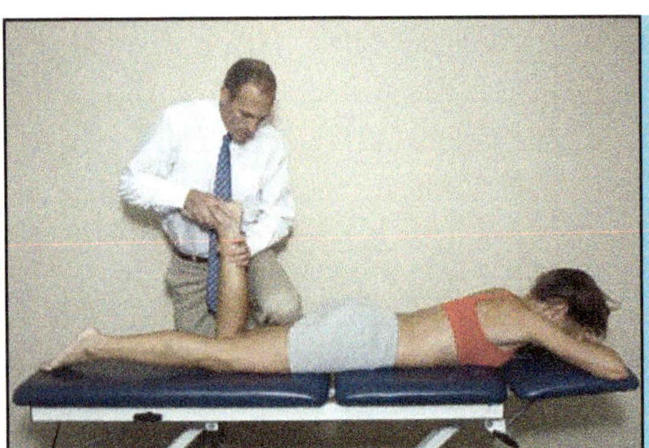

5) The examiner then leans on the patient's foot, providing a compressive force to the tibia and again rotates the tibia.

6) A positive test for a meniscus tear is indicated by more pain in compression than with distraction.

UTILITY SCORE 2

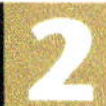

Study	Reliability	Sensitivity	Specificity	LR+	LR−	QUADAS Score (0–14)
Karachalios et al.[55] (Medial) (Lateral)	0.95 0.95	41 41	93 86	5.9 2.9	0.63 0.69	9
Kurosaka et al.[64] (Combined)	NT	13	90	1.3	0.97	10
Fowler & Lubliner[36] (Combined)	NT	16	80	0.80	1.1	10
Pookarnjanamorakot et al.[101] (Combined)	NT	16	100	NA	NA	11
Jaddue et al.[50] (Medial)	NT	81	56	1.84	0.33	11

Comments: The original description of Apley's Test[8] is a bit confusing with the narrative being different from the illustrations of the test. However, as originally described, distraction was the first force applied followed by compression force. Pain reproduced with distraction and rotation was diagnosed as a "rotation sprain" of soft tissue including collateral ligaments and/or capsule. The Karachalios et al.[55] study employs a case-control design, which dramatically overstates the diagnostic accuracy of a test. The remaining three studies seem to show, according to the likelihood ratios, that there is no value in Apley's Test[8] to detect a torn meniscus. Some may find value in Apley's Test[8] as a specific test to rule in a meniscus tear when positive.

TESTS FOR A TORN TIBIAL MENISCUS

Thessaly Test at 20 Degrees/Disco Test

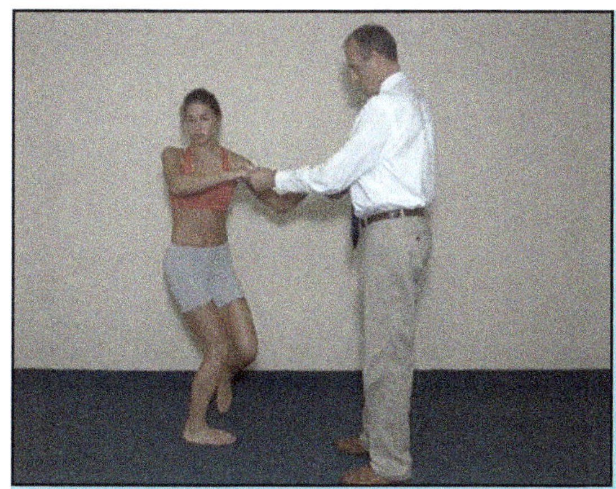

1) The patient stands on one leg facing the examiner and grasps the examiner's hands.

2) The patient flexes the knee to 20 degrees (partial squat) and rotates his or her body, first to the left and then to the right.

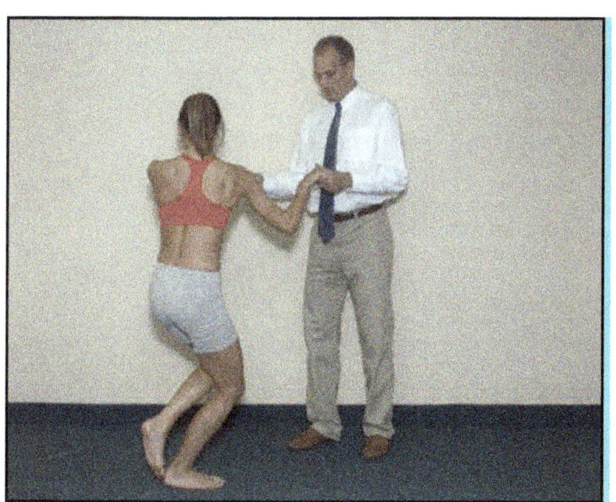

3) Step 2 is repeated three times in each direction.

4) A positive test for meniscus tear is indicated by joint-line discomfort and possibly a sense of locking or catching.

UTILITY SCORE 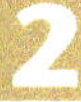

Study	Reliability	Sensitivity	Specificity	LR+	LR−	QUADAS Score (0–14)
Karachalios et al.[55] (Medial)	0.95	89	97	29.7	0.11	9
(Lateral)	0.95	92	96	23	0.08	9
Mirzatolooei et al.[86]	NT	79	40	1.3	0.51	10
Harrison et al.[45]	κ = 0.86	90	97	30.0	0.10	10
Konan et al.[62] (Medial)	NT	59	67	1.79	0.61	8
(Lateral)		31	95	6.20	0.73	
(Medial + ACL)		44	86	3.14	0.65	
(Lateral + ACL)		50	94	8.33	0.53	

Comments: There is reason to doubt the original numbers put forth by Karachalios et al.[55] because these authors employed a case-control design and used MRI as the diagnostic criterion standard, 2 major sources of bias. One newer study[86] employed a stronger design and the Thessaly Test was far less accurate. The Harrison et al.[45] study showed almost perfect reliability of this test which is encouraging. Losee[75] reported the use of this test (calling it the "Disco Test") to reproduce apprehension of the patient with a torn anterior cruciate ligament. No data is available on the Disco Test.

TESTS FOR A TORN TIBIAL MENISCUS

Thessaly Test at 5 Degrees

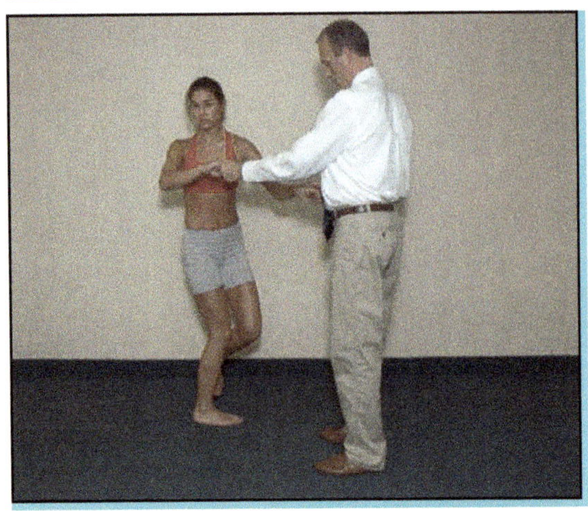

1) The patient stands on one leg facing the examiner and grasps the examiner's hands.

2) The patient flexes the knee to 5 degrees (partial squat) and rotates his or her body, first to the left and then to the right.

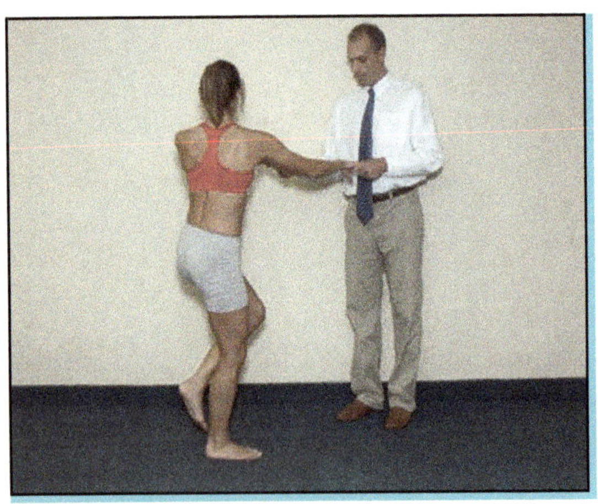

3) Step 2 is repeated three times in each direction.

4) A positive test for meniscus tear is indicated by joint-line discomfort and possibly a sense of locking or catching.

UTILITY SCORE 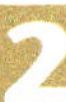

Study	Reliability	Sensitivity	Specificity	LR+	LR−	QUADAS Score (0–14)
Karachalios et al.[55] (Medial) (Lateral)	0.95 0.95	66 81	96 91	16.5 9.0	0.35 0.21	9 9
Pookarnjanamorakot et al.[101] (Merke's—Combined)	NT	27	96	6.8	0.76	11

Comments: The Karachalios et al.[55] study employs a case-control design, which dramatically overstates the diagnostic accuracy of a test. Furthermore, the use in that study of MRI and not arthroscopy as a criterion standard may bias the results. More research needs to be performed to corroborate the statistics of the original authors. This test, when performed in full knee extension, is sometimes referred to as Merke's Sign.

TESTS FOR A TORN TIBIAL MENISCUS

Ege's Test

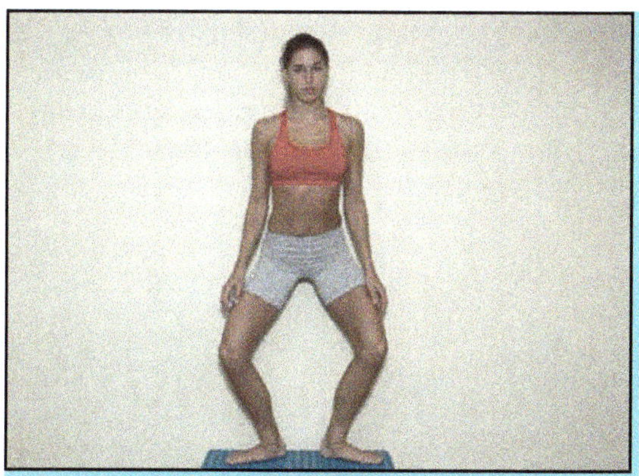

1) The patient stands with feet 30–40 cm apart and knees in full extension.

2) To test the medial meniscus, the patient externally rotates the lower legs to end range and slowly squats then stands up.

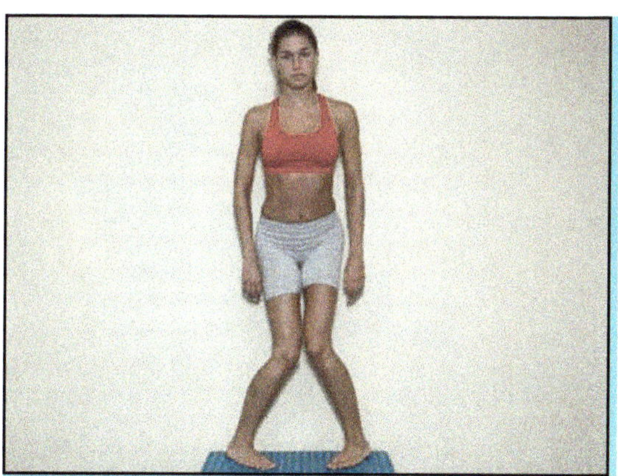

3) To test the lateral meniscus, the patient internally rotates the lower legs to end range and slowly squats then stands up.

4) A positive test for a torn meniscus is indicated by concordant pain and/or a click.

UTILITY SCORE 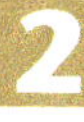

Study	Reliability	Sensitivity	Specificity	LR+	LR−	QUADAS Score (0–14)
Akseki et al.[2] (Medial)	NT	67	81	3.5	0.41	11
(Lateral)	NT	64	90	6.4	0.40	11
Comments: Ege's Test improves the posttest probability of detecting a torn meniscus by a small to moderate amount. Further research needs to be performed to corroborate the statistics reported in this study.						

TESTS FOR A TORN TIBIAL MENISCUS

Axial Pivot-Shift Test

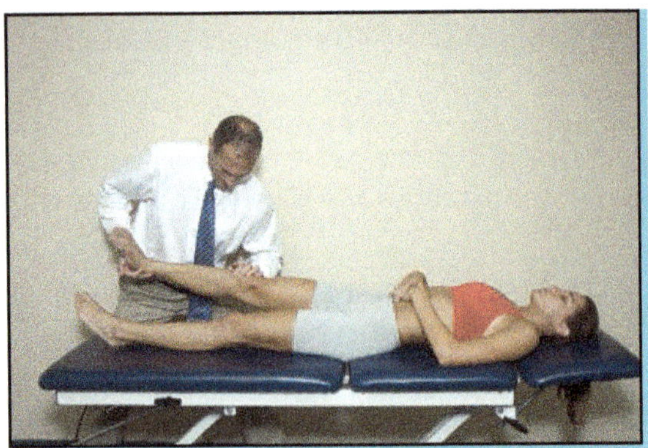

1) The patient is supine with the knee in full extension.

2) The examiner cradles the patient's leg and applies a valgus and internal rotation force to the proximal tibia.

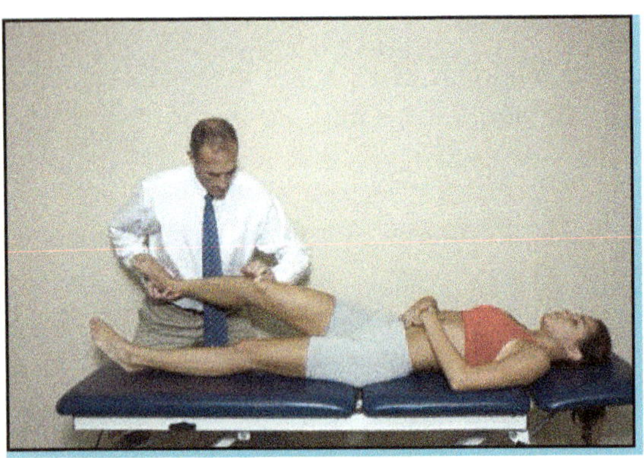

3) Axial compression is applied and the knee flexed to 30 and 45 degrees of flexion.

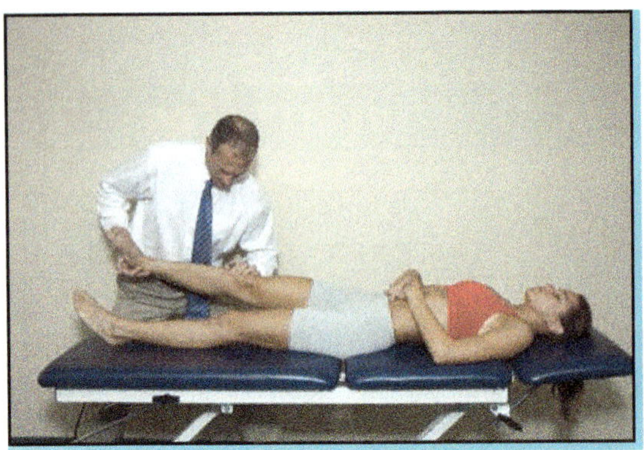

4) The valgus, internal rotation, and axial compression forces are maintained as the knee is returned to full extension.

5) A positive test for a torn meniscus is indicated by concordant joint-line pain and/or a click felt by the examiner.

UTILITY SCORE 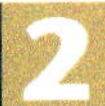

Study	Reliability	Sensitivity	Specificity	LR+	LR−	QUADAS Score (0–14)
Kurosaka et al.[64] (Combined)	NT	71	83	4.2	0.35	10
Comments: The Axial Pivot-Shift Test improves the posttest probability of detecting a torn meniscus by a small amount in patients who have had symptoms for longer than 8 weeks. More research is needed to confirm this conclusion.						

TESTS FOR A TORN TIBIAL MENISCUS

Steinmann I Sign

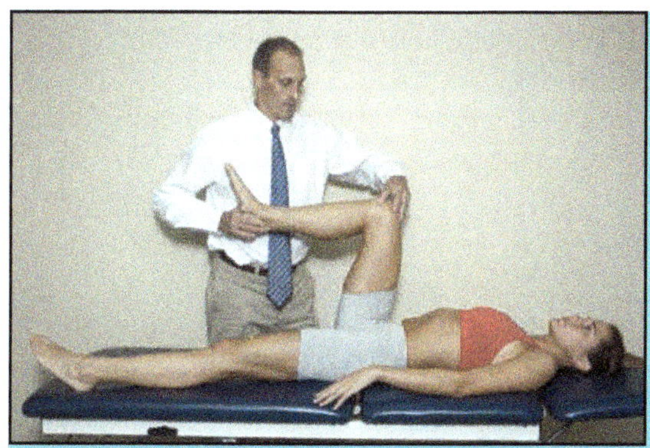

1) The patient assumes a supine position. The examiner stands to the side of the patient's involved knee.

2) The examiner grasps the patient's heel and flexes the knee and hip while using the thumb and index finger of the other hand to palpate the medial and lateral tibiofemoral joint line.

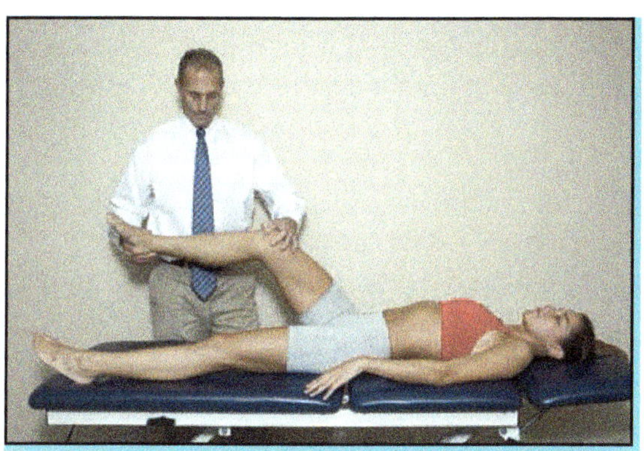

3) The examiner internally and externally rotates the tibia at various degrees of knee flexion but the knee should not be moving with any part of the test.

4) A positive test for a meniscus tear is indicated by joint-line pain.

UTILITY SCORE 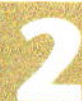

Study	Reliability	Sensitivity	Specificity	LR+	LR−	QUADAS Score (0–14)
Dervin et al.[26]	$\kappa = 0.05$	NT	NT	NA	NA	NA
Pookarnjanamorakot et al.[101]	NT	29	100	NA	NA	11
Jaddue et al.[50] (Medial)	NT	66	83	3.88	0.41	11
Sae-Jung et al.[108] (KKU Test)	NT	86	88	7.17	0.16	9

Comments: The Steinmann I/KKU Test appears to have moderate diagnostic ability.

TESTS FOR A TORN TIBIAL MENISCUS

Dynamic Test

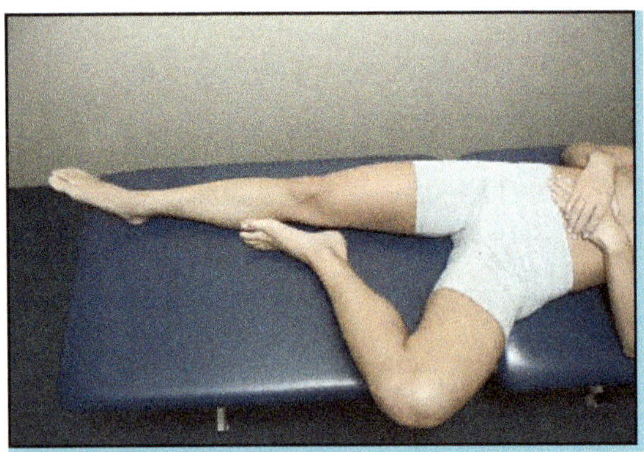

1) The patient is supine with the hip abducted 60 degrees, flexed, and externally rotated 45 degrees; the knee is flexed to 90 degrees, the lateral border of the foot resting on the examination table.

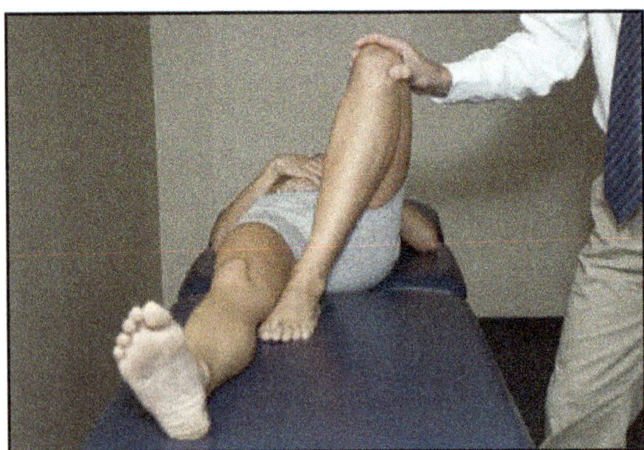

2) The examiner palpates the lateral joint-line then slowly adducts the hip while maintaining the knee in 90 degrees of flexion.

3) A positive test for a torn lateral meniscus is indicated by either an increase of pain above that elicited by lateral joint-line palpation or a sharp pain at the end of hip adduction.

UTILITY SCORE

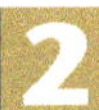

Study	Reliability	Sensitivity	Specificity	LR+	LR−	QUADAS Score (0–14)
Mariani et al.[80] (Lateral)	κ = 0.61–0.85	85	90	8.5	0.17	9
Comments: The Dynamic Test has moderate diagnostic accuracy and the interobserver agreement is substantial. Further research needs to be performed to corroborate the statistics reported in this study.						

TESTS FOR A TORN TIBIAL MENISCUS

History of Mechanical Symptoms

1) The patient reports locking or giving way during daily activities.

UTILITY SCORE 3

Study	Reliability	Sensitivity	Specificity	LR+	LR−	QUADAS Score (0–14)
Lowery et al.[77]	NT	20	94	3.33	0.85	8
Comment: This commonly used clinical sign has surprisingly limited research to support it, but patient report of mechanical symptoms may have a small ability to contribute to the diagnosis of a torn meniscus.						

Medial-Lateral Grind Test

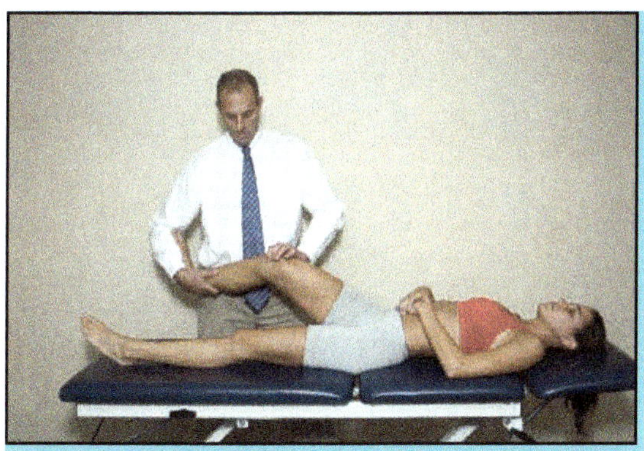

1) The patient is supine.

2) The examiner cradles the patient's affected lower extremity in one hand and, using the thumb and index finger, palpates the anterior tibiofemoral joint line.

3) A valgus stress is applied as the knee is flexed to 45 degrees.

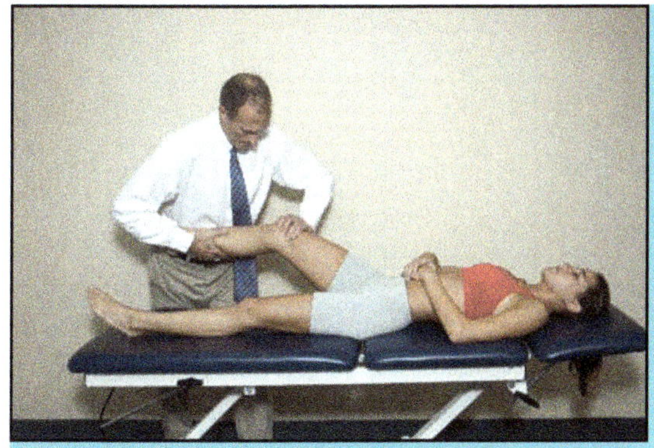

4) A varus stress is applied as the knee is extended, producing a circular motion of the knee.

5) A positive test for a torn meniscus is indicated by a palpable "grinding" sensation.

UTILITY SCORE 

Study	Reliability	Sensitivity	Specificity	LR+	LR−	QUADAS Score (0–14)
Anderson & Lipscomb[6] (Combined)	NT	70	67	2.12	0.45	9
Comments: The Medial-Lateral Grind Test improves the posttest probability of detecting a torn meniscus by a small amount. Further research needs to be performed to corroborate the statistics reported in this study as it possesses some design bias.						

TESTS FOR A TORN TIBIAL MENISCUS

Joint-Line Tenderness

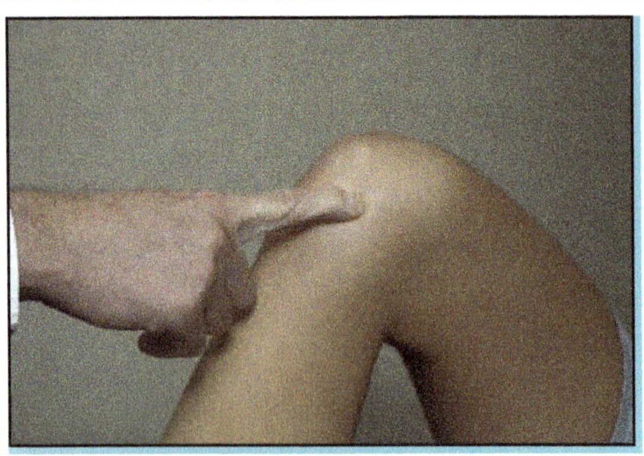

1) The patient is supine with the affected knee flexed to 90 degrees.

2) The examiner palpates the medial and lateral tibiofemoral joint line.

3) A positive test for meniscus tear is indicated by reproduction of the patient's pain (concordant sign).

UTILITY SCORE  3

Study	Reliability	Sensitivity	Specificity	LR+	LR−	QUADAS Score (0–14)
Karachalios et al.[55] (Medial)	0.95	71	87	5.5	0.33	9
(Lateral)	0.95	78	90	7.8	0.24	9
Akseki et al.[2] (Medial)	NT	88	44	1.6	0.27	11
(Lateral)	NT	67	80	3.4	0.41	11
Eren[30] (Medial)	NT	86	67	2.6	0.21	9
(Lateral)	NT	93	97	31.0	0.07	9
Kurosaka et al.[64] (Combined)	NT	55	67	1.7	0.67	10
Shelbourne et al.[115] (Medial)	NT	58	53	1.2	0.79	9
(Lateral)	NT	38	71	1.3	0.87	9
Saengnipanthkul et al.[109] (Medial)	NT	58	74	2.2	0.57	8
Boeree & Ackroyd[13] (Medial)	NT	64	69	2.1	0.52	8
(Lateral)	NT	28	87	2.2	0.83	8
Abdon et al.[1] (Medial)	NT	78	54	1.7	0.41	8
(Lateral)	NT	78	92	9.8	0.24	8
Fowler & Lubliner[36] (Combined)	κ = 0.15	85	30	1.2	0.50	10
Dervin et al.[26] (Medial)	κ = 0.21	NT	NT	NT	NT	NA
(Lateral)	κ = 0.25	NT	NT	NT	NT	NA
Barry et al.[11] (Combined)	NT	86	43	1.5	0.33	7
Noble & Erat[94] (Combined)	NT	72	13	0.83	2.2	9
Pookarnjanamorakot et al.[101]	NT	27	96	6.8	0.76	11
Lowery et al.[77]	NT	65	65	1.86	0.54	8
Wadey et al.[131]	κ = 0.48	84	31	1.2	0.49	10
Mirzatolooei[86]	NT	92	63	2.5	0.12	10

(continued)

TESTS FOR A TORN TIBIAL MENISCUS

Study	Reliability	Sensitivity	Specificity	LR+	LR−	QUADAS Score (0–14)
Konan et al.[62] (Medial) (Lateral) (Medial + ACL) (Lateral + ACL)	NT	83 68 56 57	76 97 89 94	3.46 22.67 5.09 9.50	0.22 0.33 0.49 0.46	8
Jaddue et al.[50] (Medial)	NT	84	72	3.00	0.22	11
Comments: The study by Eren[30] had 104 subjects, all of whom were male military recruits, which limits the applicability of these findings. Furthermore, the Karachalios et al.[55] study employs a case-control design, which dramatically overstates the diagnostic accuracy of the test and the 0.95 is an estimate of agreement. Research shows this test to be sensitive in the hands of some and specific in the hands of others. Finally, the interobserver agreement of joint-line tenderness is fair at best.						

Forced Extension/Extension Block/Bounce Home Test

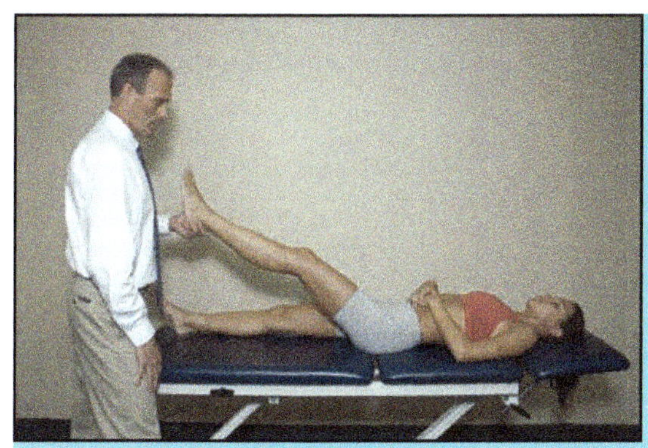

1) The patient is supine.

2) The examiner extends the affected knee to end range.

3) A positive test for meniscus tear is indicated by a block preventing full extension or pain at end-range extension.

UTILITY SCORE 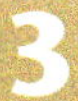 3

Study	Reliability	Sensitivity	Specificity	LR+	LR−	QUADAS Score (0–14)
Kurosaka et al.[64] (Combined)	NT	47	67	1.4	0.79	10
Dervin et al.[26] (Combined)	$\kappa = 0.07$	NT	NT	NA	NA	NA
Noble & Erat[94] (Combined)	NT	38	67	1.2	0.93	9
Fowler & Lubliner[36] (Combined)	$\kappa = 0.29$	44	85	2.9	0.66	10
Lowery et al.[77]	NT	36	86	2.57	0.74	8
Comments: Neither pain at full extension nor an extension block seems to indicate a torn meniscus. No data is specifically available for the Bounce Home Test.						

TESTS FOR A TORN TIBIAL MENISCUS

Squat/Duck Waddle/Childress Test

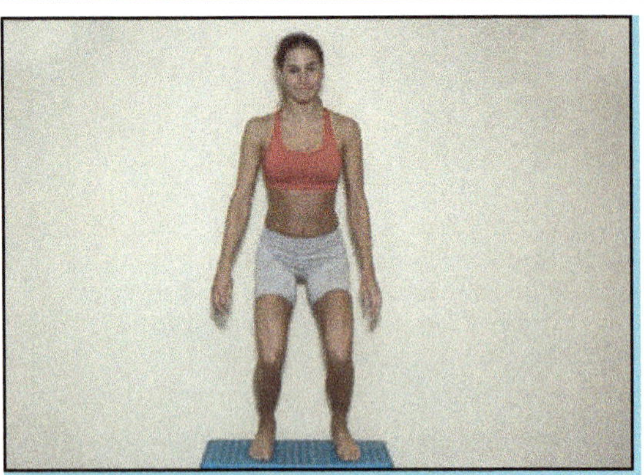

1) The patient is standing and then squats.

2) If no pain is reproduced, the patient is asked to "duck walk" in the squatting position.

3) A positive test for meniscus tear is indicated by a block preventing full flexion or pain at end-range flexion.

UTILITY SCORE 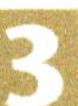

Study	Reliability	Sensitivity	Specificity	LR+	LR−	QUADAS Score (0–14)
Noble & Erat[94] (Combined)	NT	55	67	1.7	0.67	9
Pookarnjanamorakot et al.[101] (Combined)	NT	68	60	1.7	0.53	11
Comments: Neither pain with squatting nor with a "duck waddle" seems to indicate a torn meniscus.						

Flexion Block/Forced Flexion

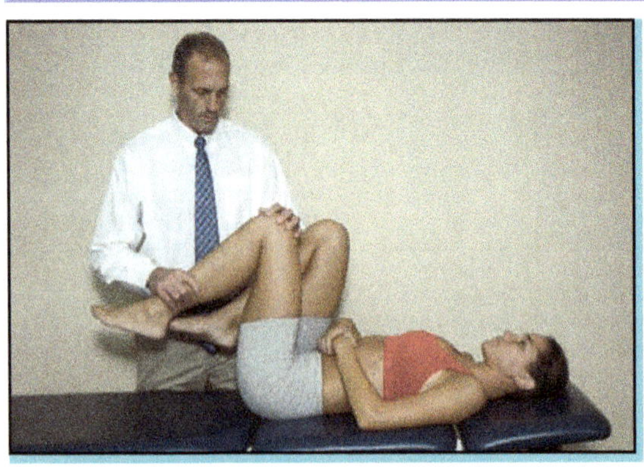

1) The patient is standing and then squats or the patient is supine and the examiner flexes the patient's knee to end-range.

2) In either case, a positive test for meniscus tear is indicated by a block preventing full flexion or pain at end-range flexion.

UTILITY SCORE 

Study	Reliability	Sensitivity	Specificity	LR+	LR−	QUADAS Score (0–14)
Noble & Erat[94] (Combined)	NT	44	57	1.0	0.98	9
Fowler & Lubliner[36] (Combined)	$\kappa = 0.18$	50	68	1.6	0.74	10
Wagemakers et al.[132]	NT	77	41	1.3	0.6	11
Lowery et al.[77]	NT	48	59	1.17	0.88	8
Comments: A flexion block does not appear to indicate a torn meniscus.						

TESTS FOR A TORN TIBIAL MENISCUS

Effusion

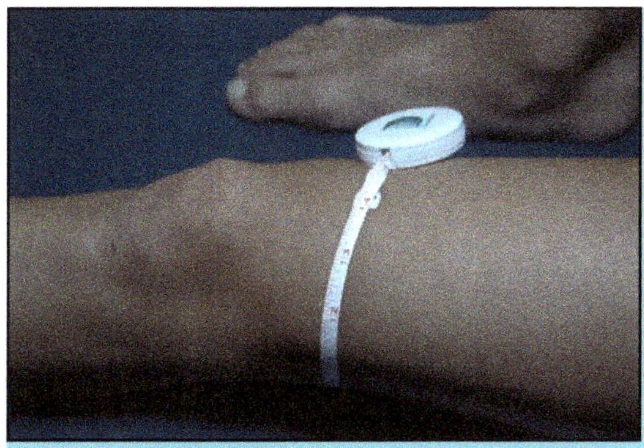

1) The examiner looks for or measures swelling about the knee.

2) A positive test for meniscus tear is indicated by more swelling/girth on the affected knee than the unaffected knee.

UTILITY SCORE 3

Study	Reliability	Sensitivity	Specificity	LR+	LR−	QUADAS Score (0–14)
Noble & Erat[94] (Combined)	NT	53	54	1.2	0.87	9
Comments: Effusion does not appear to differentiate a torn meniscus.						

Figure 4 Test (Popliteomeniscal Fascicle Tears of the Lateral Meniscus)

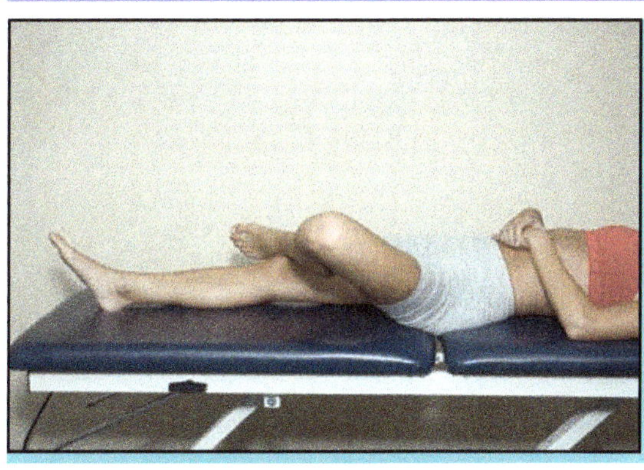

1) The patient lies supine and places the foot of the affected knee on the contralateral knee, forming a "figure 4."

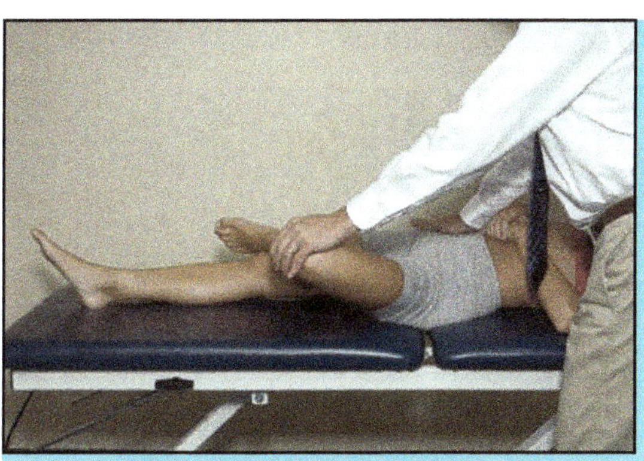

2) The examiner pushes the affected knee toward the examining table.

3) A positive test is indicated by concordant pain over the lateral joint line at the popliteal hiatus.

(continued)

TESTS FOR A TORN TIBIAL MENISCUS

UTILITY SCORE 3

Study	Reliability	Sensitivity	Specificity	LR+	LR−	QUADAS Score (0–14)
LaPrade & Konowalchuk[65]	NT	100	0	NA	NA	9
Comments: The Figure 4 Test[65] was developed to detect popliteomeniscal fascicle tears, which create instability of the lateral meniscus. This original article, while provocative, had only six patients with prolonged lateral knee pain and therefore indicates only the need for more research with this test.						

Payr Sign

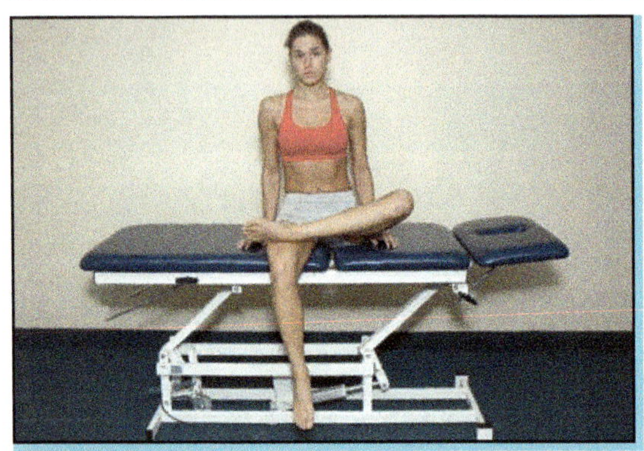

1) The patient sits and places the foot of the affected knee on the contralateral knee, forming a "figure 4."

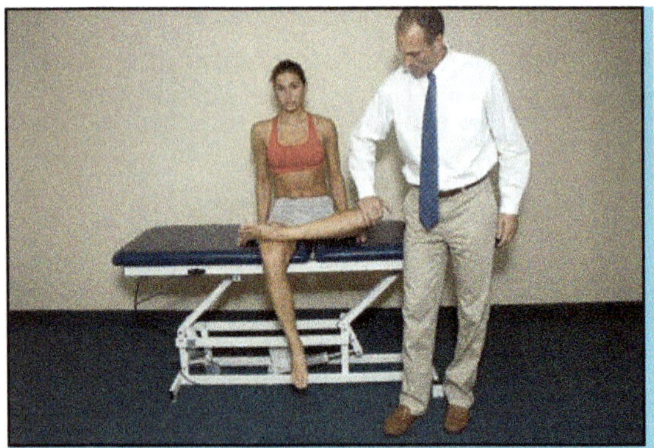

2) The examiner pushes the affected knee toward the floor.

3) A positive test for a posterior horn lesion of the medial meniscus is indicated by concordant pain over the medial joint line.

UTILITY SCORE 3

Study	Reliability	Sensitivity	Specificity	LR+	LR−	QUADAS Score (0–14)
Jerosch & Riemer[53]	NT	54	44	0.96	1.05	11
Comments: This test has as much effect on the posttest probability of detecting a torn tibial meniscus as a coin flip.						

TESTS FOR A TORN TIBIAL MENISCUS

Steinmann II Sign

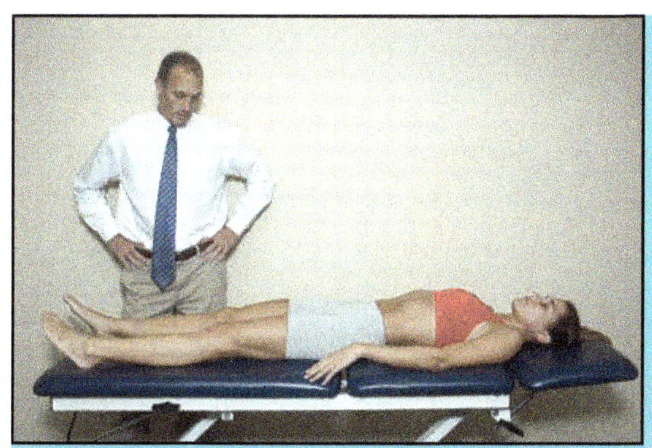

1) The patient presents with anterior tibiofemoral joint-line pain with the knee in full extension. The patient assumes a supine position. The examiner stands to the side of the patient's involved knee.

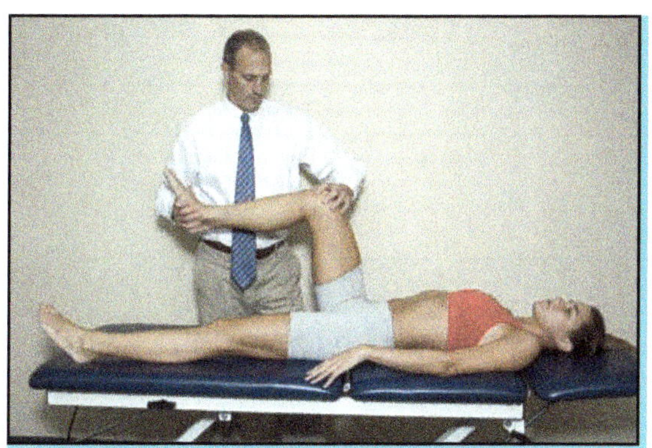

2) The examiner grasps the patient's heel and flexes the knee and hip while using the thumb and index finger of the other hand to palpate the medial and lateral tibiofemoral joint line.

3) A positive test for a meniscus tear is indicated by joint-line pain that moves in a posterior direction toward the collateral ligaments with knee flexion. If the pain doesn't move with knee flexion, the patient supposedly has a ligamentous issue.

UTILITY SCORE 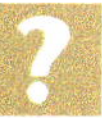

Study	Reliability	Sensitivity	Specificity	LR+	LR−	QUADAS Score (0–14)
Not tested	NT	NT	NT	NA	NA	NA
Comments: There have been no English-language studies that report the reliability or diagnostic accuracy of the Steinmann II Sign.						

TESTS FOR TORN ANTERIOR CRUCIATE LIGAMENT (ACL) AND ANTERIOR ROTARY INSTABILITY

Composite Physical Exam (ACL Tear)

UTILITY SCORE 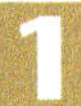

Study	Reliability	Sensitivity	Specificity	LR+	LR−	QUADAS Score (0–14)
O'Shea et al.[97]	NT	97	100	NA	NA	9
Rose & Gold[105]	NT	100	100	NA	NA	10
Simonsen et al.[119]	NT	62	75	2.5	0.51	12
Kocabey et al.[60]	NT	100	100	NA	NA	10
Kocher et al.[61]	NT	81	91	9.0	0.21	11
Jackson et al.[49]	NT	74	95	15	0.27	NA
Rayan et al.[103] (unspecified history, Lachman's, anterior drawer)	NT	77	100	NA	NA	8
Loo et al.[71] (giving way or instability and anterior drawer or Lachman's)	NT	73	79	3.5	0.34	6
Wagemakers et al.[133]—complete lesion (History: effusion, popping, giving way; Exam: anterior drawer)	NT					11
3 from history		18	98	9.0	0.84	
3 history + anterior drawer		19	99	19.9	0.80	
Oberlander et al.[98]	NT	63	99	63.0	0.37	9
Yoon et al.[138]	NT	76	97	25.33	0.25	9
Esmaili et al.[31]	NT	86	96	21.50	0.15	8

Comments: The composite physical examination for a torn ACL is highly accurate in adults with 8 of 10 studies showing sensitivities and specificities either at or near 100. The Kocher et al.[61] study would seem to indicate similar diagnostic accuracy for ACL tears in athletic children. Apparently, none of the physical examinations were performed in the acute stage of injury. The Jackson et al.[49] study is a meta-analysis and combines the data of 18 studies for ACL tear.

TESTS FOR TORN ANTERIOR CRUCIATE LIGAMENT (ACL) AND ANTERIOR ROTARY INSTABILITY

Lachman's Test (ACL Tear)

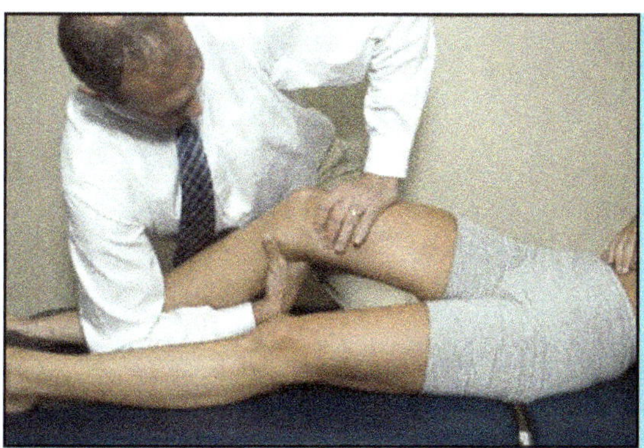

1) The patient is supine with the knee flexed to 15 degrees.

2) The examiner stabilizes the distal femur with one hand and grasps behind the proximal tibia with the other hand.

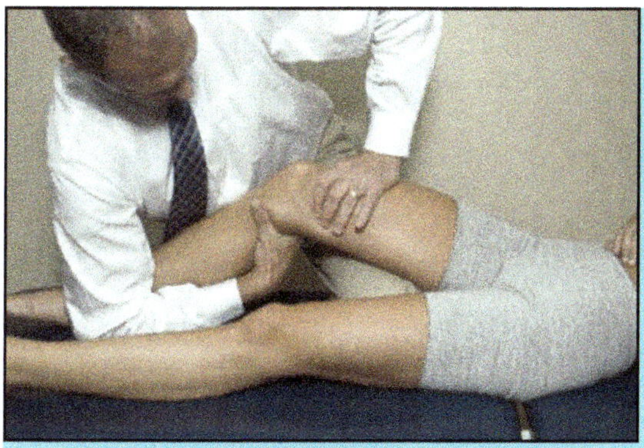

3) The examiner then applies an anterior tibial force to the proximal tibia.

4) A positive test for a torn ACL is indicated by greater anterior tibial displacement on the affected side when compared to the unaffected side.

(*continued*)

TESTS FOR TORN ANTERIOR CRUCIATE LIGAMENT (ACL) AND ANTERIOR ROTARY INSTABILITY

UTILITY SCORE 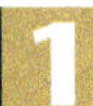

Study	Reliability	Sensitivity	Specificity	LR+	LR−	QUADAS Score (0–14)
Bomberg & McGinty[14]	NT	86	60	2.15	0.23	9
Hardaker et al.[41]	NT	74	NT	NA	NA	8
Torg et al.[130]	NT	96	100	NA	NA	7
Learmonth[68]	NT	68	94	11.3	0.38	6
Rubinstein et al.[106]	NT	96*	100*	NA	NA	9
Boeree & Ackroyd[13]	NT	63	90	6.3	0.41	8
Donaldson et al.[28]	NT	99	NT	NA	NA	8
Lee et al.[69]	NT	91	100	NA	NA	8
Liu et al.[70]	NT	95	NT	NA	NA	8
Cooperman et al.[22]	$\kappa = 0.38$	65***	42***	NA	NA	6
	$\kappa = 0.35$	77**	50**	NA	NA	6
Butt et al.[18]	NT	63	93	9.5	0.39	7
Jain et al.[51]	NA	79	100	NA	NA	8

Comments: The Lachman Test improves the posttest probability of detecting a torn ACL by a moderate to large amount. However, the weighted kappa coefficient reported in the Cooperman et al.[22] study indicates that the test is performed with only fair inter observer agreement by both orthopedic surgeons and physical therapists when grading the amount of translation.
*Data are the mean result of five orthopedic surgeons.
**Data are the sum of the results from two physical therapists.
***Data are the sum of the results from two orthopedic surgeons.

Anterior Drawer Test (ACL Tear)

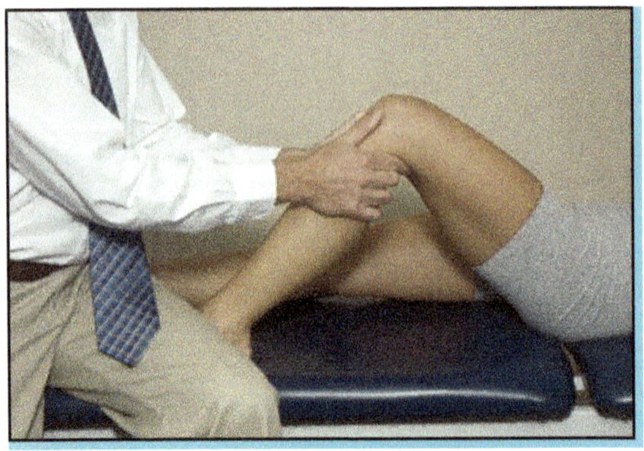

1. The patient is supine with the knee flexed to 90 degrees so that the foot is flat.

2. The examiner sits on the patient's foot and grasps behind the proximal tibia with thumbs palpating the tibial plateau and index fingers palpating the tendons of the hamstring muscle group medially and laterally.

TESTS FOR TORN ANTERIOR CRUCIATE LIGAMENT (ACL) AND ANTERIOR ROTARY INSTABILITY

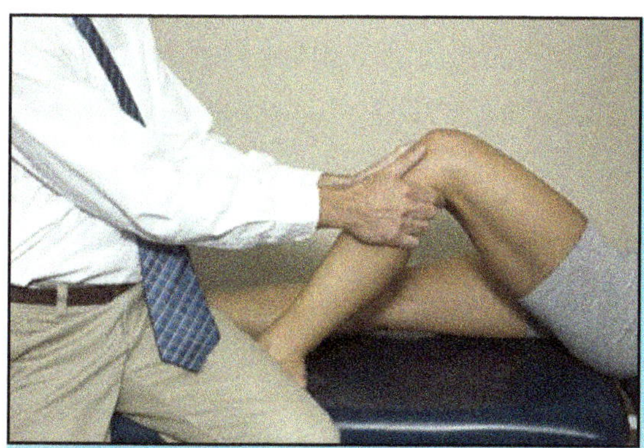

3) An anterior tibial force is applied by the examiner.

4) A positive test for a torn ACL is indicated by greater anterior tibial displacement on the affected side when compared to the unaffected side.

UTILITY SCORE 2

Study	Reliability	Sensitivity	Specificity	LR+	LR−	QUADAS Score (0–14)
Hardaker et al.[41]	NT	18	NT	NA	NA	8
Bomberg & McGinty[14]	NT	41	100	NA	NA	9
Rubinstein et al.[106]	NT	76*	86*	NA	NA	9
Jonsson et al.[54] [Acute (A)] [Chronic (C)]	NT NT	33 95	NT NT	NA NA	NA NA	8 8
Boeree & Ackroyd[13]	NT	56	92	7.0	0.48	8
Torg et al.[130]	NT	52	100	NA	NA	7
Donaldson et al.[28]	NT	70	NT	NA	NA	8
Lee et al.[69]	NR	78	100	NA	NA	8
Sandberg et al.[110]	NT	39	78	1.8	0.78	10
Noyes et al.[96]	NT	25	96	6.2	0.78	10
Liu et al.[70]	NT	63	NT	NA	NA	8
Anderson & Lipscomb[7]	NT	27	NT	NA	NA	12
Braunstein[16]	NT	91	89	8.3	0.10	10
Warren & Marshall[134,135]	NT	71	77	3.1	0.38	7
Wagemakers et al.[133] (Complete lesion) (Partial or complete lesion)	NT	88 83	55 57	1.9 1.6	0.20 0.60	11
Jain et al.[51]	NA	89	100	NA	NA	8

Comments: The Anterior Drawer Test appears to be a specific test helpful at ruling in a torn ACL when the test is positive. The Anterior Drawer Test may become more sensitive in nonacute patients and less specific in general practice compared to a specialty setting.
*Data is the mean result of five orthopedic surgeons.

TESTS FOR TORN ANTERIOR CRUCIATE LIGAMENT (ACL) AND ANTERIOR ROTARY INSTABILITY

Pivot-Shift Test (ACL Tear, Anterolateral Instability, Rotational Instability)

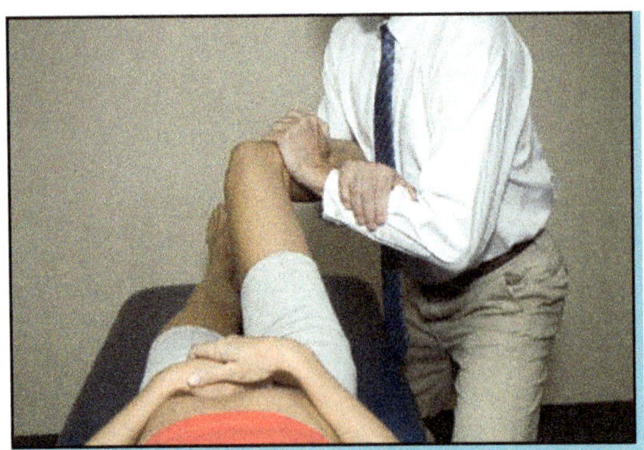

1) The patient assumes a supine position. The examiner stands to the side of the patient's involved knee.

2) The examiner wraps one arm around the patients leg pinning it firmly and flexes the knee to 90 degrees while using the palm of the other hand to medially rotate the tibia, effectively subluxing the lateral tibial plateau.

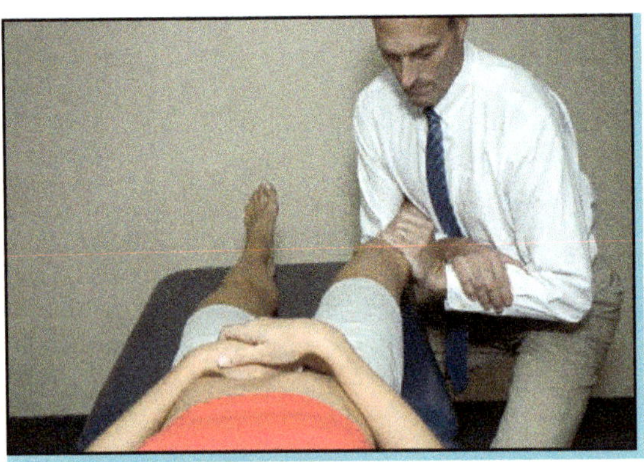

3) The examiner slowly extends the knee, maintaining rotation of the tibia.

4) As the patient's knee reaches full extension, the tibial plateau will relocate.

5) A positive test traditionally is indicated by an audible or palpable "thud" or "click."

UTILITY SCORE 2

Study	Reliability	Sensitivity	Specificity	LR+	LR−	QUADAS Score (0–14)
Anderson & Lipscomb[7]	NT	42	NT	NA	NA	12
Bomberg & McGinty[14]	NT	9	100	NA	NA	9
Hardaker et al.[41]	NT	29	NT	NA	NA	8
Rubenstein[106]	NT	93*	89*	NA	NA	9
Torg[130]	NT	9	100	NA	NA	7
Sandberg et al.[110]	NT	6	100	NA	NA	10
Boeree & Ackroyd[13]	NT	31	97	10.3	.71	8
Liu et al.[70]	NT	71	NT	NA	NA	8
Jain et al.[51]	NT	75	100	NA	NA	8

Comments: The Pivot-Shift Test appears to be a specific test helpful at ruling in a torn ACL when the test is positive.
*Data are the mean of five orthopedic surgeons. Galway & MacIntosh,[38] Hughston et al.,[47] Losee,[74] Slocum et al.,[120] Noyes et al.,[95] Bach et al.,[9] Martens and Mulier,[81] and Anderson and Lipscomb[7]—all have versions of the pivot-shift maneuver.

TESTS FOR TORN ANTERIOR CRUCIATE LIGAMENT (ACL) AND ANTERIOR ROTARY INSTABILITY

Anterior Drawer Test in External Rotation (ACL Tear, Anteromedial Instability)

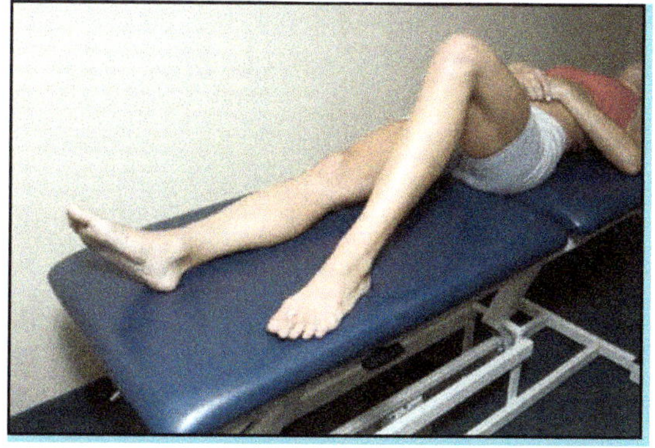

1) The patient is supine with the knee flexed to 90 degrees and the tibia in 15 degrees of external rotation.

2) The examiner sits on the patient's foot and grasps behind the proximal tibia with thumbs palpating the tibial plateau and index fingers palpating the tendons of the hamstring muscle group medially and laterally.

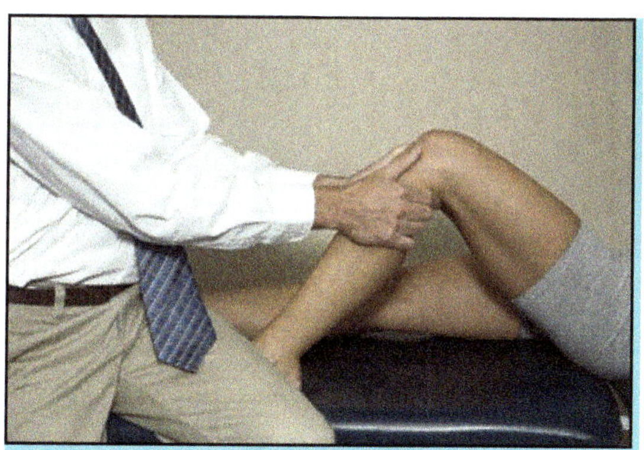

3) An anterior tibial force is applied by the examiner and more movement on the medial side will be detected.

4) A positive test for a torn ACL is indicated by greater anterior tibial displacement on the affected side when compared to the unaffected side.

UTILITY SCORE 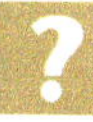

Study	Reliability	Sensitivity	Specificity	LR+	LR−	QUADAS Score (0–14)
Larson[67]	NT	NT	NT	NA	NA	NA
Comments: No data regarding the reliability or diagnostic accuracy of the Anterior Drawer in External Rotation is available.						

TESTS FOR TORN ANTERIOR CRUCIATE LIGAMENT (ACL) AND ANTERIOR ROTARY INSTABILITY

Anterior Drawer Test in Internal Rotation (ACL Tear, Anterolateral Instability)

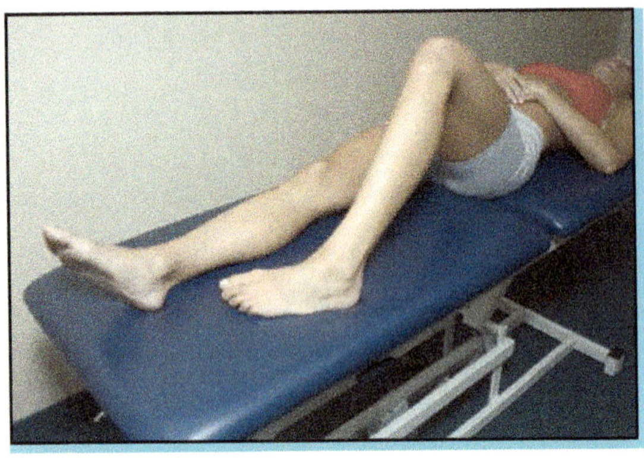

1) The patient is supine with the knee flexed to 90 degrees and the tibia in 30 degrees of internal rotation.

2) The examiner sits on the patient's foot and grasps behind the proximal tibia with thumbs palpating the tibial plateau and index fingers palpating the tendons of the hamstring muscle group medially and laterally.

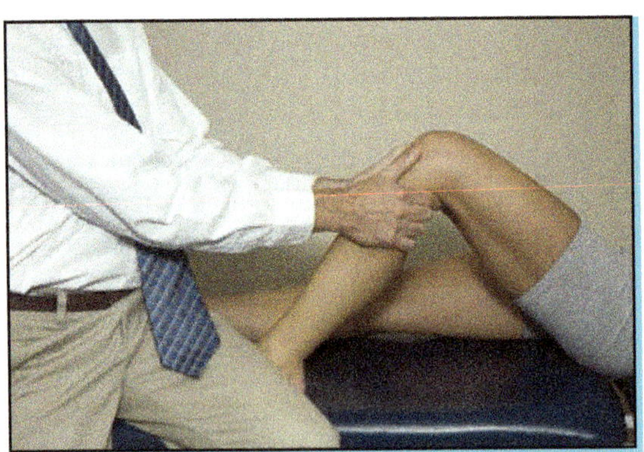

3) An anterior tibial force is applied by the examiner and greater movement of the lateral tibia is detected.

4) A positive test for a torn ACL is indicated by greater anterior tibial displacement on the affected side when compared to the unaffected side.

UTILITY SCORE

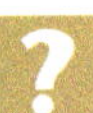

Study	Reliability	Sensitivity	Specificity	LR+	LR−	QUADAS Score (0–14)
Larson[67]	NT	NT	NT	NA	NA	NA
Comments: No data regarding the reliability or diagnostic accuracy of the Anterior Drawer in Internal Rotation is available.						

Active Lachman's Test (ACL Tear)

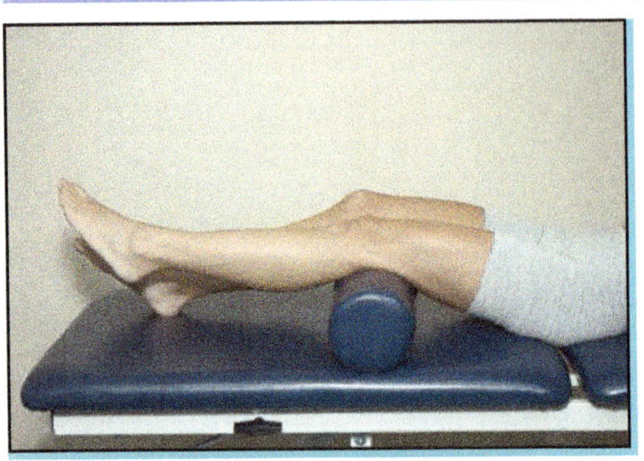

1) The patient assumes a supine position with a bolster under the distal femur so that the knee is flexed to 30–40 degrees.

2) The patient is asked to actively extend the involved knee and then to relax back to the starting position.

3) A positive test for a torn ACL is indicated by anterior glide of the proximal tibia.

UTILITY SCORE 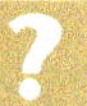

Study	Reliability	Sensitivity	Specificity	LR+	LR−	QUADAS Score (0–14)
Cross et al.[24]	NT	NT	NT	NA	NA	NA
Comments: The one study to examine the Active Lachman's Test[24] did not report reliability or diagnostic accuracy.						

Fibular Head Sign (ACL Tear, Anterolateral Instability)

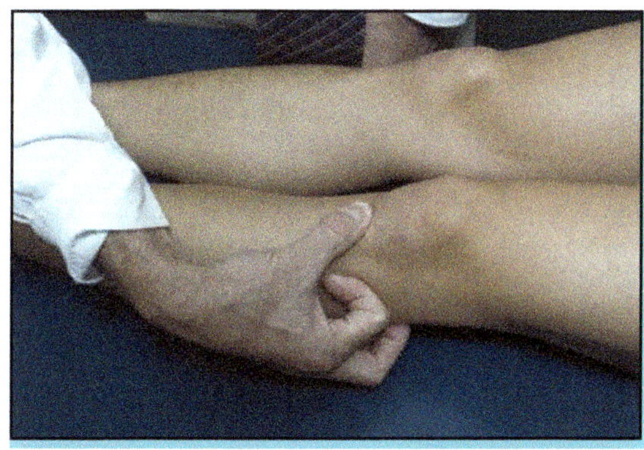

1. The patient is supine with both knees in extension and lower limbs in neutral rotation.
2. The examiner places his or her thumb on the tibial tubercle and the middle finger posterior to the fibular head. The examiner should feel the biceps femoris tendon between the middle finger and fibular head.

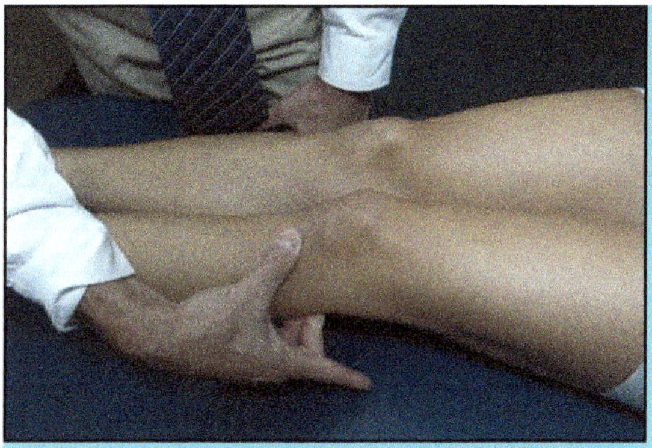

3. The examiner then extends his or her fingers to further palpate the fibular head.
4. A positive test for ACL tear is the inability to feel the biceps tendon between the middle finger and the fibular head.
5. Compare with the uninvolved knee.

UTILITY SCORE 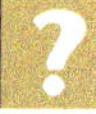

Study	Reliability	Sensitivity	Specificity	LR+	LR−	QUADAS Score (0–14)
al-Duri[3]	NT	NT	NT	NA	NA	NA
Comments: The one study to examine the Fibular Head Sign[3] did not report reliability or diagnostic accuracy and the test description was less than clear.						

TESTS FOR TORN POSTERIOR CRUCIATE LIGAMENT (PCL) AND POSTERIOR ROTARY INSTABILITY

Composite Physical Exam

UTILITY SCORE 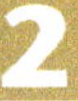

Study	Reliability	Sensitivity	Specificity	LR+	LR−	QUADAS Score (0–14)
O'Shea et al.[97]	NT	100	99	NA	NA	9
Simonsen et al.[119]	NT	91	80	4.6	0.11	12
Jackson et al.[49]	NT	81	95	16.2	0.20	NA
Esmaili et al[31]	NT	100	100	NT	NT	8

Comments: The higher numbers in the O'Shea et al.[97] article may be due to limited sample size (only 4 of 156 patients with a torn PCL) and patient population (male military personnel). The composite physical examination for a torn PCL is highly accurate, according to the Jackson et al.[49] meta-analysis, which combined the data from the Simonsen et al.[119] and O'Shea et al.[97] studies. The utility score of 2 reflects the weakness of the O'Shea et al.[97] article and the fact that only 3 articles have studied the composite exam for the PCL.

Posterior Drawer Test (PCL Tear)

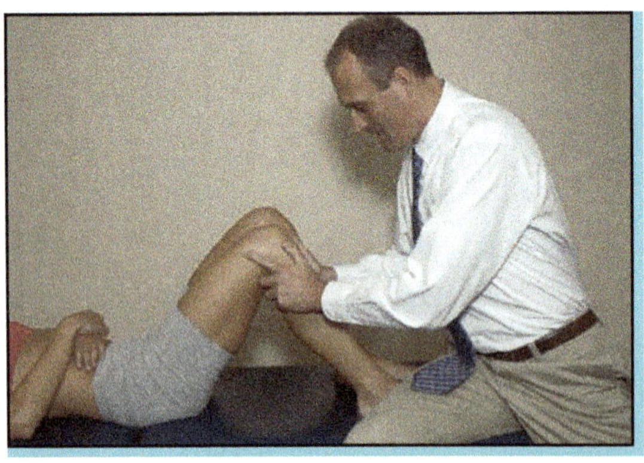

1) The patient is supine with the knee flexed to 90 degrees, the hip flexed at 45 degrees, and a neutral foot angle.

2) The examiner sits on the patient's foot to stabilize the extremity.

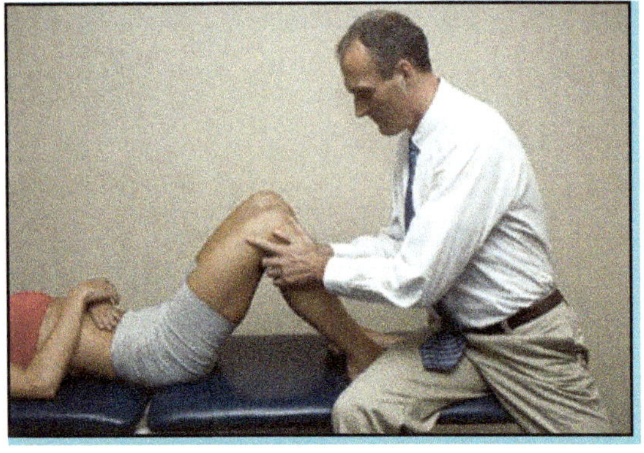

3) The examiner places both hands on the proximal anterior tibia with the thumbs on the medial and lateral joint lines.

4) The proximal tibia is translated in a posterior direction and the amount of motion is estimated. This test is then repeated with the foot internally and then externally rotated and compared to the contralateral side.

5) A positive test for PCL tear is dependent on the amount of posterior motion of the tibia, Grade 1+ (0–5 mm), grade 2+ (6–10 mm), and grade 3+ (11 mm+).

TESTS FOR TORN POSTERIOR CRUCIATE LIGAMENT (PCL) AND POSTERIOR ROTARY INSTABILITY

UTILITY SCORE 2

Study	Reliability	Sensitivity	Specificity	LR+	LR−	QUADAS Score (0–14)
Clendenin et al.[19]	NT	100	NT	NA	NA	9
Harilainen[43]	NT	33	NT	NA	NA	6
Harilainen et al.[44]	NT	25	NT	NA	NA	8
Fowler & Messieh[37]	NT	100	NT	NA	NA	10
Hughston et al.[46]	NT	22	NT	NA	NA	6
Moore & Larson[88]	NT	67	NT	NA	NA	8
Loos et al.[73]	NT	51	NT	NA	NA	6
Rubinstein et al.[106]	NT	90	99	90	0.10	9

Comments: In the higher-quality studies, the Posterior Drawer Test[25] appears to have value as a sensitive test where a negative result would rule out a PCL tear. However, some studies show that detection of the drawer sign can be difficult in the acute injury secondary to muscle guarding. Hughston et al.[46] reports that a PCL injury can occur without stress on the arcuate complex, thus preventing a positive posterior drawer sign in the acute injury. Several of the studies were done retrospectively, were not blinded, and included very small sample sizes (< 10).

Posterior Sag Sign or Godfrey's Test (PCL Tear)

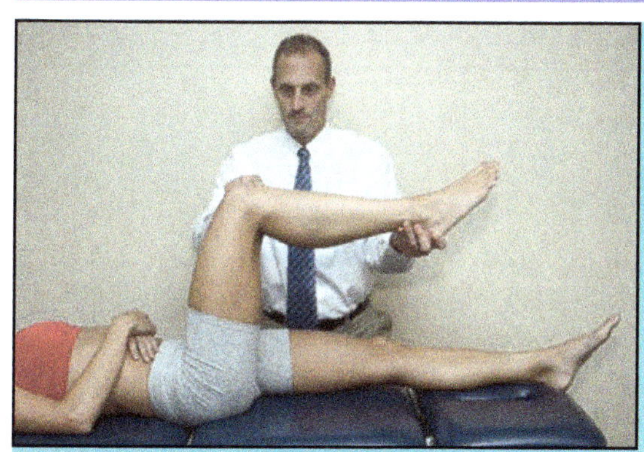

1) The patient is supine with the knee flexed to 90 degrees and the hip placed in 90 degrees of flexion.

2) The examiner supports the leg under the lower calf/heel, suspending the leg in the air.

3) A positive test for a PCL tear is posterior sagging of the tibia secondary to gravitational pull.

UTILITY SCORE 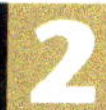

Study	Reliability	Sensitivity	Specificity	LR+	LR−	QUADAS Score (0–14)
Clendenin et al.[19]	NT	90	NT	NA	NA	9
Fowler & Messieh[37]	NT	100	NT	NA	NA	10
Staubli & Jakob[122]	NT	83	NT	NA	NA	10
Loos et al.[73]	NT	46	NT	NA	NA	6
Rubinstein et al.[106]	NT	79	100	NA	NA	9

Comments: The Sag Sign can be dependent upon the examiner's ability to detect a posterior shift of the tibia, which may or may not be obvious and may also be unreliable in the cases of multiple injuries. The Godfrey's Test[25] differs from the Posterior Sag Sign because it includes a further step where the patient is asked to raise the foot and the anterior translation of the proximal tibia indicates a positive result. The Posterior Sag may have some value as a screening test when negative due to its high sensitivity.

TESTS FOR TORN POSTERIOR CRUCIATE LIGAMENT (PCL) AND POSTERIOR ROTARY INSTABILITY

Quadriceps Active Test (PCL Tear)

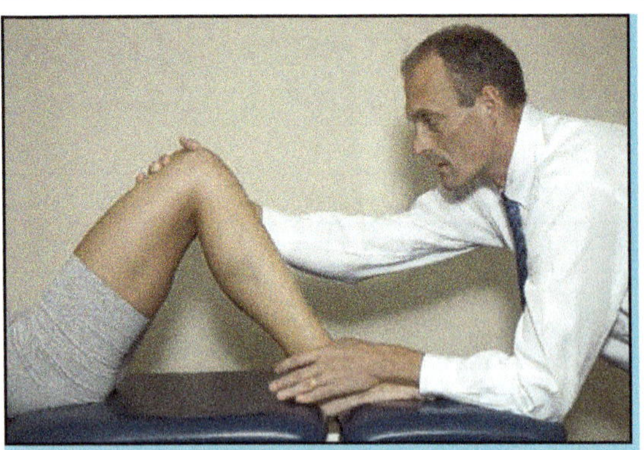

1) The patient is supine with the knee flexed to 90 degrees.

2) Keeping the eyes at the level of the subject's flexed knee, the examiner supports the subject's thigh and confirms the thigh muscles are relaxed while the foot is stabilized by the examiner's other hand.

3) The subject is asked to slide the foot gently down the table.

4) A positive test for PCL tear is anterior tibial displacement resulting from the quadriceps contraction.

UTILITY SCORE 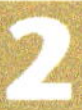

Study	Reliability	Sensitivity	Specificity	LR+	LR−	QUADAS Score (0–14)
Daniel et al.[25]	NT	98	100	NA	NA	8
Staubli & Jakob[122]	NT	75	NT	NA	NA	10
Rubinstein et al.[106]	NT	54	97	18	0.47	9
Comments: This test appears to have some value as a specific test to detect a torn PCL when positive. However, the studies are of a quality that makes any conclusions about diagnostic accuracy tentative.						

Reverse Pivot-Shift Test [PCL Tear, Posterolateral Rotary Instability (PLRI) Tear]

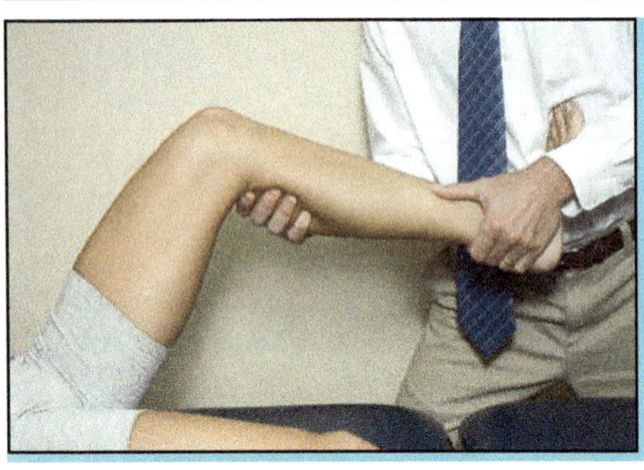

1) The patient lies supine with the knee flexed to 70–80 degrees. External rotation of the foot and leg is applied.

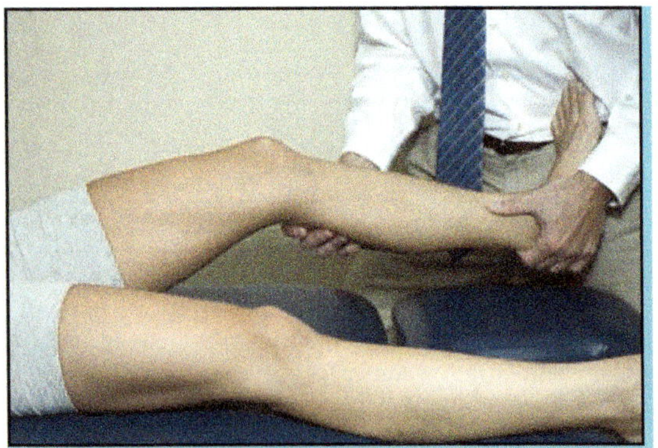

2) The knee is now allowed to straighten using nothing more than the weight of the leg. The examiner leans slightly against the foot, transmitting an axial load through the leg and a valgus stress applied to the knee using the iliac crest as a fulcrum.

3) As the knee approaches 20 degrees of flexion, one can feel and observe the lateral tibial plateau moving anteriorly with a jerk-like shift from a position of posterior subluxation and external rotation into a position of reduction and neutral rotation. This reduction is indicative of a positive test.

TESTS FOR TORN POSTERIOR CRUCIATE LIGAMENT (PCL) AND POSTERIOR ROTARY INSTABILITY

UTILITY SCORE 2

Study	Reliability	Sensitivity	Specificity	LR+	LR−	QUADAS Score (0–14)
Jakob et al.[52]	NT	NT	NT	NA	NA	NA
Fowler & Messieh[37]	NT	23	NT	NA	NA	10
LaPrade & Wentorf[66]	NT	NT	NT	NA	NA	NA
Shelbourne et al.[114]	NT	NT	NT	NA	NA	NA
Rubinstein et al.[106] (Dynamic Posterior Shift)	NT	58	94	9.67	.47	9
Rubinstein et al.[106] (Reverse Pivot-Shift)	NT	26	95	5.2	.78	9

Comments: Fowler and Messieh[37] report the Reverse Pivot-Shift Test as an occasional finding for an isolated tear of the PCL. Shelbourne et al.[114] and Rubinstein et al.[106] describe a modification of the Reverse Pivot-Shift and call the test the Dynamic Posterior Shift Test. Rubinstein et al.[106] differentiate between the Dynamic Posterior Shift and the Reverse Pivot-Shift representing the two sets of data, the first being the Dynamic Posterior Shift and the second the Reverse Pivot-Shift. The main difference between the two tests is that the Dynamic Posterior Shift Test controls rotation of the femur and tightens the hamstrings, providing axial loading across the knee joint. The Dynamic Posterior Shift accentuates the "clunk" as the knee nears extension. The test appears specific for ruling in a torn PCL if the test is positive but the quality of research studies is moderate.

Reverse Lachman's Test or Trillat's Test (PCL Tear)

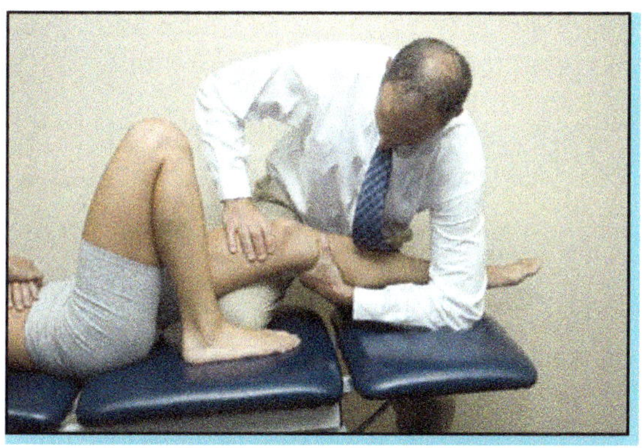

1) The patient is supine with the knee flexed to 20–30 degrees.

2) The examiner stabilizes the distal femur with one hand and grasps behind the proximal tibia with the other hand.

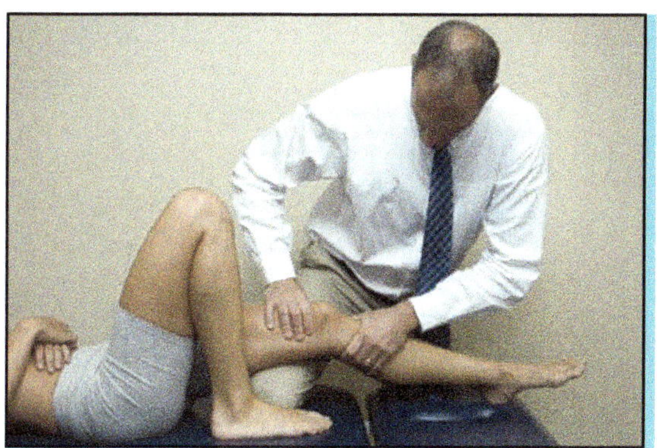

3) The examiner then applies an anterior tibial force followed by a posterior tibial force to the proximal tibia.

4) A positive test for a PCL tear is a soft or absent end point in the posterior direction compared to the contralateral side.

(continued)

TESTS FOR TORN POSTERIOR CRUCIATE LIGAMENT (PCL) AND POSTERIOR ROTARY INSTABILITY

UTILITY SCORE 3

Study	Reliability	Sensitivity	Specificity	LR+	LR−	QUADAS Score (0–14)
Rubinstein et al.[106]	NT	62	89	5.64	0.43	9
Comments: The Reverse Lachman's Test[25] is not a true reverse Lachman and examines both anterior and posterior translation of the tibia. Rubinstein et al.[106] also report sensitivity and specificity values for the Reverse Lachmans End-Point Test, although no description of the test could be found.						

Varus/Valgus Instability at 0 Degrees (PCL Tear)

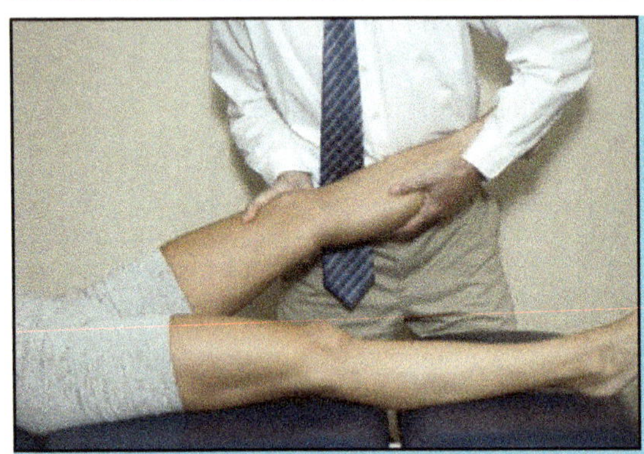

1) The patient is supine with the knee in full extension.

2) The examiner stands lateral to the patient's leg and cradling the lower leg in one hand, places the other hand over the lateral tibiofemoral joint line.

3) The examiner applies a lateral to medial force at the tibiofemoral joint line.

4) The test is repeated from the medial side of the patient's leg, providing a medial to lateral force wherein varus laxity is tested.

5) A positive test for a PCL tear is increased valgus and varus laxity when compared to the unaffected extremity.

UTILITY SCORE 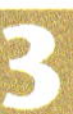

Study	Reliability	Sensitivity	Specificity	LR+	LR−	QUADAS Score (0–14)
Hughston et al.[46]	NT	94	100	NA	NA	6
Loos et al.[73]	NT	59	NT	NA	NA	6
Comments: Typically the valgus/varus instability tests are used to detect tears of the medial and lateral collateral ligaments if performed at 20–30 degrees of knee flexion. However, a conclusion regarding the valgus test performed at 0 degrees detecting an associated rupture of the PCL cannot be made due to the low quality of the studies.						

TESTS FOR TORN POSTERIOR CRUCIATE LIGAMENT (PCL) AND POSTERIOR ROTARY INSTABILITY

External Rotation Recurvatum Test

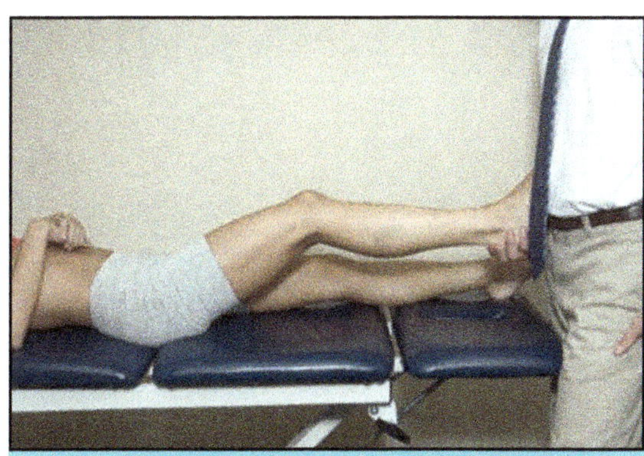

1) The patient lies supine with the examiner holding the heel of the leg in 30 degrees of knee flexion.

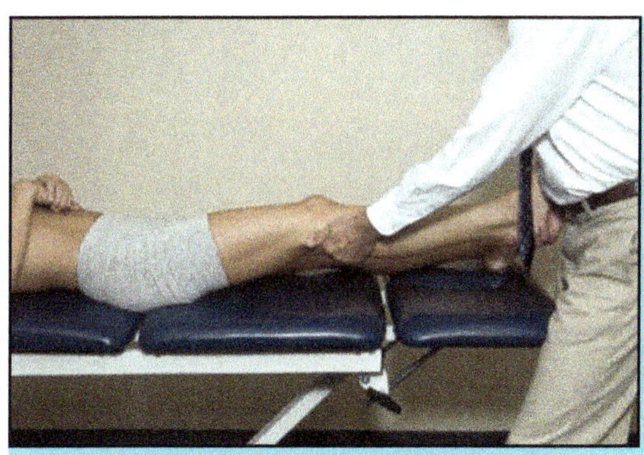

2) The examiner gradually extends the knee from 30 degrees of flexion while the opposite hand gently grasps the posterolateral aspect of the knee joint.

3) A positive test is the relative hyperextension and external rotation felt by the examiner compared to the opposite knee.

UTILITY SCORE 

Study	Reliability	Sensitivity	Specificity	LR+	LR−	QUADAS Score (0–14)
Hughston et al.[46]	NT	39	NT	NA	NA	6
Hughston & Norwood[48]	NT	NT	NT	NA	NA	NA
LaPrade & Wentorf[66]	NT	NT	NT	NA	NA	NA
Loos et al.[73]	NT	22	NT	NA	NA	6
Rubinstein et al.[106]	NT	3	99	3.0	.98	9

Comments: The low utility score reflects the poor quality of the articles. In the Hughston et al.[46] article, the majority of the patients had tears of both the ACL and PCL. The value of a positive test to rule in PLRI needs to be confirmed by more than one study.

TESTS FOR TORN POSTERIOR CRUCIATE LIGAMENT (PCL) AND POSTERIOR ROTARY INSTABILITY

Anterior Abrasion Sign (PCL Tear)

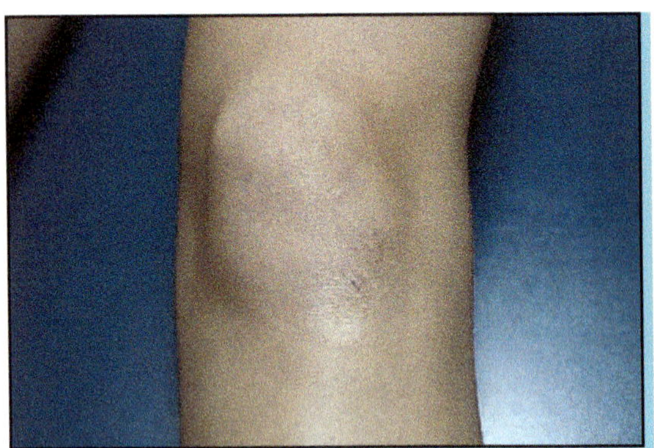

1) A positive test is an abrasion present on the anterior tibia.

UTILITY SCORE 

Study	Reliability	Sensitivity	Specificity	LR+	LR−	QUADAS Score (0–14)
Loos et al.[73]	NT	14	NT	NA	NA	6
Fowler & Messieh[37]	NT	7	NT	NA	NA	10

Comments: Fowler and Messieh[37] report their data as occasional findings for the positive skin abrasion test as they were primarily looking at the posterior drawer and sag sign. This is a poor sign to detect a torn PCL.

Fixed Posterior Subluxation (PCL Tear)

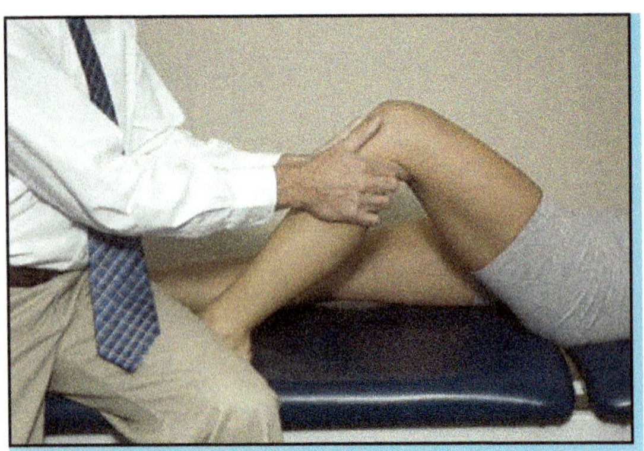

1) The patient lies supine with the knee flexed to 90 degrees.

2) The patient shows obvious posterior sagging.

3) A positive test is the inability to reduce the tibia to a neutral position during anterior tibial translation.

TESTS FOR TORN POSTERIOR CRUCIATE LIGAMENT (PCL) AND POSTERIOR ROTARY INSTABILITY

UTILITY SCORE 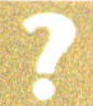

Study	Reliability	Sensitivity	Specificity	LR+	LR−	QUADAS Score (0–14)
Strobel et al.[127]	NT	NT	NT	NA	NA	NA
Comments: The one study to examine the Fixed Posterior Subluxation[127] sign did not report reliability or diagnostic accuracy.						

Proximal Tibial Percussion Test (PCL Tear)

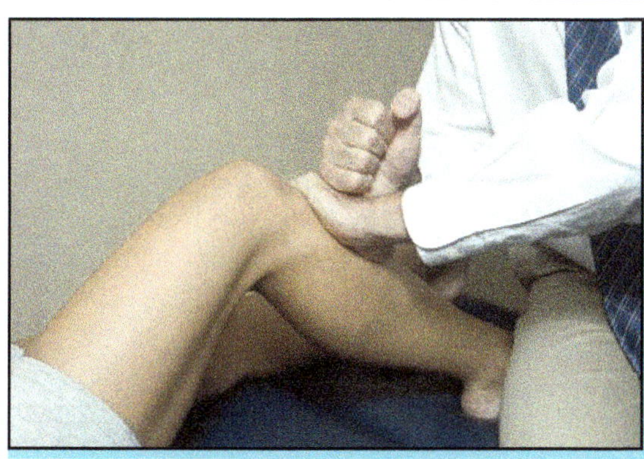

1) The patient lies supine with the hip flexed to 45 degrees and the knee in 90 degrees flexion and the examiner sitting on the patient's foot to stabilize it.

2) One of the examiner's hands is placed over the anterior-proximal tibia at the level of the tibial tubercle.

3) While the patient is relaxed, the examiner's other hand provides a blunt force to the back of the pre-positioned hand.

4) A positive test is significant posterior joint pain similar to that of original injury.

UTILITY SCORE 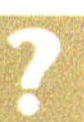

Study	Reliability	Sensitivity	Specificity	LR+	LR−	QUADAS Score (0–14)
Feltham & Albright[33]	NT	NT	NT	NA	NA	NA
Comments: The one study to examine the Proximal Tibial Percussion Test[33] did not report reliability or diagnostic accuracy. Due to the significant pain generated during this test, and the lack of evidence behind it, a clinician should question whether this test has any value.						

TESTS FOR TORN POSTERIOR CRUCIATE LIGAMENT (PCL) AND POSTERIOR ROTARY INSTABILITY

Posterior Functional Drawer Test (PCL Tear)

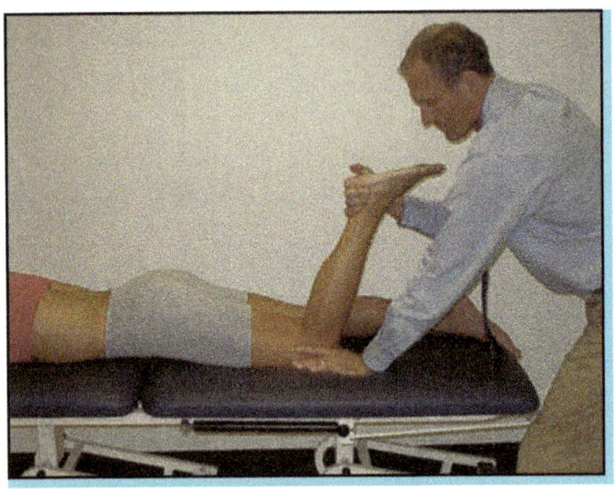

Prone

1) The patient lies prone with the knee flexed to 90 degrees, hip at 0 degrees flexion at the edge of the examining table.

2) The examiner maximally resists knee flexion and compares posterior pain and strength to the contralateral side.

3) Resistance is repeated at 20–30 degrees of knee flexion and compared to contralateral side.

4) A positive test is posterior pain and significant hamstring weakness at 90 degrees that is eliminated or reduced at 20–30 degrees when compared to the contralateral side.

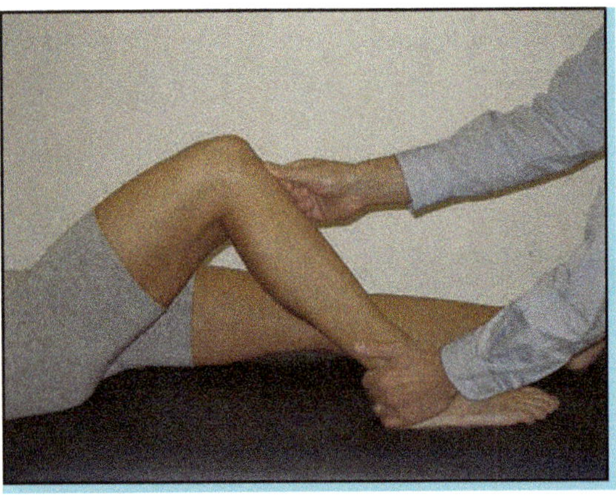

Supine

1) The patient is placed at 45 degrees hip flexion and 90 degrees knee flexion.

2) The examiner uses one hand to resist knee flexion at the heel and the other to palpate the anterior tibial plateau.

3) The examiner compares the strength of the hamstrings and patient report of posterior pain to the contralateral side.

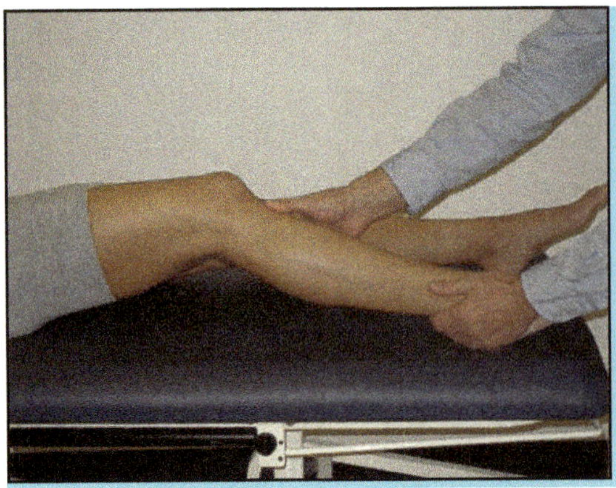

4) The test is repeated with the knee in 20–30 degrees flexion.

5) The examiner compares the strength of the hamstrings and patient report of posterior pain to the contralateral side and to exam finding at 90 degrees knee flexion.

TESTS FOR TORN POSTERIOR CRUCIATE LIGAMENT (PCL) AND POSTERIOR ROTARY INSTABILITY

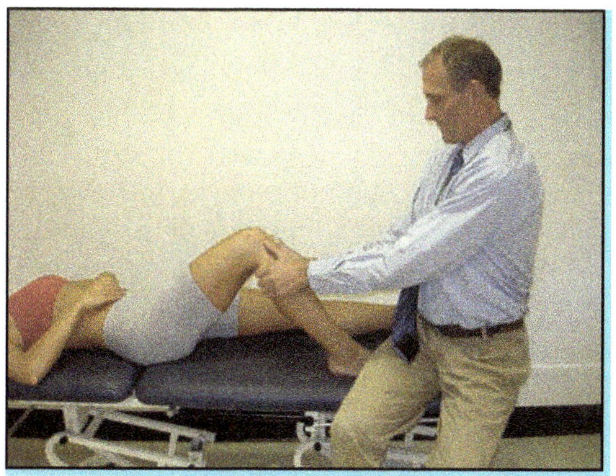

6) The examiner then applies an anterior drawer to the proximal tibia at 90 degrees knee flexion and the test is repeated.

7) A positive test is if an anterior drawer significantly reduced the pain and weakness is found in the first part of the exam.

UTILITY SCORE 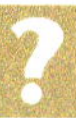

Study	Reliability	Sensitivity	Specificity	LR+	LR−	QUADAS Score (0–14)
Feltham & Albright[33]	NT	NT	NT	NA	NA	NA

Comments: The one study to examine the Posterior Functional Drawer test[33] did not report reliability or diagnostic accuracy. This test can reportedly be used in cases with partial tears or isolated PCL tears with minimal laxity for acute injuries. Post-rehabilitation, a positive test was associated with failure to return to high-level sports.

Modified Posterolateral Drawer Test or Loomer's Test (PCL Tear/PLRI)

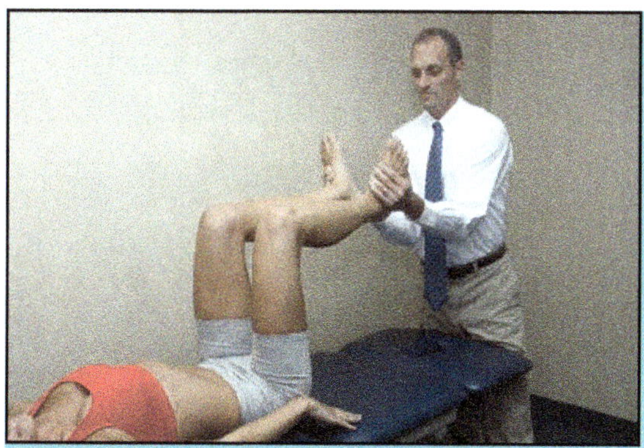

1) The patient lies supine with the hips and knees flexed to 90 degrees.

2) The examiner grasps the patient's feet and maximally externally rotates both feet.

3) A positive test has three interpretations:
   - Posterior sag of the tibia in neutral + no excessive rotation = isolated PCL tear
   - No posterior sag in neutral but excessive external rotation and posterior sag at the end of rotation = isolated PLRI
   - Posterior sag in neutral + excessive external rotation = PLRI and PCL tear.

UTILITY SCORE 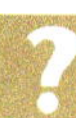

Study	Reliability	Sensitivity	Specificity	LR+	LR−	QUADAS Score (0–14)
Loomer[72]	NT	NT	NT	NA	NA	NA

Comments: The original research of this test[40] was with cadavers. The value of this test in diagnosis of PCL injury or PLRI is unknown.

TESTS FOR TORN POSTERIOR CRUCIATE LIGAMENT (PCL) AND POSTERIOR ROTARY INSTABILITY

Posterolateral Rotation Test or Dial Test (PCL Tear/PLRI)

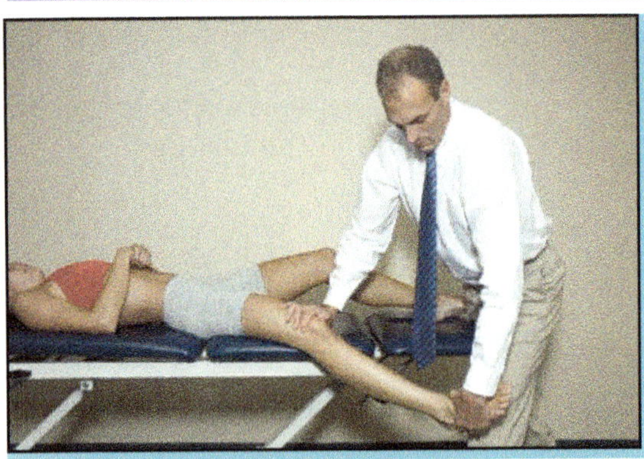

1) The patient lies either prone, where both knees can be tested concurrently, or supine, where each knee is tested separately. If the patient is supine (pictured), then the patient's lower extremity hangs off the side of the plinth.

2) The knee(s) is/are flexed to 30 degrees. An external rotation force is then applied. The amount of external rotation is noted and compared to the other lower leg.

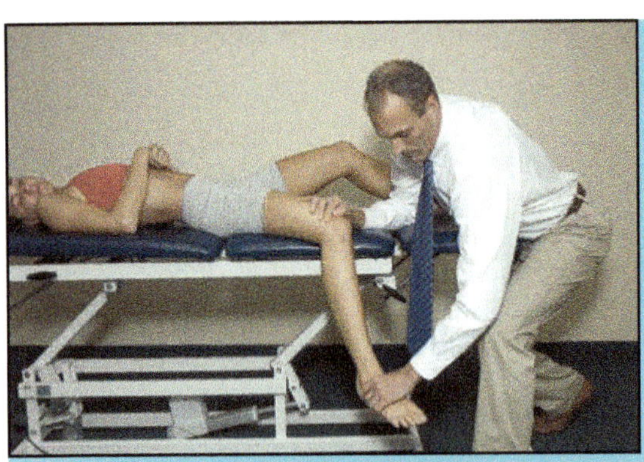

3) The knee(s) is/are now flexed to 90 degrees and, again, an external rotation force is applied. The amount of external rotation is noted and compared to the other lower leg.

4) A positive test has three interpretations:
- More external rotation at 30 degrees than 90 degrees on the same leg = posterolateral corner injury
- More external rotation at 90 degrees than 30 = PCL tear
- Excessive external rotation in both positions when compared to the uninvolved leg = PCL and/or posterolateral corner tear.

UTILITY SCORE 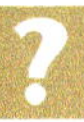

Study	Reliability	Sensitivity	Specificity	LR+	LR−	QUADAS Score (0–14)
LaPrade & Wentorf[66]	NT	NT	NT	NA	NA	NA
Allen et al.[4]	NT	NT	NT	NA	NA	NA
Comments: LaPrade & Wentorf,[66] Allen et al.,[4] and Quarles & Hosey[102] report on modifications of the dial test. No study reports on the diagnostic accuracy or reliability of this test.						

TESTS FOR TORN POSTERIOR CRUCIATE LIGAMENT (PCL) AND POSTERIOR ROTARY INSTABILITY

Posterolateral Drawer Test (PLRI)

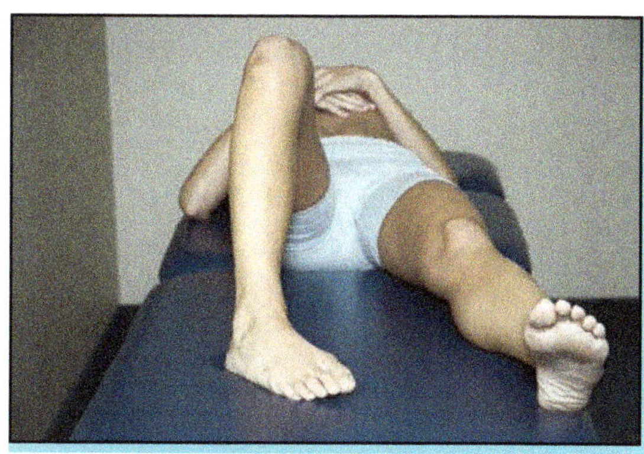

1) The patient lies supine with the hip flexed at 45 degrees and the knee flexed to 90 degrees.

2) The Posterior Drawer Test of the knee is now performed in neutral, external, and internal tibial rotation of 15 degrees.

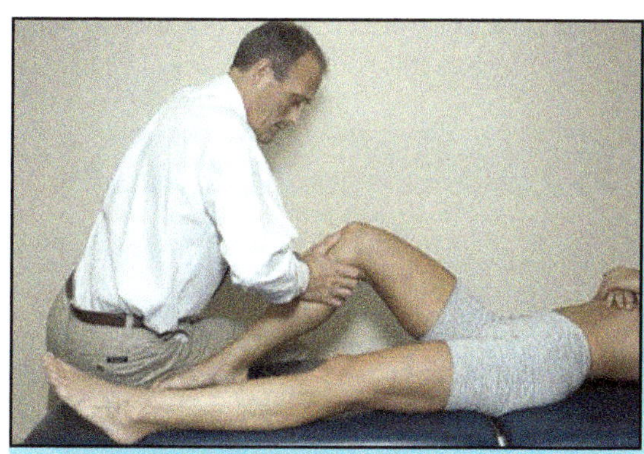

3) A positive test for PLRI is indicated by a relative posterior appearance of the lateral tibial condyle during the push phase of the drawer test when compared with the medial tibial condyle.

UTILITY SCORE 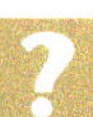

Study	Reliability	Sensitivity	Specificity	LR+	LR−	QUADAS Score (0–14)
Hughston & Norwood[48]	NT	NT	NT	NA	NA	NA

Comments: Hughston & Norwood[48] suggest that internal rotation of the knee tightens the intact fibers of the PCL, which will not allow for anterior-posterior motion on the Posterior Drawer Test. If there is any posterior motion in complete internal rotation, then there must be an injury to the PCL. If the PCL is torn, the tibial rotation of the PLRI will not be present because the PCL pivot for rotation is absent. Shino et al.,[117] LaPrade & Wentorf,[66] and Quarles & Hosey[102] all report modifications of the Posterolateral Drawer Test, and none of themm present any data on the test.

TESTS FOR TORN POSTERIOR CRUCIATE LIGAMENT (PCL) AND POSTERIOR ROTARY INSTABILITY

Standing Apprehension Test (PLRI)

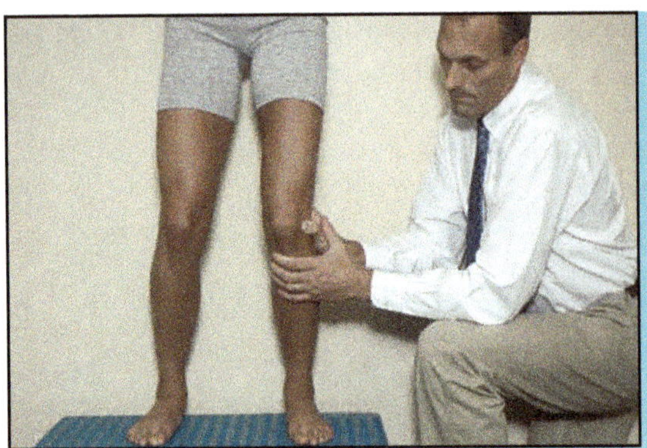

1) With the patient standing and bearing weight on the affected leg, the tip of the examiner's thumb is placed on the anterolateral femoral condyle with the rest of the thumb resting on the anterolateral tibia and joint line.

2) The patient is asked to flex the knee slightly while the examiner pushes the femoral condyle with the thumb. Increased rotation is felt as the tip of the thumb moves with the femur and the proximal portion of the thumb remains in contact with the lateral tibia.

3) A positive test for PLRI is a feeling of "giving way" experienced by the patient and movement of the femoral condyle on the tibial plateau felt by the examiner.

UTILITY SCORE 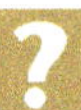

Study	Reliability	Sensitivity	Specificity	LR+	LR−	QUADAS Score (0–14)
Ferrari et al.[34]	NT	NT	NT	NA	NA	NA
Comments: The one article describing the Standing Apprehension Test[34] did not report on any diagnostic accuracy or reliability values.						

TESTS FOR TORN POSTERIOR CRUCIATE LIGAMENT (PCL) AND POSTERIOR ROTARY INSTABILITY

Posterior Medial Displacement of the Medial Tibial Plateau with Valgus Stress [Posteromedial Rotatory Instability (PMRI)]

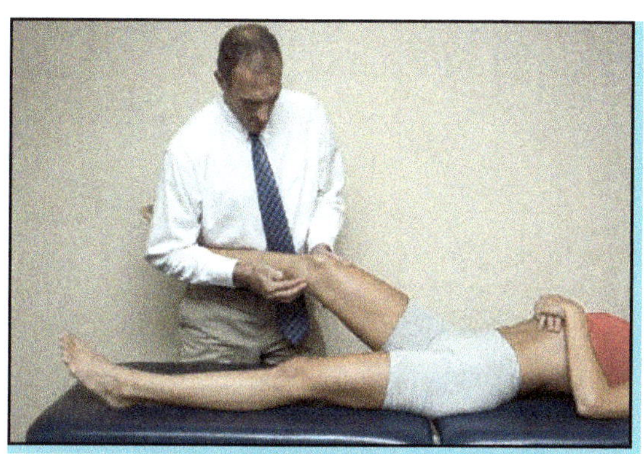

1. The patient lies supine with the knee extended.
2. The examiner produces hyperextension at the knee with a valgus force.
3. A positive test for isolated PMRI is sagging of the medial aspect of the tibia in the posteromedial corner. If the PCL is torn, the entire tibia will displace posteriorly.

UTILITY SCORE 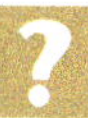

Study	Reliability	Sensitivity	Specificity	LR+	LR−	QUADAS Score (0–14)
Larson[67]	NT	NT	NT	NA	NA	NA
Comments: The one study[67] to examine the Posterior Medial Displacement of Medial Tibial Plateau with Valgus Stress Test did not report reliability or diagnostic accuracy.						

TESTS FOR TORN COLLATERAL LIGAMENT

Composite Physical Exam [Medial Collateral Ligament (MCL) Tear]

UTILITY SCORE 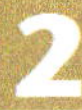

Study	Reliability	Sensitivity	Specificity	LR+	LR−	QUADAS Score (0–14)
Simonsen et al.[119]	NT	88	73	3.3	.16	12
Kastelein et al.[57] 1. History 1 of 2 (Trauma by external force to leg, Rotational trauma) + Laxity with valgus stress at 30 degrees + pain with valgus at 30 degrees	NT	56	91	6.4	0.50	11
2. History 1 of 2 (Trauma by external force to leg, Rotational trauma) + pain with valgus stress at 30 degrees		56	88	4.8	0.50	
Comments: Combining elements of history and clinical exam appears to be specific for a torn medial collateral ligament. More research is still warranted.						

TESTS FOR TORN COLLATERAL LIGAMENT

Valgus Stress Test (MCL Tear)

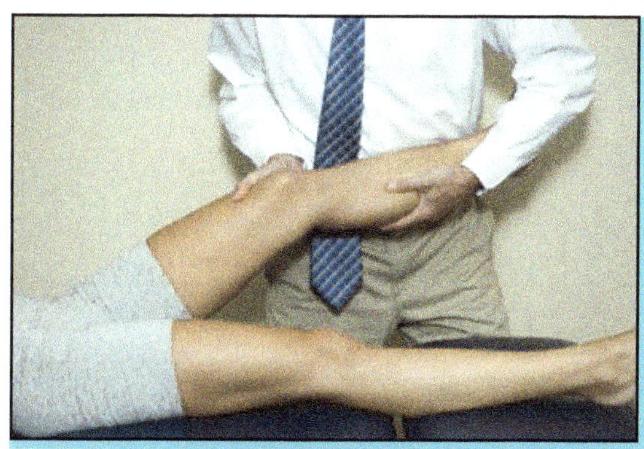

1) The patient is supine with hip slightly abducted and extended so the thigh is resting on the surface of the table.

2) The knee is flexed 30 degrees over the side of the table and the examiner places one hand about the lateral aspect of the knee while the other hand grasps the lower leg.

3) Gently apply a lateral to medial force to the knee, while the hand at the ankle externally rotates the leg slightly.

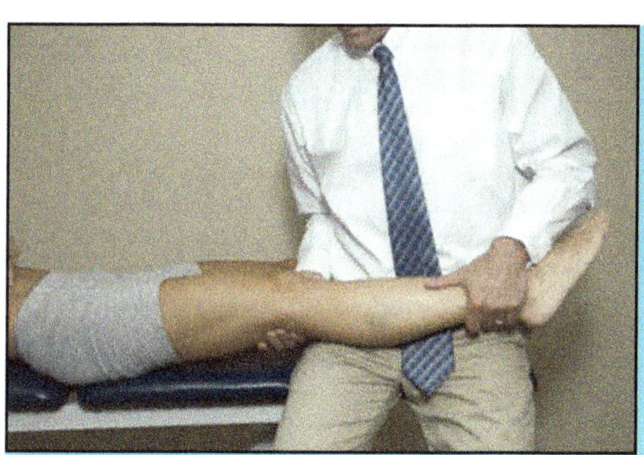

4) Repeat test with knee in full extension.

5) A positive test is excessive medial opening and concordant pain when compared to the uninvolved knee. If the test is positive at 30 degrees, the MCL is implicated. If the test is positive at 0 degrees, then the ACL/PCL and/or the joint capsule is implicated.

UTILITY SCORE 

Study	Reliability	Sensitivity	Specificity	LR+	LR−	QUADAS Score (0–14)
Harilainen[43]	NT	86	NT	NA	NA	6
Harilainen et al.[44]	NT	100	NT	NA	NA	8
McClure et al.[82] (Extension)	κ = .06	NT	NT	NA	NA	NA
(30 degrees Flexion)	κ = .16	NT	NT	NA	NA	NA
Sandberg et al.[110]	NT	80	NT	NA	NA	8
Hughston et al.[46]	NT	94	100	NA	NA	6
Kastelein et al.[57] Pain	NT	78	67	2.3	0.30	11
Laxity		91	49	1.8	0.20	

Comments: In both studies by Harilainen[43] and Harilainen et al.,[44] valgus testing was performed in 20 degrees of knee flexion. Because testing in extension was not done in these studies, a tear of the PCL could not be ruled out. In general, the Valgus Stress Test appears somewhat sensitive in ruling out a tear of the MCL when the test is negative but the quality of research makes this conclusion tenuous. The one high quality study[125] performed seems to show that laxity during valgus stress testing is a sensitive (negative test rules out MCL tear) sign for a torn MCL. More research is needed on the diagnostic accuracy and reliability of clinical tests with regard to the collateral ligaments.

TESTS FOR TORN COLLATERAL LIGAMENT

Composite Physical Exam [Lateral Collateral Ligament (LCL) Tear]

UTILITY SCORE 3

Study	Reliability	Sensitivity	Specificity	LR+	LR−	QUADAS Score (0–14)
Simonsen et al.[119]	NT	100	20	NA	NA	12

Comments: Only one article has examined the composite exam for the LCL and the low utility score reflects the limited sample size of the Simonsen et al.[119] article (only one LCL lesion).

Varus Stress Test (LCL Tear)

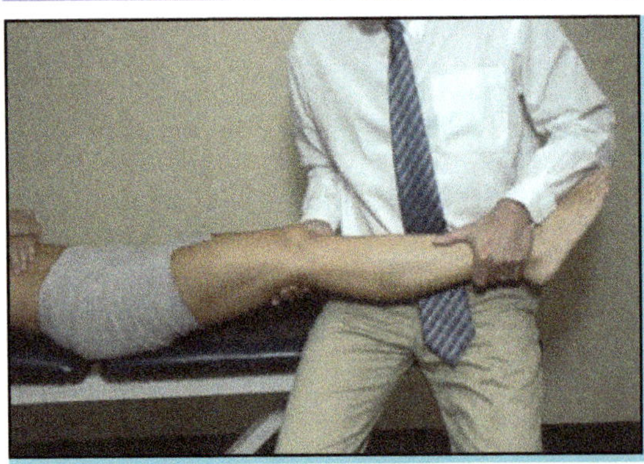

1) The patient is supine with hip slightly abducted and extended so the thigh is resting on the surface of the table.

2) The knee is flexed 30 degrees over the side of the table and the examiner places one hand about the medial aspect of the knee while the other hand grasps the foot/ankle.

3) Gently apply a medial to lateral force to the knee, while the hand at the ankle externally rotates the leg slightly.

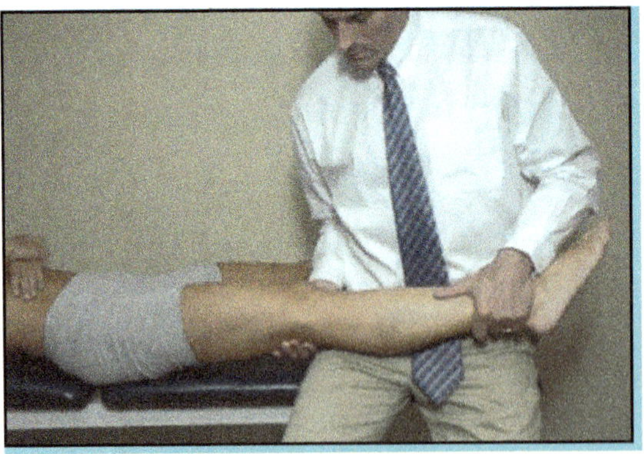

4) Repeat test with knee in full extension.

5) A positive test is excessive medial opening and concordant pain when compared to the uninvolved knee. If the test is positive at 30 degrees, the MCL is implicated. If the test is positive at 0 degrees, then the ACL//PCL and/or the joint capsule is implicated.

UTILITY SCORE 

Study	Reliability	Sensitivity	Specificity	LR+	LR−	QUADAS Score (0–14)
Harilainen[43]	NT	25	NT	NA	NA	6
Harilainen et al.[44]	NT	0	NT	NA	NA	8

Comments: In the Harilainen[43] and Harilainen et al.[44] studies, only four and one patient, respectively, were diagnosed with LCL tears confirmed by arthroscopy. Varus testing was performed in 20 degrees of knee flexion and testing in extension was not done, thus a tear of the PCL could not be ruled out. More research is needed to evaluate the diagnostic accuracy and reliability of the Varus Stress Test.

TESTS FOR PATELLOFEMORAL DYSFUNCTION

Patellar Apprehension Test or Fairbank's Apprehension Test

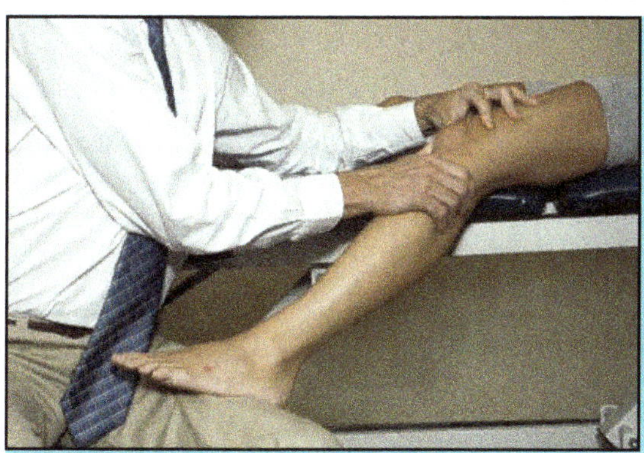

1) The patient is positioned in supine with a relaxed knee passively flexed to 30 degrees over the side of the examining table, foot resting on the examiner.

2) The examiner presses both thumbs on the medial aspect of the patella to exert a lateral force.

3) A positive test occurs when the patient shows signs of apprehension (resists the lateral force and attempts to extend the knee) or pain is reproduced.

UTILITY SCORE 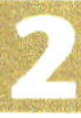

Study	Reliability	Sensitivity	Specificity	LR+	LR−	QUADAS Score (0–14)
Nijs et al.[91]	NT	32	86	2.3	0.79	9
Haim et al.[40]	NT	7	92	0.87	1.0	8
Niskanen et al.[92]	NT	37	70	1.2	0.90	9
Comments: This test, as used for patellar dislocation, appears to be more specific than sensitive, meaning a positive test would help rule in patellofemoral instability.						

TESTS FOR PATELLOFEMORAL DYSFUNCTION

Pain During Functional Activity (Patellofemoral Pain Syndrome)

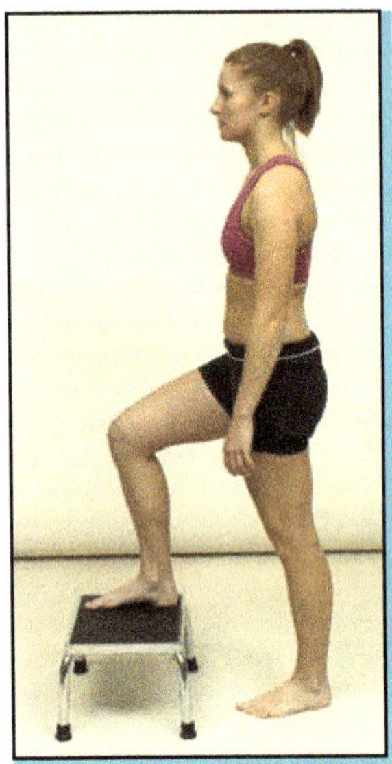

1) The patient is either queried about or asked to perform a component of function.

2) A positive test is indicated by patient report of pain with functional activities or actual reproduction of the patient's pain.

UTILITY SCORE 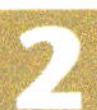

Study	Reliability	Sensitivity	Specificity	LR+	LR−	QUADAS Score (0–14)
Cook et al.[20] (Squatting Stair climbing Kneeling)	NT	91 75 84	50 43 50	1.8 1.3 1.7	0.20 0.60 0.30	10
Naslund et al.[90] (Squatting Stairclimbing)	NT	94 94	46 45	1.74 1.71	0.13 0.13	9
Comments: Studies seem to support pain with squatting, stair climbing, or kneeling as sensitive tests that can rule out patellofemoral dysfunction when negative.						

TESTS FOR PATELLOFEMORAL DYSFUNCTION

Resisted Knee Extension (Patellofemoral Pain Syndrome)

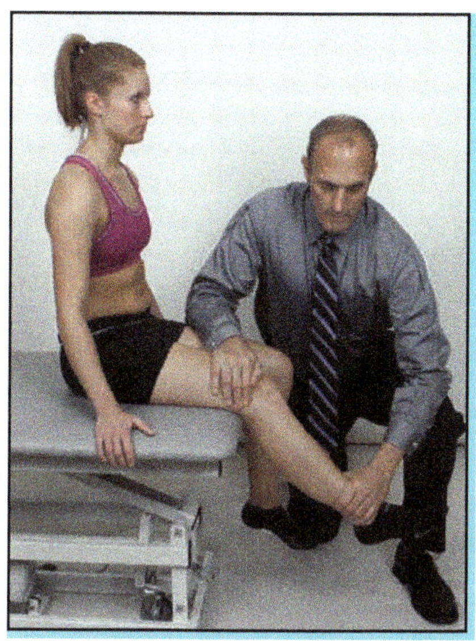

1) The patient is placed in the seated position with feet off the ground and the knees flexed.

2) The examiner resists knee extension.

3) A positive test is indicated by reproduction of the patient's pain.

UTILITY SCORE 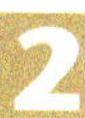

Study	Reliability	Sensitivity	Specificity	LR+	LR−	QUADAS Score (0–14)
Cook et al.[20]	NT	39	82	2.2	0.75	10
Elton et al.[29]	NT	21	95	4.2	0.83	9
Comments: Literature seems to support resisted knee extension as a specific sign to rule in patellofemoral dysfunction when positive.						

TESTS FOR PATELLOFEMORAL DYSFUNCTION

Waldron Test (Patellofemoral Joint Pathology)

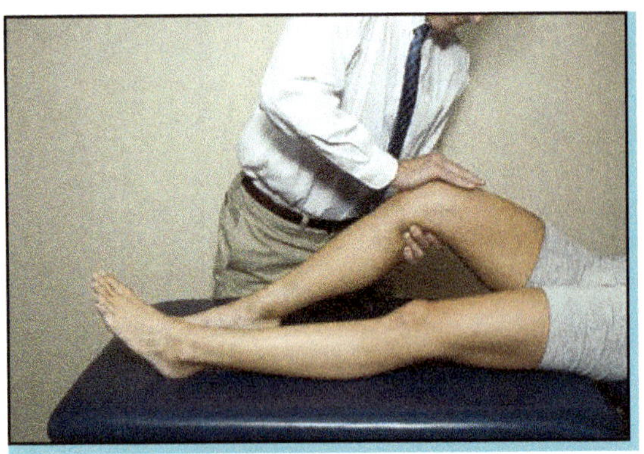

Phase I

1) The patient is positioned in supine with the knees extended.

2) The examiner presses the patella against the femur while performing passive knee flexion with the other hand.

3) A positive test is crepitus and pain reproduction during part of the range of motion.

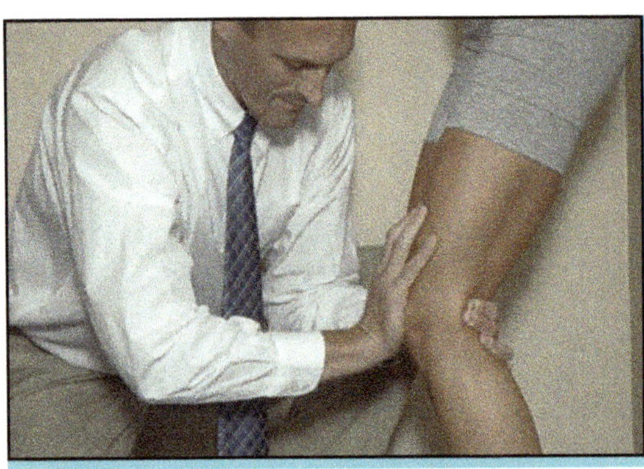

Phase II

1) The patient is positioned in standing.

2) The examiner places his hand on the patella and applies gentle compression of the patella against the femur as the patient performs a slow, full squat.

3) A positive test is crepitus and pain reproduction during the test.

UTILITY SCORE 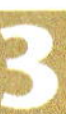

Study	Reliability	Sensitivity	Specificity	LR+	LR−	DOR	QUADAS Score (0–14)
Nijs et al.[91]—Phase I	NT	45	68	1.41	0.81	1.7	9
Nijs et al.[91]—Phase II	NT	18	83	1.05	0.99	1.1	9
Comments: Nijs et al.[91] reported unimpressive positive and negative likelihood ratios for both Phase I and II.							

TESTS FOR PATELLOFEMORAL DYSFUNCTION

Passive Patellar Tilt Test (Patellofemoral Joint Instability)

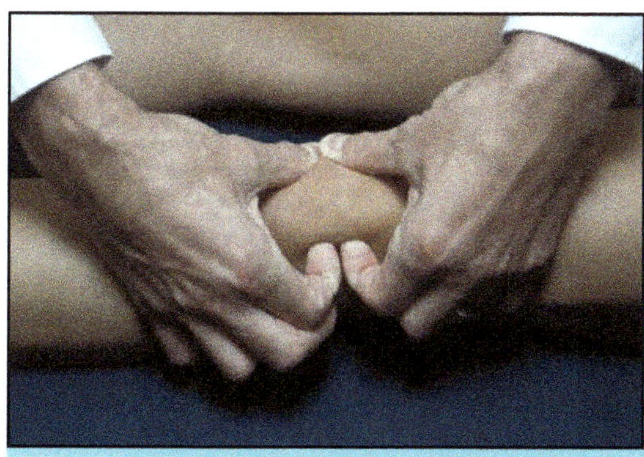

1) The patient is positioned in supine with knees extended and quadriceps relaxed.

2) The examiner stabilizes the extremity at the ankle in neutral rotation.

3) The examiner lifts the lateral edge of the patella from the lateral femoral condyle using the thumb and index finger on both hands.

4) A positive test occurs if the patella moves out of the trochlear groove and laterally subluxes.

UTILITY SCORE 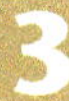 3

Study	Reliability	Sensitivity	Specificity	LR+	LR−	DOR	QUADAS Score (0–14)
Watson et al.[136]	κ = 0.2–0.35*	NT	NT	NA	NA	NA	NA
Nissen et al.[93]	NT	NT	NT	NA	NA	NA	NA
Haim et al.[40]	NT	43	92	5.4	0.62	8.7	8
Watson et al.[137]	κ = 0.19**	NT	NT	NA	NA	NA	NA

Comments: The Watson et al.[136] article categorized subjects' patellae as having positive, negative, or neutral angle with respect to the horizon. Nissen et al.[93] described the Patellar Tilt Test as elevating the lateral patellar border while depressing the medial patellar border. Haim et al.[40] reported data on military recruits in which the examiner who conducted both clinical and radiological evaluations was not masked to the group's assignments.
*Three senior physical therapy students were included in the interobserver agreement. Intraobserver agreement varied from 0.44–0.50 for this test.
**Watson et al.[137] reports on two senior physical therapy students who performed medial/lateral patellar tilts in coordinates with McConnell's Test. Intraobserver agreement varied between 0.28 and 0.33.

TESTS FOR PATELLOFEMORAL DYSFUNCTION

Clarke's Sign/Patellar Grind/Patellar Tracking with Compression (Patellofemoral Joint Pathology)

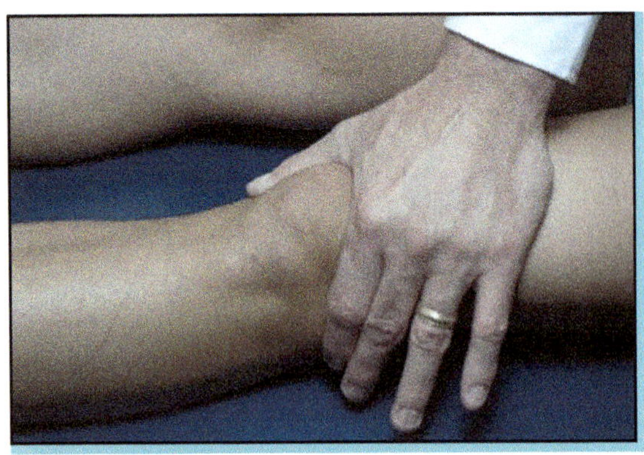

1) The patient is positioned in supine with both knees supported by a knee pad or bolster.

2) The examiner places a hand on the superior border of the patella and presses the patella distally while the patient is relaxed.

3) The patient is then asked to contract the quadriceps.

4) A positive test is pain and reproduction of symptoms.

UTILITY SCORE 

Study	Reliability	Sensitivity	Specificity	LR+	LR−	QUADAS Score (0–14)
Nijs et al.[91]	NT	49	75	1.94	0.69	9
Niskanen et al.[92]	NT	29	67	0.88	1.06	9
Solomon et al.[121]	NT	NT	NT	NA	NA	NA
Malanga et al.[78]	NT	NT	NT	NA	NA	NA
Doberstein et al.[27]	NT	39	67	1.2	0.90	7
Elton et al.[29]	NT	37	95	7.4	0.66	9

Comments: Nijs et al.[91] do not clearly describe the angle of knee flexion for this test. Niskanen et al.[92] described a variation of Clarke's[91] Sign, which was called the Patellar Inhibition Test. Variations of this test have also been described by Solomon et al.[121] and Malanga et al.[78] This test does not appear to be useful in diagnosing patellofemoral joint pathology but the quality of the studies is generally low.

Lateral Pull Test (Patellofemoral Tracking/Instability)

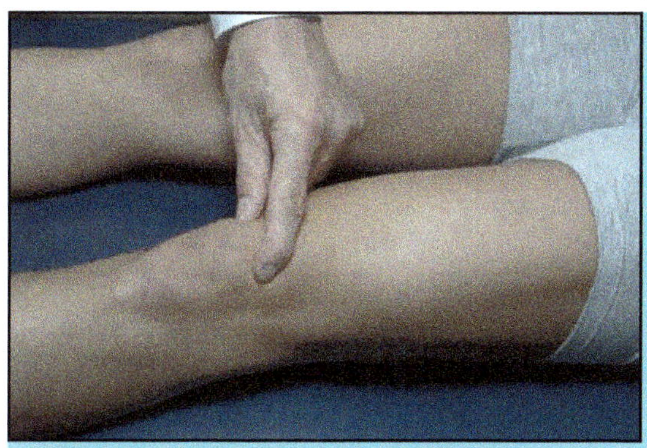

1) The patient is positioned in supine with knees extended and quadriceps relaxed.

2) The examiner stabilizes the extremity in neutral rotation at the ankle.

3) The patient was instructed to perform an isometric quadriceps femoris contraction, while the examiner observed the tracking of the patella with and without light palpation at the superior patellar pole.

4) A positive test was given when the patella tracked more laterally than superiorly.

UTILITY SCORE 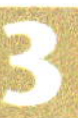

Study	Reliability	Sensitivity	Specificity	LR+	LR−	QUADAS Score (0–14)
Watson et al.[136]	κ = 0.31*	NT	NT	NA	NA	NA
Haim et al.[40]	NT	25	100	NA	NA	8

Comments: Watson et al.[136] described a negative finding as superior or equidistant superior and lateral patellar tracking. The Lateral Pull Test conducted by Haim et al.[40] was labeled the active instability test and placed the patients supine with the knee flexed to 15 degrees prior to observing the tracking of the patella with an isometric quadriceps contraction. Haim et al.[40] described a positive test if the patella moved more than 3 mm laterally.
*Two senior physical therapy students were included in the calculation of interobserver agreement. Intraobserver agreement varied from 0.39–0.47.

TESTS FOR PATELLOFEMORAL DYSFUNCTION

Patella Alta Test

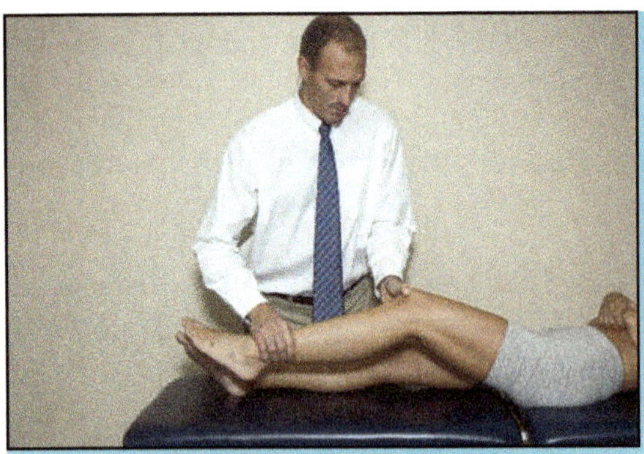

1) The patient is positioned in supine with the knee fully extended.

2) The examiner applies pressure over the lower pole of the patella of the extended knee and then flexes.

3) A positive test for patella alta is indicated when pain occurs during flexion.

UTILITY SCORE 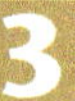

Study	Reliability	Sensitivity	Specificity	LR+	LR−	QUADAS Score (0–14)
Haim et al.[40]	NT	49	72	1.75	0.71	8
Comments: Ironically, the likelihood ratios indicate that the Patella Alta Test[40] does not improve the posttest probability of detecting patella alta.						

Vastus Medialis Coordination Test (Patellofemoral Tracking)

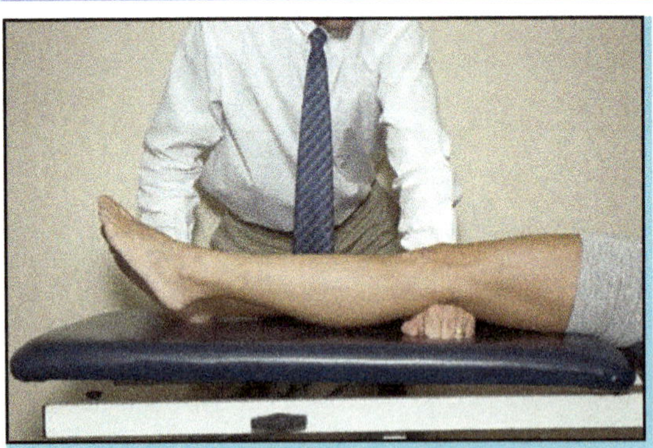

1) The patient is positioned in supine with the knee extended.

2) The examiner places his or her fist under the subject's knee and asks the patient to slowly extend the knee to full extension without pressing down or lifting away from the examiner's fist.

3) A positive test occurs when the patient has difficulty extending, does not extend the knee smoothly, or substitutes hip flexors to reach terminal extension.

UTILITY SCORE 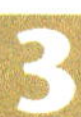

Study	Reliability	Sensitivity	Specificity	LR+	LR−	QUADAS Score (0–14)
Nijs et al.[91]	ND	17	93	2.26	0.90	9
Comments: Although this test has a high reported specificity, which would make a positive finding valuable in ruling in vastus medialis incoordination, one study does not a physical exam test make.						

Eccentric Step Test (Patellofemoral Joint Dysfunction)

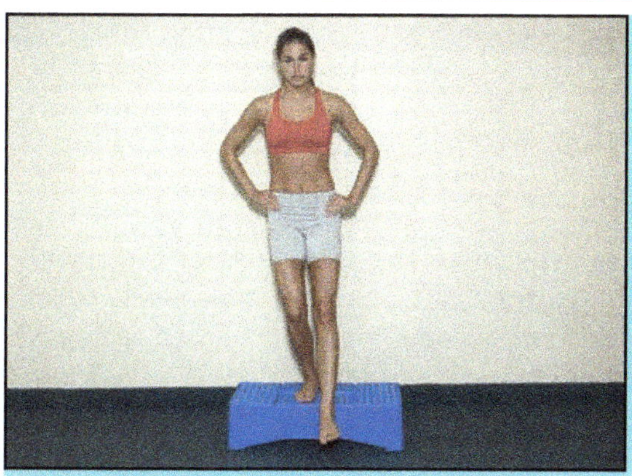

1) The patient is positioned in standing with bare feet and knees exposed, hands on hips, and up on an elevated platform.

2) The examiner gives a standard demonstration of the test and verbal instructions.*

3) The patient then preforms the test with one leg, and then repeats it on the other leg (no warmup or practice trials are allowed).

4) A positive test occurs when the patient reports knee pain during the test.

UTILITY SCORE 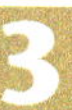

Study	Reliability	Sensitivity	Specificity	LR+	LR−	QUADAS Score (0–14)
Nijs et al.[91]	NT	42	82	2.34	0.71	9
Loudon et al.[76]	ICC = 0.94**	NT	NT	NA	NA	NA

Comments: *The verbal instructions given to the patient included: "Stand on the step, put your hands on your hips, and step down from the step as slowly and as smoothly as you can." (Nijs et al.[91]).
**Loudon et al.[76] reported intratester reliability. Selfe et al.[113] described a similar test utilizing a video analysis to determine the critical knee angle and angular velocity.

McConnell Test for Patellar Orientation (Patellofemoral Joint)

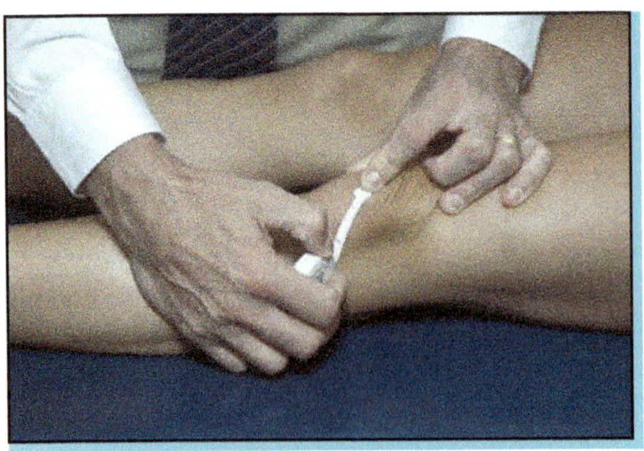

Medial/Lateral Glide

1) The patient is supine with knees extended and quadriceps relaxed.

2) The examiner determines the mid-point of the patella and then measures the distance from mid-patella to lateral femoral epicondyle and mid-patella to medial femoral epicondyle using a tape measure.

3) A positive test (score of 1) is given when distance from mid-patella to medial femoral epicondyle is > 0.5 cm from lateral measurement. A score of 0 is equal medial and lateral distances.

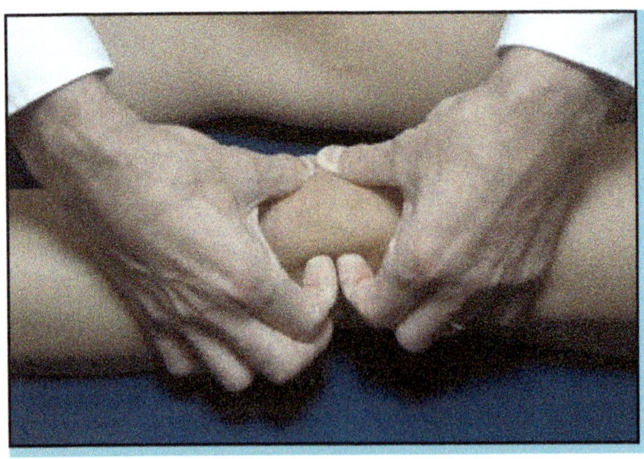

Medial/Lateral Tilt

1) The patient is supine with knees extended and quadriceps relaxed.

2) The examiner attempts to palpate the underside of the patellar borders.

3) A score of 0 is recorded when both the medial and lateral borders can be palpated. A score of 1 is given when > 50% of lateral border, but not the posterior surface, can be palpated. A score of 2 is given when < 50% of lateral border can be palpated.

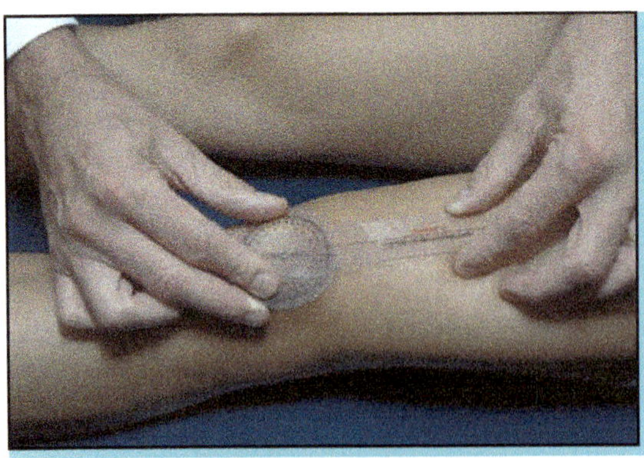

Patellar Rotation

1) The patient is supine with knees extended and quadriceps relaxed.

2) The examiner marks the superior and inferior aspects of the patella and draws a line between the two points and marks the medial and lateral aspects of the patella and creates a line. The long axis of the femur is also visualized and marked. A goniometer is used to evaluate the relationship of the two lines.

3) A score of 0 is given if two lines are parallel. A score of 1 is given if the inferior pole is lateral to femoral axis (obtuse angle of med/lat to femur). A score of – 1 is given if inferior pole is medial to femoral axis (acute angle of med/lat to femur).

TESTS FOR PATELLOFEMORAL DYSFUNCTION

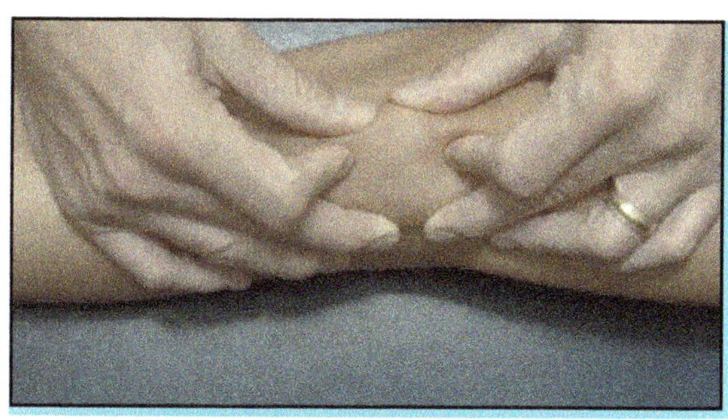

Anterior/Posterior Tilt

1. The patient is supine with knees extended and quadriceps relaxed.

2. The examiner palpates the inferior, superior, medial, and lateral aspects of the patella.

3. A score of 0 is given when distal 1/3 of patella is as easily palpated as proximal 1/3. A score of 1 is given when distal 1/3 is not as clearly palpable as proximal 1/3. A score of 2 is given when the distal 1/3 of the patella and inferior pole are not clearly palpable compared to proximal 1/3.

UTILITY SCORE 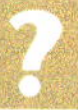

Study	Reliability	Sensitivity	Specificity	LR+	LR−	QUADAS Score (0–14)
Watson et al.[137] (M/L Glide)	κ = 0.02*	NT	NT	NA	NA	NA
Tomsich et al.[129] (M/L Glide)	κ = 0.03**	NT	NT	NA	NA	NA
Watson et al.[137] (M/L Tilt)	κ = 0.19*	NT	NT	NA	NA	NA
Tomsich et al.[129] (M/L Tilt)	κ = 0.18**	NT	NT	NA	NA	NA
Watson et al.[137] (Rotation)	κ = – 0.03*	NT	NT	NA	NA	NA
Tomsich et al.[129] (Rotation)	κ = – 0.03**	NT	NT	NA	NA	NA
Watson et al.[137] (A/P Tilt)	κ = 0.04*	NT	NT	NA	NA	NA
Tomsich et al.[129] (S/I Tilt)	κ = 0.30**	NT	NT	NA	NA	NA

Comments: *Watson et al.[137] reported interobserver agreement of two senior physical therapy students. The interobserver agreement ranged from 0.11–0.35 for med/lat glide, 0.28–0.33 for med/lat tilt, – 0.06–0.00 for rotation, and 0.03–0.23 for ant/post tilt. McConnell[83] also reported on a test for chondromalacia patellae involving quadriceps contraction at varying degrees of knee flexion and medial patellar glides, but there has been no research regarding that tests's diagnostic accuracy either.
**Tomsich et al.[129] described slight variations in testing protocols and names for the McConnell measurements. Additionally, they reported interobserver agreement for three physical therapists and intraobserver agreement of medio/lateral glide (k = 0.40), medio/lateral tilt (k = 0.57), rotation (k = 0.41), and superior/inferior tilt (k = 0.50).

TESTS FOR PATELLOFEMORAL DYSFUNCTION

Zohler's Sign (Patellofemoral Joint Dysfunction)

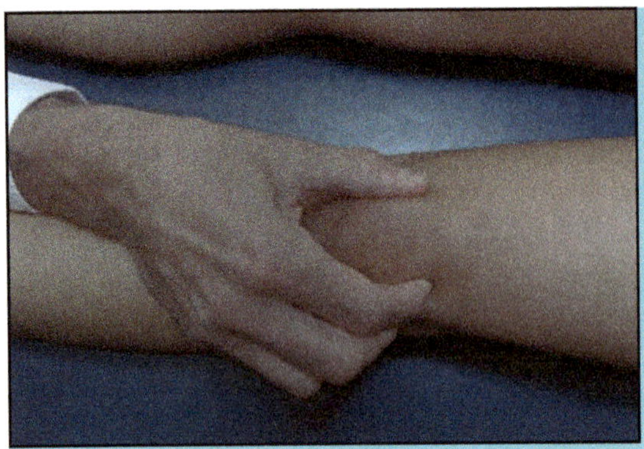

1) The patient lies supine with the knees extended.
2) The examiner pulls the patella distally and holds it in this position.
3) The patient is asked to contract the quadriceps.
4) A positive sign is pain.

UTILITY SCORE

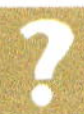

Study	Reliability	Sensitivity	Specificity	LR+	LR−	QUADAS Score (0–14)
Strobel & Stedtfeld[126]	NT	NT	NT	NA	NA	NA
Comments: The one study to examine Zohler's Sign[126] did not report reliability or diagnostic accuracy.						

Tubercle Sulcus Test (Patellofemoral Joint Alignment)

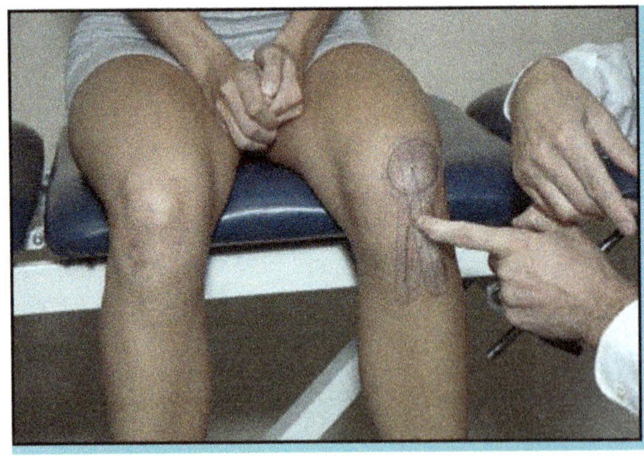

1) The patient is positioned in sitting with the knee flexed to 90 degrees and foot positioned in zero degrees of rotation.
2) The examiner draws a line from the center of the tibial tubercle to the inferior patellar pole. Another line is drawn from the femoral sulcus down the tibia perpendicular to the floor.
3) A positive test is an angle greater than 8 degrees.

UTILITY SCORE

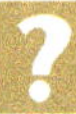

Study	Reliability	Sensitivity	Specificity	LR+	LR−	QUADAS Score (0–14)
Nissen et al.[93]	NT	NT	NT	NA	NA	NA
Comments: The study[93] that reported on this test did not report reliability or diagnostic accuracy.						

TESTS FOR PATELLOFEMORAL DYSFUNCTION

Q-Angle (Patellofemoral Joint Alignment)

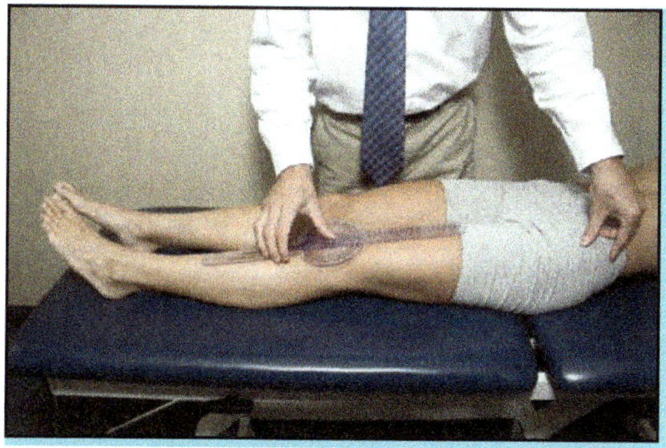

1) The patient is positioned in supine with the knee in full extension.

2) The examiner draws a line between the anterior superior iliac spine of the pelvis to the middle of the patella. Another line is drawn from the middle of the patella to the middle of the tibial tubercle.

3) A positive test is an angular value of greater than 10 degrees for males and greater than 15 degrees for females.

UTILITY SCORE 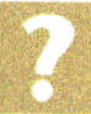

Study	Reliability	Sensitivity	Specificity	LR+	LR−	QUADAS Score (0–14)
Nissen et al.[93]	NT	NT	NT	NA	NA	NA
Haim et al.[40]	NT	NT	NT	NA	NA	NA
Greene et al.[39]	ICC = .17–.29*	NT	NT	NA	NA	NA
**Tomsich et al.[129]	ICC = .23	NT	NT	NA	NA	NA
Naslund et al.[90]	NT	76	63	2.05	0.38	9

Comments: Evidence from one study[90] of moderate quality fails to support the use of the Q-Angle to diagnose PFPS. Nissen et al.[93] recommended the test be repeated in supine and in standing with 20 degrees of knee flexion and maximal internal, neutral, and external rotation. Haim et al.[40] described this test being performed at 90 degrees of knee flexion.
*Greene et al.[39] reported the interobserver measurements for three testers.
**Tomsich et al.[129] reported intertester measurements for three physical therapists and ICC values for intratester measurements of 0.63.

TESTS FOR PATELLOFEMORAL DYSFUNCTION

Lateral Patellar Glide (Patellofemoral Joint Instability)

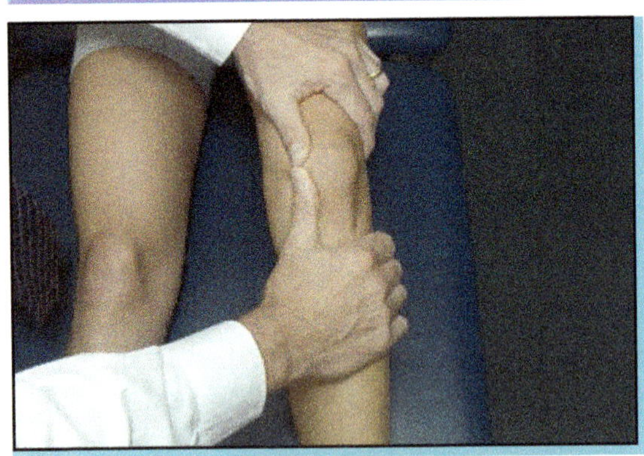

1. The patient is positioned in supine with the knee in full extension.
2. The examiner's thumbs are placed on the medial aspect of the patella, providing a lateral force on the patella.
3. The test is repeated at 20 and 45 degrees of knee flexion.
4. A positive test occurs when the patella laterally glides greater than one-half of the width of the patella.

UTILITY SCORE 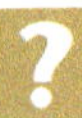

Study	Reliability	Sensitivity	Specificity	LR+	LR−	QUADAS Score (0–14)
Nissen et al.[93]	NT	NT	NT	NA	NA	NA
Haim et al.[40]	NT	NT	NT	NA	NA	NA
Watson et al.[137]	κ = 0.02*	NT	NT	NA	NA	NA
Comments: Nissen et al.[93] describe the positive test as indicative of laxity in the medial restraints. *Watson et al.[137] report on two senior physical therapy students. No information on the diagnostic accuracy of this test is available.						

TESTS FOR PATELLOFEMORAL DYSFUNCTION

Medial Patellar Glide (Patellofemoral Joint Instability)

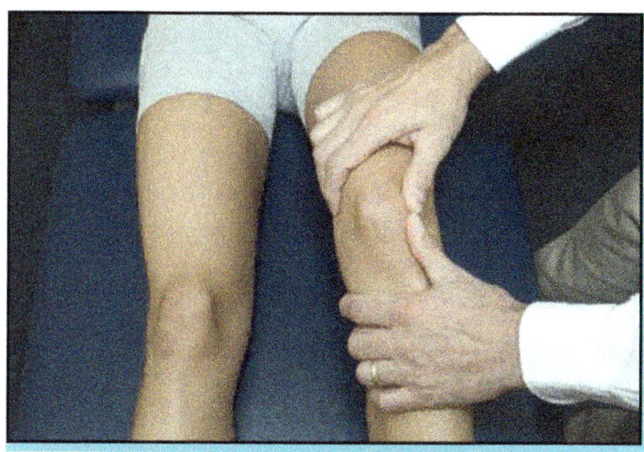

1. The patient is positioned in supine with the knee in full extension.
2. The examiner's thumbs are placed on the lateral aspect of the patella, providing a medial force on the patella.
3. The test is repeated at 20 and 45 degrees of knee flexion.
4. A positive test occurs when the patella medially glides greater than 30–40% of the width of the patella or greater than 10 mm.

UTILITY SCORE

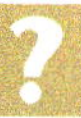

Study	Reliability	Sensitivity	Specificity	LR+	LR−	QUADAS Score (0–14)
Nissen et al.[93]	NT	NT	NT	NA	NA	NA
Haim et al.[40]	NT	NT	NT	NA	NA	NA
Watson et al.[137]	$\kappa = 0.02$*	NT	NT	NA	NA	NA

Comments: In this study, Nissen et al.[93] report that the Medial Glide Test is measured in either percentages or millimeters, where 30–40% of the width of the patella or 6–10 mm of medial glide is considered normal. A glide of less than 6 mm indicates a tight lateral retinaculum and a medial glide greater than 10 mm most commonly indicated a hypermobile patella.
*Watson et al.[137] report on two senior physical therapy students who performed medial/lateral glides.

TESTS FOR PATELLOFEMORAL DYSFUNCTION

Patella Mobility Testing (Patellofemoral Pain Syndrome)

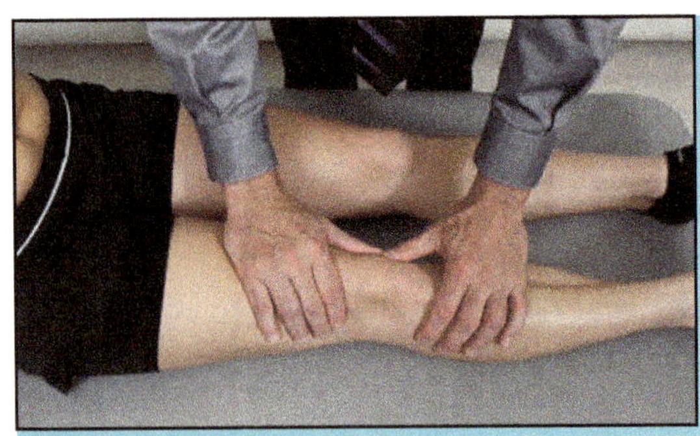

1) The patient is positioned in the long seated position with the knees slightly flexed.

2) The patella can be pushed medially/laterally or superiorly/inferiorly, or the examiner can assess the mobility of the patellar tendon, or the examiner can perform a tilt of the inferior patellar pole.

3) A positive test is indicated by decreased motion when compared to the uninvolved side.

UTILITY SCORE 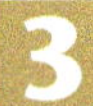

Study	Reliability	Sensitivity	Specificity	LR+	LR−	QUADAS Score (0–14)
Sweitzer et al.[128]						
(Medial-Lateral)	κ = .59	54	69	1.8	0.70	7
(Superior-Inferior)	κ = .55	63	56	1.4	0.70	
(Inferior Pole Tilt)	κ = .48	19	83	1.1	0.90	
(Patellar Tendon)	κ = .45	49	83	2.9	0.60	
Comments: Using a battery of motion tests does not appear to be diagnostic of PFPS.						

TESTS FOR PATELLOFEMORAL DYSFUNCTION

Palpation (Patellofemoral Pain Syndrome)

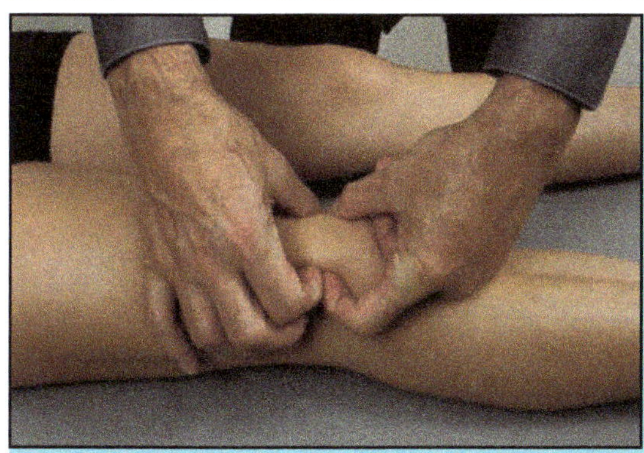

1. The patient is positioned in the long seated position with the knees extended.
2. The patella can be pushed medially or laterally but the examiner palpates named structure.
3. A positive test is indicated by reproduction of the patient's pain.

UTILITY SCORE 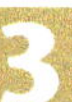 3

Study	Reliability	Sensitivity	Specificity	LR+	LR−	QUADAS Score (0–14)
Brushoj et al.[17] (Peripatellar)	NT	83	NT	NA	NA	3
Brushoj et al.[17] (Hoffa's Fat Pad)	NT	40	NT	NA	NA	3
Brushoj et al.[17] (Medial Plica)	NT	27	NT	NA	NA	3
Cook et al.[20] (Lateral)	NT	47	68	1.5	0.80	10
Naslund et al.[90]	NT					9
(Medial)		30	73	1.11	0.96	
(Lateral)		30	76	1.25	0.92	
Comments: Two recent studies seem not to support the diagnostic capability of peripatellar palpation.						

TESTS FOR PATELLOFEMORAL DYSFUNCTION

Patellar Compression Test (Patellofemoral Pain Syndrome)

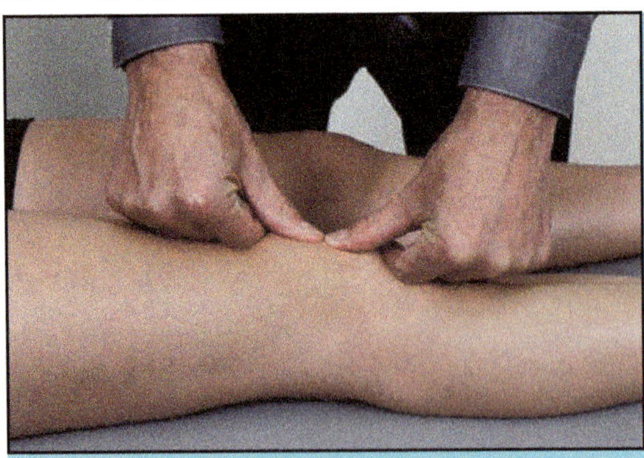

1) The patient is positioned in the long seated position with the knees extended.

2) The patella is pushed directly into the trochlea.

3) A positive test is indicated by reproduction of the patient's pain.

UTILITY SCORE 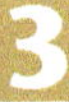 3

Study	Reliability	Sensitivity	Specificity	LR+	LR−	QUADAS Score (0–14)
Brushoj et al.[17]	NT	27	NT	NA	NA	3
Cook et al.[20]	NT	68	54	1.5	0.60	10
Naslund et al.[90]	NT	82	54	1.78	0.33	9
Comments: Three recent studies seem not to support the diagnostic capability of the Patellar Compression Test.						

Historical Elements (Patellofemoral Dysfunction)

1) The patient is queried about painful activities.

2) A positive test is indicated by patient report of pain with certain activities or positions.

UTILITY SCORE 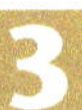 3

Study	Reliability	Sensitivity	Specificity	LR+	LR−	QUADAS Score (0–14)
Cook et al.[20] (Prolonged sitting)	NT	72	57	1.7	0.50	10
Naslund et al.[90]	NT	82	57	1.91	0.32	9
Elton et al History of:[29] (Peripatellar pain Pain with stairs or prolonged flexion Pain with with squatting)	NT	58 58 27	98 95 95	19.0 11.6 5.4	0.43 0.44 0.66	9
Comments: Literature is mixed about the value of historical findings in PFPS.						

TESTS FOR PATELLOFEMORAL DYSFUNCTION

Palpation for Tendinopathy (Jumper's Knee)

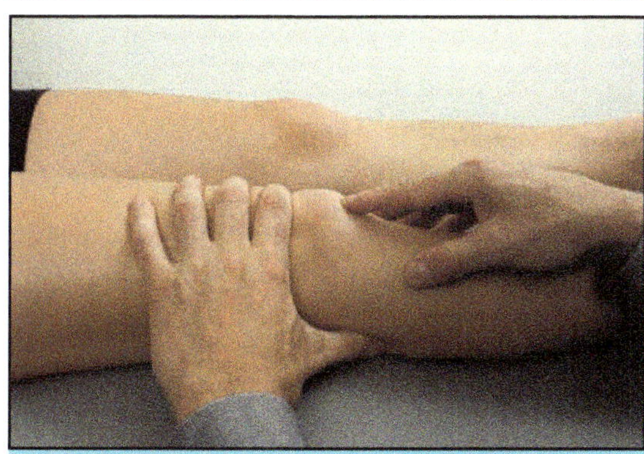

1) The examiner tilts the inferior pole of the patella anteriorly.
2) The examiner palpates on and around the inferior pole of the patella.
3) A positive sign is indicated by reproduction of the patient's knee pain.

UTILITY SCORE 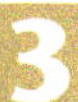

Study	Reliability	Sensitivity	Specificity	LR+	LR−	QUADAS Score (0–14)
Cook et al.[21] (Any pain) (Moderate or severe pain)	0.82	56 37	47 83	1.01 2.18	0.94 0.76	12
Comments: Pain with palpation of the patellar tendon is of little use, by itself, in diagnosing patellar tendinopathy.						

TESTS FOR PATELLOFEMORAL DYSFUNCTION

Clusters of Findings

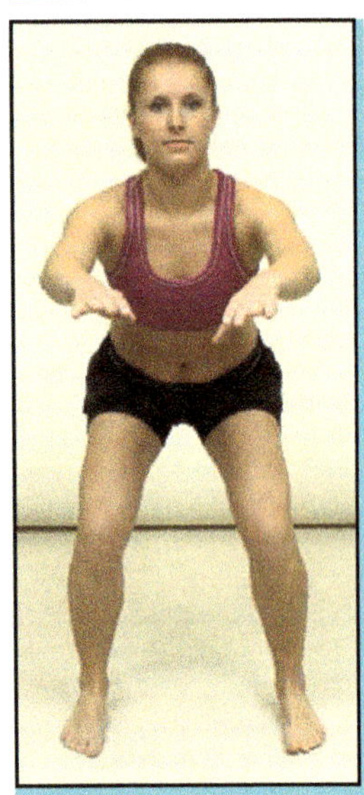

UTILITY SCORE 2

Study	Reliability	Sensitivity	Specificity	LR+	LR−	QUADAS Score (0–14)
Cook et al.[20]						
1. Pain with resisted knee extension and squatting	NT	35	89	3.3	0.79	10
2. 2 of 3 (pain with resisted knee extension, squatting, peripatellar palpation)		60	85	4.0	0.50	
3. 3 of 3 (pain with resisted knee extension, squatting, kneeling)		33	89	3.1	0.70	
Pihlajamaki et al.[99]						
Anterior knee pain + crepitus or pain with manual examination of the patella	NT	72	42	1.24	0.67	8

Comments: Pain with combinations of functional activities and resisted knee extension appear to have moderate value in diagnosing patellofemoral pain syndrome/patellofemoral dysfunction.[20] The same may not be true of actual chondromalacia (softening of patellar articular cartilage) confirmed by arthroscopy.[99]

TESTS FOR PLICA SYNDROME

Composite Examination/Clusters of Findings

UTILITY SCORE 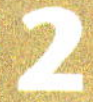

Study	Reliability	Sensitivity	Specificity	LR+	LR−	QUADAS Score (0–14)
Oberlander et al.[98]	NT	70	98	35.0	0.31	9
Yoon et al.[138]	NT	70	99	70.0	0.30	9
Shetty et al.[116]	NT	100	NA	NA	NA	8
Comments: Clinical examination appears to be diagnostic for knee plica, but there are some design faults in all of these studies so further research is necessary.						

MPP Test (Medial Patellar Plica Syndrome)

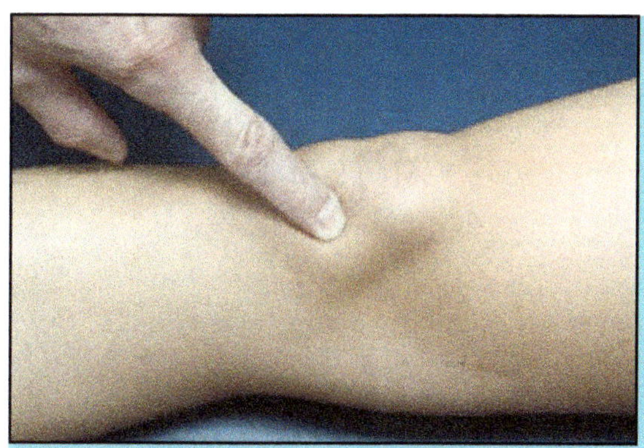

1) The patient assumes a supine position with knee in full extension. The examiner stands to the side of the patient's involved knee.

2) The examiner applies manual pressure to the plica at the inferomedial patellar border to force the plica between the medial femoral condyle and the joint line.

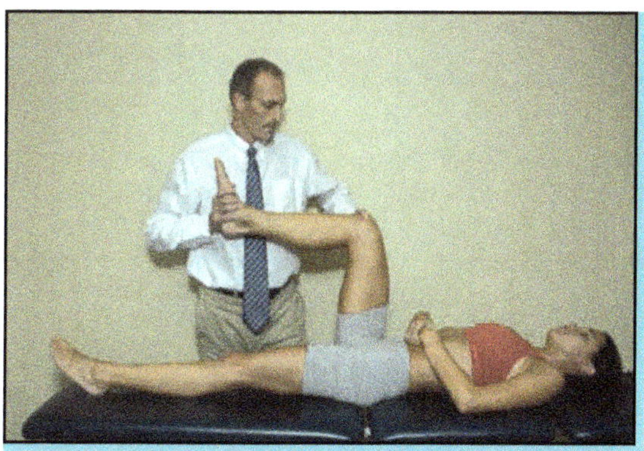

3) The examiner flexes the patient's knee to 90 degrees.

4) A positive test for a symptomatic medial patellar plica is indicated by more pain in extension than at 90 degrees flexion.

5) The painful knee is compared to the opposite side.

(*continued*)

TESTS FOR PLICA SYNDROME

UTILITY SCORE 2

Study	Reliability	Sensitivity	Specificity	LR+	LR−	QUADAS Score (0–14)
Kim et al.[58]	NT	NT	NT	NA	NA	NA
Kim et al.[59]	NT	90	89	8.18	0.11	9

Comments: The one study to examine the diagnostic accuracy of the MPP Test[59] did not report reliability. This diagnosis and a torn medial meniscus are often confused with each other but the symptomatic plica is thought to be a greater issue in active teenage individuals. A similar-sounding test was described by Flanagan et al.[35] in 1994. More research is needed to confirm the solid statistics of the Kim et al[59] study.

Medial Plica Shelf Test (Medial Patellar Plica Syndrome)

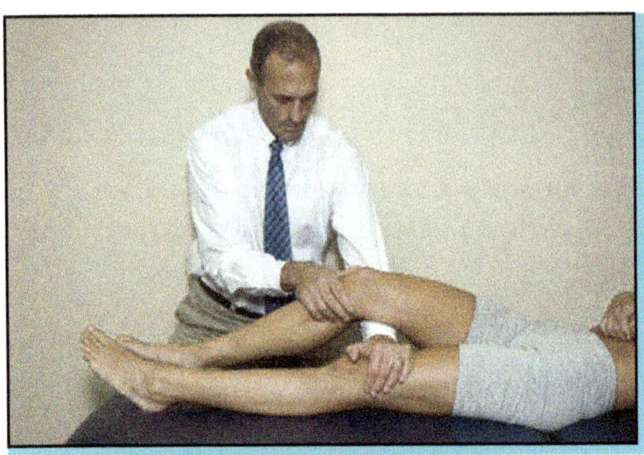

1) The patient assumes a supine position with knee flexed to 30 degrees. The examiner stands to the side of the patient's involved knee and reaches under that knee grasping the opposite thigh.

2) With the examiner's forearm acting as a bolster to maintain 30 degrees knee flexion, the examiner applies manual pressure to the lateral border of the patella with the opposite hand, causing a medial patellar glide.

3) A positive test for a symptomatic medial patellar plica is indicated by pain with the medial patellar glide.

UTILITY SCORE 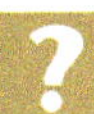

Study	Reliability	Sensitivity	Specificity	LR+	LR−	QUADAS Score (0–14)
Mital & Hayden[87]	NT	NT	NT	NA	NA	NA

Comments: The one study to examine the Medial Plica Shelf Test[87] did not report reliability or diagnostic accuracy. This diagnosis and a torn medial meniscus are often confused with each other but the symptomatic plica is thought to be a greater issue in active teenage individuals.

TESTS FOR PLICA SYNDROME

Medial Plica Test (Medial Patellar Plica Syndrome)

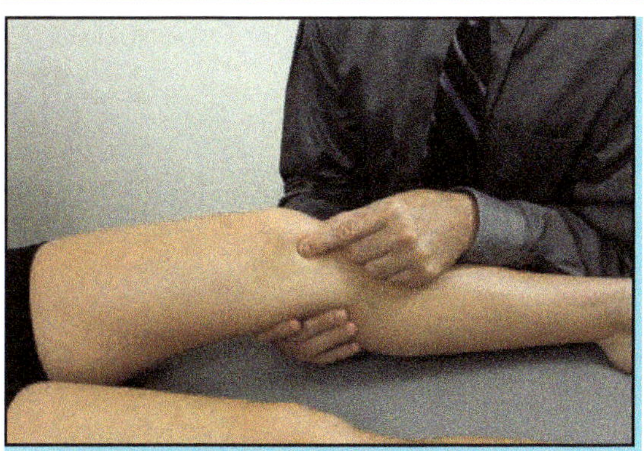

1) The patient assumes a supine position. The examiner stands to the side of the patient's involved knee.

2) The examiner palpates the medial femoral condyle while moving the patient's knee through flexion and extension.

3) A positive test for a symptomatic medial patellar plica is indicated by palpable crepitation.

UTILITY SCORE 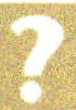

Study	Reliability	Sensitivity	Specificity	LR+	LR−	QUADAS Score (0–14)
Hardaker et al.[42]	NT	NT	NT	NA	NA	NA
Comments: The one study to examine the Medial Plica Test[42] did not report reliability or diagnostic accuracy. This diagnosis and a torn medial meniscus are often confused with each other but the symptomatic plica is thought to be a greater issue in active teenage individuals.						

Rotation Valgus Test (Medial Patellar Plica Syndrome)

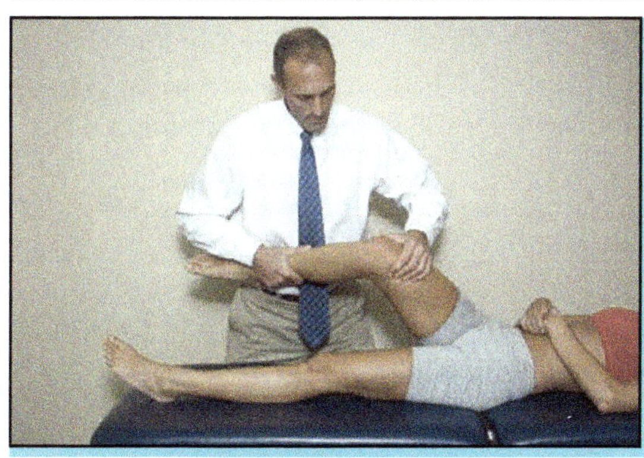

1) The examiner flexes the patient's knee while concurrently providing a valgus force, a medial patellar glide, and either internal or external tibial rotation.

2) A positive test for a symptomatic medial patellar plica is indicated by more pain either with or without a palpable medial click.

UTILITY SCORE 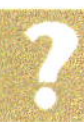

Study	Reliability	Sensitivity	Specificity	LR+	LR−	QUADAS Score (0–14)
Koshino & Okamoto[63]	NT	NT	NT	NA	NA	NA
Comments: The one study to examine the Rotation Valgus Test[63] did not report reliability or diagnostic accuracy. This diagnosis and a torn medial meniscus are often confused with each other but the symptomatic plica is thought to be a greater issue in active teenage individuals.						

TESTS FOR PLICA SYNDROME

Holding Test (Medial Patellar Plica Syndrome)

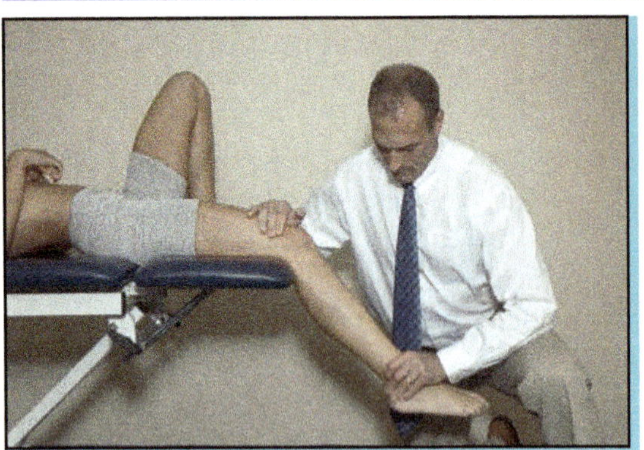

1) The patient is supine with the knee, foot, and ankle off the end of the examining table.

2) The patient extends his or her knee fully.

3) While the knee is in full extension, the examiner attempts to push the knee into flexion. The patient resists the force.

4) A positive test for a symptomatic medial patellar plica is indicated by medial pain either with or without a palpable medial click.

UTILITY SCORE 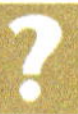

Study	Reliability	Sensitivity	Specificity	LR+	LR−	QUADAS Score (0–14)
Koshino & Okamoto[63]	NT	NT	NT	NA	NA	NA
Comments: The one study to examine the Holding Test[63] did not report reliability or diagnostic accuracy. Medial patellar plica syndrome and a torn medial meniscus are often confused with each other but the symptomatic plica is thought to be a greater issue in active teenage individuals. A combination of the Holding Test and the Rotation Valgus Test was reported by Amatuzzi et al.[5] in 1990 but no reliability or accuracy data were reported.						

Patellar Stutter Test (Suprapatellar Plica Syndrome)

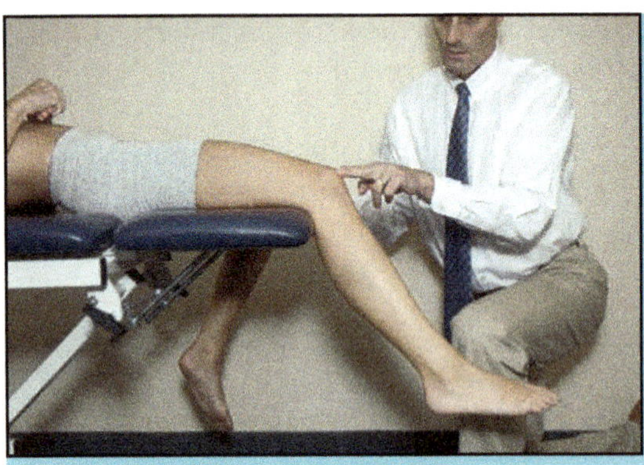

1) The patient is sitting with the knee flexed to 90 degrees, with foot and ankle off the end of the examining table.

2) The examiner places one finger on the patella while the patient slowly extends his or her knee.

3) Somewhere between 60 and 45 degrees of flexion, the patella stutters or jumps. This stutter is a positive test.

4) The author describes this test as best performed in the morning.

UTILITY SCORE 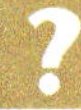

Study	Reliability	Sensitivity	Specificity	LR+	LR−	QUADAS Score (0–14)
Pipkin[100]	NT	NT	NT	NA	NA	NA
Comments: The one study to examine the Patellar Stutter Test[100] did not report reliability or diagnostic accuracy. This diagnosis and anterior knee pain from chondromalacia patella are often confused with each other.						

TESTS FOR PROXIMAL TIBIOFIBULAR JOINT INSTABILITY

Fibular Head Translation Test

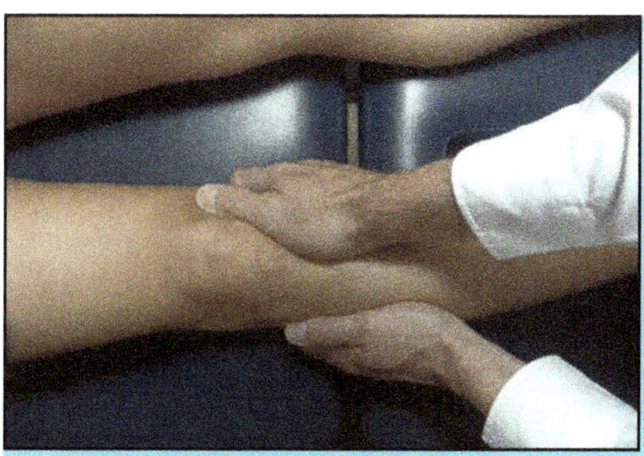

1) The examiner grasps the fibular head and provides a translatory force both in the anterior and the posterior directions.

2) A positive test is reproduction of the patient's pain and/or apprehension.

UTILITY SCORE 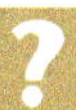

Study	Reliability	Sensitivity	Specificity	LR+	LR−	QUADAS Score (0–14)
Sijbrandij[118]	NT	NT	NT	NA	NA	NA
Comments: The one study to examine the Fibular Head Translation Test[118] did not report reliability or diagnostic accuracy.						

Radulescu Sign

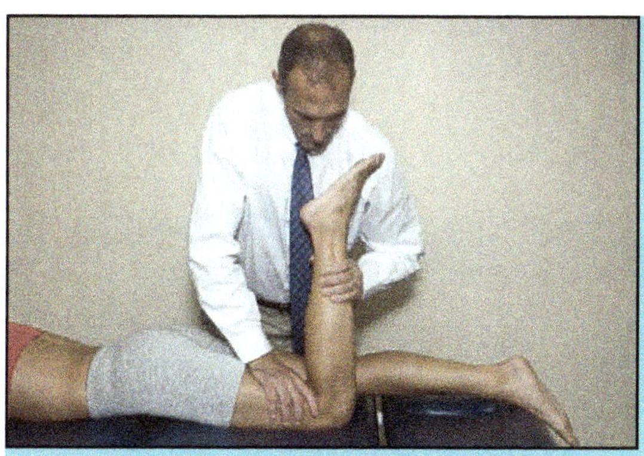

1) The patient lies prone with the knee flexed to 90 degrees.

2) The examiner stabilizes the patient's thigh with one hand while internally rotating the tibia with the other hand in an attempt to sublux the fibular head in an anterior direction.

3) A positive test is reproduction of the patient's pain, subluxation, and/or apprehension.

UTILITY SCORE 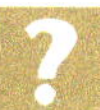

Study	Reliability	Sensitivity	Specificity	LR+	LR−	QUADAS Score (0–14)
Baciu et al.[10]	NT	NT	NT	NA	NA	NA
Comments: The one study to examine the Radulescu Sign[10] did not report reliability or diagnostic accuracy.						

TESTS FOR KNEE EFFUSION

Ballottement Test

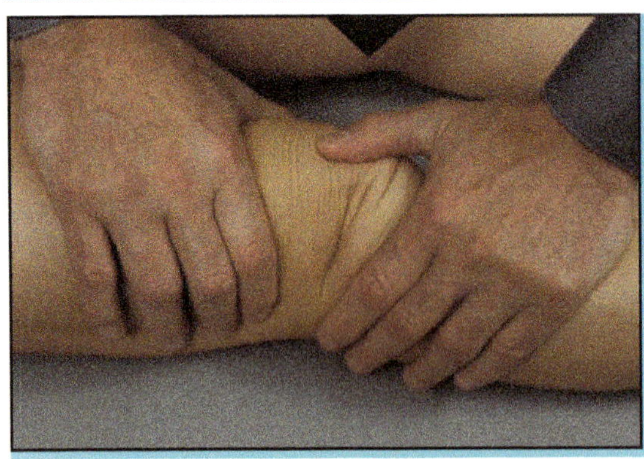

1) The patient is in the long seated position.

2) The examiner places one hand above the knee and one below moving both hands toward the knee.

3) The examiner pushes the patella into the trochlea and observes the return of the patella to its original position.

4) A positive sign is indicated by the feel of the patella flowing back to its original position.

UTILITY SCORE 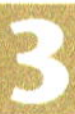

Study	Reliability	Sensitivity	Specificity	LR+	LR−	QUADAS Score (0–14)
Kastelein et al.[56]	NT	83	49	1.6	0.30	13
Comments: The Ballottement Test is of limited diagnostic value in patients with acute (less than 5 weeks) knee complaints of traumatic onset.						

Patient Report of Noticed Swelling

1) The patient is queried about swelling.

2) A positive sign is indicated by the patient reporting that they have noticed knee swelling.

UTILITY SCORE 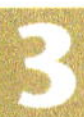

Study	Reliability	Sensitivity	Specificity	LR+	LR−	QUADAS Score (0–14)
Kastelein et al.[56]	NT	80	45	1.5	0.40	13
Comments: Patient report of swelling is of limited diagnostic value in patients with acute (less than 5 weeks) knee complaints of traumatic onset.						

Clusters of Findings for Effusion

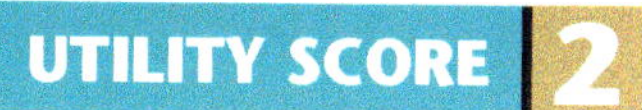

Study	Reliability	Sensitivity	Specificity	LR+	LR−	QUADAS Score (0–14)
Kastelein et al.[56] Ballottement test + Patient report of noticed swelling	NT	67	82	3.6	0.40	13
Comments: Patient report of swelling combined with the Ballottement Test is of clinical significance in patients with acute (less than 5 weeks) knee complaints of traumatic onset. Further the Kastelein et al.[56] study showed that knee swelling was associated with internal derangement of the knee.						

TESTS FOR OSTEOCHONDRAL LESIONS

Composite Examination/Clusters of Findings for Osteoarthritis (OA)/Degenerative Joint Disease (DJD)

UTILITY SCORE 2

Study	Reliability	Sensitivity	Specificity	LR+	LR−	QUADAS Score (0–14)
Oberlander et al.[98]	NT	63	99	63.0	0.37	9
Yoon et al.[138]	NT	76	97	25.33	0.25	9
Comments: Clinical examination appears to be diagnostic for knee OA but there are some design faults in these 2 studies so further research is necessary.						

Composite Examination/Clusters of Findings for Loose Bodies

UTILITY SCORE 2

Study	Reliability	Sensitivity	Specificity	LR+	LR−	QUADAS Score (0–14)
Oberlander et al.[98]	NT	65	99	65.0	0.35	9
Yoon et al.[138]	NT	67	98	33.50	0.34	9
Comments: Clinical examination appears to be diagnostic for loose bodies but there are some design faults in these 2 studies so further research is necessary.						

Composite Examination/Clusters of Findings for Chondral Fracture

UTILITY SCORE

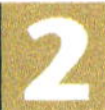

Study	Reliability	Sensitivity	Specificity	LR+	LR−	QUADAS Score (0–14)
Oberlander et al.[98]	NT	15	98	7.5	0.87	9
Yoon et al.[138]	NT	14	99	14.0	0.87	9
Comments: Clinical examination appears to be specific for chondral fractures but there are some design faults in these 2 studies so further research is necessary.						

Key Points

1. Both the Ottawa Rules and the Pittsburgh Rules appear to be strong tools to screen for a knee fracture because a negative test would rule out a fracture and a positive test would lead to referral for an x-ray.

2. For meniscus tears:
   - The composite physical exam modifies posttest probability of detecting a lateral tear by a large amount.
   - The composite physical exam modifies posttest probability of detecting a medial tear by a small amount.
   - There is no single clear physical sign or test that is accurate in diagnosing a meniscus tear, although some of the newer weightbearing tests are intriguing.

3. For the ACL:
   - The composite physical examination has strong diagnostic accuracy in the nonacute patient.
   - The Lachman Test has the best diagnostic accuracy of any single physical exam test.
   - Both the pivot-shift and anterior drawer are specific tests valuable at ruling in a torn ACL when positive.

4. There are no substantiated tests for symptomatic plica or proximal tibiofibular joint instability.

5. For the PCL:
   - The composite physical exam has potential for high diagnostic predictive values in detecting PCL tears. However, more studies need to be conducted to make the accuracy generalizable.
   - There is no all-or-none sign or test that is consistently accurate in diagnosing a torn PCL.
   - A positive Valgus or Varus Stress Test performed at 0 degrees may be indicative of a torn PCL.

6. For the MCL:
   - The value of the composite physical exam for a torn MCL is unknown.
   - The Valgus Stress Test is sensitive and has value in ruling out a torn MCL when the test is negative.
   - The Valgus Stress Test can be performed at both 0 degrees and 30 degrees of knee flexion to determine an isolated MCL tear (30 degrees) versus a combined PCL/MCL tear (0 degrees).

7. For the LCL:
   - The accuracy of the composite exam cannot be determined as only one article has been examined and the sample size only included one PCL lesion.
   - There are no proven tests to diagnose a torn LCL.

8. For the patellofemoral joint:
   - Although many tests have been described to clinically diagnose patellofemoral symptoms, the diagnostic accuracy and reliability of the majority are questionable.
   - Studies seem to support pain with squatting, stair climbing, or kneeling as sensitive tests that can rule out patellofemoral dysfunction when negative.
   - Literature seems to support resisted knee extension as a specific sign to rule in patellofemoral dysfunction when positive.

9. Physical examination appears to be able to detect plica syndrome although research in this area is of moderate quality and poorly describes of what the physical examination consists. The MPP test shows promise in both ruling in and ruling out plica syndrome but only 1 study has investigated the diagnostic accuracy of this test.

10. The Ballottement Test combined with a patient report of feeling like their knee is swollen has a moderate ability to detect knee effusion in acutely injured patients and this effusion may be related to internal derangement.

11. The physical examination seems specific for osteochondral lesions of the knee, including OA, but this information comes from only 2 studies of moderate quality.

References

1. Abdon P, Lindstrand A, Thorngren KG. Statistical evaluation of the diagnostic criteria for meniscal tears. *Int Orthop.* 1990;14(4):341–345.
2. Akseki D, Ozcan O, Boya H, Pinar H. A new weight-bearing meniscal test and a comparison with McMurray's test and joint line tenderness. *Arthroscopy.* Nov 2004;20(9):951–958.
3. al-Duri Z. Relation of the fibular head sign to other signs of anterior cruciate ligament insufficiency. A follow-up letter to the editor. *Clin Orthop Relat Res.* Feb 1992(275):220–225.
4. Allen CR, Kaplan LD, Fluhme DJ, Harner CD. Posterior cruciate ligament injuries. *Curr Opin Rheumatol.* Mar 2002;14(2):142–149.
5. Amatuzzi MM, Fazzi A, Varella MH. Pathologic synovial plica of the knee. Results of conservative treatment. *Am J Sports Med.* Sep–Oct 1990;18(5):466–469.
6. Anderson AF, Lipscomb AB. Clinical diagnosis of meniscal tears. Description of a new manipulative test. *Am J Sports Med.* Jul–Aug 1986;14(4):291–293.
7. Anderson AF, Lipscomb AB. Preoperative instrumented testing of anterior and posterior knee laxity. *Am J Sports Med.* May–Jun 1989;17(3):387–392.
8. Apley AG. The diagnosis of meniscus injuries; some new clinical methods. *J Bone Joint Surg Am.* Jan 1947; 29(1):78–84.
9. Bach BR, Jr., Warren RF, Wickiewicz TL. The pivot shift phenomenon: results and description of a modified clinical test for anterior cruciate ligament insufficiency. *Am J Sports Med.* Nov–Dec 1988;16(6):571–576.
10. Baciu CC, Tudor A, Olaru I. Recurrent luxation of the superior tibio-fibular joint in the adult. *Acta Orthop Scand.* 1974;45(5):772–777.
11. Barry OC, Smith H, McManus F, MacAuley P. Clinical assessment of suspected meniscal tears. *Ir J Med Sci.* Apr 1983;152(4):149–151.
12. Bauer SJ, Hollander JE, Fuchs SH, Thode HC, Jr. A clinical decision rule in the evaluation of acute knee injuries. *J Emerg Med.* Sep–Oct 1995;13(5):611–615.
13. Boeree NR, Ackroyd CE. Assessment of the menisci and cruciate ligaments: an audit of clinical practice. *Injury.* Jul 1991;22(4):291–294.
14. Bomberg BC, McGinty JB. Acute hemarthrosis of the knee: indications for diagnostic arthroscopy. *Arthroscopy.* 1990;6(3):221–225.
15. Bonamo JJ, Shulman G. Double contrast arthrography of the knee. A comparison to clinical diagnosis and arthroscopic findings. *Orthopedics.* Jul 1988;11(7):1041–1046.
16. Braunstein EM. Anterior cruciate ligament injuries: a comparison of arthrographic and physical diagnosis. *AJR Am J Roentgenol.* Mar 1982;138(3):423–425.
17. Brushoj C, Holmich P, Nielsen MB, Albrecht-Beste E. Acute patellofemoral pain: aggravating activities, clinical examination, MRI and ultrasound findings. *Br J Sports Med.* Jan 2008;42(1):64–67; discussion 67.
18. Butt MF, Farooq M, Dhar SA, Gani N, Hussain A, Mumtaz I. Clinical evaluation of the knee for medial meniscal lesion and anterior cruciate ligament tears: An assessment of clinical reliability. *J Orthopaedics* 2007;4:e7.
19. Clendenin MB, DeLee JC, Heckman JD. Interstitial tears of the posterior cruciate ligament of the knee. *Orthopedics.* 1980;3:764–772.
20. Cook C, Hegedus E, Hawkins R, Scovell F, Wyland D. Diagnostic accuracy and association to disability of clinical test findings associated with patellofemoral pain syndrome. *Physiother Can.* Winter 2010;62(1):17–24.
21. Cook JL, Khan KM, Kiss ZS, Purdam CR, Griffiths L. Reproducibility and clinical utility of tendon palpation to detect patellar tendinopathy in young basketball players. Victorian Institute of Sport tendon study group. *Br J Sports Med.* Feb 2001;35(1):65–69.
22. Cooperman JM, Riddle DL, Rothstein JM. Reliability and validity of judgments of the integrity of the anterior cruciate ligament of the knee using the Lachman's test. *Phys Ther.* Apr 1990;70(4):225–233.
23. Corea JR, Moussa M, al Othman A. McMurray's test tested. *Knee Surg Sports Traumatol Arthrosc.* 1994; 2(2):70–72.
24. Cross MJ, Schmidt DR, Mackie IG. A no-touch test for the anterior cruciate ligament. *J Bone Joint Surg Br.* Mar 1987; 69(2):300.
25. Daniel DM, Stone ML, Barnett P, Sachs R. Use of the quadriceps active test to diagnose posterior cruciate-ligament disruption and measure posterior laxity of the knee. *J Bone Joint Surg Am.* Mar 1988;70(3):386–391.
26. Dervin GF, Stiell IG, Wells GA, Rody K, Grabowski J. Physicians' accuracy and interrator reliability for the diagnosis of unstable meniscal tears in patients having osteoarthritis of the knee. *Can J Surg.* Aug 2001;44(4):267–274.
27. Doberstein ST, Romeyn RL, Reineke DM. The diagnostic value of the Clarke sign in assessing chondromalacia patella. *J Athl Train.* Apr–Jun 2008;43(2):190–196.
28. Donaldson WF, 3rd, Warren RF, Wickiewicz T. A comparison of acute anterior cruciate ligament examinations. Initial versus examination under anesthesia. *Am J Sports Med.* Jan–Feb 1985;13(1):5–10.
29. Elton K, McDonough K, Savinar-Nogue E, Jensen GM. A preliminary investigation: History, physical, and isokinetic exam results versus arthroscopic diagnosis of chondromalacia patella. *J Orthop Sports Phys Ther.* 1985;7(3):115–123.
30. Eren OT. The accuracy of joint line tenderness by physical examination in the diagnosis of meniscal tears. *Arthroscopy.* Oct 2003;19(8):850–854.
31. Esmaili Jah AA, Keyhani S, Zarei R, Moghaddam AK. Accuracy of MRI in comparison with clinical and arthroscopic findings in ligamentous and meniscal injuries of the knee. *Acta Orthop Belg.* Apr 2005; 71(2):189–196.

32. Evans PJ, Bell GD, Frank C. Prospective evaluation of the McMurray test. *Am J Sports Med.* Jul–Aug 1993; 21(4):604–608.

33. Feltham GT, Albright JP. The diagnosis of PCL injury: literature review and introduction of two novel tests. *Iowa Orthop J.* 2001;21:36–42.

34. Ferrari DA, Ferrari JD, Coumas J. Posterolateral instability of the knee. *J Bone Joint Surg Br.* Mar 1994; 76(2):187–192.

35. Flanagan JP, Trakru S, Meyer M, Mullaji AB, Krappel F. Arthroscopic excision of symptomatic medial plica. A study of 118 knees with 1–4 year follow-up. *Acta Orthop Scand.* Aug 1994;65(4):408–411.

36. Fowler PJ, Lubliner JA. The predictive value of five clinical signs in the evaluation of meniscal pathology. *Arthroscopy.* 1989;5(3):184–186.

37. Fowler PJ, Messieh SS. Isolated posterior cruciate ligament injuries in athletes. *Am J Sports Med.* Nov–Dec 1987;15(6):553–557.

38. Galway HR, MacIntosh DL. The lateral pivot shift: a symptom and sign of anterior cruciate ligament insufficiency. *Clin Orthop Relat Res.* Mar–Apr 1980;147:45–50.

39. Greene CC, Edwards TB, Wade MR, Carson EW. Reliability of the quadriceps angle measurement. *Am J Knee Surg.* Spring 2001;14(2):97–103.

40. Haim A, Yaniv M, Dekel S, Amir H. Patellofemoral pain syndrome: validity of clinical and radiological features. *Clin Orthop Relat Res.* Oct 2006;451:223–228.

41. Hardaker WT, Jr., Garrett WE, Jr., Bassett FH, 3rd. Evaluation of acute traumatic hemarthrosis of the knee joint. *South Med J.* Jun 1990;83(6):640–644.

42. Hardaker WT, Whipple TL, Bassett FH, 3rd. Diagnosis and treatment of the plica syndrome of the knee. *J Bone Joint Surg Am.* Mar 1980;62(2):221–225.

43. Harilainen A. Evaluation of knee instability in acute ligamentous injuries. *Ann Chir Gynaecol.* 1987;76:269–273.

44. Harilainen A, Myllynen P, Rauste J, Silvennoinen E. Diagnosis of acute knee ligament injuries: the value of stress radiography compared with clinical examination, stability, under anaesthesia and arthroscopic or operative findings. *Ann Chir Gynaecol.* 1986;75:37–43.

45. Harrison BK, Abell BE, Gibson TW. The Thessaly test for detection of meniscal tears: validation of a new physical examination technique for primary care medicine. *Clin J Sport Med.* Jan 2009;19(1):9–12.

46. Hughston JC, Andrews JR, Cross MJ, Moschi A. Classification of knee ligament instabilities. Part I. The medial compartment and cruciate ligaments. *J Bone Joint Surg Am.* Mar 1976;58(2):159–172.

47. Hughston JC, Andrews JR, Cross MJ, Moschi A. Classification of knee ligament instabilities. Part II. The lateral compartment. *J Bone Joint Surg Am.* Mar 1976; 58(2):173–179.

48. Hughston JC, Norwood LA, Jr. The posterolateral drawer test and external rotational recurvatum test for posterolateral rotatory instability of the knee. *Clin Orthop Relat Res.* Mar–Apr 1980;147:82–87.

49. Jackson JL, O'Malley PG, Kroenke K. Evaluation of acute knee pain in primary care. *Ann Intern Med.* Oct 7 2003;139(7):575–588.

50. Jaddue DAK, Tawfiq FH, Sayed-Noor AS. The utility of clinical examination in the diagnosis of medial meniscus injury in comparison with arthroscopic findings. *Eur J Orthop Surg Traumatol.* 2010; online before print.

51. Jain DK, Amaravati R, Sharma G. Evaluation of the clinical signs of anterior cruciate ligament and meniscal injuries. *Indian J Orthop.* Oct 2009;43(4):375–378.

52. Jakob RP, Hassler H, Staeubli HU. Observations on rotatory instability of the lateral compartment of the knee. Experimental studies on the functional anatomy and the pathomechanism of the true and the reversed pivot shift sign. *Acta Orthop Scand Suppl.* 1981;191:1–32.

53. Jerosch J, Riemer S. [How good are clinical investigative procedures for diagnosing meniscus lesions?]. *Sportverletz Sportschaden.* Jun 2004;18(2):59–67.

54. Jonsson T, Althoff B, Peterson L, Renstrom P. Clinical diagnosis of ruptures of the anterior cruciate ligament: a comparative study of the Lachman test and the anterior drawer sign. *Am J Sports Med.* Mar–Apr 1982;10(2):100–102.

55. Karachalios T, Hantes M, Zibis AH, Zachos V, Karantanas AH, Malizos KN. Diagnostic accuracy of a new clinical test (the Thessaly test) for early detection of meniscal tears. *J Bone Joint Surg Am.* May 2005;87(5):955–962.

56. Kastelein M, Luijsterburg PA, Wagemakers HP, et al. Diagnostic value of history taking and physical examination to assess effusion of the knee in traumatic knee patients in general practice. *Arch Phys Med Rehabil.* Jan 2009;90(1):82–86.

57. Kastelein M, Wagemakers HP, Luijsterburg PA, Verhaar JA, Koes BW, Bierma-Zeinstra SM. Assessing medial collateral ligament knee lesions in general practice. *Am J Med.* Nov 2008;121(11):982–988 e982.

58. Kim SJ, Jeong JH, Cheon YM, Ryu SW. MPP test in the diagnosis of medial patellar plica syndrome. *Arthroscopy.* Dec 2004;20(10):1101–1103.

59. Kim SJ, Lee DH, Kim TE. The relationship between the MPP test and arthroscopically found medial patellar plica pathology. *Arthroscopy.* Dec 2007;23(12):1303–1308.

60. Kocabey Y, Tetik O, Isbell WM, Atay OA, Johnson DL. The value of clinical examination versus magnetic resonance imaging in the diagnosis of meniscal tears and anterior cruciate ligament rupture. *Arthroscopy.* Sep 2004;20(7):696–700.

61. Kocher MS, DiCanzio J, Zurakowski D, Micheli LJ. Diagnostic performance of clinical examination and selective magnetic resonance imaging in the evaluation of intraarticular knee disorders in children and adolescents. *Am J Sports Med.* May–Jun 2001;29(3):292–296.

62. Konan S, Rayan F, Haddad FS. Do physical diagnostic tests accurately detect meniscal tears? *Knee Surg Sports Traumatol Arthrosc.* Jul 2009;17(7):806–811.

63. Koshino T, Okamoto R. Resection of painful shelf (plica synovialis mediopatellaris) under arthroscopy. *Arthroscopy.* 1985;1(2):136–141.

64. Kurosaka M, Yagi M, Yoshiya S, Muratsu H, Mizuno K. Efficacy of the axially loaded pivot shift test for the diagnosis of a meniscal tear. *Int Orthop.* 1999;23(5):271–274.

65. LaPrade RF, Konowalchuk BK. Popliteomeniscal fascicle tears causing symptomatic lateral compartment knee pain: diagnosis by the figure-4 test and treatment by open repair. *Am J Sports Med.* Aug 2005;33(8):1231–1236.

66. LaPrade RF, Wentorf F. Diagnosis and treatment of posterolateral knee injuries. *Clin Orthop Relat Res.* Sep 2002;402:110–121.

67. Larson RL. Physical examination in the diagnosis of rotatory instability. *Clin Orthop Relat Res.* Jan–Feb 1983(172):38–44.

68. Learmonth DJ. Incidence and diagnosis of anterior cruciate injuries in the accident and emergency department. *Injury.* Jul 1991;22(4):287–290.

69. Lee JK, Yao L, Phelps CT, Wirth CR, Czajka J, Lozman J. Anterior cruciate ligament tears: MR imaging compared with arthroscopy and clinical tests. *Radiology.* Mar 1988;166(3):861–864.

70. Liu SH, Osti L, Henry M, Bocchi L. The diagnosis of acute complete tears of the anterior cruciate ligament. Comparison of MRI, arthrometry and clinical examination. *J Bone Joint Surg Br.* Jul 1995;77(4):586–588.

71. Loo WL, Liu YB, Lee YH, Hoong Y, Soon M. A comparison of accuracy between clinical history, physical examination and magnetic resonance imaging and arthroscopy in the diagnosis of meniscal and anterior cruciate ligament tears. *J Orthopaedics.* 2008;5:e8.

72. Loomer RL. A test for knee posterolateral rotatory instability. *Clin Orthop Relat Res.* Mar 1991(264):235–238.

73. Loos WC, Fox JM, Blazina ME, Del Pizzo W, Friedman MJ. Acute posterior cruciate ligament injuries. *Am J Sports Med.* Mar–Apr 1981;9(2):86–92.

74. Losee RE. Concepts of the pivot shift. *Clin Orthop Relat Res.* Jan–Feb 1983(172):45–51.

75. Losee RE. Diagnosis of chronic injury to the anterior cruciate ligament. *Orthop Clin North Am.* Jan 1985; 16(1):83–97.

76. Loudon JK, Wiesner D, Goist-Foley HL, Asjes C, Loudon KL. Intrarater reliability of functional performance tests for subjects with patellofemoral pain syndrome. *J Athl Train.* Sep 2002;37(3):256–261.

77. Lowery DJ, Farley TD, Wing DW, Sterett WI, Steadman JR. A clinical composite score accurately detects meniscal pathology. *Arthroscopy.* Nov 2006;22(11):1174–1179.

78. Malanga GA, Andrus S, Nadler SF, McLean J. Physical examination of the knee: a review of the original test description and scientific validity of common orthopedic tests. *Arch Phys Med Rehabil.* Apr 2003;84(4):592–603.

79. Manzotti A, Baiguini P, Locatelli A, et al. Statistical evaluation of McMurray's test in the clinical diagnosis of meniscus injuries. *Journal of Sports Traumatology and Related Research* 1997;19:83–89.

80. Mariani PP, Adriani E, Maresca G, Mazzola CG. A prospective evaluation of a test for lateral meniscus tears. *Knee Surg Sports Traumatol Arthrosc.* 1996;4(1):22–26.

81. Martens MA, Mulier JC. Anterior subluxation of the lateral tibial plateau. A new clinical test and the morbidity of this type of knee instability. *Arch Orthop Trauma Surg.* 1981;98(2):109–111.

82. McClure PW, Rothstein JM, Riddle DL. Intertester reliability of clinical judgments of medial knee ligament integrity. *Phys Ther.* Apr 1989;69(4):268–275.

83. McConnell J. The management of chondromalacia patella. *Aust J Physiother.* 1986;32:215–223.

84. McMurray TP. The semilunar cartilages. *Br J Surg.* 1942; 29:407–414.

85. Miao Y, Yu JK, Ao YF, Zheng ZZ, Gong X, Leung KKM. Diagnostic values of 3 methods for evaluating meniscal healing status after meniscal repair: comparison among second-look arthroscopy, clinical assessment, and magnetic resonance imaging. *Am J Sports Med.* 2011; online before print.

86. Mirzatolooei F, Yekta Z, Bayazidchi M, Ershadi S, Afshar A. Validation of the Thessaly test for detecting meniscal tears in anterior cruciate deficient knees. *Knee.* Jun 2010;17(3):221–223.

87. Mital MA, Hayden J. Pain in the knee in children: the medial plica shelf syndrome. *Orthop Clin North Am.* Jul 1979;10(3):713–722.

88. Moore HA, Larson RL. Posterior cruciate ligament injuries. Results of early surgical repair. *Am J Sports Med.* Mar–Apr 1980;8(2):68–78.

89. Muellner T, Weinstabl R, Schabus R, Vecsei V, Kainberger F. The diagnosis of meniscal tears in athletes. A comparison of clinical and magnetic resonance imaging investigations. *Am J Sports Med.* Jan–Feb 1997;25(1):7–12.

90. Naslund J, Naslund UB, Odenbring S, Lundeberg T. Comparison of symptoms and clinical findings in subgroups of individuals with patellofemoral pain. *Physiother Theory Pract.* Jun 2006;22(3):105–118.

91. Nijs J, Van Geel C, Van der auwera C, Van de Velde B. Diagnostic value of five clinical tests in patellofemoral pain syndrome. *Man Ther.* Feb 2006;11(1):69–77.

92. Niskanen RO, Paavilainen PJ, Jaakkola M, Korkala OL. Poor correlation of clinical signs with patellar cartilaginous changes. *Arthroscopy.* Mar 2001;17(3):307–310.

93. Nissen CW, Cullen MC, Hewett TE, Noyes FR. Physical and arthroscopic examination techniques of the patellofemoral joint. *J Orthop Sports Phys Ther.* Nov 1998;28(5):277–285.

94. Noble J, Erat K. In defence of the meniscus. A prospective study of 200 meniscectomy patients. *J Bone Joint Surg Br.* Feb 1980;62-B(1):7–11.

95. Noyes FR, Grood ES, Cummings JF, Wroble RR. An analysis of the pivot shift phenomenon. The knee motions and subluxations induced by different examiners. *Am J Sports Med.* Mar–Apr 1991;19(2):148–155.

96. Noyes FR, Paulos L, Mooar LA, Signer B. Knee sprains and acute knee hemarthrosis: misdiagnosis of anterior cruciate ligament tears. *Phys Ther.* Dec 1980; 60(12):1596–1601.

97. O'Shea KJ, Murphy KP, Heekin RD, Herzwurm PJ. The diagnostic accuracy of history, physical examination, and radiographs in the evaluation of traumatic knee disorders. *Am J Sports Med.* Mar–Apr 1996;24(2): 164–167.

98. Oberlander MA, Shalvoy RM, Hughston JC. The accuracy of the clinical knee examination documented by arthroscopy. A prospective study. *Am J Sports Med.* Nov–Dec 1993;21(6):773–778.

99. Pihlajamaki HK, Kuikka PI, Leppanen VV, Kiuru MJ, Mattila VM. Reliability of clinical findings and magnetic resonance imaging for the diagnosis of chondromalacia patellae. *J Bone Joint Surg Am.* Apr 2010;92(4):927–934.

100. Pipkin G. Knee injuries: the role of the suprapatellar plica and suprapatellar bursa in simulating internal derangements. *Clin Orthop Relat Res.* Jan 1971;74:161–176.

101. Pookarnjanamorakot C, Korsantirat T, Woratanarat P. Meniscal lesions in the anterior cruciate insufficient knee: the accuracy of clinical evaluation. *J Med Assoc Thai.* Jun 2004;87(6):618–623.

102. Quarles JD, Hosey RG. Medial and lateral collateral injuries: prognosis and treatment. *Prim Care.* Dec 2004;31(4):957–975, ix.

103. Rayan F, Bhonsle S, Shukla DD. Clinical, MRI, and arthroscopic correlation in meniscal and anterior cruciate ligament injuries. *Int Orthop.* Feb 2009;33(1):129–132.

104. Richman PB, McCuskey CF, Nashed A, et al. Performance of two clinical decision rules for knee radiography. *J Emerg Med.* Jul–Aug 1997;15(4):459–463.

105. Rose NE, Gold SM. A comparison of accuracy between clinical examination and magnetic resonance imaging in the diagnosis of meniscal and anterior cruciate ligament tears. *Arthroscopy.* Aug 1996;12(4):398–405.

106. Rubinstein RA, Jr., Shelbourne KD, McCarroll JR, VanMeter CD, Rettig AC. The accuracy of the clinical examination in the setting of posterior cruciate ligament injuries. *Am J Sports Med.* Jul–Aug 1994; 22(4):550–557.

107. Ryan PJ, Reddy K, Fleetcroft J. A prospective comparison of clinical examination, MRI, bone SPECT, and arthroscopy to detect meniscal tears. *Clin Nucl Med.* Dec 1998;23(12):803–806.

108. Sae-Jung S, Jirarattanaphochai K, Benjasil T. KKU knee compression-rotation test for detection of meniscal tears: a comparative study of its diagnostic accuracy with McMurray test. *J Med Assoc Thai.* Apr 2007;90(4):718–723.

109. Saengnipanthkul S, Sirichativapee W, Kowsuwon W, Rojviroj S. The effects of medial patellar plica on clinical diagnosis of medial meniscal lesion. *J Med Assoc Thai.* Dec 1992;75(12):704–708.

110. Sandberg R, Balkfors B, Henricson A, Westlin N. Stability tests in knee ligament injuries. *Arch Orthop Trauma Surg.* 1986;106(1):5–7.

111. Seaberg DC, Jackson R. Clinical decision rule for knee radiographs. *Am J Emerg Med.* Sep 1994;12(5):541–543.

112. Seaberg DC, Yealy DM, Lukens T, Auble T, Mathias S. Multicenter comparison of two clinical decision rules for the use of radiography in acute, high-risk knee injuries. *Ann Emerg Med.* Jul 1998;32(1):8–13.

113. Selfe J, Harper L, Pederson I, Breen-Turner J, Waring J. Four outcome measures for patellofemoral joint problems. Part I. Development and validity. *Physiotherapy.* 2001;87:507–515.

114. Shelbourne KD, Benedict F, McCarroll JR, Rettig AC. Dynamic posterior shift test. An adjuvant in evaluation of posterior tibial subluxation. *Am J Sports Med.* Mar–Apr 1989;17(2):275–277.

115. Shelbourne KD, Martini DJ, McCarroll JR, VanMeter CD. Correlation of joint line tenderness and meniscal lesions in patients with acute anterior cruciate ligament tears. *Am J Sports Med.* Mar–Apr 1995;23(2):166–169.

116. Shetty VD, Vowler SL, Krishnamurthy S, Halliday AE. Clinical diagnosis of medial plica syndrome of the knee: a prospective study. *J Knee Surg.* Oct 2007;20(4):277–280.

117. Shino K, Horibe S, Ono K. The voluntarily evoked posterolateral drawer sign in the knee with posterolateral instability. *Clin Orthop Relat Res.* Feb 1987(215): 179–186.

118. Sijbrandij S. Instability of the proximal tibio-fibular joint. *Acta Orthop Scand.* Dec 1978;49(6):621–626.

119. Simonsen O, Jensen J, Mouritsen P, Lauritzen J. The accuracy of clinical examination of injury of the knee joint. *Injury.* Sep 1984;16(2):96–101.

120. Slocum DB, James SL, Larson RL, Singer KM. Clinical test for anterolateral rotary instability of the knee. *Clin Orthop Relat Res.* Jul–Aug 1976(118):63–69.

121. Solomon DH, Simel DL, Bates DW, Katz JN, Schaffer JL. The rational clinical examination. Does this patient have a torn meniscus or ligament of the knee? Value of the physical examination. *JAMA.* Oct 3 2001;286(13):1610–1620.

122. Staubli HU, Jakob RP. Posterior instability of the knee near extension. A clinical and stress radiographic analysis of acute injuries of the posterior cruciate ligament. *J Bone Joint Surg Br.* Mar 1990;72(2):225–230.

123. Stiell IG, Greenberg GH, Wells GA, et al. Prospective validation of a decision rule for the use of radiography in acute knee injuries. *JAMA.* Feb 28 1996; 275(8):611–615.

124. Stiell IG, Greenberg GH, Wells GA, et al. Derivation of a decision rule for the use of radiography in acute knee injuries. *Ann Emerg Med.* Oct 1995;26(4):405–413.

125. Stiell IG, Wells GA, Hoag RH, et al. Implementation of the Ottawa Knee Rule for the use of radiography in acute knee injuries. *JAMA.* Dec 17 1997;278(23):2075–2079.

126. Strobel MJ, Stedtfeld HW, eds. *Diagnostic Evaluation of the Knee.* Berlin: Springer-Verlag; 1990.

127. Strobel MJ, Weiler A, Schulz MS, Russe K, Eichhorn HJ. Fixed posterior subluxation in posterior cruciate ligament-deficient knees: diagnosis and treatment of a new clinical sign. *Am J Sports Med.* Jan–Feb 2002;30(1):32–38.

128. Sweitzer BA, Cook C, Steadman JR, Hawkins RJ, Wyland DJ. The inter-rater reliability and diagnostic accuracy of patellar mobility tests in patients with anterior knee pain. *Phys Sportsmed.* Oct 2010;38(3):90–96.

129. Tomsich DA, Nitz AJ, Threlkeld AJ, Shapiro R. Patellofemoral alignment: reliability. *J Orthop Sports Phys Ther.* Mar 1996;23(3):200–208.

130. Torg JS, Conrad W, Kalen V. Clinical diagnosis of anterior cruciate ligament instability in the athlete. *Am J Sports Med.* Mar–Apr 1976;4(2):84–93.

131. Wadey VM, Mohtadi NG, Bray RC, Frank CB. Positive predictive value of maximal posterior joint-line tenderness in diagnosing meniscal pathology: a pilot study. *Can J Surg.* Apr 2007;50(2):96–100.

132. Wagemakers HP, Heintjes EM, Boks SS, et al. Diagnostic value of history-taking and physical examination for assessing meniscal tears of the knee in general practice. *Clin J Sport Med.* Jan 2008;18(1):24–30.

133. Wagemakers HP, Luijsterburg PA, Boks SS, et al. Diagnostic accuracy of history taking and physical examination for assessing anterior cruciate ligament lesions of the knee in primary care. *Arch Phys Med Rehabil.* Sep 2010;91(9):1452–1459.

134. Warren RF, Marshall JL. Injuries of the anterior cruciate and medial collateral ligaments of the knee. A long-term follow-up of 86 cases—part II. *Clin Orthop Relat Res.* Oct 1978(136):198–211.

135. Warren RF, Marshall JL. Injuries of the anterior cruciate and medial collateral ligaments of the knee. A retrospective analysis of clinical records—part I. *Clin Orthop Relat Res.* Oct 1978(136):191–197.

136. Watson CJ, Leddy HM, Dynjan TD, Parham JL. Reliability of the lateral pull test and tilt test to assess patellar alignment in subjects with symptomatic knees: student raters. *J Orthop Sports Phys Ther.* Jul 2001; 31(7):368–374.

137. Watson CJ, Propps M, Galt W, Redding A, Dobbs D. Reliability of McConnell's classification of patellar orientation in symptomatic and asymptomatic subjects. *J Orthop Sports Phys Ther.* Jul 1999;29(7):378–385; discussion 386–393.

138. Yoon YS, Rah JH, Park HJ. A prospective study of the accuracy of clinical examination evaluated by arthroscopy of the knee. *Int Orthop.* 1997;21(4):223–227.

PEARSON **myhealthprofessionskit**™

Use this address to access the Companion Website created for this textbook. Simply select "Physical Therapy" from the choice of disciplines. Find this book and log in using your username and password to access video clips of selected tests.

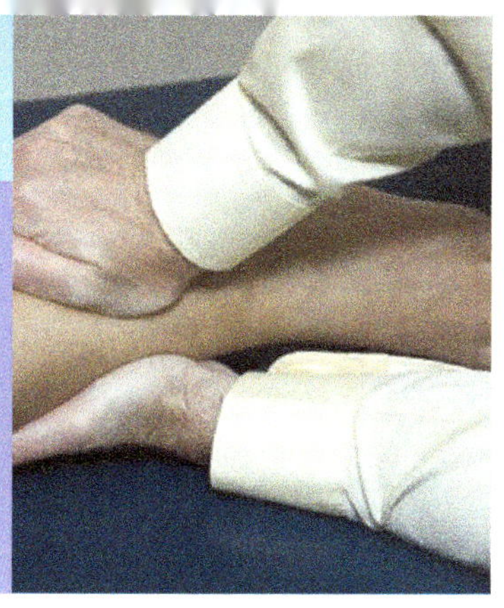

Physical Examination Tests for the Lower Leg, Ankle, and Foot

Chad E. Cook

Please refer to the chapter "Introduction to Diagnostic Accuracy" before reading this chapter.

Index of Tests

Test for Lateral Ligament Integrity

Medial Talar Tilt Stress Test

Test for Achilles Tendon Integrity

Thompson Test

Test for Tarsal Tunnel Syndrome

Tinel's Sign

Tests for Anterior Ankle Impingement

Forced Dorsiflexion Test

Clinical Prediction Rule of Impingement

Test for Ankle Swelling

Figure-8 Test

Tests for Stress Fracture or Interdigital Neuroma

Morton's Test (Foot Squeeze Test)

Web Space Tenderness

Plantar Percussion Test

Toe Tip Sensation Deficit

Tuning Fork

Tests for Deep Vein Thrombosis

Well's Clinical Prediction Rule for Deep Vein Thrombosis

Calf Swelling

Homan's Sign

Calf Tenderness

Popkin's Sign

Test for Surgical Stabilization Required with Fractured Fibula

Clinical Prediction Rule for Surgical Stabilization

Test for Foot and Ankle Fractures

Ottawa Ankle Rules

TEST FOR FIRST RAY MOBILITY

Manual Examination of the First Ray

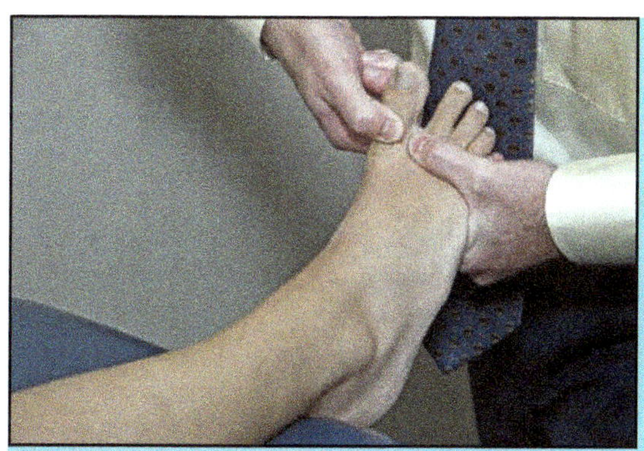

1) The patient lies in a supine position.

2) The second through fifth digits are stabilized by one hand of the examiner while the other hand stabilizes the first ray. The stabilization is held just distal to the metatarsal-phalangeal joint.

3) The examiner applies a dorsal and a plantar force to the first ray to determine first ray mobility. Typically, movement is considered normal or hypomobile.

4) A positive test is reduction of motion into dorsiflexion or plantarflexion.

UTILITY SCORE 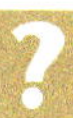

Study	Reliability	Sensitivity	Specificity	LR+	LR−	QUADAS Score (0–14)
Glasoe et al.[10]	0.16 kappa	NT	NT	NA	NA	NA
Glasoe et al.[11] (use of a ruler)	0.05 ICC	NT	NT	NA	NA	NA
Shirk et al.[26]	0.03 kappa	NT	NT	NA	NA	NA
Comments: This test demonstrates poor agreement and unknown diagnostic accuracy.						

TESTS FOR SYNDESMOTIC ANKLE SPRAINS

Fibular Translation Test

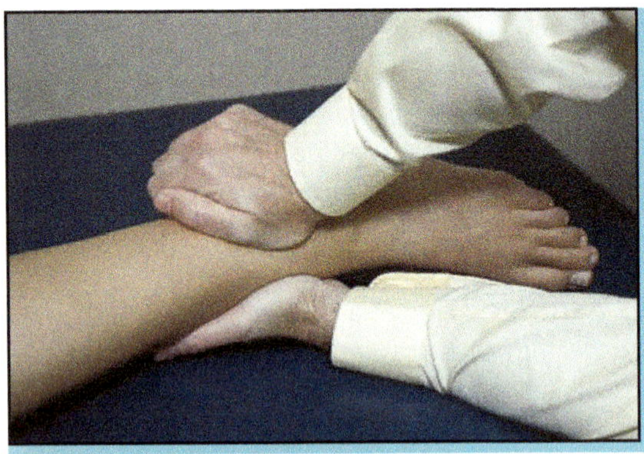

1) The patient lies in a sidelying position.

2) The examiner applies anterior and posterior forces on the fibula at the level of the syndesmosis.

3) A positive test is pain during translation and more displacement to the fibula than the compared side.

UTILITY SCORE 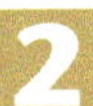

Study	Reliability	Sensitivity	Specificity	LR+	LR−	QUADAS Score (0–14)
Beumer et al.[3]	NT	82	88	6.8	0.2	8
Comments: Beumer et al.[3] only found increased translation when all ligaments were removed in cadavers.						

External Rotation Test

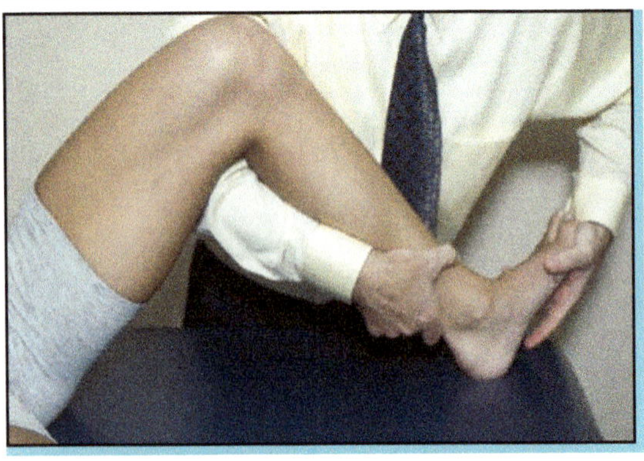

1) The patient lies in a supine position; the knee of the patient is flexed to 90 degrees.

2) The examiner holds the ankle in a neutral position then applies an externally rotated movement to the ankle.

3) A positive test is reproduction of concordant symptoms during movement.

UTILITY SCORE 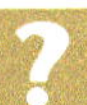

Study	Reliability	Sensitivity	Specificity	LR+	LR−	QUADAS Score (0–14)
Alonso et al.[1]	0.75 kappa	NT	NT	NA	NA	NA
Beumer et al.[3]	NT	NT	95	NA	NA	8
Comments: Beumer et al.[3] found significant displacement with this test in cadavers with ligaments individually sectioned.						

TESTS FOR SYNDESMOTIC ANKLE SPRAINS

Cotton Test

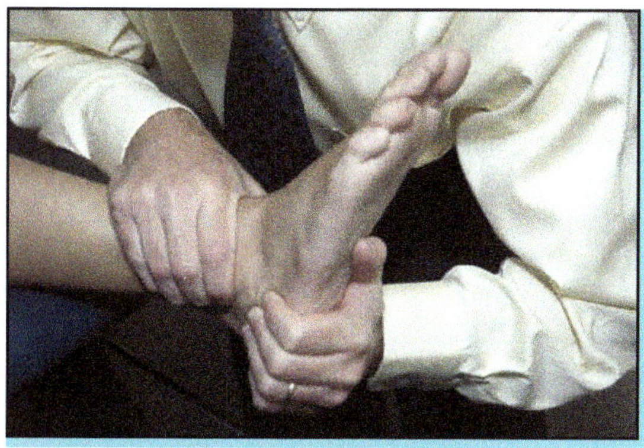

1) The patient lies in a supine position.
2) The examiner stabilizes the tibia with one hand and applies a lateral force to the ankle with the other. Occasionally, dorsiflexion is added to improve the sensitivity of the test.
3) A positive test is lateral translation of the ankle.

UTILITY SCORE 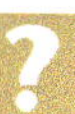

Study	Reliability	Sensitivity	Specificity	LR+	LR−	QUADAS Score (0–14)
Beumer et al.[4]	NT	NT	NT	NA	NA	NA
Beumer et al.[3]	NT	46	NT	NA	NA	8
Comments: To translate the foot on the tibia effectively, the tibia requires appropriate stabilization. Consider stabilizing the tibia on the plinth.						

Syndesmosis Squeeze Test

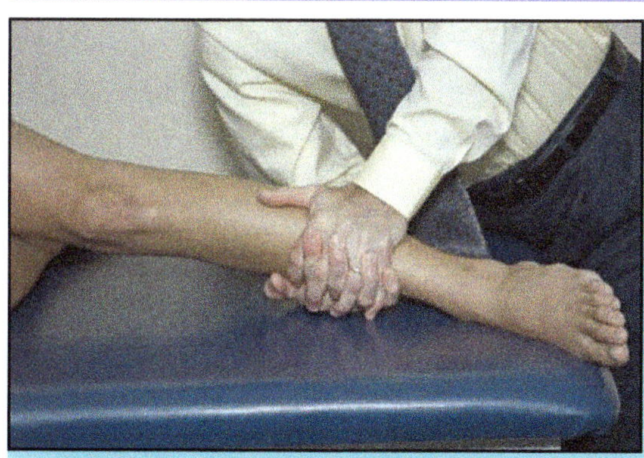

1) The patient lies in a supine or sidelying position.
2) The examiner applies a manual squeeze, pushing the fibula into the tibia, applying a force at the midpoint of the calf.
3) The test is considered positive if the proximal force causes distal pain near the syndesmosis.

UTILITY SCORE 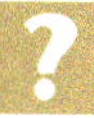

Study	Reliability	Sensitivity	Specificity	LR+	LR−	QUADAS Score (0–14)
Alonso et al.[1]	0.50 kappa	NT	NT	NA	NA	NA
Comments: This test is also described as the squeeze test of the leg and, occasionally, as the distal tibiofibular compression test if performed distal to the mid-point of the lower leg. Some describe a positive finding as pain when the squeeze is released.						

TESTS FOR ANTERIOR TALUS DISPLACEMENT RELATIVE TO THE TIBIA

Anterior Drawer Test

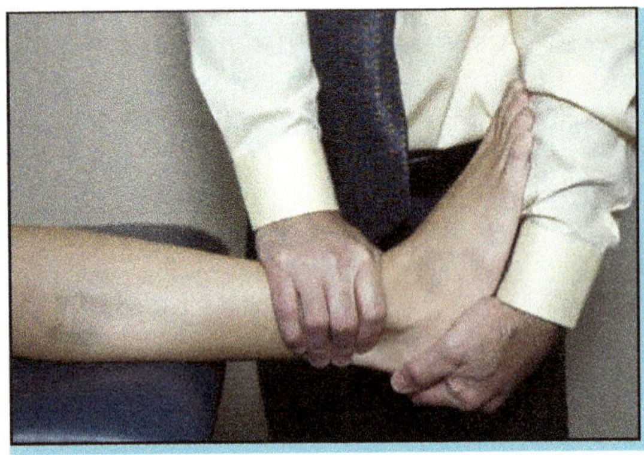

1) The patient lies in a supine position. The ankle is prepositioned into slight plantarflexion.

2) The examiner provides an anterior glide of the calcaneus and talus on the stabilized tibia.

3) A positive test is excessive translation of one side in comparison to the opposite extremity.

UTILITY SCORE 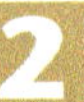

Study	Reliability	Sensitivity	Specificity	LR+	LR−	QUADAS Score (0–14)
Hertel et al.[13]	NT	78	75	3.1	0.29	8
Phisitkul et al.[22]	NT	100	100	Inf	Inf	7

Comments: The test is designed to measure damage to the anterior talofibular ligament. The examiner should observe the presence of a dimple or sulcus sign near the region of the anterior talofibular ligament. Phistikul's study used cadavers and was poorly performed.

Anterior Lateral Drawer Test

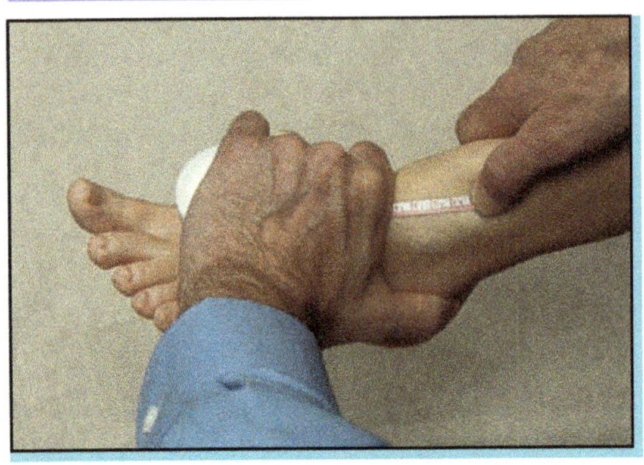

1) The patient assumes a sitting position.

2) The examiner stabilizes the lower leg just above the ankle. The other hand provides an anterior directed force, measurement of talar translation, and control of ankle plantarflexion.

3) A positive test is 3 millimeters or more of translation.

UTILITY SCORE 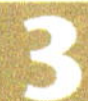

Study	Reliability	Sensitivity	Specificity	LR+	LR−	QUADAS Score (0–14)
Phisitkul et al.[22]	NT	75	50	1.5	0.50	7

Comments: The study used cadavers and was poorly performed.

TEST FOR SUBTALAR JOINT STABILITY

Medial Subtalar Glide Test

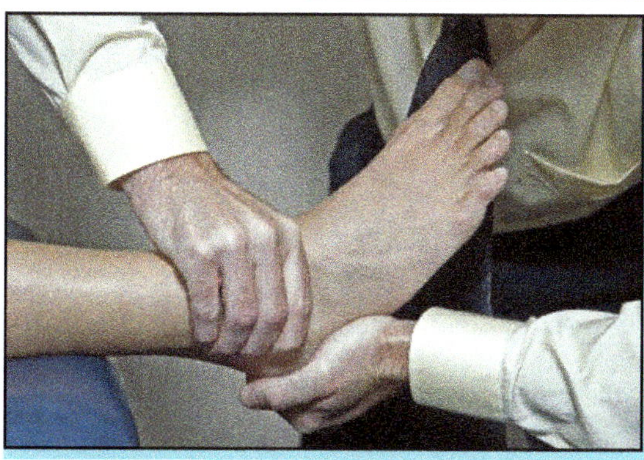

1) The patient lies in a supine position.
2) The examiner stabilizes the talus superiorly while gripping the calcaneus at the plantar aspect of the foot.
3) The examiner applies a medial glide of the calcaneus on the fixed talus.
4) A positive test is gross laxity during the procedure.

UTILITY SCORE 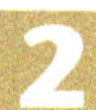

Study	Reliability	Sensitivity	Specificity	LR+	LR−	QUADAS Score (0–14)
Hertel et al.[13]	NT	78	75	3.1	0.29	8
Comments: Actual subtalar movement is minimal, subsequently gross laxity during assessment should be indicative of instability.						

TEST FOR SUBTALAR JOINT PRONATION

Subtalar Joint Neutral (Open and Closed Chain)

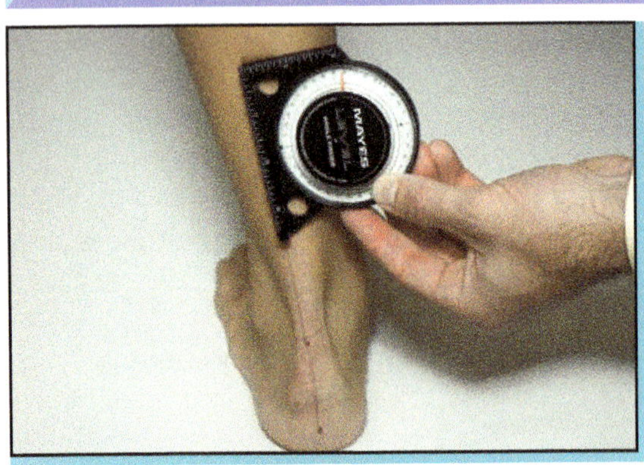

1) The patient stands.

2) The examiner places the patient in a subtalar neutral position. Subtalar neutral is found by palpation of the patient's tali in which both medial and lateral aspects are felt equally by the examiner.

3) Often, subtalar neutral is examined by measuring the position of the calcaneus using an inclinometer.

4) A positive test is excessive pronation or supination during obtained subtalar neutral.

UTILITY SCORE 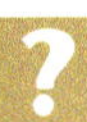

Study	Reliability	Sensitivity	Specificity	LR+	LR−	QUADAS Score (0–14)
Picciano et al.[23] (Open Chain)	0.00 ICC	NT	NT	NA	NA	NA
Picciano et al.[23] (Closed Chain)	0.15 ICC	NT	NT	NA	NA	NA
Comments: Many question the benefit of finding subtalar neutral. Note the exceptionally poor reliability in detecting subtalar joint neutral.						

TESTS FOR MIDTARSAL JOINT PRONATION

Navicular Drop Test

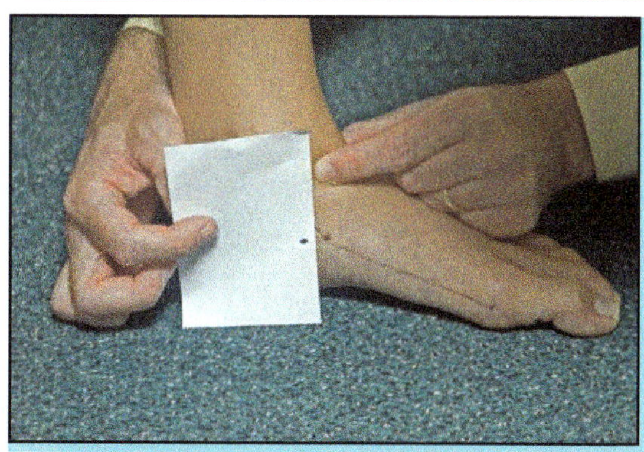

1) The patient stands. The examiner places the patient in a subtalar neutral position. Subtalar neutral is found by palpation of the patient's tali in which both medial and lateral aspects are felt equally by the examiner.

2) The most prominent aspect of the navicular bone is palpated and marked with a pen.

3) The examiner marks the height of the "neutral" position on a 3 × 5 note card. The patient is then instructed to stand normally.

4) Once the patient stands normally, the navicular height is again measured using the 3 × 5 card. The difference of the two measures is taken. The process is repeated for the opposite foot.

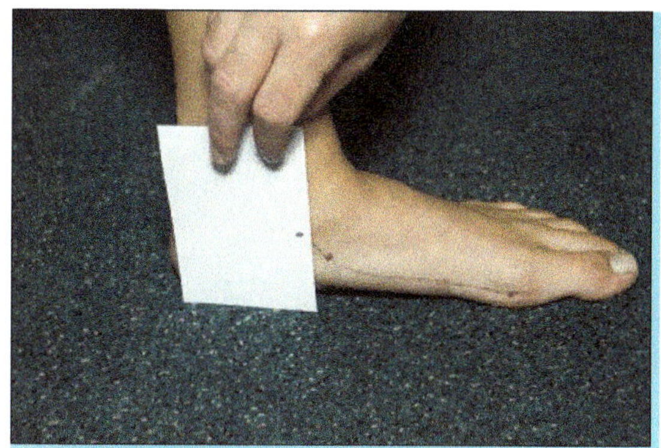

5) A significant difference of one side in comparison to the opposite is considered a positive finding.

UTILITY SCORE 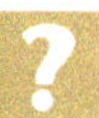

Study	Reliability	Sensitivity	Specificity	LR+	LR−	QUADAS Score (0–14)
Smith et al.[27] (Left Foot)	0.72 ICC	NT	NT	NA	NA	NA
Smith et al.[27] (Right Foot)	0.82 ICC	NT	NT	NA	NA	NA
Loudon & Bell[16] (Right Foot)	0.87 kappa	NT	NT	NA	NA	NA
Picciano et al.[23]	0.57 ICC	NT	NT	NA	NA	NA
Sell et al.[24] (Resting)	0.95 ICC	NT	NT	NA	NA	NA
Sell et al.[24] (Neutral)	0.92 ICC	NT	NT	NA	NA	NA
Sell et al.[24] (Measurement of Difference)	0.83 ICC	NT	NT	NA	NA	NA
Vinicombe et al.[30]	0.33 ICC	NT	NT	NA	NA	NA
Comments: It is questionable whether a significant drop is also indicative of dysfunction. The measurement does appear to be somewhat consistent.						

TESTS FOR MIDTARSAL JOINT PRONATION

Feiss Line (Longitudinal Arch Angle)

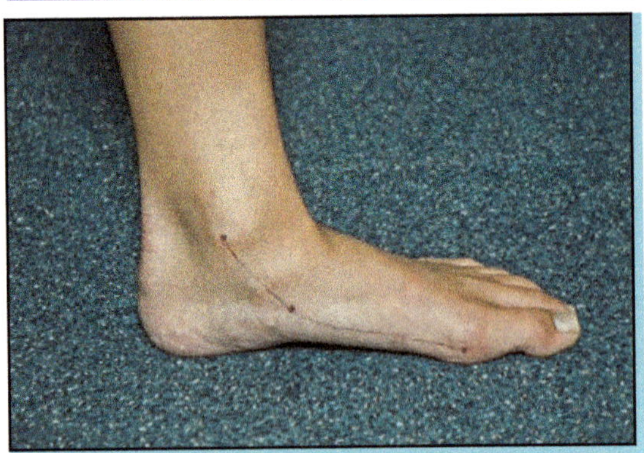

1) The patient is placed in a standing position.

2) Three marks are made on the patient's foot. One mark is made on the medial aspect of the malleolus, another at the navicular tubercle, and another at the medial aspect of the first metatarsal head.

3) The examiner places the patient in subtalar weight-bearing neutral.

4) The patient is instructed to weight-bear normally. A positive test is a dramatic drop (increased angle) of the Feiss line. Normal values would be 130 to 150 degrees and below 130 degrees is considered to be associated with foot pathology.

UTILITY SCORE 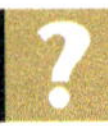

Study	Reliability	Sensitivity	Specificity	LR+	LR−	QUADAS Score (0–14)
Hegedus et al.[12]	NT	NT	NT	NA	NA	NA
Comments: It is likely that one will see a high amount of false positives with this test.						

TESTS FOR MIDTARSAL JOINT PRONATION

Arch Ratio

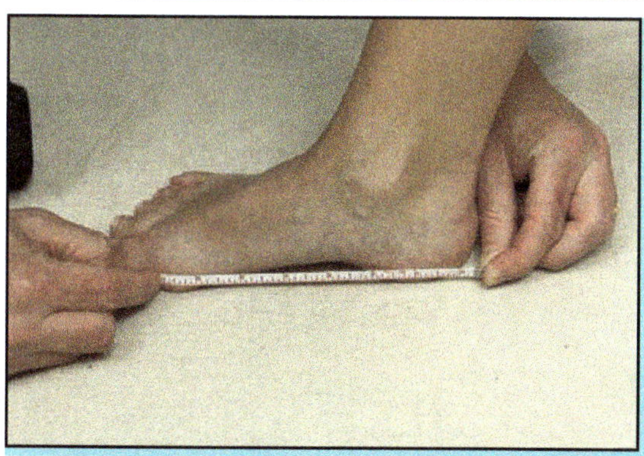

1) The patient is placed in a standing position.

2) To calculate the arch ratio, the height of the foot at midpoint is divided by the individual's truncated foot (posterior aspect of calcaneus to the first metatarsal phalangeal joint).

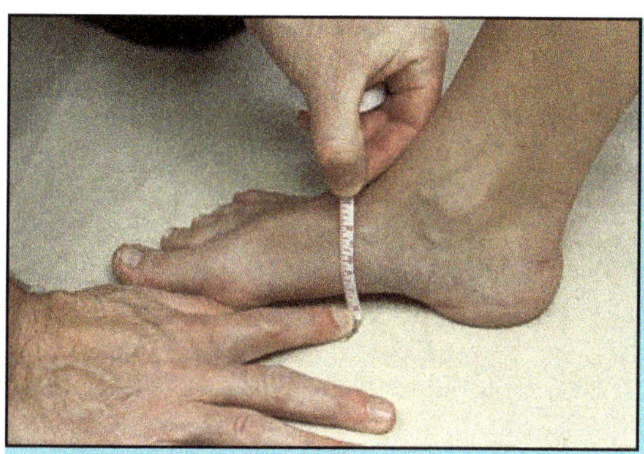

3) High arch is 0.35 or higher whereas low arch is 0.275 or lower.

4) A positive finding is extremes outside these limits.

UTILITY SCORE 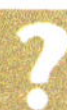

Study	Reliability	Sensitivity	Specificity	LR+	LR−	QUADAS Score (0–14)
Hegedus et al. [12]	NT	NT	NT	NA	NA	NA
Comments: It is likely that one will see a high amount of false positives with this test.						

TEST FOR REARFOOT VARUS AND VALGUS

Calcaneal Position Technique

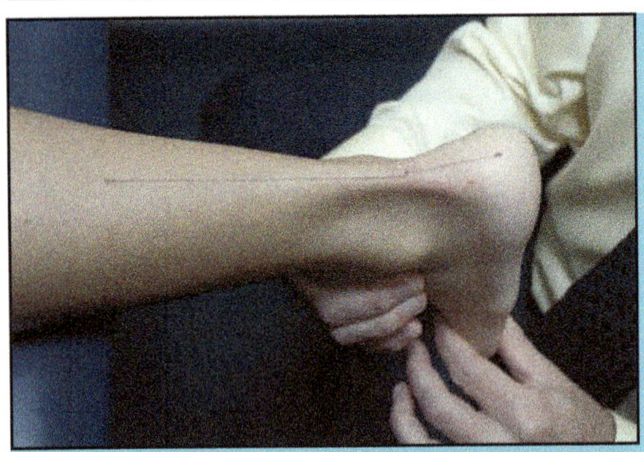

1) The patient lies in a prone position with both legs hanging over the plinth.

2) The calcaneus is palpated medially and laterally and bisected by placing dots in the inferior aspect and middle aspect of the calcaneus. A line is drawn to connect the dots.

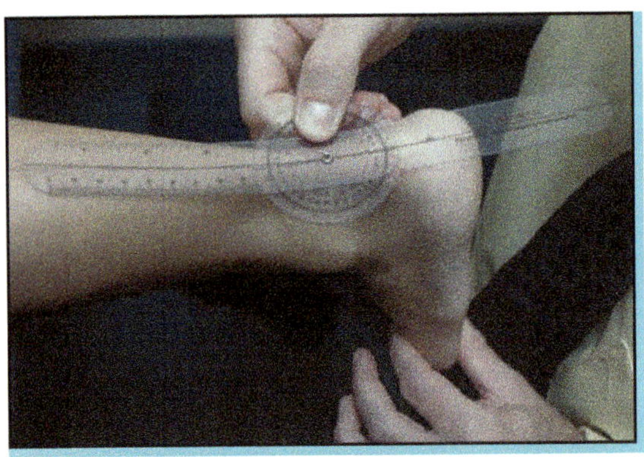

3) The examiner then finds subtalar neutral by palpating the patient's tali in which both medial and lateral aspects are felt equally by the examiner.

4) A goniometer is used to measure the varus or valgus of the calcanei.

5) A positive test is substantial rearfoot inversion or eversion during subtalar neutral.

UTILITY SCORE

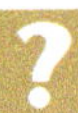

Study	Reliability	Sensitivity	Specificity	LR+	LR−	QUADAS Score (0–14)
Sell et al.[24] (Neutral)	0.85 ICC	NT	NT	NA	NA	NA
Sell et al.[24] (Resting)	0.85 ICC	NT	NT	NA	NA	NA
Comments: This test differs from the subtalar joint neutral assessment in that it is performed in non-weight-bearing versus standing.						

TESTS FOR MEDIAL LIGAMENT INTEGRITY

Lateral Talar Tilt Stress Test

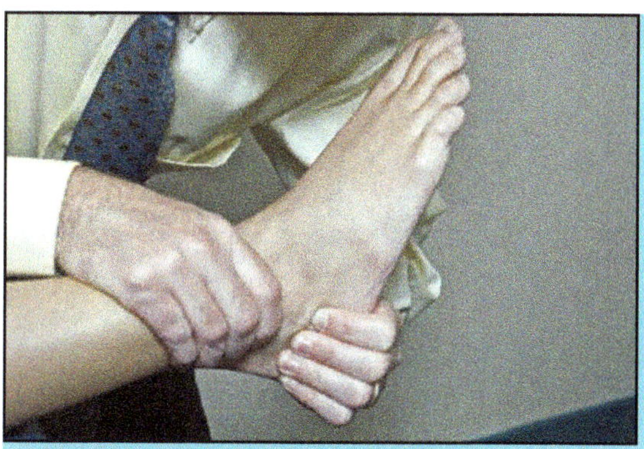

1) The patient is placed in a sitting or supine position.
2) The examiner grasps the ankle of the patient at the malleoli.
3) The examiner applies a quick lateral thrust to the calcaneus.
4) A positive test is excessive laxity when compared to the opposite side.

UTILITY SCORE 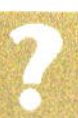

Study	Reliability	Sensitivity	Specificity	LR+	LR−	QUADAS Score (0–14)
Not tested	NT	NT	NT	NA	NA	NA
Comments: The test remains unstudied.						

Medial Tenderness

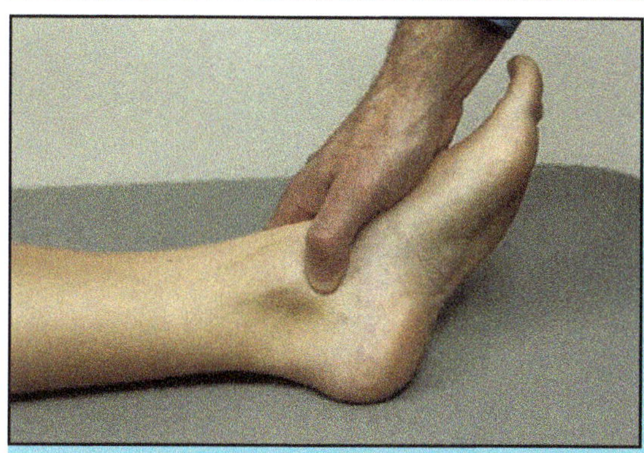

1) The patient is placed in a sitting or supine position.
2) The examiner places pressure in the area of the deltoid ligament.
3) A positive test is presence of pain during pressure placement.

UTILITY SCORE 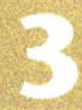

Study	Reliability	Sensitivity	Specificity	LR+	LR−	QUADAS Score (0–14)
DeAngelis et al.[7]	NT	57	59	1.4	0.72	NA
Comments: The test is designed to detect medial ligament (deep deltoid ligament) incompetence. All subjects were adults with ankle fractures.						

TEST FOR LATERAL LIGAMENT INTEGRITY

Medial Talar Tilt Stress Test

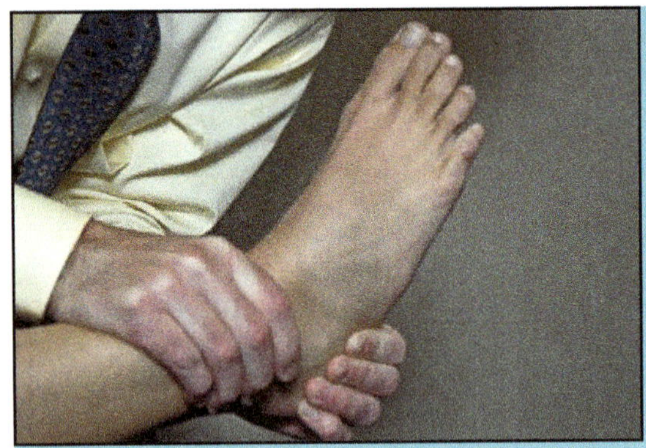

1) The patient is placed in a sitting or supine position.

2) The examiner grasps the ankle of the patient at the malleoli.

3) The examiner applies a quick medial thrust to the calcaneus.

4) A positive test is excessive laxity when compared to the opposite side.

UTILITY SCORE 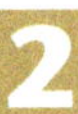

Study	Reliability	Sensitivity	Specificity	LR+	LR−	QUADAS Score (0–14)
Hertel et al.[13]	NT	67	75	2.7	0.44	8
Comments: Expect positive findings after inversion sprains.						

TEST FOR ACHILLES TENDON INTEGRITY

Thompson Test

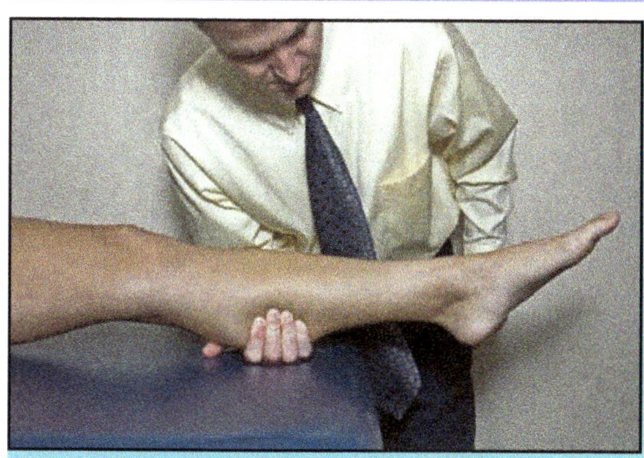

1) The patient lies in a supine position.
2) The examiner applies a squeeze to the calf of the patient's affected leg.
3) A positive test is a nonresponse during the squeeze test.

UTILITY SCORE 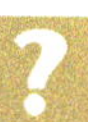

Study	Reliability	Sensitivity	Specificity	LR+	LR−	QUADAS Score (0–14)
Thompson & Doherty[29]	NT	40	NT	NA	NA	7
Comments: The test has surprisingly low sensitivity. Concurrent patient history is essential when performing this test.						

TEST FOR TARSAL TUNNEL SYNDROME

Tinel's Sign

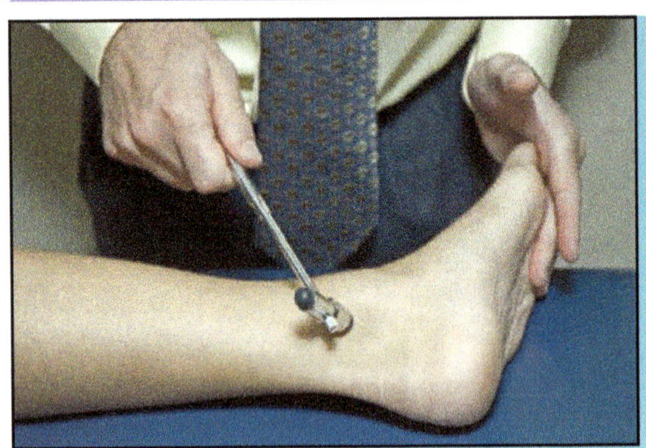

1. The patient assumes a sidelying position.
2. The examiner applies a tapping force to the posteromedial aspect of the ankle.
3. A positive finding is reproduction of tingling during the test.

UTILITY SCORE 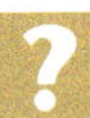

Study	Reliability	Sensitivity	Specificity	LR+	LR−	QUADAS Score (0–14)
Oloff & Schulhofer[19]	NT	58	NT	NA	NA	5
Comments: Like all Tinel's tests throughout the body, the test provides only marginal sensitivity.						

TESTS FOR ANTERIOR ANKLE IMPINGEMENT

Forced Dorsiflexion Test

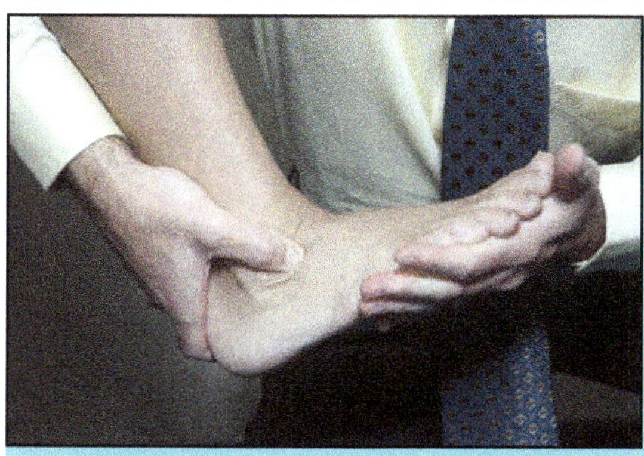

1) The patient assumes a sitting position.

2) The examiner stabilizes the distal aspect of the tibia and places his or her thumb on the anterolateral aspect of the talus near the lateral gutter. Pressure is applied.

3) The examiner applies a forceful dorsiflexion movement.

4) A positive test is reproduction of pain at the anterolateral aspect of the foot during forced dorsiflexion.

UTILITY SCORE 2

Study	Reliability	Sensitivity	Specificity	LR+	LR−	QUADAS Score (0–14)
Alonso et al.[1]	0.36 kappa	NT	NT	NA	NA	NA
Molloy et al.[17]	NT	95	88	7.9	0.06	8

Comments: Alonso et al.[1] tested for a syndesmosis injury. Although the diagnostic values for the test are strong, the quality of the study and the reliability among examiners is poor.

TESTS FOR ANTERIOR ANKLE IMPINGEMENT

Clinical Prediction Rule of Impingement

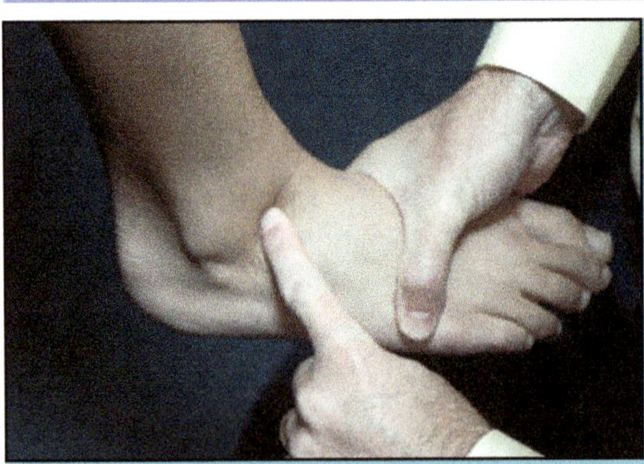

Five of six symptoms below are considered positive for anterior ankle impingement:

1) Anterolateral ankle joint tenderness.
2) Anterolateral ankle joint swelling.
3) Pain with forced dorsiflexion.
4) Pain with single-leg squat on the affected side.
5) Pain with activities.
6) Absence of ankle instability.

UTILITY SCORE 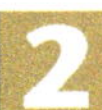

Study	Reliability	Sensitivity	Specificity	LR+	LR−	QUADAS Score (0–14)
Liu et al.[15]	NT	94	75	3.8	0.08	7
Comments: Some disagreement exists whether absence of ankle instability should be a rule for impingement. The quality of the single study is suspect.						

TEST FOR ANKLE SWELLING

Figure-8 Test

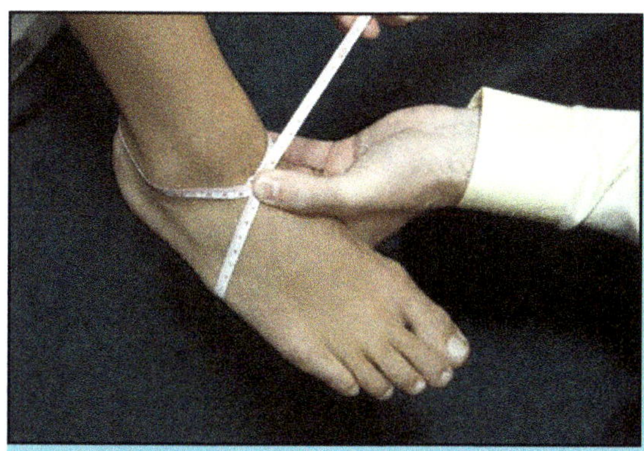

1) The patient lies in a supine or sitting position.

2) Using a flexible tape measure, and starting at the mid-point of the anterior aspect of the ankle, the examiner winds the tape measure around both the medial and lateral malleolus (but distal to each) and under the foot. The final winding should replicate a figure 8.

3) The examiner measures the distance of the excursion.

4) The test is a measurement of the girth of one limb to another. A substantial difference from one side to another a positive finding.

UTILITY SCORE 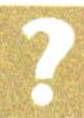

Study	Reliability	Sensitivity	Specificity	LR+	LR−	QUADAS Score (0–14)
Petersen et al.[21]	0.98 ICC	NT	NT	NA	NA	NA
Tatro-Adams et al.[28]	0.99 ICC	NT	NT	NA	NA	NA
Comments: It is essential to identify the same landmarks to perform the figure-8 tests when comparing both sides.						

TESTS FOR STRESS FRACTURE OR INTERDIGITAL NEUROMA

Morton's Test (Foot Squeeze Test)

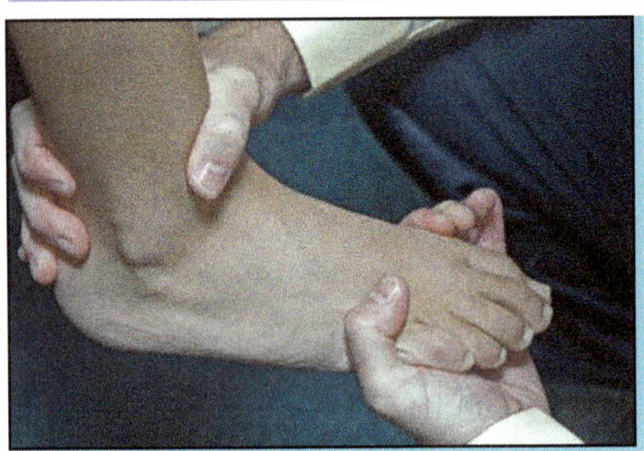

1) The patient assumes a supine or sitting position.
2) The examiner applies a squeeze to the metatarsal heads from lateral to medial toward mid-line.
3) A positive test is reproduction of patient symptoms.

UTILITY SCORE 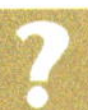

Study	Reliability	Sensitivity	Specificity	LR+	LR−	QUADAS Score (0–14)
Owens et al.[20]	NT	88	NT	NA	NA	7
Comments: A false positive is possible in patients with metatarsalgia.						

Web Space Tenderness

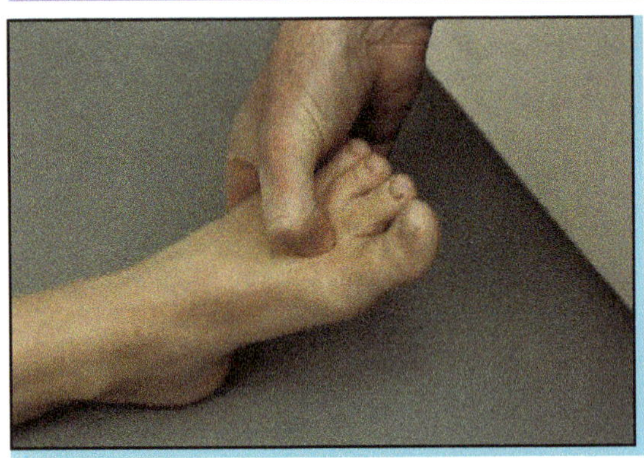

1) The patient assumes a supine or sitting position.
2) The examiner applies a force between the 2nd and 3rd metatarsals using the end of his or her thumb.
3) A positive test is reproduction of patient symptoms.

UTILITY SCORE 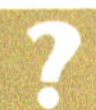

Study	Reliability	Sensitivity	Specificity	LR+	LR−	QUADAS Score (0–14)
Owens et al.[20]	NT	95	NT	NA	NA	7
Comments: A false positive is possible in patients with metatarsalgia.						

TESTS FOR STRESS FRACTURE OR INTERDIGITAL NEUROMA

Plantar Percussion Test

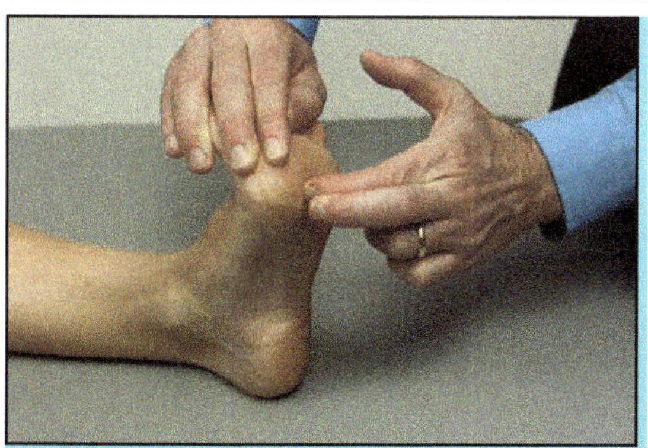

1) The patient assumes a supine or sitting position.
2) The examiner extends the toes to full range. The examiner taps the region between the 2nd and 3rd metatarsal head.
3) A positive test is reproduction of tingling (neurological findings).

UTILITY SCORE 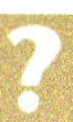

Study	Reliability	Sensitivity	Specificity	LR+	LR−	QUADAS Score (0–14)
Owens et al.[20]	NT	62	NT	NA	NA	7
Comments: A false positive is possible in patients with metatarsalgia.						

Toe Tip Sensation Deficit

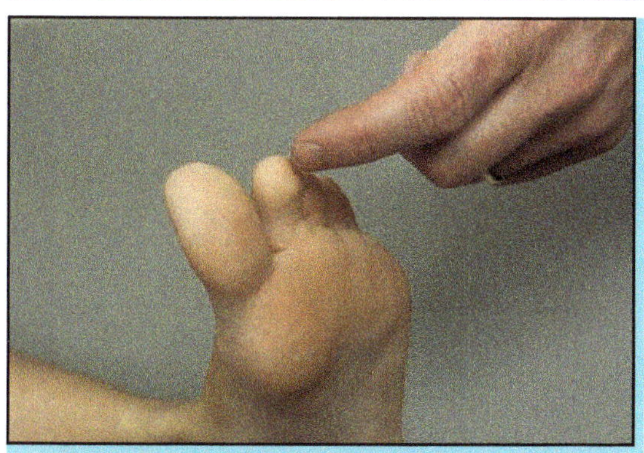

1) The patient assumes a supine or sitting position.
2) The examiner applies a light touch sensibility assessment to the patient's 2nd and 3rd toes.
3) A positive test is paresthesia or anesthesia.

UTILITY SCORE 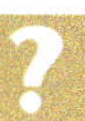

Study	Reliability	Sensitivity	Specificity	LR+	LR−	QUADAS Score (0–14)
Owens et al.[20]	NT	49	NT	NA	NA	7
Comments: A false positive is possible in patients with metatarsalgia.						

TESTS FOR STRESS FRACTURE OR INTERDIGITAL NEUROMA

Tuning Fork

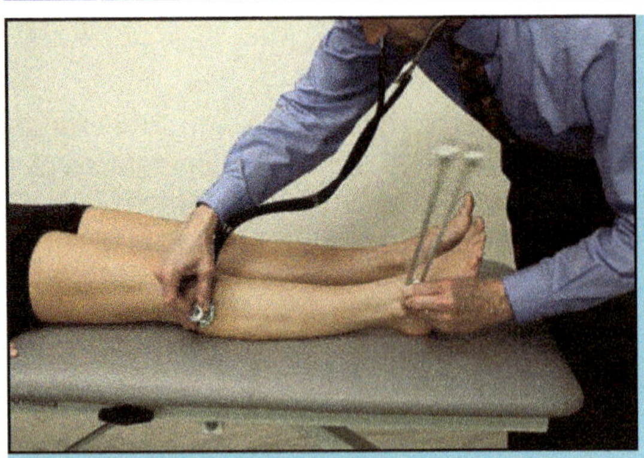

1) The patient lies in a supine position.

2) The examiner places a stethoscope on the fibular head and the tuning fork on the lateral malleolus.

3) A positive test is a change in "tone" (sound) during the assessment.

UTILITY SCORE 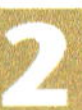

Study	Reliability	Sensitivity	Specificity	LR+	LR−	QUADAS Score (0–14)
Moore[18] (over the boney landmark)	NT	83	80	4.2	0.21	5
Moore[18] (over the swollen region)	NT	83	92	10.4	0.18	5
Comments: There were a number of cases involving different forms of fractures, some of which were in the upper extremity. Use caution, this study was done poorly.						

TESTS FOR DEEP VEIN THROMBOSIS

Well's Clinical Prediction Rule for Deep Vein Thrombosis

1) Query or assess the patient for the following major criteria:
   - Active cancer within the last 6 months
   - Paralysis
   - Recently bedridden
   - Localized tenderness
   - Thigh and calf are swollen
   - Strong family history of DVT

2) Query or assess the patient for the following minor criteria:
   - History of recent trauma
   - Pitting edema
   - Dilated superficial veins
   - Hospitalized within last 6 months
   - Erythema

3) A positive test is > 3 of the major criteria and > 2 of the minor criteria.

UTILITY SCORE 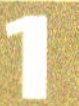

Study	Reliability	Sensitivity	Specificity	LR+	LR−	QUADAS Score (0–14)
Wells et al.[31]	NT	78	98	39	0.22	8
Comments: At present, only one fairly designed study has examined these criteria; otherwise, the findings are promising.						

TESTS FOR DEEP VEIN THROMBOSIS

Calf Swelling

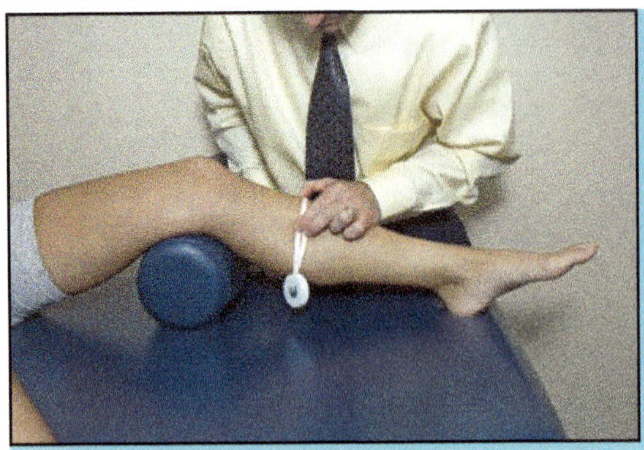

1. The patient lies in a supine position with the knee slightly flexed.
2. The examiner performs a circumferential measure of the calf and compares the size to the opposite side.
3. A positive test is a difference of 15 mm for men and 12 mm for women.

UTILITY SCORE 2 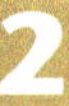

Study	Reliability	Sensitivity	Specificity	LR+	LR−	QUADAS Score (0–14)
Cranley et al.[5]	NT	90	92	11.3	0.11	7
Shafer & Duboff[25]	NT	NT	NT	NA	NA	NA
Comments: This special test would benefit from further examination.						

Homan's Sign

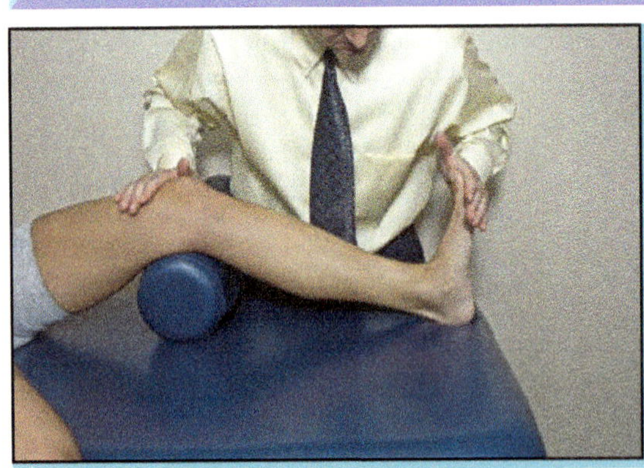

1. The patient lies in a supine position with the knee slightly flexed.
2. The examiner applies a forceful dorsiflexion maneuver.
3. A positive test is popliteal pain and calf pain.

UTILITY SCORE 3 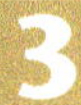

Study	Reliability	Sensitivity	Specificity	LR+	LR−	QUADAS Score (0–14)
Cranley et al.[5]	NT	48	41	0.81	1.27	7
Knox[14]	NT	35	NT	NA	NA	4
Comments: A number of conditions may lead to false positives. The test does not appear to be diagnostic.						

TESTS FOR DEEP VEIN THROMBOSIS

Calf Tenderness

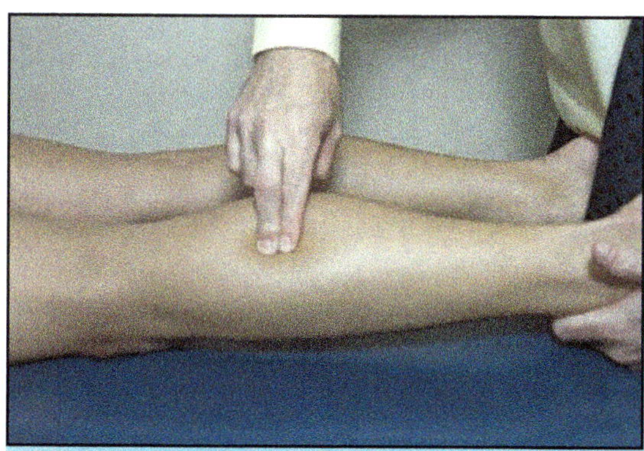

1) The patient is queried regarding an aching or pain in the calf along with a feeling of fullness.

2) A positive test is a report of these symptoms, specifically if reproduced during manual compression of the calf.

UTILITY SCORE 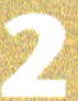

Study	Reliability	Sensitivity	Specificity	LR+	LR−	QUADAS Score (0–14)
Cranley et al.[5]	NT	82	72	2.9	0.25	7
Shafer & Duboff[25]	NT	35	NT	NA	NA	4
Comments: It is likely the fair to moderate diagnostic value from the Cranley et al.[5] study was associated with testing bias.						

Popkin's Sign

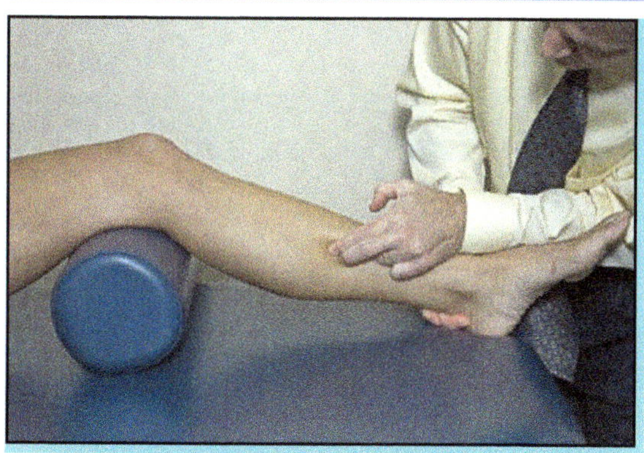

1) The patient lies in a supine position with the knee slightly flexed.

2) The examiner applies pressure with his or her index finger over the anterior medial aspect of the lower extremity.

3) A positive test is reproduction of pain or patient grimacing.

UTILITY SCORE 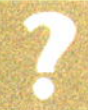

Study	Reliability	Sensitivity	Specificity	LR+	LR−	QUADAS Score (0–14)
Shafer & Duboff[25]	NT	NT	NT	NA	NA	NA
Comments: Untested and somewhat unbelievable.						

TEST FOR SURGICAL STABILIZATION REQUIRED WITH FRACTURED FIBULA

Clinical Prediction Rule for Surgical Stabilization

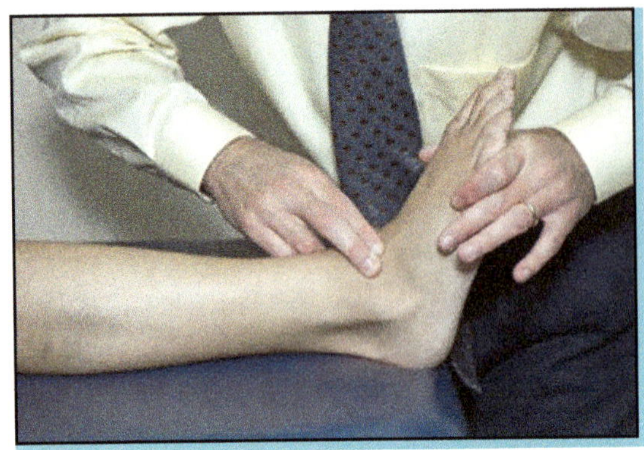

1) The patient lies in a supine position.

2) The examiner observes and palpates the ankle for swelling.

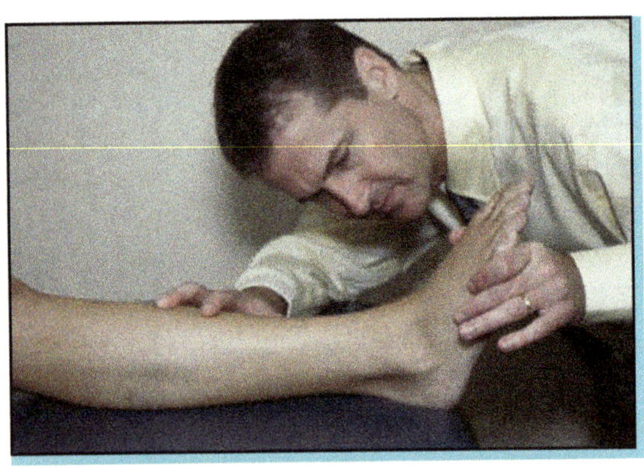

3) The examiner further observes the ankle for tenderness and ecchymosis.

4) A positive test is identified by positive stress x-rays in addition to clinical findings.

UTILITY SCORE 

Study	Reliability	Sensitivity	Specificity	LR+	LR−	QUADAS Score (0–14)
Egol et al.[6] (Medial Tenderness)	NT	56	80	2.8	0.55	8
Egol et al.[6] (Swelling)	NT	55	71	1.9	0.63	8
Egol et al.[6] (Ecchymosis)	NT	26	91	2.9	0.81	8
Egol et al.[6] (Tenderness and Swelling)	NT	39	91	4.3	0.67	8
Egol et al.[6] (Tenderness and Ecchymosis)	NT	20	97	6.7	0.82	8
Egol et al.[6] (Swelling and Ecchymosis)	NT	21	91	2.3	0.87	8
Comments: The test demonstrates strong specificity and is likely not a good screen.						

TEST FOR FOOT AND ANKLE FRACTURES

Ottawa Ankle Rules

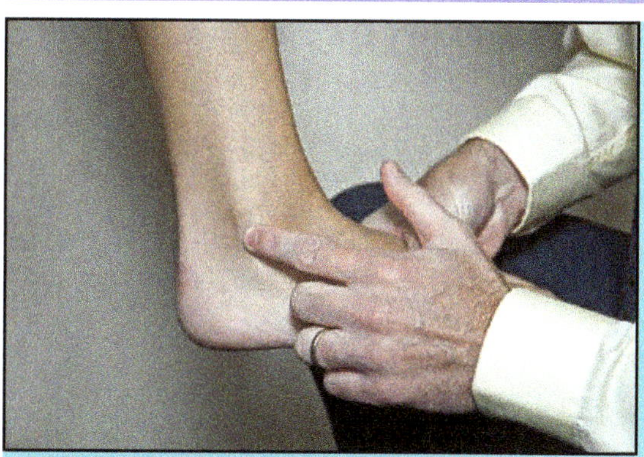

1) An ankle x-ray is required if there is any pain in the anterior aspect of the medial and lateral malleoli and anterior talar dome region, and any of the following findings:
   - Bone tenderness at the posterior aspects of the medial malleolus
   - Bone tenderness at the lateral malleolus
   - Inability to weight-bear immediately after the injury and in the emergency room

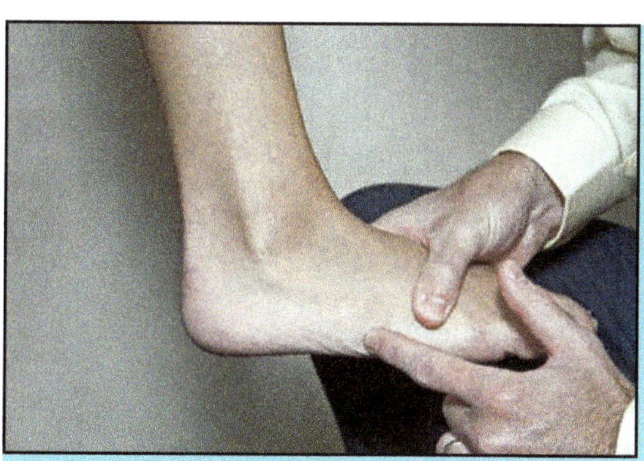

2) A foot x-ray series is required if there is any pain in the dorsal medial and lateral aspect of the mid-foot and any of the following findings:
   - Bone tenderness at the base of the fifth metatarsal
   - Bone tenderness at the navicular
   - Inability to weight-bear immediately after the injury and in the emergency room

UTILITY SCORE 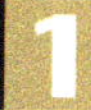

Study	Reliability	Sensitivity	Specificity	LR+	LR−	QUADAS Score (0–14)
Bachmann et al.[2] (all subjects) (meta-analysis)	NT	98	32	1.4	0.07	NA
Dowling et al.[9] (for children) (meta-analysis)	NT	98.5	7.9–50	NR	0.11	NA
Dissmann and Han[8] (use of a tuning fork to improve specificity) (tip of lateral malleolus)	NT	100	62	2.59	Inf	6
Dissmann and Han[8] (use of a tuning fork to improve specificity) (Distal Fibular Shaft)	NT	100	95	22	Inf	6
Comments: A positive test requires radiographic assessment. Pooled results included studies that demonstrated QUADAS scores of 9 to 12. The test is an excellent screen. Dissmann's work shows that adding a tuning fork may improve specificity but the design was poor.						

Key Points

1. Clinical special tests of the lower leg, ankle, and foot are woefully understudied.
2. Most of the clinical special tests of the lower leg, ankle, and foot have been studied using poor designs and are hampered by internal bias.
3. Commonly used tests for deep vein thrombosis tend to be more specific than sensitive (occasionally) and lack proper study design.
4. The Ottawa rules include pooled analysis of 27 different studies with moderate to good methodology. The rules are excellent screens for ruling out the need for an x-ray among adults and children.
5. Although several syndesmosis tests exist, only a few have been studied for diagnostic accuracy.
6. The commonly used talar stress tests have been poorly tested. It is likely that results depend on the vigor of the stress used by the examiner.
7. The navicular drop test appears to be a moderately reliable test for pronation; however, the contribution of the findings of the test to pathology is untested.

References

1. Alonso A, Khoury L, Adams R. Clinical tests for ankle syndesmosis injury: reliability and prediction of return to function. *J Orthop Sports Phys Ther.* 1998;27(4):276–284.
2. Bachmann LM, Kolb E, Koller MT, Steurer J, ter Riet G. Accuracy of Ottawa ankle rules to exclude fractures of the ankle and mid-foot: systematic review. *BMJ.* 2003;326(7386):417.
3. Beumer A, Swierstra BA, Mulder PG. Clinical diagnosis of syndesmotic ankle instability: evaluation of stress tests behind the curtains. *Acta Orthop Scand.* 2002;73(6):667–669.
4. Beumer A, van Hemert WL, Swierstra BA, Jasper LE, Belkoff SM. A biomechanical evaluation of clinical stress tests for syndesmotic ankle instability. *Foot Ankle Int.* 2003;24(4):358–363.
5. Cranley JJ, Canos AJ, Sull WJ. The diagnosis of deep venous thrombosis: fallibility of clinical symptoms and signs. *Arch Surg.* 1976;111(1):34–36.
6. Egol KA, Amirtharajah M, Tejwani NC, Capla EL, Koval KJ. Ankle stress test for predicting the need for surgical fixation of isolated fibular fractures. *J Bone Joint Surg Am.* 2004;86-A(11): 2393–2398.
7. DeAngelis N, Eskander MS, French BG. Does medial tenderness predict deep deltoid ligament incompetence in supination-external rotation type ankle fractures? *J Orthop Trauma.* 2007;21:244–247.
8. Dissmann PD, Han KH. The tuning fork test—a useful tool for improving specificity in "Ottawa positive" patients after ankle inversion injury. *Emerg Med J.* 2006;23:788–790.
9. Dowling S, Spooner CH, Liang Y, et al. Accuracy of Ottawa ankle rules to exclude fractures of the ankle and midfoot in children: a meta-analysis. *Acad Emerg Med.* 2009;16:277–287.
10. Glasoe WM, Allen MK, Saltzman CL, Ludewig PM, Sublett SH. Comparison of two methods used to assess first-ray mobility. *Foot Ankle Int.* 2002;23(3):248–252.
11. Glasoe WM, Grebing BR, Beck S, Coughlin MJ, Saltzman CL. A comparison of device measures of dorsal first ray mobility. *Foot Ankle Int.* 2005;26(11):957–961.
12. Hegedus EJ, Cook C, Fiander C, Wright A. Measures of arch height and their relationship to pain and dysfunction in people with lower limb impairments. *Physiother Res Int.* 2010;15(3):160–166.
13. Hertel J, Denegar CR, Monroe MM, Stokes WL. Talocrural and subtalar joint instability after lateral ankle sprain. *Med Sci Sports Exerc.* 1999;31(11):1501–1508.
14. Knox FW. The clinical diagnosis of deep vein thrombophlebitis. *Practitioner.* 1965;195:214–216.
15. Liu SH, Nuccion SL, Finerman G. Diagnosis of anterolateral ankle impingement: comparison between magnetic resonance imaging and clinical examination. *Am J Sports Med.* 1997;25(3):389–393.
16. Loudon JK, Bell SL. The foot and ankle: an overview of arthrokinematics and selected joint techniques. *J Athl Train.* 1996;31(2):173–178.
17. Molloy S, Solan MC, Bendall SP. Synovial impingement in the ankle: a new physical sign. *J Bone Joint Surg Br.* 2003;85(3):330–333.
18. Moore M. The use of tuning fork and stethoscope to identify fractures. *J Athl Train.* 2009;44:272–274.
19. Oloff LM, Schulhofer SD. Flexor hallucis longus dysfunction. *J Foot Ankle Surg.* 1998;37(2):101–109.
20. Owens R, Gougoulias N, Guthrie H, Sakellariou A. Morton's neuroma: clinical testing and imaging in 76 feet, compared to a control group. *Foot Ankle Surg.* 2010 (E pub ahead of print).
21. Petersen EJ, Irish SM, Lyons CL, Miklaski SF, Bryan JM, Henderson NE, Masullo LN. Reliability of water volumetry and the figure eight method on patients with ankle joint swelling. *J Orthop Sports Phys Ther.* 1999;29(10):609–615.
22. Phisitkul P, Chaichankul C, Sripongsai R, Prasitdamrong I, Tengtrakulcharoen P, Suarchawaratana S. Accuracy

of anterolateral drawer test in lateral ankle instability: A cadaveric study. *Foot Ankle Internat.* 2009;30:690–695.

23. Picciano AM, Rowlands MS, Worrell T. Reliability of open and closed kinetic chain subtalar joint neutral positions and navicular drop test. *J Orthop Sports Phys Ther.* 1993;18(4):553–558.
24. Sell KE, Verity TM, Worrell TW, Pease BJ, Wigglesworth J. Two measurement techniques for assessing subtalar joint position: a reliability study. *J Orthop Sports Phys Ther.* 1994;19(3):162–167.
25. Shafer N, Duboff S. Physical signs in the early diagnosis of thrombophlebitis. *Angiology.* 1971;22(1):18–30.
26. Shirk C, Sandrey MA, Erickson M. Reliability of first ray position and mobility measurements in experienced and inexperienced examiners. *J Athl Train.* 2006;41:93–101.
27. Smith J, Szczerba JE, Arnold BL, Perrin DH, Martin DE. Role of hyperpronation as a possible risk factor for anterior cruciate ligament injuries. *J Athl Train.* 1997;32(1):25–28.
28. Tatro-Adams D, McGann SF, Carbone W. Reliability of the figure-of-eight method of ankle measurement. *J Orthop Sports Phys Ther.* 1995;22(4):161–163.
29. Thompson TC, Doherty JH. Spontaneous rupture of tendon of Achilles: a new clinical diagnostic test. *J Trauma.* 1962;2:126–129.
30. Vinicombe A, Raspovic A, Menz HB. Reliability of navicular displacement measurement as a clinical indicator of foot posture. *J Am Podiatr Med Assoc.* 2001; 91(5):262–268.
31. Wells PS, Hirsh J, Anderson DR, Lensing AW, Foster G, Kearon C, Weitz J, D'Ovidio R, Cogo A, Prandoni P. Accuracy of clinical assessment of deep-vein thrombosis. *Lancet.* 1995;345(8961):1326–1330.

PEARSON
myhealthprofessionskit™

Use this address to access the Companion Website created for this textbook. Simply select "Physical Therapy" from the choice of disciplines. Find this book and log in using your username and password to access video clips of selected tests.

Index

Page references followed by "f" indicate illustrated figures or photographs; followed by "t" indicates a table.

T

U

V

W

X